TEXTBOOK OF ANATOMY
ABDOMEN AND LOWER LIMB

TEXTBOOK OF ANATOMY
ABDOMEN AND LOWER LIMB
Volume II

Second Edition

Vishram Singh, MS, PhD, FASI
Professor and Head, Department of Anatomy
Professor-in-Charge, Medical Education Unit
Santosh Medical College, Ghaziabad
Editor-in-Chief, Journal of the Anatomical Society of India
Member, Academic Council and Core Committee PhD Course, Santosh University
Member, Editorial Board, Indian Journal of Otology
Medicolegal Advisor, ICPS, India
Consulting Editor, ABI, North Carolina, USA

Formerly at: GSVM Medical College, Kanpur
King George's Medical College, Lucknow
Al-Arab Medical University, Benghazi (Libya)
All India Institute of Medical Sciences, New Delhi

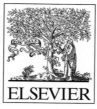

ELSEVIER

ELSEVIER
A Division of RELX India Private Limited (Formerly Reed Elsevier India Private Limited)

Textbook of Anatomy: Abdomen and Lower Limb, Volume II, 2e

Vishram Singh

First edition 2011
Second edition 2014
Reprinted 2015, 2016

ISBN: 978-81-312-3728-1
e-book ISBN: 978-81-312-3626-0

Notices

Knowledge and best practice in this field are constantly changing. As new research and experience broaden our understanding, changes in research methods, professional practices, or medical treatment may become necessary.

Practitioners and researchers must always rely on their own experience and knowledge in evaluating and using any information, methods, compounds, or experiments described herein. In using such information or methods they should be mindful of their own safety and the safety of others, including parties for whom they have a professional responsibility.

With respect to any drug or pharmaceutical products identified, readers are advised to check the most current information provided (i) on procedures featured or (ii) by the manufacturer of each product to be administered, to verify the recommended dose or formula, the method and duration of administration, and contraindications. It is the responsibility of practitioners, relying on their own experience and knowledge of their patients, to make diagnoses, to determine dosages and the best treatment for each individual patient, and to take all appropriate safety precautions.

To the fullest extent of the law, neither the Publisher nor the authors, contributors, or editors, assume any liability for any injury and/or damage to persons or property as a matter of products liability, negligence or otherwise, or from any use or operation of any methods, products, instructions, or ideas contained in the material herein.

Please consult full prescribing information before issuing prescription for any product mentioned in this publication.

The Publisher

Published by RELX India Private Limited (Formerly Reed Elsevier India Private Limited)
Registered Office: 818, Indraprakash Building, 21, Barakhamba Road, New Delhi 110 001
Corporate Office: 14th Floor, Building No. 10B, DLF Cyber City, Phase II, Gurgaon-122 002, Haryana, India

Senior Project Manager-Education Solutions: Shabina Nasim
Content Strategist: Renu Rawat
Project Coordinator: Goldy Bhatnagar
Senior Operations Manager: Sunil Kumar
Production Manager: NC Pant
Sr. Production Executive: Ravinder Sharma
Sr. Graphic Designer: Milind Majgaonkar

Typeset by Chitra Computers, New Delhi

Printed and bound at Repro India Ltd., Navi Mumbai

Dedicated to

My Mother
Late Smt Ganga Devi Singh Rajput
an ever guiding force in my life for achieving knowledge through education

My Wife
Mrs Manorama Rani Singh
for tolerating my preoccupation happily during the preparation of this book

My Children
Dr Rashi Singh and **Dr Gaurav Singh**
for helping me in preparing the manuscript

My Teachers
Late Professor (Dr) AC Das
for inspiring me to be multifaceted and innovative in life
Professor (Dr) A Halim
for imparting to me the art of good teaching

My Students, Past and Present
for appreciating my approach to teaching anatomy and
transmitting the knowledge through this book

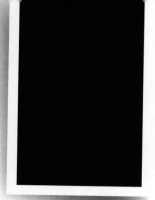

Preface to the Second Edition

It is with great pleasure that I express my gratitude to all students and teachers who appreciated, used, and recommended the first edition of this book. It is because of their support that the book was reprinted three times since its first publication in 2011.

The huge success of this book reflects appeal of its clear, unclustered presentation of the anatomical text supplemented by perfect simple line diagrams, which could be easily drawn by students in the exam and clinical correlations providing the anatomical, embryological, and genetic basis of clinical conditions seen in day-to-day life in clinical practice.

Based on a large number of suggestions from students and fellow academicians, the text has been extensively revised. Many new line diagrams and halftone figures have been added and earlier diagrams have been updated.

I greatly appreciate the constructive suggestions that I received from past and present students and colleagues for improvement of the content of this book. I do not claim to absolute originality of the text and figures other than the new mode of presentation and expression.

Once again, I whole heartedly thank students, teachers, and fellow anatomists for inspiring me to carry out the revision. I sincerely hope that they will find this edition more interesting and useful than the previous one. I would highly appreciate comments and suggestions from students and teachers for further improvement of this book.

"To learn from previous experience and change
accordingly, makes you a successful man."

Vishram Singh

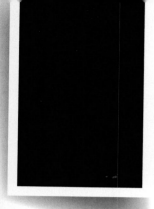

Preface to the First Edition

This textbook on abdomen and lower limb has been carefully planned for the first year MBBS students. It follows the revised anatomy curriculum of the Medical Council of India. Following the current trends of clinically-oriented study of Anatomy, I have adopted a parallel approach – that of imparting basic anatomical knowledge to students and simultaneously providing them its applied aspects.

To help students score high in examinations the text is written in simple language. It is arranged in easily understandable small sections. While anatomical details of little clinical relevance, phylogenetic discussions, and comparative analogies have been omitted, all clinically important topics are described in detail. Brief accounts of histological features and developmental aspects have been given only where they aid in understanding of gross form and function of organs and appearance of common congenital anomalies. The tables and flowcharts summarize important and complex information into digestible knowledge-capsules. Multiple choice questions have been given chapter-by-chapter at the end of the book to test the level of understanding and memory recall of the students. The numerous simple 4-color illustrations further assist in fast comprehension and retention of complicated information. All the illustrations are drawn by the author himself to ensure accuracy.

Throughout the preparation of this book one thing I have kept in mind is that anatomical knowledge is required by clinicians and surgeons for physical examination, diagnostic tests, and surgical procedures. Therefore, topographical anatomy relevant to diagnostic and surgical procedures is clinically correlated throughout the text. Further, Clinical Case Study is provided at the end of each chapter for problem-based learning (PBL) so that the students could use their anatomical knowledge in clinical situations. Moreover, the information is arranged regionally since while assessing lesions and performing surgical procedures, the clinicians encounter region-based anatomical features. Due to propensity of fractures, dislocations, and peripheral nerve lesions in the lower limb there is in-depth discussion on joints and peripheral nerves. Similarly due to high incidence of abdominal hernias and tumors involving abdominopelvic viscera, the inguinal region and abdominal viscera are described in detail.

As a teacher, I have tried my best to make the book easy to understand and interesting to read. For further improvement of this book I would greatly welcome comments and suggestions from the readers.

Vishram Singh

Preface to the First Edition

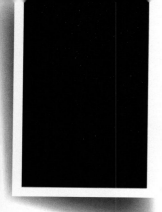

Acknowledgments

At the outset, I express my gratitude to Dr P Mahalingam, CMD; Dr Sharmila Anand, DMD; and Dr Ashwyn Anand, CEO, Professor VK Arora, Vice Chancellor, Santosh University, Ghaziabad, for providing an appropriate academic atmosphere in the university and encouragement which helped me in preparing this book.

I am also thankful to Dr Usha Dhar, Dean Santosh Medical College for her cooperation. I highly appreciate the good gesture shown by Dr Deepa Singh and Dr Preeti Srivastava for checking the final proofs.

I sincerely thank my colleagues in the Department, especially Professor Nisha Kaul and Dr Ruchira Sethi for their assistance.

I gratefully acknowledge the feedback and support of fellow colleagues in Anatomy, particularly,

- Professors AK Srivastava (Head of the Department), PK Sharma, and Dr Punita Manik, King George's Medical College, Lucknow.
- Professor NC Goel (Head of the Department), Hind Institute of Medical Sciences, Barabanki, Lucknow.
- Professor Kuldeep Singh Sood (Head of the Department), SGT Medical College, Budhera, Gurgaon, Haryana.
- Professor Poonam Kharb, Sharda Medical College, Greater Noida, UP.
- Professor TC Singel (Head of the Department), MP Shah Medical College, Jamnagar, and Professor Suresh P Rathod (Head of the Department), Pandit Deendayal Upadhyay Medical College, Rajkot, Gujarat.
- Professor TS Roy (Head of the Department), AIIMS, New Delhi.
- Professors RK Suri (Head of the Department), Gayatri Rath, and Dr Hitendra Loh, Vardhman Mahavir Medical College and Safdarjang Hospital, New Delhi.
- Professor Veena Bharihoke (Head of the Department), Rama Medical College, Hapur, Ghaziabad.
- Professors SL Jethani (Dean and Head of the Department) and RK Rohtagi, Dr Deepa Singh and Dr Akshya Dubey, Himalayan Institute of Medical Sciences, Jolly Grant, Dehradun.
- Professors Anita Tuli (Head of the Department), Shipra Paul, and Shashi Raheja, Lady Harding Medical College, New Delhi.
- Professor SD Joshi (Dean and Head of the Department), Sri Aurobindo Institute of Medical Sciences, Indore, MP.

Lastly, I eulogize the patience of my wife Mrs Manorama Rani Singh, daughter Dr Rashi Singh, and son Dr Gaurav Singh for helping me in the preparation of this manuscript.

I would also like to acknowledge with gratitude and pay my regards to my teachers Prof AC Das and Prof A Halim and other renowned anatomists of India, viz. Prof Shamer Singh, Prof Inderbir Singh, Prof Mahdi Hasan, Prof AK Dutta, Prof Inder Bhargava, etc. who inspired me during my student life.

I gratefully acknowledge the help and cooperation received from the staff of Elsevier, a division of Reed Elsevier India Pvt. Ltd., especially Ganesh Venkatesan (Director Editorial and Publishing Operations), Shabina Nasim (Senior Project Manager-Education Solutions), Renu Rawat (Content Strategist), and Goldy Bhatnagar (Project Coordinator).

Vishram Singh

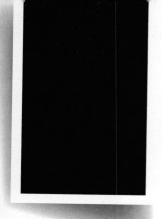

Contents

Introduction and Overview of the Abdomen

The abdomen is the lower part of the trunk below the diaphragm. Its walls surround a large cavity called the **abdominal cavity**. The abdominal cavity is much more extensive than what it appears from the outside. It extends upward deep to the costal margin up to the diaphragm and downward within the bony pelvis. Thus, a considerable part of the abdominal cavity is overlapped by the lower part of the thoracic cage above and by the bony pelvis below.

The abdominal cavity is subdivided by the plane of the pelvic inlet into a larger upper part, i.e., the **abdominal cavity proper**, and a smaller lower part, i.e., the **pelvic cavity**.

Clinically the term abdominal cavity stands for abdominal cavity proper.

Clinically the importance of the abdomen is manifold. To the physician, the physical examination of the patient is never complete until he/she thoroughly examines the abdomen.

To the surgeon, the abdomen remains an enigma because in number of cases the cause of abdominal pain and nature of abdominal lump remains inconclusive even after all possible investigations. To the obstetrician and gynecologist, the examination of the pelvis and perineum is extremely important. To the venereologist, the main territory of examination is confined to the external genitalia. To summarize, many branches of medicine such as general surgery, gastroenterology, nephrology, urology, obstetrics, gynecology, and venereology are all confined to the abdomen.

ABDOMINAL CAVITY (Fig. 1.1)

The abdominal cavity is the largest cavity of the body. Its boundaries and contents are as follows:

BOUNDARIES

The boundaries of the abdominal cavity are:

Superiorly: Diaphragm, which separates it from the thoracic cavity.

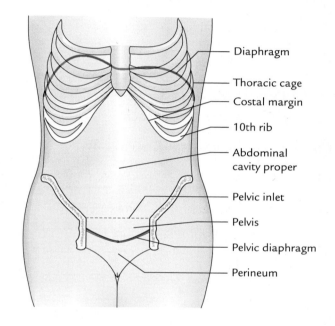

Fig. 1.1 Abdominal cavity.

Inferiorly: Continues with the pelvic cavity at the pelvic inlet.

Anteriorly: Anterior abdominal wall, formed by muscles.

Posteriorly: Posterior abdominal wall, formed by lumbar vertebrae and muscles.

Laterally: Lower ribs and parts of muscles of the anterior abdominal wall.

N.B.

- The diaphragm forming the superior boundary moves up and down with respiration.
- The anterior abdominal wall is firm and elastic.
- Firmness of anterior abdominal wall protects the abdominal viscera and its elasticity allows the expansion of the abdominal viscera.
- The posterior abdominal wall is osteomuscular and rigid. Its rigidity provides support to the abdominal organs.

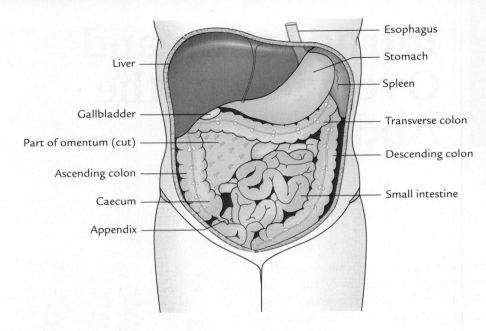

Fig. 1.2 Organs occupying the anterior part of the abdominal cavity.

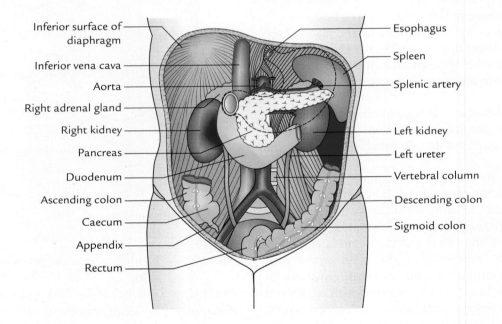

Fig. 1.3 Organs occupying the posterior part of the abdominal cavity. (The broken line shows the position of the stomach.)

CONTENTS (Figs 1.2 and 1.3)

The organs and glands of the digestive and urinary systems occupy most of the abdominal cavity. These organs and glands are listed below:

1. Stomach, small intestine, and most of the large intestine.
2. Liver, gallbladder, and pancreas.
3. Two kidneys and upper part of the ureters.
4. Adrenal glands (also known as suprarenal glands).
5. Other structures include blood vessels, lymph vessels, nerves, spleen, and lymph nodes.

PELVIC CAVITY

The pelvic cavity is roughly funnel shaped. Its boundaries and contents are as follows:

BOUNDARIES

The boundaries of the pelvic cavity are:

Superiorly: Continuous with the abdominal cavity at the pelvic inlet.
Inferiorly: Pelvic diaphragm.
Posteriorly: Sacrum and coccyx.
Anteriorly: Pubic bones.
Laterally: Hip bones.

N.B. The part of pelvis below the pelvic diaphragm is termed *perineum* (Fig. 1.1).

CONTENTS (Figs 1.4 and 1.5)

The pelvic cavity contains the following structures:

1. Loops of the small intestine.
2. Sigmoid colon, rectum, and anal canal.
3. Urinary bladder, lower part of the ureters, and urethra.

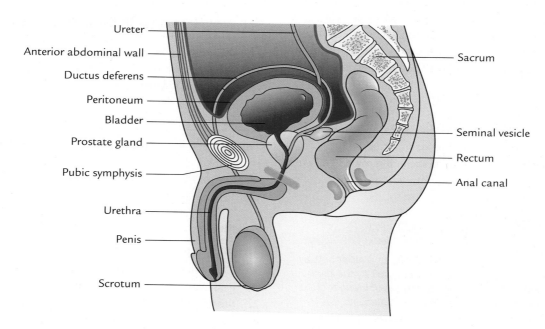

Fig. 1.4 Structures present in the male pelvis.

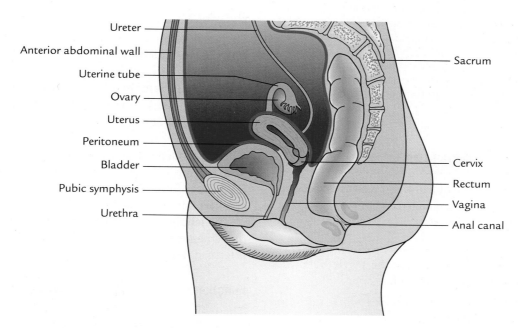

Fig. 1.5 Structures present in the female pelvis.

4. Reproductive organs:
    (a) Prostate gland, seminal vesicles, vas deferens, and ejaculatory ducts in male.
    (b) Uterus, uterine tubes, ovaries, and vagina in female.

N.B. The pelvic and urogenital diaphragms forming the inferior boundary of the pelvic cavity support the pelvic viscera and regulate the act of defecation, micturition, and parturition.

The walls of the abdominal cavity and most of the viscera present within it are covered or enclosed by an extensive serous membrane called **peritoneum**. The peritoneum consists of parietal and visceral layers, which are continuous with each other and enclose a potential space called **peritoneal cavity**.

N.B.
- All the abdominal viscera are intra-abdominal but extraperitoneal except the ovaries in female.
- The peritoneal cavity is a closed sac in the male but in the female it is an open sac and communicates to the exterior through the openings of the uterine tubes.

Clinical correlation

- The upper part of the abdominal cavity is overlapped by the lower thoracic region and the lower part by the gluteal region. Therefore, the penetrating wounds of these regions frequently involve the abdominal viscera also.
- The upper abdominal contents such as liver and spleen fill the concavity of the diaphragm. Therefore, it is easy for the surgeons to reach these organs through the thorax and diaphragm or through the anterior abdominal wall.
- The mobile diaphragm forms the upper boundary/limit of the abdominal cavity; the abdominal contents descend with it on deep inspiration. This is made use of in clinical examination of certain organs, such as liver and enlarged spleen, which can be palpated through the anterior abdominal wall, inferior to the costal margin on deep inspiration, though hidden by the thoracic cage in quiet respiration.

PERINEUM

It is a region at the lower end of trunk and seen as a diamond-shaped area when thighs are abducted.

BOUNDARIES

The perineum is an area outlined by the pelvic outlet. Its boundaries and contents are as follows:
The boundaries of perineum are:
Anteriorly: Pubic symphysis.
Posteriorly: Coccyx.

Laterally: Ischiopubic rami (anteriorly) and sacrotuberous ligaments (posteriorly).
The **roof** of perineum is formed by the pelvic diaphragm and its **floor** is formed by the skin.

CONTENTS

The contents of perineum are external genitalia (penis and scrotum with its contents in male and vulva in female) and anus.

ABDOMINAL VISCERA

The abdominal viscera includes stomach and intestines, their associated glands (liver and pancreas), blood and lymph vessels, spleen, kidney, and suprarenal glands.

STOMACH

The stomach is the most dilated part of the digestive tube. It is J-shaped and located in the abdominal cavity below the diaphragm slightly to the left of the midline. The capacity of the stomach is about 1500 ml in the adult.

Functions

The main functions of the stomach are as follows:
1. Churning and breaking of food and mixing it with the gastric juice secreted by specialized glands in its mucosa.
2. Storing the food temporarily.
3. Secreting intrinsic factor needed for absorption of vitamin B_{12}.

SMALL INTESTINE

The small intestine is a convoluted tube connecting stomach with the large intestine. It is about 6 m in length and extends from the pyloric sphincter to the ileocecal junction. The small intestine is located in the central and lower parts of the abdominal cavity surrounded by the large intestine. It consists of three parts: (a) duodenum, (b) jejunum, and (c) ileum.

The **duodenum** is proximal short curved (c-shaped) portion and is about 25 cm long. It is the widest and most fixed part of the small intestine. The ducts from gallbladder and liver and pancreas enter it.

The **jejunum** is the name given to the upper two-fifth of the remainder of the small intestine and the lower three-fifth is termed **ileum**.

Functions

The main functions of the small intestine are digestion of food and absorption of nutrients.

LARGE INTESTINE

The large intestine begins at the end of the ileum as caecum and terminates at the anus. It is about 1.5 m long and forms an arch around the coiled up small intestine. For descriptive purposes, it is divided into following seven parts:

1. Caecum and appendix.
2. Ascending colon.
3. Transverse colon.
4. Descending colon.
5. Sigmoid colon.
6. Rectum.
7. Anal canal.

Functions

The main functions of the large intestine are as follows:

1. Absorption of water and salts.
2. Formation and excretion of feces.

LIVER

The liver is the largest gland of the body. It is located in the upper right part of the abdominal cavity. It has two main lobes: right and left. The right lobe is much larger than the left lobe.

Functions

Some important functions of the liver are as follows:

1. Metabolism of carbohydrate, fat, and protein.
2. Detoxification of drugs and poisons.
3. Storage of glycogen and fat-soluble vitamins (ADEK).
4. Secretion of bile.

GALLBLADDER

The gallbladder is a pear-shaped organ located on the under surface of the right lobe of the liver. It receives bile from the liver, which it stores and concentrates. When fatty food enters the duodenum, the bile is poured into the intestine through the bile duct by the contraction of the walls of the bladder.

Clinical correlation

Jaundice: It is a clinical condition characterized by yellowing of the skin and sclera of the eyes. It occurs when bile enters the blood in liver diseases such as hepatitis or cirrhosis of the liver where the liver cells break down and release bile into the blood. Bile also enters into the blood when outlet of bile from the gallbladder to intestine through the bile duct is blocked.

PANCREAS

The pancreas is an elongated, soft, pale, and finely lobulated grey gland. It is about 12–15 cm in length and lies transversely across the posterior abdominal wall. It consists of broad head, neck, body, and a narrow tail. The head of the gland lies within the curve of the duodenum, the body behind the stomach and tail in front of the left kidney. The tail extends as far as the spleen.

Functions

The pancreas is an exo-endocrine gland. The function of exocrine pancreas is to produce pancreatic juice containing enzymes that digest carbohydrates, proteins, and fats.

The function of endocrine pancreas is to secrete hormones, insulin and glucagon, which control the blood glucose level.

Clinical correlation

Diabetes mellitus: Deficiency of insulin results in diabetes mellitus. The blood sugar level rises above the renal threshold and glucose is lost in the urine.

SPLEEN

The spleen is a large wedge-shaped mass of vascular and lymphoid tissue. It is purplish-red in colour and lies high up at the back of the abdominal cavity on the left side behind the stomach.

Functions

The main functions of the spleen are as follows:

1. Destruction of red blood cells.
2. Production of fresh lymphocytes for the blood stream.

KIDNEYS

The kidneys are two bean-shaped organs situated on the posterior abdominal wall, one on each side of the vertebral column, behind the peritoneum. The right kidney usually lies at a slightly lower level than the left.

Function

The main function of the kidney is to secrete and excrete urine.

N.B. The composition of blood must not vary beyond certain limits if the tissues of the body are to remain healthy. This regulation depends on the removal of harmful waste products and maintenance of water and electrolyte balance.

URETERS

The ureters are two tubes, which connect the kidneys to the urinary bladder. Each ureter is usually 25 cm long with a diameter of about 3 mm.

Function

The ureters transport urine from the kidneys to the urinary bladder.

ADRENAL GLANDS (SUPRARENAL GLANDS)

There are two suprarenal glands—right and left. Each gland caps the upper pole of the corresponding kidney. The right gland is triangular whereas the left gland is semilunar in shape. Each gland consists of two parts: cortex and medulla.

Functions

The function of the cortex is to secrete a number of steroid hormones, which are responsible for: (a) maintenance of electrolyte and water balance, (b) maintenance of blood sugar concentration and of liver and muscle glycogen, and (c) control of inflammatory reactions.

The function of medulla is to secrete adrenaline and noradrenaline in the blood, which serve as neurotransmitters.

PELVIC VISCERA

The pelvic viscera in males are urinary bladder, prostate, and rectum; and in females are urinary bladder, uterus, and rectum.

URINARY BLADDER

The urinary bladder is a reservoir of urine. Its size, shape, and position vary with the amount of urine it contains. When empty it lies in the pelvic cavity, but when distended with urine it expands upward and forward into the abdominal cavity. The bladder can hold up to 500 ml (rarely 600 ml) of urine, though this would cause pain. The desire to empty the bladder is normally felt when it contains around 250–300 ml of urine.

The two ureters enter into it through its posterior wall. The urethra leaves the bladder at its neck. The neck of the bladder is the lowest and most fixed part of the urinary bladder. A thickening of smooth muscle called internal urethral sphincter surrounds the opening of the urethra.

Function

The urinary bladder stores urine and expels it into the urethra.

URETHRA

The urethra is a narrow canal that extends from the **internal urethral orifice** in the urinary bladder to the **external urethral orifice.**

In a male, the urethra is about 18–20 cm long and in a female, it is about 4 cm long.

Functions

In a male, the urethra serves as a common passage for both semen and urine whereas in a female, the urethra discharges urine from the body.

PROSTATE GLAND

The prostate is a fibromusculoglandular organ, which surrounds the commencement of the urethra in the male. It is situated in the pelvic cavity behind the pubic symphysis and in front of the rectum. It is about the size of a chestnut and is traversed by the urethra and ejaculatory ducts.

Function

The function of the prostate is to secrete a thin, milky fluid, which forms about 30% of the semen, and gives it a milky appearance. The prostatic secretion is alkaline in nature and provides nourishment to the sperms.

SEMINAL VESICLES

The seminal vesicles are two small fibromuscular pouches lying between the base of the bladder and the rectum.

Function

The seminal vesicles secrete an alkaline fluid containing nutrients for the sperms and forms about 60% of the seminal fluid.

EJACULATORY DUCTS

The ejaculatory ducts are two narrow tubes about 1 cm long. The duct of seminal vesicle and ductus deferens unite to form ejaculatory duct. They traverse the prostate gland to open into the urethra within the gland (prostatic part of urethra).

Function

The ejaculatory ducts expel the secretions of testes and seminal vesicles into the prostatic urethra.

UTERUS

The uterus is a hollow, thick-walled, muscular organ situated in the pelvic cavity between the urinary bladder and the rectum. It is pear shaped and flattened anteroposteriorly. In the majority of women it leans forward (**anteflexion**) and bends forward (**anteversion**) almost at a right angle to the vagina. In the erect posture, the uterus lies in an almost horizontal position.

The uterus is divided from above downward into following three parts: (a) fundus, (b) body, and (c) cervix. The cervix protrudes into the vagina through its anterior wall and opens into it at the *external os*.

Above on either side, it communicates with the uterine tubes, which open into it. Below it communicates with the vagina.

Functions

The functions of the uterus after puberty are:

1. Responsible for menstrual cycle (MC).
2. Provides implantation to zygote in its wall.
3. Allows growth and development of the embryo and fetus.

VAGINA

The vagina is a fibromuscular tube, which extends obliquely downward and forward from the uterus to the vestibule of vagina — the elliptical space between the labia. It is situated between the urinary bladder in front, and the rectum and anal canal behind. The vagina has no secretory glands though it is kept moist by the cervical secretions.

Functions

The functions of the vagina are as follows:

1. Acts as a receptacle for penis during coitus.
2. Provides an elastic passage to the baby during childbirth.

UTERINE TUBES

There are two uterine tubes. Each tube is about 10 cm long, which extends from the side of the uterus (between the fundus and body) to the ovary where it opens into the peritoneal cavity.

It is divided into the following parts from distal to the proximal end: (a) infundibulum, (b) ampulla, (c) isthmus, and (d) intramural.

Functions

The functions of uterine tubes are as follows:

1. Transport the ovum from ovary to its lumen and provides an ideal site for fertilization.
2. Transport the fertilized ovum to uterine cavity for implantation.

OVARIES

The ovaries are female gonads. Each ovary is about the size and shape of an almond and is situated in a shallow fossa on

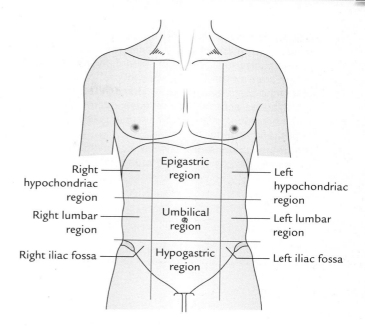

Fig. 1.6 Regions of the abdominal cavity.

the lateral wall of the pelvic cavity behind and below the distal end of the uterine tube.

Functions

The ovaries begin to function at puberty and continue to discharge ova at monthly intervals from about the age of 13 years to about the age of 45 years.

REGIONS OF THE ABDOMEN

The abdominal cavity is conventionally divided by the clinicians into nine regions (Fig. 1.6). This facilitates the description and position of the organs present in the abdominal cavity during clinical examination.

Clinical correlation

Disorders of the abdomen: The disorders of the abdomen and pelvis are numerous; the important ones are as follows:
(a) **Hernia:** It is the protrusion of an organ through the wall, which contains/retains it. The common abdominal hernias are inguinal, umbilical, femoral, and incisional; the order reflecting their frequency.
(b) **Abdominal pain:** Many intra-abdominal diseases present with pain only. The two important features of an abdominal pain are its **site** and its **nature**. If a clinician knows about these features, he/she has a good chance of making a correct diagnosis. In general: (i) The upper abdominal pain mostly occurs due to involvement of gallbladder, stomach, duodenum, and pancreas. (ii) The central abdominal pain usually occurs due to involvement of small bowel and kidneys. (iii) The lower abdominal pain occurs due to involvement of urinary bladder, uterus, caecum, and sigmoid colon.

(c) **Abdominal mass:** The common causes of abdominal masses are: hepatomegaly (enlargement of liver), splenomegaly (enlargement of spleen), hydronephrosis (enlargement of the kidney), pseudocyst of pancreas, mesenteric cysts, carcinoma of stomach, enlargement of gallbladder, accumulation of feces, retention of urine in urinary bladder, ovarian cyst, pregnant uterus, uterine fibroids, and appendicular mass.

(d) **Abdominal distension:** The six common causes of abdominal distension are **Fetus, Flatus** (gas in intestine), **Feces** (impaction of feces in bowel), **Fat, Fluid** (ascites), and **Fibroids**.

The names of six conditions that cause abdominal distension start with the letter "F."

The distension (**prominent abdomen**) is normal in infants and young children due to the following reasons:

– Their gastrointestinal tract contains a considerable amount of air.
– Their liver is relatively large in size.
– Their abdominal muscles are relatively less toned.

Golden Facts to Remember

➤ Largest gland in the body	Liver
➤ Most dilated part of the digestive tube	Stomach
➤ Pelvic organ with thickest muscular walls	Uterus
➤ Most of the abdominal cavity is occupied by	Organs and glands of the digestive system
➤ Bulk of semen is formed by	Secretion of seminal vesicles
➤ Commonest cause of abdominal distension in a married female	Pregnancy

Osteology of the Abdomen

The osteology of abdomen deals with the bones of the abdomen and pelvis.

The bones of the abdomen and pelvis are as follows (Fig. 2.1):

1. Lower ribs and costal cartilages.
2. Lumbar vertebrae.
3. Sacrum.
4. Coccyx.
5. Hip or innominate bone.

LOWER RIBS AND COSTAL CARTILAGES

The ribs and costal cartilages are described in detail in *Textbook of Anatomy: Upper Limb and Thorax,* 2nd Edition by Vishram Singh. The costal cartilages of 7th, 8th, 9th, and 10th

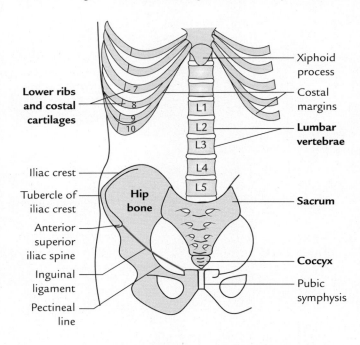

Fig. 2.1 Bones of the abdomen and pelvis.

Labels (from figure): Lower ribs and costal cartilages · 7 · 8 · 9 · 10 · Iliac crest · Tubercle of iliac crest · Anterior superior iliac spine · Inguinal ligament · Pectineal line · Hip bone · L1 · L2 · L3 · L4 · L5 · Xiphoid process · Costal margins · Lumbar vertebrae · Sacrum · Coccyx · Pubic symphysis

ribs articulate with each other to form the **costal margin.** The 11th and 12th ribs are shorter and do not articulate either with the transverse processes of 11th and 12th thoracic vertebrae or with the adjacent costal cartilages. As a result they can move independently, hence are termed **floating ribs.**

LUMBAR VERTEBRAE

The lumbar vertebrae consist of the same elements as the thoracic vertebrae but are more massive in keeping with the greater load, which they have to transmit. There are five lumbar vertebrae out of which first four (L1 to L4) are typical and fifth (L5) is atypical.

Identifying features of the lumbar vertebrae are as follows:

1. Massive reniform bodies.
2. Absence of costal facets on the body.
3. Absence of foramina transversaria in the transverse processes.
4. Presence of accessory and mammillary processes.
5. Thick quadrilateral spinous processes.

FEATURES OF TYPICAL LUMBAR VERTEBRAE (L1, L2, L3, L4)

General Features (Fig. 2.2)

Body

1. The body is massive and reniform.
2. Its transverse diameter is more than the anteroposterior diameter.
3. It is constricted in front and at the sides.
4. The size of the body increases progressively from first to fifth lumbar vertebra.
5. The length of the body is slightly greater anteriorly. This contributes to the forward convexity of the lumbar vertebral column.
6. The body has no costal facets on its sides.

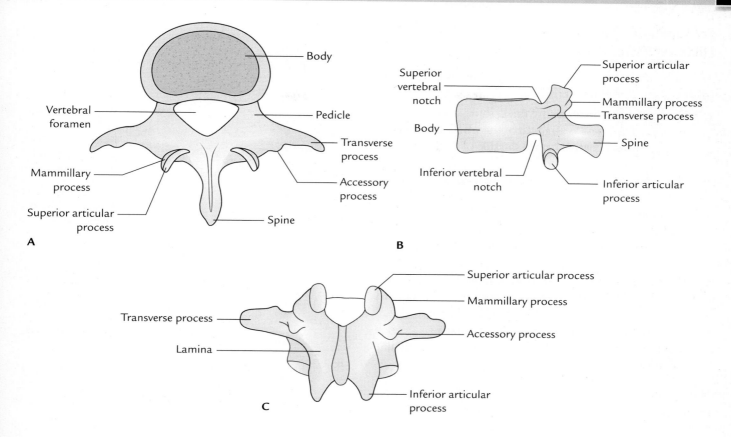

Fig. 2.2 Typical lumbar vertebra: **A**, superior view; **B**, lateral view; **C**, posterior view.

Vertebral Foramen

1. It is triangular in shape.
2. It is larger than in the thoracic vertebrae but smaller than in the cervical vertebrae.

Vertebral Arch

Pedicles

- The pedicles are short and strong processes.
- They project backward from the upper parts of the body; as a result, the inferior vertebral notches are much deeper than the superior ones.

Laminae

- The laminae are short, thick, and broad plates.
- They are directed posteromedially.
- The overlapping between the laminae of the adjoining vertebrae is minimal.

Spine

- The spine is quadrilateral in shape.
- It projects almost backward.

Transverse processes

- The transverse processes are thin and tapering.
- They are homologous to the ribs in the thoracic region.
- The posteroinferior aspect of each transverse process presents a small rough elevation called **accessory process**. This represents the true transverse process of the vertebra.
- A vertical ridge near the tip marks the anterior surface of each transverse process.

Superior articular processes

- The facets on the superior articular processes are concave, which project backward and medially.
- The superior articular processes lay farther apart than the inferior articular processes.
- Their posterior borders are marked by a rough elevation called **mammillary process.**

Inferior articular processes

- The inferior articular processes lie nearer to each other than the superior articular processes.
- They bear convex articular facets, which face forward and laterally.

FEATURES OF ATYPICAL FIFTH LUMBAR VERTEBRA (L5)

The fifth lumbar vertebra presents the following atypical (distinguishing) features (Fig. 2.3):

1. **The transverse processes** are thick, short, and pyramidal in shape. Their base is attached to the whole thickness of the pedicle and encroaches on the side of the body. They seem to be turned upward.
2. The **spine** is small, short, least substantial, and rounded at the tip.
3. The **body** is largest of all lumbar vertebrae. The vertical height of the anterior surface of the body is more than that of the posterior surface. This difference is responsible for sharp/prominent lumbosacral angle (120°).
4. The **superior articular facets** look more backward than medially and **inferior articular facets** look more forward than laterally as compared to typical lumbar vertebrae.
5. The distance between the **inferior articular processes** is equal or more than that between the **superior articular processes**.

N.B. *Fawcett's rule for identification of individual lumbar vertebrae* (Fig. 2.4): According to this rule, an individual lumbar vertebra can be identified if it is looked from behind. A four-sided figure can be constructed by joining the four articular processes. The quadrangular figure thus constructed differs in different lumbar vertebrae as given in the box below.

Shape of quadrangular figure	Vertebra
Trapezium with top broader than base	1st/2nd lumbar vertebra
Rectangle with long vertical lines	3rd lumbar vertebra
Square	4th lumbar vertebra
Rectangle with long horizontal lines	5th lumbar vertebra

The characteristic features of typical lumbar vertebrae are summarized in Table 2.1.

Table 2.1 Characteristic features of the lumbar vertebrae

Part	Characteristics
Body	Massive and kidney shaped
Vertebral foramen	Triangular and relatively smaller than in cervical vertebrae
Transverse process	Long and slender with **accessory process** on the posterior surface of base of each process
Articular processes	• Superior articular facets directed posteromedially • Inferior articular facets directed anterolaterally
Spinous process	Short, thick, broad, and hatchet shaped

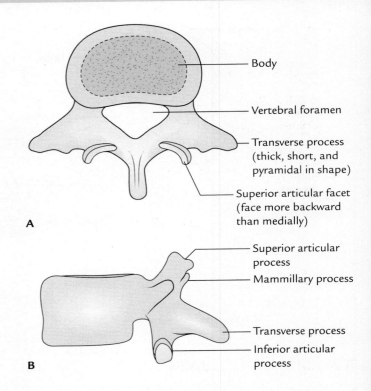

Fig. 2.3 Fifth lumbar vertebra: **A**, as seen from above; **B**, as seen from the side.

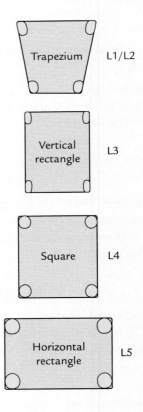

Fig. 2.4 Quadrangular figures formed by joining the articular process of lumbar vertebra (H.E. Fawcett, 1932).

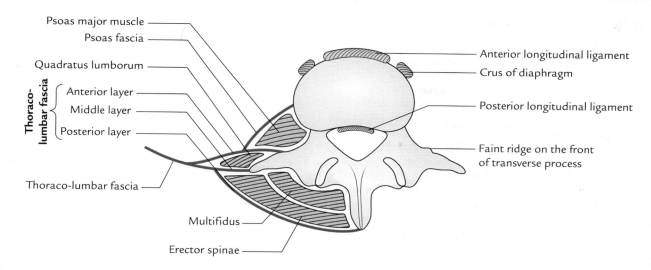

Fig. 2.5 Attachments of the lumbar vertebra.

SPECIAL FEATURES OF LUMBAR VERTEBRAE (Fig. 2.5)

The special features include attachment of muscles and ligaments, which are described below:

1. **Anterior longitudinal ligament** is attached on the upper and lower borders of lumbar vertebral bodies anteriorly.
2. **Posterior longitudinal ligament** is attached on the upper and lower borders of lumbar vertebral bodies posteriorly.
3. **Right crus of diaphragm** is attached on the front of upper three lumbar vertebral bodies.
4. **Left crus of diaphragm** is attached on the front of upper two lumbar vertebral bodies.
5. **Psoas major** arises by fleshy slips from upper and lower borders of all lumbar vertebrae.
6. **Tendinous arches of psoas major** are attached across the constricted parts of the bodies on each side.
7. **Ligamenta flava** are attached to the laminae of adjacent vertebrae.
8. **Posterior layer of thoraco-lumbar fascia** is attached to the spinous processes of lumbar vertebrae.
9. **Supraspinous** and **interspinous ligaments** are attached to the spinous processes of lumbar vertebrae.
10. **Erector spinae** and **multifidus muscles** are attached to the spinous processes of lumbar vertebrae.
11. **Middle layer of thoraco-lumbar fascia** is attached to the tips of transverse processes of the all lumbar vertebrae.
12. **Medial** and **lateral arcuate ligaments** of diaphragm are attached to the tips of transverse processes of L1 vertebra.
13. **Anterior layer of thoraco-lumbar fascia** is attached to the faint ridge on the front of transverse processes.
14. **Multifidus** and **intertransverse muscles** are attached to the mammillary processes.
15. **Iliolumbar ligaments** are attached to the tips of the transverse processes of the fifth lumbar vertebra.
16. **Accessory** and **mammillary processes** provide attachment to the medial intertransverse muscles.

OSSIFICATION

A lumbar vertebra ossifies from three *primary centres* and five *secondary centres*. The sites of appearance and age of fusion are given in Table 2.2.

Table 2.2 Ossification of a lumbar vertebra

Ossification centres	Fusion
Primary centres (appear between 7th and 8th week of intrauterine life) • One for body • Two for two halves of the vertebral arch	• Two halves of the vertebral arch fuse during the 1st year • Vertebral arch fuses with the body during the 6th year
Secondary centres (appear at about puberty) • Two for annular epiphysis of the upper and lower surfaces of the body • Two for tips of the transverse processes • Two for mammillary processes • One for the tip of the spine	The portions derived from secondary centres fuse with rest of the bone at about 25 years

Clinical correlation

- **Sacralization of the fifth lumbar vertebra:** It is the fusion of the fifth lumbar vertebra with the sacrum. The fusion may be complete or incomplete. The transverse process of L5 may articulate with ala of sacrum and/or ilium and compress the L5 spinal nerve. This condition occurs in about 5% of normal individuals.
- **Spina bifida:** It occurs due to non fusion of two halves of the vertebral arch. In this condition the meninges and spinal cord are exposed and may herniate out in the midline through the gap (for details, see *Clinical and Surgical Anatomy,* 2nd Edition by Vishram Singh).
- **Spondylolysis:** In this condition, there is a separation of body of 5th lumbar vertebra from vertebral arch bearing inferior articular process on one side only. Inferior articular processes of L5 vertebra normally interlock with the articular processes of the sacrum (Fig. 2.6).
- **Spondylolisthesis:** It is the forward slipping of the fifth lumbar vertebra over the sacrum. Sometimes the inferior articular processes, laminae, and spine of L5 vertebra are separated from the rest of the vertebra, which slip forward on the sloping superior surface of the sacrum (Fig. 2.7). This condition may clinically present as backache and pain radiating along the course of the sciatic nerve—**sciatica** (also see page 470).
- **Cauda equina syndrome:** It is caused due to compression of cauda equina—a leash of nerve roots of L2 to S1 around the filum terminale. Clinically, it presents as:
  - (a) Flaccid paraplegia.
  - (b) Saddle-shaped anesthesia.
  - (c) Late bladder and bowel involvement leading to incontinence of urine and feces.
  - (d) Impotence.
  - (e) Absence of knee and ankle jerks.

SACRUM

The sacrum (Latin *sacrum*: sacred) is a large flattened triangular/wedge-shaped bone formed by the fusion of five sacral vertebrae (Fig. 2.8). The sacrum articulates on either side with the hip bone to form the sacroiliac joint. The functions of sacrum are as follows:

1. Forms posterior part of the bony pelvis.

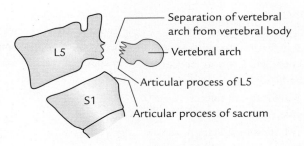

Fig. 2.6 Spondylolysis.

Labels: L5, S1, Separation of vertebral arch from vertebral body, Vertebral arch, Articular process of L5, Articular process of sacrum

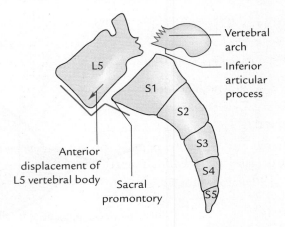

Labels: L5, S1, S2, S3, S4, S5, Vertebral arch, Inferior articular process, Anterior displacement of L5 vertebral body, Sacral promontory

Fig. 2.7 Spondylolisthesis (forward displacement of L5 vertebral body over the sacrum).

2. Supports the vertebral column.
3. Transmits the weight of the body to the pelvic girdle through the sacroiliac joints.

ANATOMICAL POSITION

To keep the sacrum in anatomical position, hold it in such a way that:

1. Its smooth pelvic surface faces downward and forward and its rough dorsal surface faces upward and backward.
2. Upper surface of the body of the first sacral vertebra slopes forward at an angle of about 30°.
3. Upper end of the sacral canal is directed almost upward and slightly backward.

N.B. In an articulated skeleton, the sacrum is placed obliquely like a wedge between the two hip bones. When lumbar vertebral column is in position, an angle is formed between L5 and L1 vertebrae. This angle is called sacrovertebral/lumbosacral angle. It measures about 210° and is being rounded by the intervening disc which is much thicker in front than behind.

GENERAL FEATURES (Fig. 2.8)

The sacrum presents the following general features:

1. Base.
2. Apex.
3. Four surfaces: pelvic, dorsal, and two lateral (right and left) surfaces.
4. Sacral canal.

Base

The base of the sacrum is directed upward and forward. It is formed by the superior surface of the first sacral vertebra. It is divided into three parts: median part and right and left lateral parts. The median part is formed by the oval upper surface of the body of the first sacral vertebra. Its anterior border is termed **sacral promontory**. The right and left lateral parts are fan shaped and represent the upper surfaces of lateral masses of sacrum called alae. The lateral masses represent the fused costal and transverse elements of the sacral vertebrae.

1. Upper surface of the body of the first sacral vertebra articulates with the fifth lumbar vertebra.
2. *Vertebral foramen* lying behind the body is triangular and leads into the **sacral canal**.
3. *Pedicles* are short and directed backward and laterally.
4. *Laminae* are quite oblique.
5. *Transverse processes* are massive and fused with the corresponding costal transverse element of lower sacral vertebrae to form the broad sloping lateral masses called *alae of sacrum*.

6. The *spinous process* forms the first *spinous tubercle*.
7. The *superior articular processes* are prominent and project upward. They flank the superior opening of sacral canal.

Apex

1. It is the lower narrow blunt extremity formed by the inferior surface of the body of the fifth sacral vertebra.
2. It bears an oval facet for articulation with the coccyx to form the **sacrococcygeal joint**.

Surfaces

Pelvic Surface (Fig. 2.8A)

The pelvic surface of sacrum is **concave** and directed downward and forward. It presents the following features:
1. *Four transverse ridges* that indicate the lines of fusion of five sacral vertebrae.

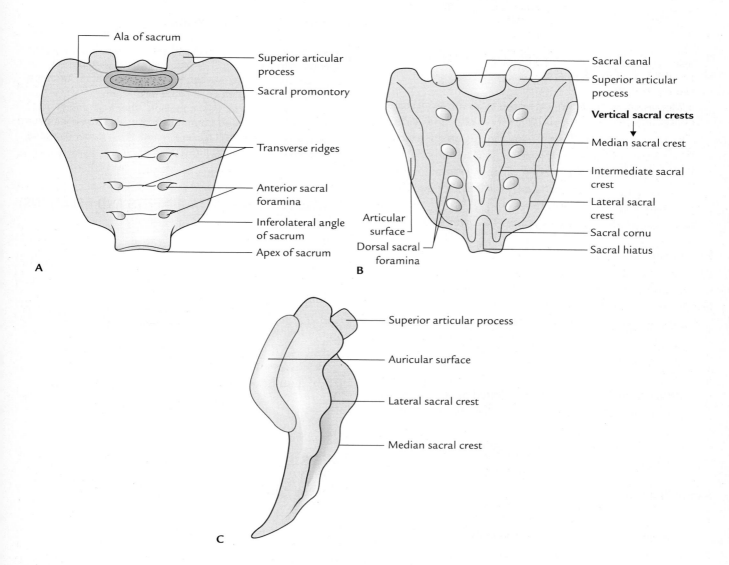

Fig. 2.8 General features of the sacrum: A, pelvic surface; B, dorsal surface; C, lateral surface.

2. Lateral to transverse ridges are *four anterior sacral foramina* through which ventral rami of upper four sacral nerves come out.
3. The part of bone lateral to foramina is the lateral mass.

Dorsal Surface (Fig. 2.8B)

The dorsal surface of sacrum is rough, irregular, and convex.

1. In the median plane, there is *median sacral crest* that bears three or four spinous tubercles representing spinous processes of fused sacral vertebrae.
2. Lateral to median crest, the posterior surface is formed by *fused laminae* of upper four sacral vertebrae.
   The laminae of the fifth sacral vertebra fail to join behind, forming a U-shaped gap called **sacral hiatus**.
3. Lateral to laminae are four *articular tubercles* in line with the superior articular process of the first sacral vertebra.
4. The inferior articular processes of the fifth sacral vertebra project downward as *sacral cornua* on either side of sacral hiatus.

N.B. The most prominent features on the dorsal surface of sacrum are presence of:
- *Five vertical crests*:
  - *Median sacral crest*, formed by the fusion of sacral spines.
  - *Two intermediate sacral crests*, one on either side of median crest, are formed by the fusion of articular processes of sacral vertebrae.
  - *Two lateral sacral crests*, one on each side of lateral to intermedial crest, are formed by the fusion of transverse processes of sacral vertebrae.
- *Sacral hiatus:* An U-shaped gap at the lower end.

Lateral Surfaces (Fig. 2.8C)

Each lateral surface is the lateral aspect of lateral mass formed by the fusion of transverse and costal elements of sacral vertebrae.

1. It is wide above and narrow below.
2. Lower narrow part turns abruptly medially to form the **inferolateral angle** of the sacrum.
3. Upper wider part bears an inverted *L-shaped* **auricular surface** anteriorly and a deeply pitted area posteriorly. The auricular surface is so called because of its resemblance to the auricle of the external ear. It extends on to the upper three or three and a half sacral vertebrae.

Sacral Canal

1. The sacral canal is formed by the superimposed vertebral foramina of the sacral vertebrae.
2. The upper end of the canal is directed upward in line with vertebral canal of lumbar vertebrae and its lower end opens at the **sacral hiatus**.

3. The sacral canal communicates with the pelvic and dorsal sacral foramina through the intervertebral foramina.

Contents of Sacral Canal

1. Lower part of cauda equina (sacral and coccygeal nerve roots).
2. Filum terminale.
3. Spinal meninges.
4. Lateral sacral vessels.

N.B. The *dural tube* and *arachnoid* mater extend up to the second sacral vertebra.

Structures Emerging through Sacral Hiatus

1. Fifth sacral (S5) nerves.
2. Coccygeal (C×1) nerves.
3. Filum terminale.

Clinical correlation

- **Sacralization:** The term sacralization means incorporation of the fifth lumbar (L5) or first coccygeal vertebra (C1) in the sacrum. In sacralization the number of sacral foramina is increased unilaterally or bilaterally.
- **Lumbarization:** In this condition, the first sacral (S1) vertebra is separated from the sacrum and fused with the fifth lumbar vertebra (L5). As a result, the number of sacral foramina is reduced to three pairs.

SPECIAL FEATURES (ATTACHMENTS AND RELATIONS)

Base

1. The upper surface of the body of the first sacral vertebra articulates with the L5 vertebra to form the lumbosacral joint.
2. The smooth medial part of the **ala** of sacrum is related to the following four structures from medial to lateral side (Fig. 2.9):
   (a) Sympathetic chain.
   (b) Lumbosacral trunk.

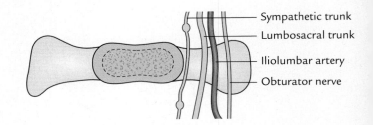

Sympathetic trunk
Lumbosacral trunk
Iliolumbar artery
Obturator nerve

Fig. 2.9 Structure related to the smooth medial part of the ala of sacrum.

(c) Iliolumbar artery.

(d) Obturator nerve.

The ventral ramus of L5 nerve is so taut that it grooves the ala.

3. The rough lateral part of the ala gives origin to **iliacus muscle** anteriorly and attachment to the **lumbosacral ligament** posteriorly.

Apex

It bears an oval facet, which articulates with the body of first coccygeal vertebra to form the sacrococcygeal joint.

Surfaces

Pelvic Surface

It presents the following particular features (Fig. 2.10A):

1. The **median sacral vessels** are related to the pelvic surface in the median plane.
2. The **sympathetic trunks** are related to the pelvic surface along the medial margins of pelvic sacral foramina.
3. The **upper two-and-half sacral vertebrae** are related to the parietal peritoneum except for the site of attachment of the medial limb of the sigmoid mesocolon.
4. The **lower two-and-half vertebrae** are related to the rectum, but separated from S3 vertebra by bifurcation of the superior rectal artery.
5. The **piriformis muscle** arises from the bodies of middle three sacral vertebrae in an E-shaped fashion.
6. The **pelvic sacral foramina** transmit ventral rami of the corresponding upper four sacral nerves and a branch from lateral sacral arteries.

Dorsal Surface

It presents the following particular features (Fig. 2.10B):

1. The four dorsal foramina transmit the dorsal rami of the corresponding **upper four sacral spinal nerves.**
2. The **erector spinae muscle** arises from an elongated U-shaped linear area involving the continuous rows of the spinous and transverse tubercles.
3. The **multifidus** arises from the area enclosed by U-shaped origin of erector spinae. The dorsal rami of upper four sacral spinal nerves reach the surface by piercing multifidus and erector spinae muscles.

Lateral Surfaces

The auricular surface/facet articulates with the corresponding auricular surface of the ilium to form sacroiliac joint.

1. The rough area behind the auricular surface gives attachment to strong **interosseous sacroiliac ligament.**
2. The lower narrow part of the lateral surface opposite the **inferolateral angle** gives attachment to four structures. From behind forward these are:
    (a) Gluteus maximus.
    (b) Sacrotuberous ligament.
    (c) Sacrospinous ligament.
    (d) Coccygeus.

The last structure (i.e., coccygeus) encroaches on the pelvic surface of the sacrum.

The differences between male and female sacrum are given in Table 2.3.

N.B. *Sacral index:* It is the ratio between the length and breadth of the sacrum and is expressed by the formula, breadth × 100/length.

The sacral index is higher in females than males. The average sacral index in a female is 116 and in a male it is 112.

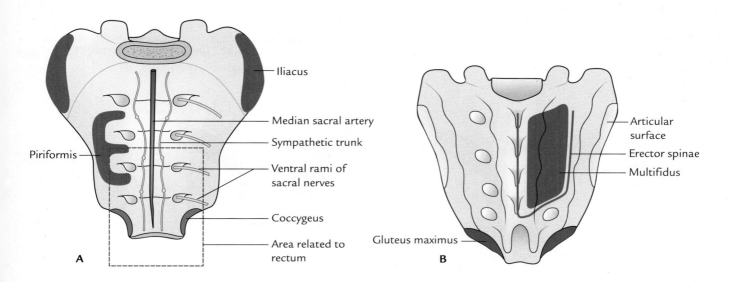

Fig. 2.10 Special features of the sacrum: A, pelvic surface; B, dorsal surface.

Table 2.3 Differences between the male and female sacrum

Features	Male	Female
Base of sacrum	Width of articular area (body of S1 vertebra)is more than the length of ala of one side, i.e., body is broad and alae are narrow	Width of articular area (body of S1 vertebra) is either equal or less than the length of ala of one side, i.e., body is narrow and alae are broad
Sacral index	Less (sacrum is relatively longer and narrower)	More (sacrum is relatively shorter and broader)
Pelvic surface	• Smoothly curved, "C" shaped (curvature of the pelvic surface is gradual from above downward) • Concavity of sacrum is shallower	• Abruptly curved, "J" shaped (lower part of the pelvic surface abruptly curves forward, curvature being most marked between S1 and S2 segments and between S3 and S5 segments) • Concavity of sacrum is deeper
Auricular surface	• Extends on to the upper 3 or 3½ of sacral vertebrae • Relatively larger and less obliquely set • Concavity of dorsal border of the auricular surface is less marked	• Extends on to the upper 2 or 2½ of the sacral vertebrae • Relatively smaller and more obliquely set • Concavity of dorsal border of the auricular surface is more marked

OSSIFICATION

The ossification of sacrum is not of much clinical interest. However, students should simply know that since the sacrum is a composite bone formed by the fusion of five sacral vertebrae, it ossifies by multiple centres.

COCCYX (Fig. 2.11)

The coccyx, or tailbone, is a small, triangular bone formed by the fusion of four rudimentary coccygeal vertebrae, which progressively reduce in size from above downward. The tip of coccyx lies at the level of the upper border of the pubic symphysis. The coccyx can be palpated in the natal cleft.

1. The word "coccyx" is derived from the Greek word "cuckoo," a bird. The tailbone was so named because its shape resembled the bird's beak.
2. Morphologically coccyx represents the tail (tailbone).
3. The number of coccygeal vertebrae may vary from three to five.

GENERAL FEATURES

The coccyx is directed downward and forward, making a continuous curve with the sacrum. It presents the following features:

1. Base.
2. Apex or tip.
3. Pelvic surface.
4. Dorsal surface.
5. Lateral margins.

SPECIAL FEATURES

Base

1. It is formed by the upper surface of the body of the first coccygeal vertebra.
2. It articulates with the apex of sacrum to form a cartilaginous sacrococcygeal joint.

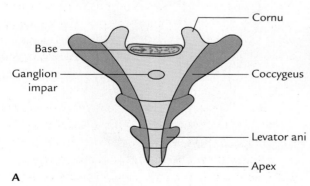
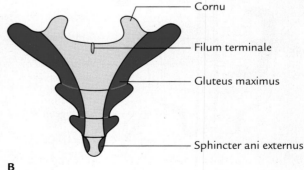

Fig. 2.11 Coccyx: **A,** pelvic surface; **B,** dorsal surface.

4. A pair of bony processes called **coccygeal cornu** project from the posterolateral aspects of the body of the first coccygeal vertebra and are connected with the sacral cornua by the **intercornual ligaments**.

5. The **fifth sacral nerves** after emerging from the sacral hiatus pass laterally through the interval between the body of the fifth sacral vertebra and the intercornual ligaments.

6. The rudimentary transverse processes of the first coccygeal vertebrae project laterally and upward from the side of the base.

Apex

1. It is formed by the body of the fourth coccygeal vertebra.
2. It lies about 4 cm behind and above the anal orifice.
3. It provides attachment to **sphincter ani externus** and **anococcygeal ligaments**.

Pelvic Surface

1. It is related to the rectum.
2. It provides attachment on each side to the **coccygeus muscle** in the upper two pieces and **levator ani** in the lower two pieces of the coccygeal vertebra.
3. The **ganglion impar**, where the sympathetic trunks of two sides meet, lies on the pelvic surface of first coccygeal vertebra deep to the rectum.
4. Anastomosis between the median sacral and inferior lateral sacral arteries and coccygeal body lies on the pelvic surface distal to ganglion impar.

Dorsal Surface

1. It provides origin on each side to **gluteus maximus**.
2. It provides origin to **sphincter ani externus** at the tip.
3. It provides attachment to **filum terminale** on the first coccygeal vertebra.

Lateral Margins

They provide attachment to sacrotuberous and sacrospinous ligaments.

OSSIFICATION

The coccyx ossifies from four primary centres, one for each segment.

HIP BONE

There are two hip bones, right and left. The hip bone is a large irregular bone which articulates in front with the corresponding bone of the opposite side. Posteriorly, two hip bones articulate with the sacrum. The **pelvic girdle** consists of the two hip bones.

PARTS (Fig. 2.12)

Each hip bone consists of three parts: ilium, ischium, and pubis, which are fused together at a cup-shaped hollow on the outer aspect of the bone called **acetabulum**.

Ilium

The ilium is the upper expanded part of the hip bone. It presents the following features:
1. Iliac crest.
2. Three surfaces.
3. Three borders.

Iliac Crest

It is the broad, flattened, sinuous ridge forming the upper limit of the ilium. The highest point of iliac crest lies at the level of intervertebral disc between L3 and L4 vertebrae.

- The anterior end of iliac crest presents a bony projection called anterior superior iliac spine, which provides attachment to the lateral end of the inguinal ligament. The **anterior superior iliac spine** is easily felt at the lateral end of the fold of the groin.
- The posterior end of iliac crest also presents a bony projection called **posterior superior iliac spine**, which lies at the level of spine of S2 vertebra and marked on the surface as a small dimple on the lower part of the back.
- The outer lip of iliac crest, about 5 cm behind the anterior superior iliac spine, presents a tubercle called **tubercle of the iliac crest**.

N.B. Morphologically, the iliac crest is divided into anterior two-third (ventral segment) and posterior one-third (dorsal segment). The ventral segment presents an inner lip, an outer lip, and an intermediate area. The dorsal segment presents inner (medial) and outer (lateral) sloping surfaces.

Surfaces

1. **Gluteal surface:** It is the outer surface of the ilium. It is divided into four areas by three gluteal lines. This surface is so named because it provides origin to gluteal muscles (gluteus maximus, medius, and minimus).
2. **Iliac fossa:** It is a large, smooth, hollowed-out area on the anterior part of inner/medial aspect of the ilium. The upper two-third of this area gives origin to the

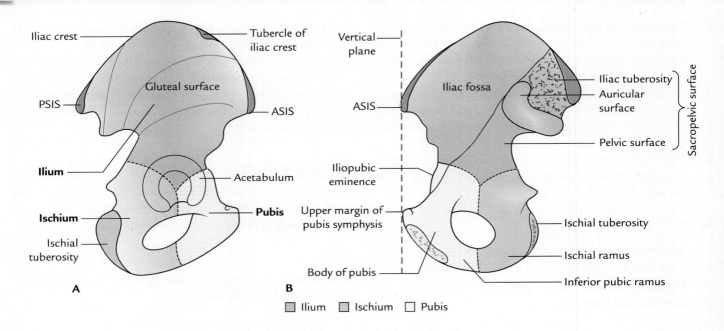

Fig. 2.12 Hip bone: **A**, lateral view; **B**, medial view (ASIS = anterior superior iliac spine, PSIS = posterior superior iliac spine).

iliacus muscle. Posterior to iliac fossa, lie the auricular surface and tuberosity of ilium.

A curved ridge called **arcuate line** of ilium separates the iliac fossa (which forms the bony wall of greater pelvis) from the part of ilium medial to acetabulum (which forms the upper part of bony wall of lesser pelvis).

3. **Sacropelvic surface:** It is situated behind the medial border of the ilium and consists of three parts: iliac tuberosity, auricular surface, and pelvic surface.
   (a) The **iliac tuberosity** is a rough area below the dorsal segment of the iliac crest.
   (b) The **auricular surface** is ear-shaped articular surface situated anteroinferior to the iliac tuberosity.
   (c) The **pelvic surface** is situated anteroinferior to the auricular surface.

Borders

1. **Anterior border:** It extends from anterior superior iliac spine to the acetabulum.
2. **Posterior border:** It extends from posterior superior iliac spine to the upper end of the posterior border of ischium. It presents posterior inferior iliac spine and greater sciatic notch.
3. **Medial border:** It extends from iliac crest to the iliopubic eminence. It separates iliac fossa from sacropelvic surface.

Pubis

The pubis is the anteroinferior part of the hip bone and articulates with the pubis of the opposite hip bone to form the **symphysis pubis**. It consists of three parts:

1. Body.
2. Superior ramus.
3. Inferior ramus.

Body

It is flattened anteroposteriorly and presents the following features:

1. Pubic crest, pubic tubercle, and three surfaces (anterior, posterior, and medial).
2. The **pubic crest** is the upper border of the body of pubis. At the lateral end of the pubic crest is the **pubic tubercle.**

Superior Ramus

It extends from the body of pubis to the acetabulum above the obturator foramen. It presents three borders (pectineal line, obturator crest, and inferior border) and three surfaces (pectineal, pelvic, and obturator).

- The **pectineal line** (also called **pecten pubis**) extends from pubic tubercle to the iliopubic eminence.
- The **obturator crest** extends from pubic tubercle to the acetabular notch.
- The **inferior border** is sharp and forms the upper margin of the obturator foramen.
- The **pectineal surface** is situated between the pectineal line and obturator crest. It is roughly triangular in shape and extends from pubic tubercle to the iliopubic eminence.
- The **pelvic surface** is situated between the pectineal line and inferior border of the superior ramus.

- The **obturator surface** is situated between the obturator crest and inferior border.

Inferior Ramus

It extends from the lower and lateral part of the body of pubis to fuse with the ramus of ischium to form conjoint **ischiopubic ramus** on the medial side of the obturator foramen.

N.B. *Arcuate line of ilium:* It is a thick, curved ridge extending from anteroinferior part of auricular surface of ilium to the iliopubic eminence.

Linea terminalis: It is formed by pubic crest, pectin pubis, iliopubic eminence, arcuate line of ilium, and anterior margin of ala of sacrum.

Ischium

The ischium is the posteroinferior part of the hip bone and forms the posterior boundary of the obturator foramen. It consists of two parts:

1. Body.
2. Ramus.

Body

- The body is thick and lies below and posterior to the acetabulum. It presents two ends (upper and lower), three borders (anterior, posterior, and lateral), and three surfaces (femoral, dorsal, and pelvic).
- The upper end of the body forms part (two-fifth) of the acetabulum, whereas its lower end forms ischial tuberosity.
- The posterior border of the body is continuous with the posterior border of the ilium and presents **ischial spine** superior to the tuberosity. The ischial spine projects posteromedially and separates the lesser **sciatic notch** of the ischium inferiorly from the greater sciatic notch on the posterior border of the ilium.

Ramus

The ramus arises from the lower part of the body and runs forward, upward, and medially. It presents two surfaces (anterior and posterior) and two borders (upper and lower).

The upper border forms the boundary of obturator foramen and lower border forms the lateral border of pubic arch.

The hip bone is described in detail in Chapter 21.

BONY PELVIS

The term pelvis is derived from the Latin word, which means basin.

The bony pelvis is formed by the following four bones (Fig. 2.13):

(a) Two hip bones, one on either side.
(b) Sacrum, behind.
(c) Coccyx, behind.

These bones are united by four joints:

(a) Two synovial sacroiliac joints (posterosuperolaterally).
(b) Two fibrocartilaginous joints (pubic symphysis anteroinferiorly and sacrococcygeal joint posteroinferiorly).

The differences between male and female bony pelvis are given in Table 2.4.

ANATOMICAL POSITION

It is the position in which pelvis lies within the body in erect posture with the upper margins of the pubic symphysis and anterior superior iliac spines in the same coronal plane.

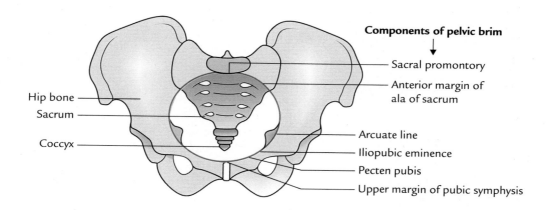

Fig. 2.13 Boundaries of the pelvic inlet (red line shows the shape of the pelvic inlet).

Table 2.4 Sex differences of the bony pelvis

Features	Male	Female
False pelvis	Narrow and deep	Wide and shallow
Pelvic inlet	Heart shaped	Transversely oval
True pelvis (pelvic cavity)	Narrow and deep	Roomy and shallow
Sacrum	Long and narrow with smoothly curved pelvic surface	Short and wide with abruptly curved pelvic surface near lower end
Subpubic angle	Narrow (70°)	Wide (90°–100°)

To keep the articulated pelvis in anatomical position, place the pelvis in such a way that the above three points touch the vertical surface.

PARTS

The pelvis is divided into two parts: greater pelvis and lesser pelvis by the pelvic inlet (superior pelvic aperture).

The **pelvic inlet** (also called pelvic brim) is bounded (Fig. 2.13):

- **Posteriorly** by sacral promontory.
- **Anteriorly** by upper margin of the pubic symphysis.
- **On either side** by linea terminalis which includes anterior margin of ala of sacrum, arcuate line, pectin pubis/pectineal line, and pubic crest.

Greater Pelvis (False Pelvis)

- It is the part of the pelvis above the pelvic brim and is formed by two iliac fossae.
- The greater pelvis forms a part of posterior abdominal wall, and contains sigmoid colon and coils of ilium.

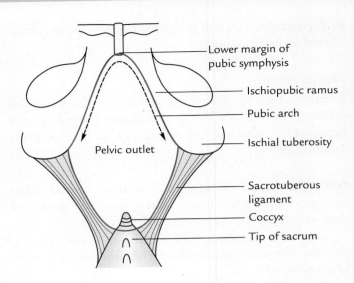

Fig. 2.14 Boundaries of the pelvic outlet (red line shows the shape of the pelvic outlet).

Lesser Pelvis (True Pelvis)

It is part of pelvis below the pelvic brim; clinically the term **pelvis** is usually applied to the lesser pelvis. The lesser pelvis is enclosed by sacrum and lower parts of the two hip bones (below the pelvic inlet).

The short anteroinferior wall of the lesser pelvis is formed by the pubic symphysis, whereas its long posterosuperior wall is formed by the sacrum and coccyx. On each side, the pelvic wall is formed by ischiopubic ramus and lower part of the ileum.

The **pelvic outlet** (also called inferior pelvic aperture) is bounded (Fig. 2.14):

- Anteriorly by lower margin of the public symphysis.
- Posteriorly by coccyx.
- On each side by ischiopubic ramus, ischial tuberosity, and sacrotuberous ligament.

The true pelvis is described in detail in Chapter 14.

Golden Facts to Remember

➤ Largest lumbar vertebra	Fifth lumbar (L5)
➤ All the lumbar vertebrae are typical *except*	Fifth lumbar vertebra which is atypical
➤ Most prominent feature on the dorsal surface of the sacrum	Presence of five vertical crests
➤ Sacred bone	Sacrum
➤ Tail bone	Coccyx

Clinical Case Study

A 65-year-old man visited a hospital and complained of low backache and pain radiating to the posterolateral aspect of the thigh. During the physical examination, on running his fingers along the lumbar spinous processes, the doctor found an abnormally prominent L5 spinous process. He suspected **spondylolisthesis**. The diagnosis was confirmed by sagittal MRI of the lumbosacral region.

Questions

1. What is spondylolysis?
2. What is spondylolisthesis?
3. In normal conditions, which parts of the fifth lumbar vertebra and sacrum interlock with each other.

Answers

1. A defect allowing part of vertebral arch of L5 vertebra to be separated from the body. In this condition there is separation of vertebral body from the part of vertebral arch bearing the inferior articular processes (Fig. 2.6).
2. When the defect is bilateral (vide supra), the body of L5 vertebra slides anteriorly on the sacrum so that it overlaps the sacral promontory. This condition is called **spondylolisthesis** (Fig. 2.7).
3. Normally inferior articular processes of L5 vertebra interlock with the articular processes of the sacrum.

Anterior Abdominal Wall

The anterior abdominal wall is a musculoaponeurotic structure confined to the anterior and lateral aspects of the abdomen. It is bounded *above* by the xiphoid process, and right and left costal margins; *below* by the anterior part of the iliac crest, fold of groin, pubic tubercle, pubic crest, and pubic symphysis; and *on each side* it is separated from the posterior abdominal wall by the midaxillary line.

The anatomy of anterior abdominal wall is clinically very important due to the following reasons:

1. The physical examination of the abdomen is mostly performed through the anterior abdominal wall.
2. Access to the abdomen and its contents is usually obtained through the incisions in the anterior abdominal wall.
3. Abdominal hernias mostly occur through the anterior abdominal wall.

N.B. Clinically the term anterior abdominal wall includes both the front and the side walls of the abdomen.

SURFACE LANDMARKS

The surface landmarks such as costal margins, umbilicus, anterior superior iliac spine, iliac tubercle, linea semilunaris, etc. are important guides in orienting the clinician to the location of the viscera in the abdominal cavity.

BONY LANDMARKS (Fig. 3.1)

Costal Margins

The cartilages of the 7th, 8th, 9th, and 10th ribs form the costal margins. The 7th costal cartilage is the lowest cartilage to reach the sternum. The right and left costal

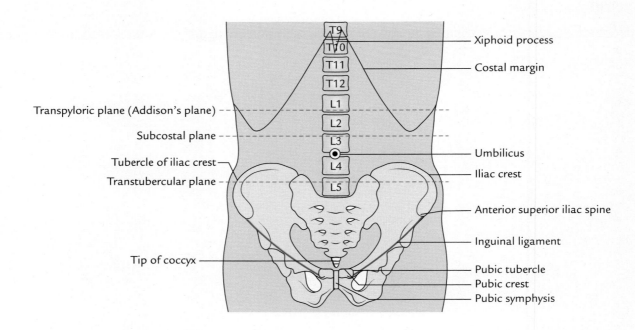

Fig. 3.1 Bony landmarks and planes of the abdomen.

margins run upward and medially toward the side of the xiphoid process and enclose between them an *infrasternal (subcostal) angle.* The costal margin reaches its lowest level in the midaxillary line.

Xiphoid Process

It forms the upper limit of anterior abdominal wall in the anterior median plane. It lies at the apex of subcostal angle and its apex is sometimes bent forward and hence easily palpable beneath the skin. The xiphoid process lies at the level of T9 vertebra.

Iliac Crest

It forms the lower limit of the anterior abdominal wall at the side and can be traced forward to the *anterior superior iliac spine.* About 5 cm behind the anterior superior iliac spine a prominent tubercle (**tubercle of iliac crest**) can be felt on the outer lip of the crest.

The highest points of iliac crests lie at the level of L4 vertebra just below the level of umbilicus.

Pubic Symphysis

It forms the lower limit of anterior abdominal wall in the anterior median plane. It is easily palpable and lies at the level of coccyx.

SOFT TISSUE LANDMARKS (Figs 3.2 and 3.3)

Groove of Groin

It is a curved linear horizontal groove which extends downward and medially from *anterior superior iliac spine* to the *pubic tubercle.* It is convex downward and overlies the inguinal/Poupart's ligament. Hence, it is also called inguinal line/Poupart's line. It is placed at the junction of the anterior abdominal wall and the front of the thigh.

Midline Furrow/Groove

It is a linear furrow/groove, which extends from the xiphoid process above to the pubic symphysis below. It corresponds to the *linea alba* — a tendinous raphe, which separates the two rectus muscles from each other. The midline linear furrow divides the anterior abdominal wall into right and left halves.

Umbilicus

It is an irregular, depressed scarred area in the linear midline furrow, a little below its midpoint (for details see page 27).

Linea Semilunaris

It is a curved furrow, which extends from tip of the 9th costal cartilage to the pubic tubercle. It lies few centimeters away from the median furrow and corresponds to the lateral margin of the rectus abdominis.

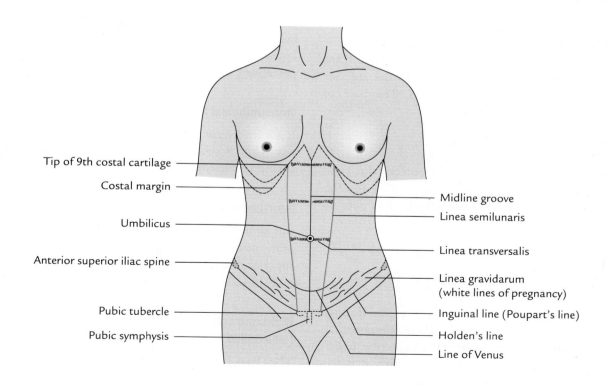

Tip of 9th costal cartilage
Costal margin
Umbilicus
Anterior superior iliac spine
Pubic tubercle
Pubic symphysis

Midline groove
Linea semilunaris
Linea transversalis
Linea gravidarum (white lines of pregnancy)
Inguinal line (Poupart's line)
Holden's line
Line of Venus

Fig. 3.2 Soft tissue landmarks on the front of abdomen.

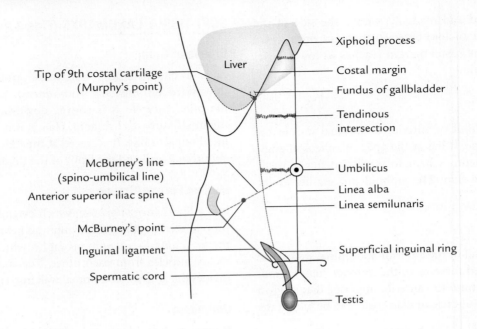

Fig. 3.3 Soft tissue landmarks of the abdomen and their relationship with gallbladder, appendix, and spermatic cord.

Spermatic Cord

It is a soft rounded cord present in the males. It can be palpated through skin as it passes downward just above the medial end of inguinal ligament to enter the scrotum.

McBurney's Point

It is a point at the junction of medial 2/3rd and lateral 1/3rd of the line extending from the umbilicus to the anterior superior iliac spine (**spinoumbilical line**). The base of appendix lies deep to this point.

Murphy's Point

It is a point where linea semilunaris meets the right subcostal margin. It corresponds to the tip of the 9th costal cartilage. The fundus of gall bladder lies deep to this point.

ABDOMINAL PLANES

Transpyloric Plane/Addison's Plane

It is an imaginary horizontal plane which passes through the midpoint of the line joining the jugular (suprasternal) notch to the symphysis pubis. It lies about one hand's breadth below the xiphisternal joint. Anteriorly it passes through the tip of the 9th costal cartilage and posteriorly through the lower border of the body of L1 vertebra. It is the **key plane of the abdomen** as it corresponds to number

of abdominal viscera, viz. pylorus of stomach, hila of kidneys, etc.

Subcostal Plane

It is an imaginary horizontal plane, which passes immediately below the costal margins. It passes anteriorly through the lowest borders of costal cartilages of the 10th rib, and posteriorly through the body of L3 vertebra.

Transumbilical Plane

It is a transverse plane that passes through the umbilicus (or navel) and lies at the level of intervertebral disc between the L3 and L4 vertebrae.

Intertubercular Plane

It is an imaginary horizontal plane which joins the tubercles of the iliac crests. It is palpable 5 cm posterior to the anterior superior iliac spines and passes through the upper part of the body of L5 vertebra.

Right and Left Vertical Planes (also called Midclavicular Planes)

They pass from the midpoint of the clavicle superiorly to the point midway between the anterior superior iliac spine and the pubic symphysis inferiorly, i.e., midinguinal point.

N.B. These planes are used to delineate the 9 regions or 4 quadrants of the abdominal cavity, which the clinicians refer, to describe the location of the abdominal viscera and pain abdomen.

These regions and quadrants are described in detail in Chapter 6, p. 74.

LAYERS OF THE ANTERIOR ABDOMINAL WALL

The anterior abdominal wall is firm and elastic. It consists of eight layers. From superficial to deep, these are:

1. Skin.
2. Superficial fascia.
3. External oblique muscle.
4. Internal oblique muscle.
5. Transversus abdominis muscle.
6. Fascia transversalis.
7. Extraperitoneal tissue.
8. Parietal layer of peritoneum.

N.B. The *deep fascia is absent in the anterior abdominal wall* to allow the bulging/distension of the abdominal wall as after taking meals, during pregnancy, etc. It is also absent in the penis, scrotum, and perineum.

SKIN

The skin of the anterior abdominal wall is thinner and more sensitive than the skin of the posterior abdominal wall.

Visible Skin Creases/Lines on the Anterior Abdominal Wall (Fig. 3.2)

1. *Midline furrows/groove* (see page 25)
2. *Linea semilunaris* (see page 25)
3. *Transverse furrows*: Two or three transverse furrows may sometimes be seen crossing the rectus abdominis muscle and corresponds to the tendinous intersections of the muscle. They are called *linea transversalis*.
4. *Line of Venus*: It is a semilunar line with concavity facing upward, seen mostly in females on the anterior abdominal wall between the umbilicus and pubic symphysis.
5. *Linea gravidarum*: In the multiparous women, the lower part of the anterior abdominal wall presents a number of irregularly branched white lines called *striae gravidarum*. They occur due to degenerative fibrosis of subcutaneous fat because of undue stretching of the anterior abdominal wall by the gravid uterus.

Cleavage Lines of Skin in the Anterior Abdominal Wall

The cleavage lines (**Langer's lines**) in the anterior abdominal wall run horizontally. Therefore, the abdominal incisions

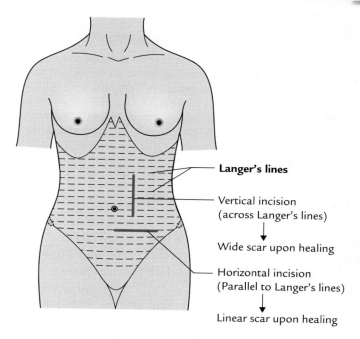

Fig. 3.4 Cleavage (Langer's) lines/crease lines on the anterior abdominal wall.

preferably should be given horizontally. So that wounds heal with invisible linear scars (Fig. 3.4).

The umbilicus is of great anatomical, embryological, and clinical importance and hence discussed in detail in the following text.

Umbilicus

1. The umbilicus is the most obvious feature of the anterior abdominal wall.
2. It is in fact a normal puckered scar in the anterior abdominal wall representing the site of attachment of the umbilical cord in the fetus.

Position
The position of umbilicus is variable:

1. *In adult*, it lies at the level of intervertebral disc between L3 and L4 vertebrae.
2. *In newborn*, it is slightly at a lower level due to poorly developed pelvic region.
3. *In old age*, it comes down to lower level due to diminished tone of the abdominal muscles.

Anatomical Significance

1. The level of umbilicus serves as water-shed line for venous and lymphatic drainage. The venous blood and lymph flow upward above the level of the umbilicus and downward below the level of the umbilicus.
2. It indicates the level of T10 dermatome, i.e., skin around the umbilicus is supplied by the 10th spinal segment.
3. It is one of the important sites of portocaval anastomosis.

- Although the umbilicus is a scar in the anterior abdominal wall, it is of immense cosmetic value particularly in the females. Therefore, the surgical incision should never be given across it.
- The skin around the umbilicus is supplied by T10 spinal segment. Therefore, visceral pain of appendicitis is referred to the umbilicus (note the appendix is supplied by T10 spinal segment).

Embryological Significance

1. It is the meeting point of four folds of embryonic plate (e.g., two lateral folds, head fold, and tail fold).
2. In embryonic life, a defect exists in the linea alba at this site called **umbilical ring**, which provides passage to the following structures:
   (a) The midgut loop herniates into the umbilical cord during fifth to tenth weeks of IUL (intrauterine life) but returns back to the abdominal cavity during tenth to twelfth week of intrauterine life.
   (b) The two endodermal tubes (allantois and vitello-intestinal duct) project into the umbilical cord. The allantois is a diverticulum of endodermal cloaca. Its proximal part gives rise to the urinary bladder and distal part to urachus. The vitello-intestinal duct is a diverticulum of midgut extending from the distal part of ileum to the umbilicus. Sometimes its proximal part persists as *Meckel's diverticulum*.
   (c) Umbilical vessels (two arteries, one vein) pass to and fro between umbilical cord and placenta. The remnants of umbilical arteries are present in adult as medial umbilical ligament and remnant of umbilical vein as ligamentum teres.

Thus, there are four important embryological remnants at the umbilicus (Fig. 3.5).

1. Ligamentum teres (remnant of left umbilical vein).
2. ⎫ Two medial umbilical ligaments (remnant of umbilical
3. ⎭ arteries).
4. Median umbilical ligament (remnant of urachus).

Congenital anomalies: The important congenital anomalies of the umbilicus are fistulae and exomphalos.
(a) **Faecal fistula:** Failure of vitello-intestinal duct to obliterate results in faecal fistula at the umbilicus.
(b) **Urinary fistula:** Failure of urachus to obliterate leads to urinary fistula at the umbilicus.
(c) **Exomphalos (or omphalocele):** Failure of midgut loop to return in the abdominal cavity results in the exomphalos. Since the intestine protrude through a defect in all layers of the abdominal wall at umbilical ring a thin transparent membrane—the amnion—covers it.
(d) **Congenital umbilical hernia (Fig. 3.6):** In this condition the intestine protrudes through the umbilicus due to weakness of umbilical scar, hence it is covered by the peritoneum (for details, see *Clinical and Surgical Anatomy*, 2nd Edition by Vishram Singh).

The umbilicus is therefore considered as **hot-bed of embryology** by the clinicians.

SUPERFICIAL FASCIA

The superficial fascia contains a variable amount of fat, maximum in the lower half of the anterior abdominal wall. The anterior abdominal wall is the major site of fat accumulation especially in the females leading to obesity.

Above the level of the line joining the two anterior superior iliac spines the superficial fascia consists of a single layer but below this line it consists of two layers (Fig. 3.7): (a) a superficial fatty layer (*Camper's fascia*) and (b) a deep membranous layer (*Scarpa's fascia*). The space between the two layers contains superficial epigastric, circumflex iliac, external pudendal vessels, and superficial inguinal lymph nodes.

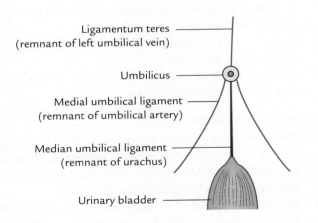

Ligamentum teres
(remnant of left umbilical vein)

Umbilicus

Medial umbilical ligament
(remnant of umbilical artery)

Median umbilical ligament
(remnant of urachus)

Urinary bladder

Fig. 3.5 Four embryological remnants at the umbilicus.

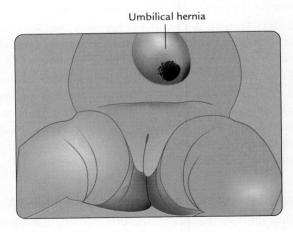

Umbilical hernia

Fig. 3.6 Congenital umbilical hernia.

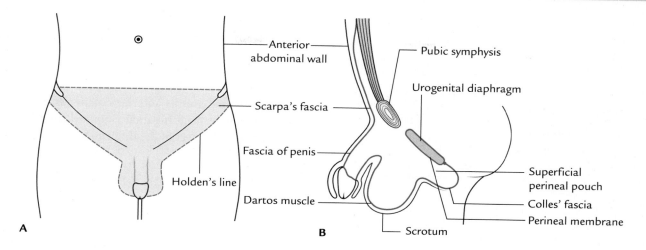

Fig. 3.7 Extent of the membranous layer of superficial fascia of the abdomen (Scarpa's fascia): **A**, as seen in anterior view; **B**, as seen in sagittal section.

Camper's Fascia (Superficial Fatty Layer)

This superficial fatty layer of superficial fascia of the abdomen is continuous with the superficial fascia of the adjoining areas of the body. Over the penis, it is devoid of fat, and in the scrotum, it is replaced by an involuntary **dartos muscle**.

Scarpa's Fascia

This deep membranous layer of superficial fascia of the abdomen is made up of elastic type of fibrous tissue. Students must remember its following features:

1. **In the midline**, it is attached to the linea alba.
2. **On each side**, it is separated from underlying external oblique muscle by a layer of loose areolar tissue, which disappears superiorly and toward the median plane.
3. **Below,**
   (a) it crosses the inguinal ligament and gets attached to the fascia lata of the thigh immediately below and parallel to the ligament.
   (b) it is prolonged over the penis to enclose it up to the base of the glans and forms the **fascia of the penis** (Buck's fascia).
   (c) it covers the scrotum where it is replaced by dartos muscle and then continues with the superficial fascia of perineum—the **Colles' fascia**. The Colles' fascia stretches across the margins of pubic arch and is attached to the posterior edge of the urogenital diaphragm/posterior border of the perineal membrane, which also stretches across the pubic arch. The space between the perineal membrane and Colles' fascia is known as **superficial perineal pouch**.

N.B.
- The line of attachment of Scarpa's fascia with the fascia lata is marked on the surface by **Holden's line**, which begins a little lateral to the pubic tubercle and extends laterally for about 8 cm.
- A potential space exists in the anterior abdominal wall between Scarpa's fascia and aponeurosis of the external oblique. It is termed **superficial inguinal space**.

Clinical correlation

Clinical significance of Scarpa's fascia: The Scarpa's fascia bears two important clinical relations:
(a) It serves as a firm unit for suturing the superficial fascia during closure of the anterior abdomen/perineum after abdominal or pelvic surgery.
(b) The attachments of Scarpa's and Colles' fasciae are such that they prevent the passage of extravasated urine due to urethral rupture backward into the ischiorectal fossae and downward into the thighs.

The line of fusion of Scarpa's fascia passes over Holden's line, body of pubis, margins of pubic arch, and posterior border of the perineal membrane/posterior edge of the urogenital diaphragm (Fig. 3.8).

Therefore, if male urethra is ruptured in the perineum, the extravasated urine collects first in the *superficial pouch of perineum* and then on to the anterior abdominal wall inferior to the umbilicus in the *superficial inguinal space* (Fig. 3.9).

The presence of urine in this confined space where Scarpa's fascia is attached makes the clinician to suspect urethral rupture due to trauma. Clinically rupture of the urethra in the perineum presents as follows:
(a) Swollen perineum.
(b) Swollen scrotum.
(c) Swollen penis.
(d) Swollen lower part of abdominal wall.

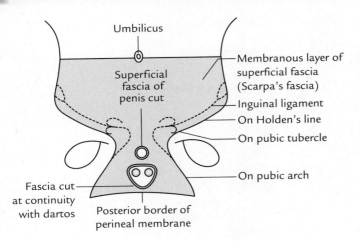

Fig. 3.8 Attachment of the membranous layer of superficial fascia.

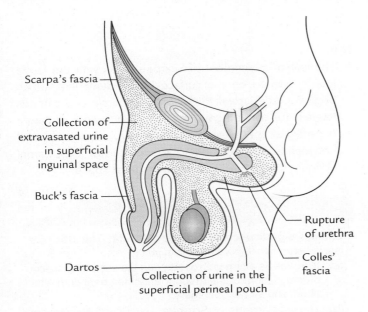

Fig. 3.9 Rupture of urethra in perineum and collection of extravasated urine in superficial perineal pouch and superficial inguinal space.

Cutaneous Nerves (Fig. 3.10)

The skin of the anterior abdominal wall is almost entirely supplied by the lower six thoracic nerves through intercostal and subcostal nerves. Only the most inferior part is supplied by the first lumbar nerve through the iliohypogastric and ilioinguinal nerves.

Anterior Cutaneous Branches

The anterior cutaneous nerves (seven in number) are derived from the lower five intercostal, subcostal, and iliohypogastric nerves. They pierce the anterior wall of the rectus sheath a short distance away from the median plane and divide into medial and lateral branches to supply the skin.

The cutaneous branches from T7 to T10 are arranged in a sequence with T7 near the xiphoid process and T10 close to the umbilicus. The anterior cutaneous branch of iliohypogastric nerve emerges 2.5 cm above the superficial inguinal ring. The ilioinguinal nerve lacks the lateral cutaneous branch and its anterior cutaneous branch passes through the superficial inguinal ring and supplies skin on the upper medial aspect of the thigh and skin of the scrotum or labium majus.

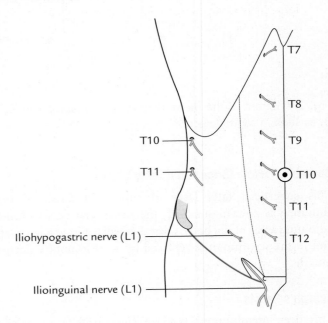

Fig. 3.10 Cutaneous nerves of the anterior abdominal wall.

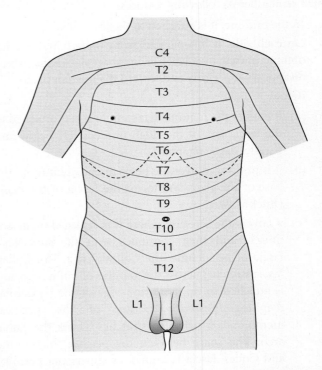

Fig. 3.11 Dermatomes on the anterior abdominal wall.

The dermatomes of the anterior abdominal wall are shown in Figure 3.11.

Lateral Cutaneous Branches

1. The lateral cutaneous branches from lower two intercostal nerves emerge through the external intercostal muscle and divide into a large anterior and small posterior branches to supply the skin.
2. The lateral cutaneous branches of subcostal and iliohypogastric nerves appear close to the iliac crest and descend over it to supply the skin in the upper anterior part of the gluteal region.

Cutaneous Arteries (Fig. 3.12)

These are as follows:

1. **The anterior cutaneous arteries are the branches of superior and inferior epigastric arteries. They** accompany the anterior cutaneous nerves.
2. **The lateral cutaneous arteries are the branches of posterior intercostal arteries. They** accompany the lateral cutaneous nerves.
3. **The three superficial inguinal arteries are the three superficial branches of femoral artery** (superficial external pudendal, superficial epigastric, and superficial circumflex iliac) and supply the skin of the abdomen below the umbilicus.
   (a) The *superficial external pudendal artery* runs medially and passes in front of the spermatic cord to supply the scrotum (or labium majus) and penis.
   (b) The *superficial epigastric artery* runs superomedially across the inguinal ligament up to the umbilicus.
   (c) The *superficial circumflex iliac artery* runs laterally below the inguinal ligament toward the anterior superior iliac spine to supply the skin of inguinal region.

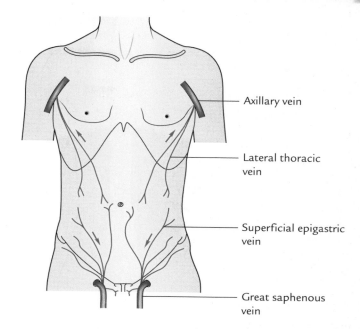

Fig. 3.13 Superficial veins of the anterior abdominal wall.

Cutaneous (Superficial) Veins (Fig. 3.13)

They accompany the cutaneous arteries and drain as follows:

1. **Below the umbilicus** they run downward and drain into the great saphenous vein in the groin and thus eventually in the inferior vena cava.
2. **Above the umbilicus** they run toward the axilla and drain into the axillary vein and thus eventually in the superior vena cava.

N.B. Small veins from the umbilicus run along the ligamentum teres to drain into the portal vein.

Clinical correlation

Clinical significance of superficial veins of the anterior abdominal wall: The superficial veins of the anterior abdominal wall anastomose freely with each other and with the small veins (paraumbilical veins) which drain the umbilicus.

- In *portal vein obstruction* (Fig. 3.14A), when the venous drainage through the liver is obstructed, the backflow of blood may occur through paraumbilical veins toward the umbilicus. As a result, the paraumbilical veins and superficial veins around the umbilicus become grossly distended and tortuous. They radiate out from the umbilicus like spokes of a wheel, producing a clinical sign called *caput medusae*. This condition is so called because of its resemblance to the serpents on the head of the Medusa, a mythical lady in Greek mythology.
- In *caval obstruction* (Fig. 3.14B) (i.e., obstructions of superior and inferior vena cavae), the *thoraco-epigastric vein* connecting the saphenous and axillary veins opens up.
- In *superior vena cava obstruction,* blood in the thoraco-epigastric vein flows downward whereas in the *inferior vena cava obstruction* it flows upward.

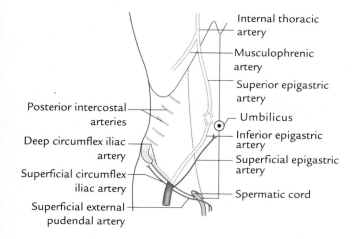

Fig. 3.12 Arteries of the anterior abdominal wall.

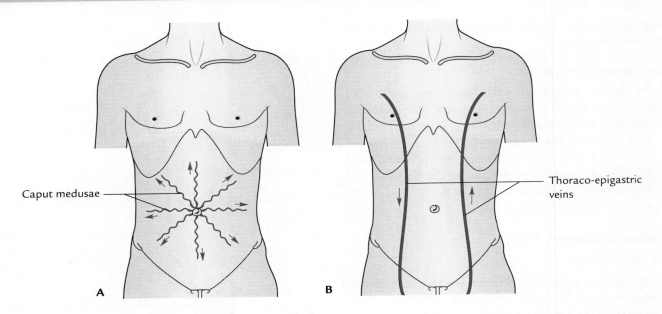

Fig. 3.14 Subcutaneous venous collateral circulation: A, formation of caput medusae in portal obstruction; B, formation of thoraco-epigastric vein in caval obstruction. (The arrows indicate the direction of blood flow in superior vena cava obstruction on the right side and in inferior vena cava obstruction on the left side.)

N.B. The *thoraco-epigastric vein* is formed by the anastomosis of lateral thoracic vein (a tributary of axillary vein) with the superficial epigastric vein (a tributary of great saphenous vein).

Cutaneous (Superficial) Lymph Vessels (Fig. 3.15)

The lymph from the skin of the abdominal wall is drained into axillary and superficial inguinal lymph nodes as follows:

1. **Above the umbilicus,** the lymph vessels run upward to drain into the *axillary lymph nodes* (anterior/pectoral group).
2. **Below the umbilicus,** the lymph vessels run downward and laterally to drain into the *superficial inguinal lymph nodes.*

Thus lymphatics faithfully follow the water-shed line at the level of the umbilicus.

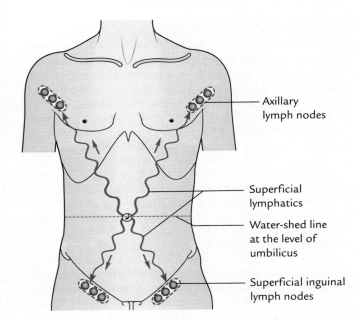

Fig. 3.15 Superficial lymphatics of the anterior abdominal wall.

> ### Clinical correlation
>
> **Clinical significance of cutaneous lymph vessels of anterior abdominal wall:** The infection or malignant tumor of the skin in the lower part of the anterior abdominal wall may cause swelling in the groin due to enlargement of superficial inguinal lymph nodes, and similar lesions in the upper part of the abdomen may produce swelling in the axilla due to enlargement of axillary lymph nodes.

MUSCLES OF THE ANTERIOR ABDOMINAL WALL

The anterior abdominal wall consists of five pairs of muscles—five on either side of midline (three flat muscles and two vertical muscles).

The three flat muscles are external oblique, internal oblique, and transversus abdominis; and two vertical muscles are rectus abdominis and pyramidalis.

All these are large muscles except pyramidalis which is a small triangular muscle.

The three flat muscles are fleshy posterolaterally and aponeurotic anteromedially. The aponeuroses of these muscles pass toward the midline to enclose the rectus abdominis and pyramidalis, and then fuse with each other and with the aponeuroses of the muscles of the opposite side in the median fibrous raphe extending from the xiphoid process to the pubic symphysis, forming the *linea alba*.

N.B. If you place your hands on either side of your abdomen with fingertips just touching in the midline, the palms of your hands lie mainly over the fleshy portions of flat muscles and fingers over their aponeuroses. Thus, anterior part of the abdominal wall is mostly aponeurotic except for the rectus abdominis and pyramidalis, which are enclosed within the aponeurosis.

FLAT MUSCLES

The three anterolateral flat muscles (external oblique, internal oblique, and transversus abdominis) form three distinct layers in the anterior abdominal wall, similar to those in the intercostal space, and as in the intercostal space the neurovascular structures lie between the internal oblique and transversus abdominis muscles.

External Oblique Muscle (Fig. 3.16)

Origin

The external oblique muscle arises from eight fleshy slips from the outer surfaces (the middle of the shaft) of lower eight ribs.

Insertion

Most of the fleshy fibres run downward, forward, and medially in the same direction as the fingers do when you put the hand inside the side pocket of your pantaloon.

The insertion occurs as follows:

1. The posterior-most fibres pass vertically downward to be inserted on to the outer lip of the anterior two-third of the iliac crest. The posterior border of muscle is thus free.

2. The remaining fibres pass downward, forward and medially to end in a broad aponeurosis, which is inserted into the linea alba extending from the xiphoid process to the pubic symphysis.

    (a) The upper border of the aponeurosis is free and overlapped by the fibres of pectoralis major muscle.

    (b) The lower border of the aponeurosis is free and jumps from anterior superior iliac spine to the pubic tubercle bridging across the muscles, nerves, and vessels that enter the thigh from the abdomen.

The free lower border of the aponeurosis is thickened and rolled inward on itself to form the *inguinal ligament.*

N.B. *Additional points of interest:*

- The upper four slips of origin interdigitate with the slips of serratus anterior and lower four slips with the slips of latissimus dorsi.
- Above the pubic symphysis the aponeurosis presents a triangular gap called *superficial inguinal ring.*

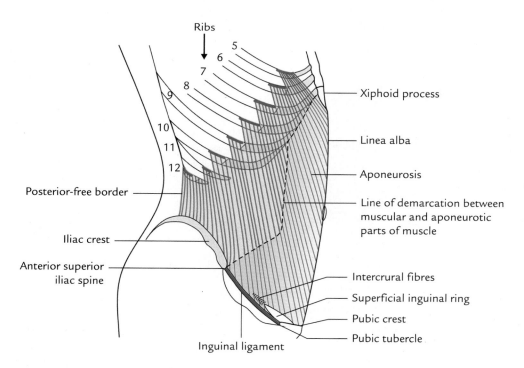

Ribs

5
6
7
8
9
10
11
12

Xiphoid process

Linea alba

Aponeurosis

Line of demarcation between muscular and aponeurotic parts of muscle

Posterior-free border

Iliac crest

Anterior superior iliac spine

Intercrural fibres

Superficial inguinal ring

Pubic crest

Pubic tubercle

Inguinal ligament

Fig. 3.16 External oblique muscle.

- Posterior-free border of muscle forms the anterior boundary of the *lumbar triangle*.
- Muscle fibres become aponeurotic approximately at the midclavicular line medially and spino-umbilical line (line extending from the umbilicus to the anterior superior iliac spine) inferiorly.

Nerve Supply
By anterior primary rami of lower six thoracic spinal nerves (T7–T12).

Internal Oblique Muscle (Fig. 3.17)
This muscle is relatively smaller and thinner than the external oblique. It lies deep to external oblique and its fibres are oriented at right angles to those of external oblique.

Origin
It arises from:

1. Lateral two-thirds of the upper surface of the inguinal ligament.
2. Anterior two-thirds of the iliac crest (intermediate area).
3. Thoraco-lumbar fascia.

Insertion
Most of the fibres run upward, forward, and medially at right angle to that of external oblique (as your fingers do when you place your hand in front of the chest).

The insertion occurs as follows:

1. Most of the fibres run upward, forward, and medially, and end in a broad aponeurosis, which is inserted into the 7th, 8th, and 9th costal cartilages, and linea alba

extending from the xiphoid process to the pubic symphysis.
2. The posterior-most fibres ascend vertically upward and inserted by fleshy fibres into the lower border of lower 3rd or 4th ribs and their costal cartilages.
3. The fleshy fibres arise from inguinal ligament arch over the inguinal canal and its contents, and then descend to be inserted on to the pubic tubercle and pecten pubis. These fibres fuse with the corresponding tendinous fibres of the transversus abdominis muscle to form **conjoint tendon** which is inserted into the pubic crest and medial part of the pecten pubis.

Nerve Supply
By the anterior primary rami of lower six thoracic nerves (T7–T12) and first lumbar nerve (L1) via iliohypogastric, and ilioinguinal nerves.

Transversus Abdominis Muscle (Fig. 3.18)
The transversus abdominis muscle is the innermost of three flat abdominal muscles. The direction of most of its fibres is horizontal/transverse.

Origin
It arises from:

1. Lateral one-third of the upper surface of the inguinal ligament.
2. Anterior two-third of the iliac crest (inner lip).
3. Thoraco-lumbar fascia.
4. Inner surfaces of the lower six ribs and their costal cartilage.

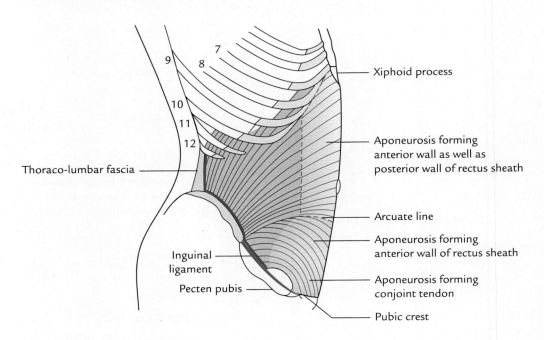

Fig. 3.17 Internal oblique muscle.

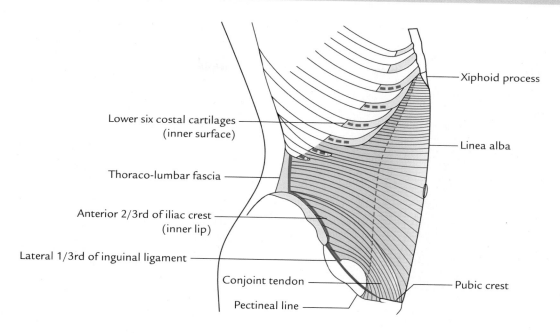

Fig. 3.18 Origin and insertion of transversus abdominis muscle.

Insertion

1. Inguinal fibres arch backward forming the roof of the inguinal canal, and then turn downward and medially forming an aponeurosis which joins similar aponeurosis of internal oblique to form conjoint tendon, through which it is inserted into the pubic crest and medial part of pecten pubis.
2. Most of the fibres run horizontally and end in a broad aponeurosis, which is inserted into the linea alba extending from the xiphoid process to the pubic symphysis.

Nerve Supply

By the anterior primary rami of lower six thoracic nerves (T7–T12), and first lumbar (L1) nerve via iliohypogastric and ilioinguinal nerves.

N.B. An important fact for students to remember is that external oblique lies superficial to the lower ribs, internal oblique attaches to the costal margin, and transversus abdominis muscle lies deep to the lower ribs.

STRUCTURES DERIVED FROM FLAT MUSCLES

The structures derived from flat muscles are as follows:
1. Inguinal ligament.
2. Conjoint tendon.
3. Cremaster muscle.

Inguinal Ligament

It is the lower-free border of external oblique aponeurosis stretching between anterior superior iliac spine and pubic tubercle (for details see page 46).

Conjoint Tendon (Falx Inguinalis)

It is formed by the fusion of lower aponeurotic fibres of internal oblique and transversus abdominis muscles which arches over the spermatic cord and is attached on to the pubic crest and medial part of the pectineal line (pecten pubis). The important features of the conjoint tendon are as follows:

1. It forms the medial half of the posterior wall of the inguinal canal and strengthens the anterior abdominal wall of the canal opposite the superficial inguinal ring.
2. Medially, it blends with the anterior wall of the rectus sheath.
3. Laterally, it may extend occasionally up to the *interfoveolar ligament*, a thickening in the fascia transversalis along the medial border of deep inguinal ring. The interfoveolar ligament extends from the lower border of transversus abdominis to the superior ramus of the pubis.

N.B. The weakening of conjoint tendon due to old age or injury of iliohypogastric and ilioinguinal nerves predisposes the occurrence of direct inguinal hernia.

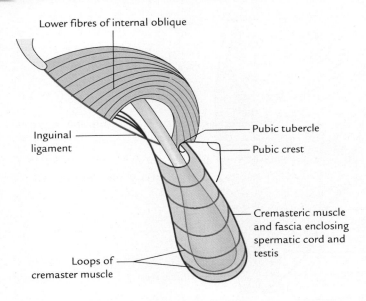

Fig. 3.19 Schematic diagram to show cremaster muscle.

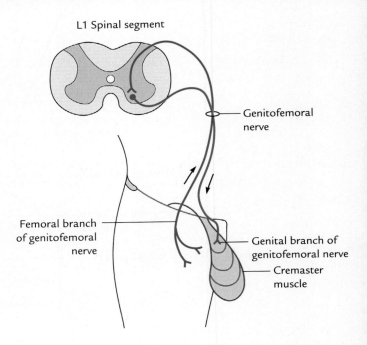

Fig. 3.20 Neural pathway for cremasteric reflex.

Cremaster Muscle (Fig. 3.19)

The cremaster muscle consists of a series of **loops of skeletal muscle fibres** joined by loose areolar tissue, the **cremaster fascia**. The loops of cremaster muscle and fascia form the covering around the spermatic cord and testis. These muscle loops are derived from lower arched fibres of internal oblique. The medial ends of loops are attached to the pubic tubercle, pubic crest, and conjoint tendon. The cremaster muscle is supplied by sympathetic fibres from L1 and L2 spinal segments through the genital branch of genitofemoral nerve and hence not under voluntary control.

The contraction of cremaster muscle pulls the testis up toward the superficial inguinal ring, which helps to plug the superficial inguinal ring. It also helps in controlling the temperature of the testis.

Clinical correlation

Cremasteric reflex (Fig. 3.20): Upon stroking the skin of the upper medial aspect of thigh, there is reflex contraction of cremaster muscle leading to reflex elevation of the testis. The reflex is more brisk in children.

The *femoral branch of genitofemoral nerve* forms the afferent limb and *genital branch of genitofemoral nerve* forms the efferent limb. The reflex centre is in L1 and L2 spinal segments.

VERTICAL MUSCLES

The two vertical muscles—rectus abdominis and pyramidalis—lie on either side of the anterior midline and are enclosed in the tendinous sheath formed by the aponeuroses of the flat muscles.

Rectus Abdominis Muscle (Fig. 3.21)

It is a long, flat strap muscle, which extends vertically upward along the linea alba from the pubic symphysis below to the costal margin above. It widens as it ascends from the pubic symphysis to the costal margin, thus it is wider above and narrows below.

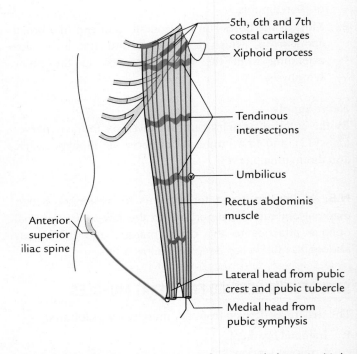

Fig. 3.21 Origin and insertion of rectus abdominis (right side).

Origin

It arises by two tendinous heads:

1. **Medial head** arises from the anterior surface of the pubic symphysis.
2. **Lateral head** arises from the lateral part of the pubic crest and pubic tubercle.

Insertion

It is inserted on the anterior thoracic wall by four fleshy slips along a horizontal line passing laterally from xiphoid process and cutting in that order, the 7th, 6th, and 5th costal cartilages.

N.B. *Additional features of interest:*

- The muscle presents three **tendinous intersections:** first at the level of tip of the xiphoid process; second at the level of the umbilicus; and third at the level midway between the above two. Sometimes a fourth intersection may be present below the umbilicus.

  Each tendinous intersection passes horizontally in a zigzag manner and is attached to the anterior wall of the rectus sheath. The tendinous intersection divides the long muscle column into shorter segments to provide more strength.
- The muscle is enclosed in the aponeurotic sheath derived from three-paired anterolateral flat muscles of the abdominal wall.

Nerve Supply

By the lower five intercostal and subcostal nerves (T7–T12).

Action

Flexion of the trunk on the pelvis.

Pyramidalis

The pyramidalis is rudimentary in human beings. It is a small triangular muscle, lying anterior to the lower part of the rectus abdominis muscle within the rectus sheath. It has its base below in front of the pubis and its apex is directed above and medially.

Origin

It arises from the front of the body of pubis and anterior pubic ligament.

Insertion

It is inserted into the linea alba midway between the umbilicus and the pubic symphysis.

Nerve Supply

By the subcostal nerve (T12).

Action

It tenses the linea alba.

N.B. The pyramidalis is absent in about 20% of people.

The origin, insertion, and nerve supply of muscles of anterior abdominal wall is summarized in Table 3.1.

FUNCTIONS OF THE ANTERIOR ABDOMINAL MUSCLES

The three main functions of the anterior abdominal muscles are:

1. To provide strong and expandable support for the abdominal viscera against gravity and protect them from injury.
2. To compress the abdominal contents to increase the intra-abdominal pressure and thus help in expulsive and expiratory acts.
3. To move the trunk to maintain the posture.

The details are as under:

Support and Protection of Abdominal Viscera

The tone of oblique and transverse muscles provides firm but elastic support to the abdominal viscera and protects them from external injury.

Compression of Abdominal Contents

The contraction of oblique and transverse muscles compresses the abdominal viscera and increases the intra-abdominal pressure, which subserve the following functions:

1. Elevates the relaxed diaphragm to expel air during respiration.
2. Is required for forceful expiratory acts such as coughing, sneezing, nose blowing, screaming, etc.
3. Produces force for expulsive acts such as defecation, micturition, and parturition.
4. Is involved in heavyweight lifting, as a result the force may sometime cause hernia.

Movements of the Trunk

1. *Flexion of trunk* especially of the lumbar region is mainly performed by the rectus abdominis muscles.
2. *Lateral flexion of trunk* is done by the unilateral contraction of oblique muscles.
3. *Rotation of trunk* produces the combined contraction of external oblique muscle of one side with internal oblique muscle of the opposite side.

RECTUS SHEATH

The rectus sheath is an aponeurotic sheath enclosing the rectus abdominis muscle (and pyramidalis muscle if present) on either side of the linea alba. It is derived from the aponeuroses of flat muscles of the anterior abdominal wall. The **functions of rectus sheath** include:

Table 3.1 Muscles of the anterior abdominal wall

Muscles	Origin	Insertion	Nerve supply
Flat muscles			
• External oblique	By eight fleshy slips from the outer surfaces of lower eight ribs (the upper four slips interdigitate with serratus anterior, and the lower four slips with latissimus dorsi)	(a) By fleshy fibres into the anterior 2/3rd of the outer lip of iliac crest (b) By aponeurosis into xiphoid process, linea alba, pubic symphysis, pubic crest, and the pectineal line	Lower six thoracic spinal nerves (anterior rami of T7–T12)
• Internal oblique	Fleshy origin from: (a) Lateral 2/3rd of the inguinal ligament (b) Anterior 2/3rd of the intermediate area of iliac crest (c) Thoraco-lumbar fascia	(a) By fleshy fibres into the inferior border of lower 3rd or 4th ribs and their cartilages (b) By aponeurosis into 7th, 8th, and 9th costal cartilages, xiphoid process, linea alba, pubic crest, and pectineal line of pubis	Lower six thoracic and first lumbar spinal nerves (anterior rami of T7–T12; L1)
• Transversus abdominis	Fleshy origin from: (a) Lateral 1/3rd of the inguinal ligament (b) Anterior 2/3rd of the inner lip of iliac crest (c) Thoraco-lumbar fascia (d) Inner surfaces of the lower six costal cartilages (these fibres interdigitate with diaphragm)	By aponeurosis into xiphoid process, linea alba, pubic crest, and pectineal line	Lower six thoracic and first lumbar spinal nerves (anterior rami of T7–T12; L1)
Vertical muscles			
• Rectus abdominis	By two tendinous heads: (a) *Lateral head* from lateral part of the pubic crest (b) *Medial head* from anterior surface of the pubic symphysis	(a) 5th, 6th, and 7th costal cartilages (along a horizontal line) (b) Xiphoid process	Lower six or seven thoracic nerves (anterior rami of T7–T12)
• Pyramidalis	(a) Anterior surface of the body of pubis (b) Anterior pubic ligament	Into linea alba	Subcostal nerve (T12)

(a) Checking the bowing of rectus abdominis muscle during its contraction and hence increasing its efficiency.
(b) Maintaining the strength of the anterior abdominal wall.

FEATURES (Figs 3.22 and 3.23)

1. The rectus sheath presents anterior and posterior walls.
2. The anterior wall is complete and covers the entire extent of muscle longitudinally from the upper end to the lower end.
3. The posterior wall is deficient above and below, and hence does not cover the entire extent of muscle longitudinally. **Above** it is attached to the costal margin (7th, 8th, and 9th costal cartilages) and thus muscle lies directly on 5th, 6th, and 7th costal cartilage. **Below** it

presents a free curved margin with concavity facing inferiorly called arcuate line (line of Douglas) between the umbilicus and pubic symphysis. Below this level, muscle lies directly on the fascia transversalis.

N.B. The anterior wall of rectus sheath is firmly adherent to the tendinous intersections of the rectus abdominis, whereas its posterior layer is free from the muscle.

FORMATION (Fig. 3.24)

The formation of rectus sheath differs from above downward as follows:

1. *Above the level of costal margin:*
   (a) *Anterior wall* is formed by the aponeurosis of external oblique only.

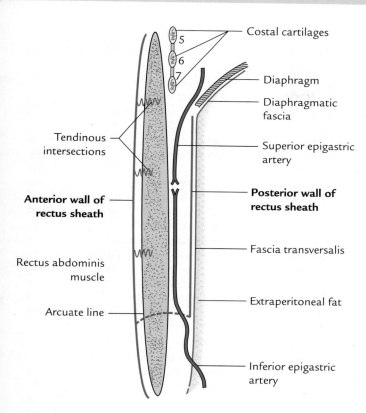

Fig. 3.22 Anterior and posterior walls of rectus sheath as seen in sagittal section. Note: Tendinous intersections are attached only to the anterior wall.

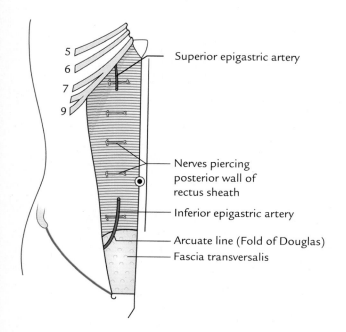

Fig. 3.23 Posterior wall of the rectus sheath.

(b) *Posterior wall* is deficient and muscle lies directly on the 5th, 6th, and 7th costal cartilages.

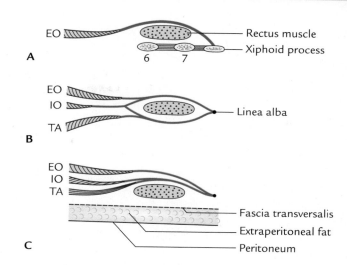

Fig. 3.24 Formation of the rectus sheath as seen in transverse sections through rectus abdominis and its sheaths at three different levels: A, above the costal margin; B, between costal margin and arcuate line; C, below the arcuate line (EO = external oblique, IO = internal oblique, TA = transversus abdominis).

2. *Between costal margin and arcuate line:*
   (a) *Anterior wall* is formed by the fusion of aponeurosis of external oblique with the anterior lamina of aponeurosis of internal oblique.
   (b) *Posterior wall* is formed by the fusion of aponeurosis of transversus abdominis with the posterior lamina of aponeurosis of internal oblique.

3. *Below the level of arcuate line:*
   (a) *Anterior wall* is formed by the aponeuroses of all the three flat muscles (the aponeuroses of transversus abdominis and internal oblique are fused but the aponeurosis of external oblique remains separate).
   (b) *Posterior wall* is deficient.

N.B. *Recent view of rectus sheath formation:* Recently it is found that the aponeuroses of all the three flat muscles (external, internal, and transversus) are bilaminar thus giving six laminae in all. The three layers form anterior wall and three layers form posterior wall of the rectus sheath. The laminae do not terminate in the linea alba but decussate with other laminae across the midline, i.e., in the region of linea alba and continue as the laminae of contralateral muscles.

CONTENTS (Fig. 3.25)

The rectus sheath contains the following structures:

1. **Two muscles:** Rectus abdominis and pyramidalis (if present).

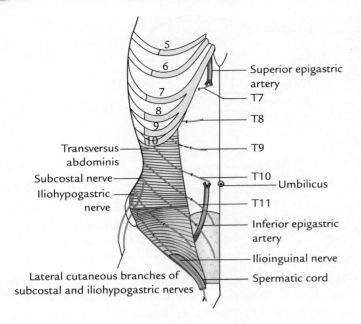

Fig. 3.25 Nerves and arteries within the rectus sheath. Also note the course taken by lower five intercostal, subcostal, iliohypogastric, and ilioinguinal nerves.

2. **Two arteries:** Superior epigastric and inferior epigastric.
3. **Two veins:** Superior epigastric and inferior epigastric.
4. **Six nerves:** Terminal parts of lower six thoracic nerves, including lower five intercostal nerves and subcostal nerve. (They are accompanied by terminal parts of posterior intercostal vessels.)

Relevant Features of Contents

The **superior epigastric artery,** a branch of internal thoracic artery, enters the rectus by passing through the gap between the costal and xiphoid slips of origin of the diaphragm and passes deep to the rectus abdominis. The **inferior epigastric artery,** a branch of external iliac artery, enters the sheath by passing in front of the arcuate line. These arteries anastomose with each other within the sheath and supply the rectus muscle.

The **superior epigastric vein** accompanies the superior epigastric artery and drains into the internal thoracic vein. The **inferior epigastric vein** accompanies the inferior epigastric artery and drains into the external iliac vein.

The **intercostal nerves** (T7–T11) pass from their intercostal spaces into the abdominal wall between the internal oblique and transversus abdominis muscles, and run in this neurovascular plane to enter the rectus sheath by piercing the posterior lamina of internal oblique aponeurosis. Within the sheath, they proceed forward deep to rectus muscle to about its midline and then enter the muscle, supply it, and emerge through the anterior wall of the sheath as the **anterior cutaneous nerves.**

- The pedicle flap of the upper part of the rectus abdominis muscle based on the superior epigastric artery is commonly used in the *reconstructive surgery of the breast*.
- **Divarication of the recti (separation of the recti abdominis muscles; Fig. 3.26):** The separation of two rectus muscles usually occur in elderly multiparous woman with weak abdominal muscles. In this condition, the aponeuroses forming the rectus sheaths become excessively stretched, consequently when the patient coughs or strains, the recti separate widely and a hernial sac containing loops of intestine protrudes forward between the medial margins of the recti.
- **Hematoma of rectus sheath:** Sometimes the superior and inferior epigastric arteries are unduly stretched during a severe bout of coughing or in later months of pregnancy and ruptures if they are exposed to blunt trauma to the anterior abdominal wall leading to the formation of hematoma within the rectus sheath. Clinically, it presents as:
  (a) Midline abdominal pain.
  (b) Tender mass confined to one rectus sheath.
- **Epigastric hernia (Fig. 3.27):** The linea alba, a midline fibrous raphe, is formed by the interlacing of aponeurotic fibres of three paired flat muscles of the anterior abdominal wall. It extends from the xiphoid process to the pubic

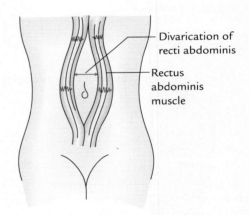

Fig. 3.26 Divarication of the recti abdominis.

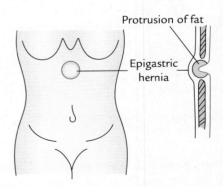

Fig. 3.27 Epigastric hernia.

symphysis. Above the umbilicus, it is wider (about 1 cm) and below the umbilicus it is very narrow. It becomes weak in elderly multiparous women and chronically ill children. When the intra-abdominal pressure is excessively raised, a small amount of extraperitoneal fat may protrude through the upper part of linea alba and eventually may drag behind it a small peritoneal sac which may contain a portion of the greater omentum forming the *epigastric hernia*.

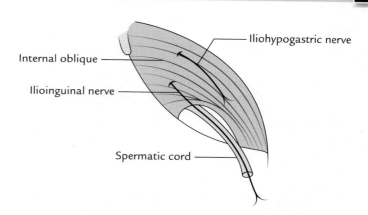

Fig. 3.28 Iliohypogastric and ilioinguinal nerves.

DEEP NERVES OF THE ANTERIOR ABDOMINAL WALL

These nerves are derived from the lower six thoracic and first lumbar segments of spinal cord and supply the anterior abdominal wall. These include the following nerves:

1. Lower five intercostal nerves (T7–T11).
2. Subcostal nerve (T12).
3. Iliohypogastric nerve (L1).
4. Ilioinguinal nerve (L1).

LOWER FIVE INTERCOSTAL NERVES

1. They leave the intercostal spaces between the slips of origin of transversus abdominis muscle and diaphragm; and enter the abdominal wall by passing behind the 7th, 8th, 9th, and 10th costal cartilages.
2. They run forward in a neurovascular plane between the internal oblique and transversus abdominis muscle; and enter the rectus sheath by piercing its posterior wall. Within the sheath they pass in front of epigastric vessels, pierce the rectus muscle and anterior wall of rectus sheath to come out as the **anterior cutaneous nerves**, which supply the skin of the anterior abdominal wall.
3. They give *muscular branches* to supply the muscles of anterior abdominal wall and give off the **lateral cutaneous nerves**, which supply the skin on the side of the abdominal wall.

SUBCOSTAL NERVE

It is the anterior primary ramus of T12 spinal nerve. It enters the anterior abdominal wall by passing behind the lateral arcuate ligament of the diaphragm and runs laterally in the neurovascular plane similar to the intercostal nerves. It supplies pyramidalis muscle and its *lateral cutaneous branch* supplies the skin of the gluteal region.

ILIOHYPOGASTRIC NERVE

It is derived from the anterior primary ramus of the L1 spinal nerve. It runs in the neurovascular plane (i.e., between the internal oblique and transversus abdominis) and pierces the internal oblique about 2.5 cm in front of the anterior superior iliac spine (Fig. 3.28). It becomes cutaneous by piercing the external oblique aponeurosis about 2.5 cm above the superficial inguinal ring.

It does not enter the rectus sheath and its *lateral cutaneous branch* supplies the skin of the gluteal region.

ILIOINGUINAL NERVE

It is the anterior primary ramus of L1 spinal nerve. It pierces the internal oblique muscle from below and enters the inguinal canal lateral to the iliohypogastric nerve, and runs along the inferolateral side of the spermatic cord. It comes out through the superficial inguinal ring. It has *no lateral cutaneous branch* (Fig. 3.28).

The deep nerves of the anterior abdominal wall are summarized in Table 3.2.

Table 3.2 Deep nerves of the anterior abdominal wall

Nerves	Root value	Motor branches	Cutaneous branches
Lower five intercostal	T7–T11	• Internal oblique • External oblique • Transversus abdominis • Rectus abdominis	• Anterior • Lateral
Subcostal	T12	Pyramidalis	• Anterior • Lateral
Iliohypogastric	L1	• Internal oblique • Transversus abdominis	• Anterior • Lateral
Ilioinguinal	L1	• Internal oblique • Transversus abdominis	• Anterior

N.B.
- *Iliohypogastric and ilioinguinal nerves* do not enter the rectus sheath.
- *Lateral cutaneous branches of subcostal and iliohypogastric nerves* supply gluteal region.
- *Ilioinguinal nerve* does not give lateral cutaneous branch.
- *All deep nerves of the anterior abdominal wall* give sensory twigs to the parietal peritoneum.

DEEP ARTERIES OF THE ANTERIOR ABDOMINAL WALL

The deep arteries supply the anterior abdominal wall. These include the following arteries (Fig. 3.12):

1. Superior epigastric artery.
2. Musculophrenic artery.
3. Inferior epigastric artery.
4. Deep circumflex iliac artery.

SUPERIOR EPIGASTRIC ARTERY

It is one of the two terminal branches of *internal thoracic artery*. It begins in the 6th intercostal space and enters the abdomen by passing between the sternal and 7th costal slips of origin of the diaphragm. It crosses the upper border of transversus abdominis and enters the rectus sheath, where it runs vertically downward on its posterior wall and ends by anastomosing with the inferior epigastric artery.

MUSCULOPHRENIC ARTERY

It is the other terminal branch of the internal thoracic artery. It runs downward and laterally; and enters the abdomen by passing through the gap between the 7th and 8th costal slips of origin of the diaphragm. It continues its course downward and laterally along the deep surface of the diaphragm as far as the 10th intercostal space.

INFERIOR EPIGASTRIC ARTERY

It arises from the external iliac artery just above the inguinal ligament. It runs upward and medially in the extraperitoneal tissue along the medial margin of the deep inguinal ring. It pierces fascia transversalis just at the lateral border of the rectus abdominis and enters the rectus sheath by crossing the arcuate line. Within the sheath, it runs on its posterior wall and ends by anastomosing with the superior epigastric artery.

N.B. The pubic branch of the inferior epigastric artery anastomoses with the pubic branch of the obturator artery. It may become the *abnormal obturator artery when* the obturator artery is very small.

DEEP CIRCUMFLEX ILIAC ARTERY

The deep circumflex iliac artery arises from the lateral side of the lower end of external iliac artery opposite to the origin of inferior epigastric artery. It runs upward and laterally along the inguinal ligament, pierces fascia transversalis and continues its course along the iliac crest up to its middle where it pierces the transversus abdominis to enter the plane between the transversus abdominis and internal oblique.

FASCIA TRANSVERSALIS

The fascia transversalis is a thin layer of fascia that lines the inner surface of the transversus abdominis muscle (Fig. 3.29).

EXTENT

Superiorly, it is continuous with the similar layer lining the inferior aspect of the diaphragm — the *diaphragmatic fascia* and inferiorly with the fascia lining the iliacus muscle — the *fascia iliaca.*

Anteriorly, it extends up to the linea alba to which it becomes adherent, and posteriorly it becomes continuous with the anterior layer of the thoraco-lumbar fascia.

IMPORTANT FEATURES

1. The fascia transversalis presents an oval opening about 1.2 cm above the midinguinal point called **deep inguinal ring** which provides passage to the spermatic cord in male and round ligament of the uterus in female.
2. It forms a tubular prolongation around the spermatic cord in the form of **internal spermatic fascia.**
3. Its prolongation into the thigh over the femoral vessels forms the anterior wall of the **femoral sheath.**
4. All the main arteries of the abdominal cavity lie deep to the fascia transversalis whereas main nerves lie outside it. This explains why femoral vessels are inside the femoral sheath and femoral nerve outside it.
5. It forms **iliopubic tract,** which is the thickened inferior margin of the fascia transversalis in the inguinal region. This tract appears as a fibrous band running parallel and posterior (deep) to the inguinal ligament.

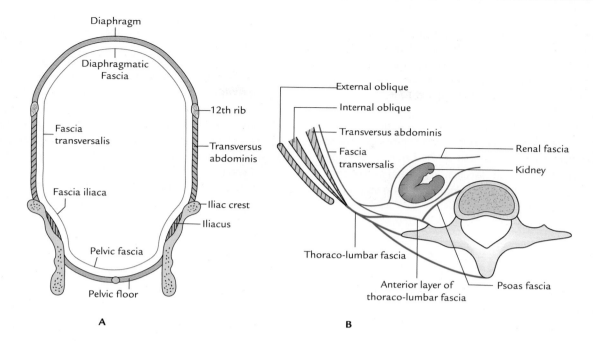

Fig. 3.29 Fascia transversalis and its continuations as seen in coronal section (A) and transverse section (B).

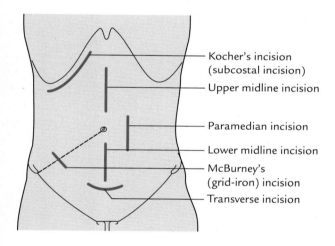

Fig. 3.30 Common abdominal incisions.

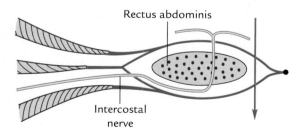

Fig. 3.31 Paramedian abdominal incision (arrow) and course of intercostal nerve.

Clinical correlation

Abdominal incisions (Fig. 3.30): The abdominal incisions are commonly given by surgeons to explore the abdominal cavity and perform the desired surgery. The undergraduate medical students should have some idea about these incisions. The abdominal incisions may sometime give rise to **incisional hernias**. A brief account of some commonly given incisions is given in the following:

1. *Midline incision:* This incision is given in the midline along the linea alba. It is easier to perform incision above the umbilicus because linea alba is wider in this region.

   The advantages of this incision are:
   (a) It is almost bloodless.
   (b) No muscle fibres are cut across.
   (c) No nerves are injured.
   (d) It gives access to both sides of the abdomen.

   The disadvantage of supra-umbilical incision is that healing is poor and may lead to incisional hernia. The infra-umbilical incision is safer because of the close approximation of recti prevents the ventral incisional hernia.

2. *Paramedian incision* (Fig. 3.31): This incision is sounder than the median incision. The anterior wall of rectus sheath is exposed and incised about 1 inch (2.5 cm) lateral and parallel to the midline. The anterior wall of the sheath is freed from the tendinous intersections. The rectus muscle is retracted laterally with its nerve supply intact and posterior wall of the sheath is exposed. The posterior wall of the sheath along with fascia transversalis and peritoneum is then incised. The wound is closed in layers. In paramedian incision, postoperative weakness and occurrence of incisional hernia is minimal. Hence, it is given most frequently.

3. *McBurney's incision/grid-iron incision:* It is commonly given for appendicectomy. An oblique incision is made in the region of the right iliac fossa about 2 inches (5 cm) above and medial to the anterior superior iliac spine at right angle to the spino-umbilical line.

The external oblique, internal oblique, and transversus abdominis muscles are incised or split in the line of their fibres and retracted to expose the fascia transversalis. Hence, it is also termed muscle-splitting incision. The transversalis fascia and parietal peritoneum are incised to open the abdominal cavity, the incision is closed in layers. This incision has no postoperative weakness.

4. *Kocher's incision (Right subcostal incision):* It is given 2 to 5 cm below and parallel to the right costal margin. This incision is used to explore the gallbladder and associated ducts.

5. *Transverse incision:* The transverse incision in the lower part of the abdomen (with slight concavity upward) is given about 2 cm below the umbilicus along the skin crease (line of Venus). It is used to explore the pelvic organs, especially in surgeries related to the uterus and ovaries.

Golden Facts to Remember

▶ Largest and most superficial flat muscle of the anterior abdominal wall	External oblique
▶ Largest content of rectus sheath	Rectus abdominis muscle
▶ Most common vertical incision given in the anterior abdominal wall	Paramedian incision
▶ Most preferred incision for appendectomy/appendicectomy	McBurney's incision
▶ Commonest site of abdominal hernias	Groin
▶ Most important soft tissue landmark on the anterior abdominal wall	
▶ Most prominent surface feature of the anterior abdominal wall	Umbilicus

Clinical Case Study

A 65-year-old obese and overweight woman visited the hospital and complained of pain and swelling around her umbilicus. On examination, the doctor noticed a lump beside the umbilicus which on pushing to one side acquired a crescent shape. The lump was firm in consistency and its surface was smooth. It was resonant on percussion and expansive on coughing. It could also be reduced easily. The "**paraumbilical hernia**" was diagnosed.

Questions

1. What is umbilical hernia?
2. What are the various types of umbilical hernias?
3. Enumerate the differences between the three types of umbilical hernias (vide supra).

Answers

1. Any hernia which is closely related to the umbilicus is called umbilical hernia.

2. The three types of umbilical hernias are: (a) congenital umbilical hernia, (b) acquired umbilical hernia, and (c) paraumbilical hernia.
3. (a) *Congenital umbilical hernia* is the protrusion of bowel through the weak scar of the umbilicus just after the fall of the atrophied umbilical cord or few months later. The umbilical scar is usually attached to the hernial sac.
   (b) *Acquired umbilical hernia* is the protrusion of abdominal contents through the umbilical scar in the adults due to raised intra-abdominal pressure. The *umbilical scar* is attached to the centre of hernial sac.
   (c) *Paraumbilical hernia* is the common acquired hernia. It appears through a defect, which is adjacent to the umbilical scar. It does not bulge through the centre of umbilical scar hence umbilical skin is not attached to the centre of the sac.

Inguinal Region/Groin

The inguinal region (groin) is the junction of the anterior abdominal wall and the anterior aspect of the thigh. It extends between the anterior superior iliac spine and the pubic tubercle. Clinically the inguinal region includes area along and around the inguinal ligament. This region is important both anatomically and clinically, anatomically because it is the region where structures exit from and enter into the abdominal cavity and clinically because the pathways of exit and entry are potential sites of herniation. Majority of abdominal hernias occur in this region, e.g., inguinal and femoral hernias; only inguinal hernias account for 75% of all hernias of the body. The key structures in this region are the inguinal ligament, inguinal canal, and femoral canal. Hence, surgically it is the most important region.

INGUINAL LIGAMENT

The inguinal ligament is a thick, fibrous band extending from anterior superior iliac spine to the pubic tubercle. It lies beneath the fold of groin. It is formed by the lower-free border of the external oblique aponeurosis, which is thickened and folded backward on itself. Thus the lower aspect of the ligament is round while its upper aspect presents a groove. The grooved upper surface of inguinal ligament forms the floor of inguinal canal (Fig. 4.1).

The strong deep fascia of the thigh (**fascia lata**) is attached to the lower aspect of the entire length of the ligament, which makes it convex inferiorly by its pull.

EXTENSIONS/EXPANSIONS

The various extensions/expansions of the inguinal ligament are:

Lacunar Ligament (or Gimbernat's Ligament)

From the medial end the deep fibres of the inguinal ligament curve horizontally backward to the medial part of the pecten pubis forming lacunar ligament. This ligament is triangular

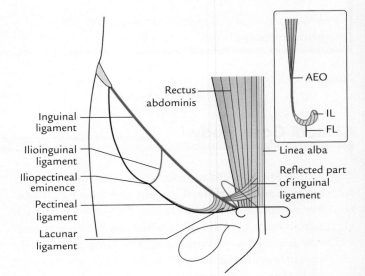

Fig. 4.1 Inguinal ligament and its extensions. Figure in the inset shows formation of inguinal ligament and its attachment to the fascia lata (AEO = aponeurosis of external oblique, IL = inguinal ligament, FL = fascia lata).

in shape with apex attached to the pubic tubercle. Its sharp lateral edge forms the medial boundary of the femoral canal, which is the site of production of a femoral hernia.

Pectineal Ligament (Ligament of Cooper)

It is the extension of the posterior part of the lacunar ligament along the pecten pubis up to the iliopectineal eminence. Some authorities regard it as a thickening in the upper part of the pectineal fascia.

Reflected Part of Inguinal Ligament

The superficial fibres from the medial end of the inguinal ligament expand upward and medially to form this ligament. It lies behind the superficial inguinal ring and in front of the conjoint tendon. Its fibres interlace with those of its counter-part of the opposite side at the linea alba.

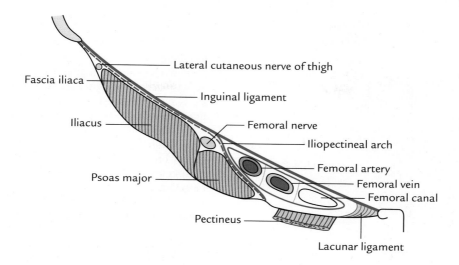

Fig. 4.2 Subinguinal space and structures passing through it.

Ilioinguinal Ligament

It is a fibrous band extending from the inferior aspect of the inguinal ligament to the iliopectineal eminence.

SUBINGUINAL SPACE (PELVIFEMORAL SPACE)

The space between the inguinal ligament and the hip bone is called pelvifemoral/subinguinal space (Fig. 4.2). The muscles (psoas major and iliacus) and neurovascular structures of posterior abdominal wall/pelvis pass into the femoral region of the thigh through this space. This space is divided by the ilioinguinal ligament/arch into two parts:

(a) Large lateral part called *lacuna musculorum*.
(b) Small medial part called *lacuna vasculorum*.

The iliacus and psoas muscles, and femoral and lateral cutaneous nerves of thigh pass through the lacuna musculorum behind the fascia iliaca.

The external iliac vessels in abdomen become femoral vessels as they pass through the medial part of the subinguinal space—the lacuna vasculorum.

The fascial lining of the abdomen is prolonged into the thigh to enclose the upper 3.75 cm of the femoral vessels forming the **femoral sheath**.

FEMORAL SHEATH

It is a funnel-shaped fascial sheath enclosing upper 3.75 cm of femoral vessels. The base of the sheath is directed upward toward the abdominal cavity and apex merges with the tunica adventitia of the femoral vessels (Fig. 4.3).

The anterior wall of the femoral sheath is formed by the downward prolongation of the fascia transversalis and the posterior wall by the downward prolongation of the fascia iliaca (Fig. 4.3).

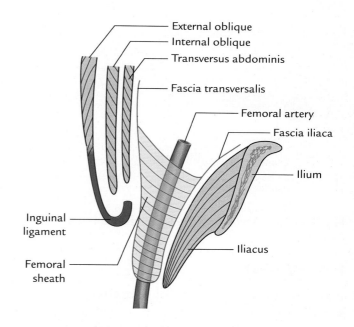

Fig. 4.3 Formation of the femoral sheath (lateral view).

The femoral sheath is not symmetrical. Its lateral wall is vertical whereas its medial wall is oblique being directed downward and laterally (Fig. 4.4).

Compartments (Fig. 4.5)

The interior of the femoral sheath is divided into three compartments by two anteroposterior fibrous septa.

1. *Lateral compartment* lodges the femoral artery and genital branch of the genitofemoral nerve.
2. *Middle compartment* contains the femoral vein.
3. *Medial compartment* is relatively empty and called **femoral canal**. It contains lymph node of Cloquet and fibrofatty tissue.

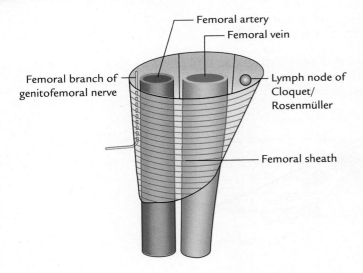

Fig. 4.4 Walls and contents of the femoral sheath (anterior view).

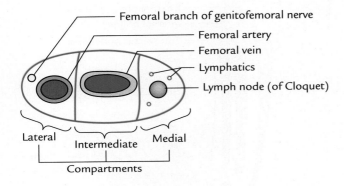

Fig. 4.5 Compartment of the femoral sheath.

FEMORAL CANAL

It is a short fascial tube (medial compartment of femoral sheath) which diminishes rapidly in width from above downward and is closed inferiorly by the fusion of its walls.

The upper end of the femoral canal, which opens into the abdominal cavity is called **femoral ring**. A fatty areolar tissue called **femoral septum** normally closes it. **Cloquet's node** is a lymph node situated in the femoral canal. The canal provides a dead space for the expansion of femoral vein during increased venous return.

Boundaries

Anterior: Inguinal ligament
Medial: Sharp edge of the lacunar ligament
Posterior: Pecten pubis
Lateral: Femoral vein

Below the inguinal ligament, the canal lies posterior to the saphenous opening and thin cribriform fascia, and anterior to the fascia covering the pectineus muscle.

Femoral hernia (Figs 4.6 and 4.7): The protrusion of abdominal contents (a loop of intestine) through the femoral canal is called **femoral hernia**. The femoral hernia presents as a globular swelling in groin inferolateral to the pubic tubercle below the inguinal ligament (Fig. 4.6).

The femoral ring is the site of potential weakness of the groin when the femoral ring is enlarged due to the abdominal distention with weakness of abdominal muscles, e.g., pregnancy. Any condition, which raises the intra-abdominal pressure, e.g., repeated forceful coughing or straining forces the loop of intestine into the femoral ring, it carries with it the peritoneal covering of the abdominal opening of the canal in front of it. This forms the hernial sac, which descends in the femoral canal posterior to the weak cribriform fascia and bulges forward through it into the superficial fascia of the thigh close to the saphenous vein (Fig. 4.7).

If hernial sac continues to enlarge, it expands superolaterally in the superficial fascia. Consequently, the entire hernia becomes U-shaped.

The femoral hernia is more common in female because the femoral ring is larger due to greater width of the pelvis.

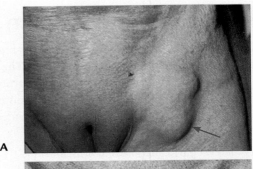

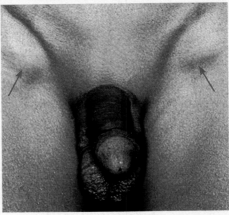

Fig. 4.6 Femoral hernia: **A,** unilateral femoral hernia on the left side in female; **B,** bilateral femoral hernia in male (rare) causing a bulging enlargement of the femoral canal. (*Source:* **A,** Fig. 17.24, Page 461–474, *Textbook of Diagnostic Sonography,* 7e, Sandra L Hagen-Ansert. Copyright Mosby Inc 2012, All rights reserved. **B,** Fig. 17-130, Page 643–692, *Atlas of Pediatric Physical Diagnosis,* 6e, Basil J Zitelli, Sara C MIntire and Andrew J Nowalk. Copyright Saunders 2012, All rights reserved.)

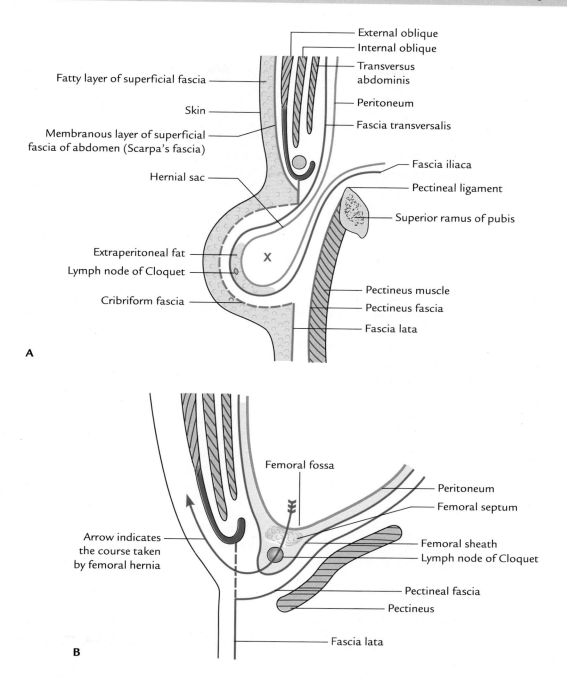

Fig. 4.7 A, Formation of the hernial sac; **B**, course of the femoral hernia.

ILIOPUBIC TRACT (Fig. 4.8)

It is the thickened inferior margin of the fascia transversalis which appears as a fibrous band running parallel and posterior to the inguinal ligament. When the inguinal region is viewed from its posterior aspect, the iliopubic tract is seen in place of the inguinal ligament.

N.B. According to Fruchaud, the inguinal ligament and iliopubic tract span an innate area of weakness in the inguinal region.

INGUINAL CANAL

The inguinal canal is an oblique intermuscular passage about 4 cm long lying above the medial half of the inguinal ligament.

EXTENT AND DIRECTION

The inguinal canal extends from **deep inguinal ring** (an oval opening in the fascia transversalis) to the **superficial inguinal**

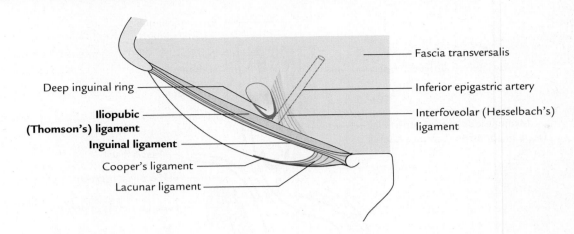

Fig. 4.8 Iliopubic tract.

ring (a triangular gap in the external oblique aponeurosis). It is directed downward, forward, and medially.

On the surface the canal is marked by two parallel lines (1 cm apart and 4 cm long) just above the medial half of the inguinal ligament. The deep inguinal ring is marked 1.2 cm above the midinguinal point as an oval opening at the lateral end of two parallel lines (vide supra). The superficial inguinal ring is marked just above the pubic tubercle as a triangular opening at the medial end of two parallel lines. The centre of superficial inguinal ring lies 1 cm above and lateral to the pubic tubercle (Fig. 4.9).

Inguinal Rings

Deep Inguinal Ring

1. The deep inguinal ring is an oval opening in the fascia transversalis and lies about 1.25 cm (1/2 inch) above the midinguinal point.
2. From its margins, the fascia transversalis is prolonged into the canal like a sleeve, the **internal spermatic fascia**, around the structures that pass through the ring.

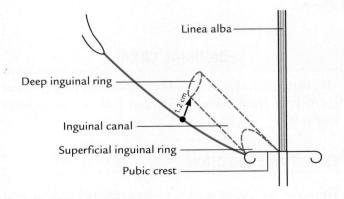

Fig. 4.9 Surface marking of the inguinal canal.

These structures constitute the spermatic cord in male.

Superficial Inguinal Ring

1. The superficial inguinal ring is a triangular gap in the aponeurosis of external oblique and lies above and lateral to the pubic crest.
2. The pubic crest forms the base of the triangle. The sides (upper/medial and lower/lateral margins) of the triangle are called **crura,** which meet laterally to form an obtuse apex. Near the apex, the two crura are united by the intercrural fibres.
3. It is 2.5 cm long and 1.2 cm broad (at the base).

Table 4.1 enumerates the structures passing through the deep and superficial inguinal rings.

Table 4.1 Structures passing through the deep and superficial inguinal rings

Deep inguinal ring	
In male	*In female*
• Ductus deferens and its artery • Testicular artery and the accompanying veins • Obliterated remains of processus vaginalis • Genital branch of genitofemoral nerve • Autonomic nerves and lymphatics	• Round ligament of uterus • Obliterated remains of processus vaginalis • Lymphatics from the uterus
Superficial inguinal ring	
In male	*In female*
• Spermatic cord • Ilioinguinal nerve*	• Round ligament of uterus • Ilioinguinal nerve*

*Ilioinguinal nerve enters the inguinal canal by piercing the wall and not through the deep inguinal ring.

BOUNDARIES

The boundaries of the inguinal canal (Fig. 4.10) are:

Anterior wall: It is formed from superficial to deep by:
    (a) Skin
    (b) Superficial fascia ⎫ in the whole extent.
    (c) External oblique ⎬
        aponeurosis ⎭
    (d) Internal oblique muscle fibres, in lateral one-third.

Posterior wall: It is formed from deep to superficial by:
    (a) Fascia transversalis, in the whole extent
    (b) Conjoint tendon, in medial two-third
    (c) Reflected part of the inguinal ligament, in medial-most part.

Roof: It is formed by the lower arched fibres of internal oblique and transversus abdominis muscles.

Floor: It is formed by:
    (a) Grooved upper surface of the inguinal ligament in the whole extent
    (b) Abdominal surface of the lacunar ligament at the medial end.

The arrangement of muscles (external oblique, internal oblique, and transversus abdominis) and fascia transversalis in relation to the inguinal canal is shown in Figure 4.11.

CONTENTS

In male: Spermatic cord and ilioinguinal nerve.
In female: Round ligament of the uterus and ilioinguinal nerve.

N.B. The ilioinguinal nerve, although a content of the inguinal canal, does not enter the canal through the deep inguinal ring. It enters the canal from side through a slit between the external and internal oblique muscles. It lies in front of the cord and passes out of canal through the superficial inguinal ring to supply the inguinal region.

Spermatic Cord

The spermatic cord is a collection of structures that pass to and fro from testis through the inguinal canal. It extends from the deep inguinal ring to the posterior border of the testis and is covered by three fascial layers.

Constituents/Contents (Fig. 4.12)

The spermatic cord consists of the following six groups of structures:

1. Ductus deferens, in the posterior part.
2. Three arteries:
    (a) Testicular artery, from abdominal aorta.

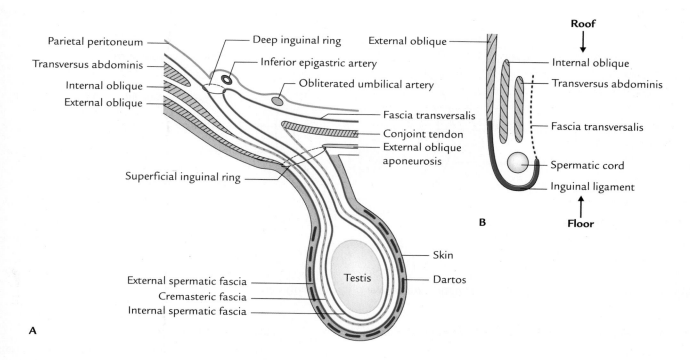

Fig. 4.10 Boundaries of the inguinal canal: A, anterior and posterior walls as seen in coronal section; B, roof and floor as seen in sagittal section.

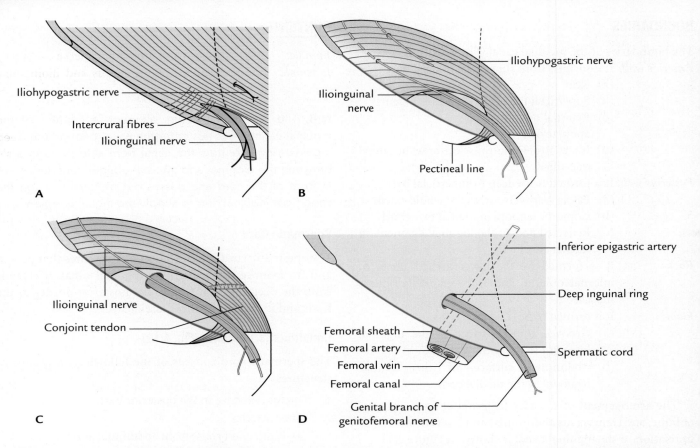

Fig. 4.11 Schematic diagrams to show the formation of the walls of inguinal canal from outside inwards: **A**, external oblique; **B**, internal oblique; **C**, transversus abdominis; **D**, fascia transversalis. The formation of anterior and posterior walls and location of inguinal rings can easily be deduced from these figures.

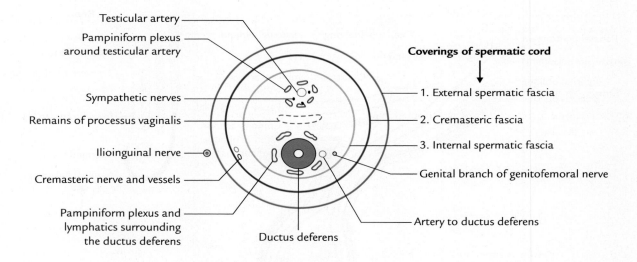

Fig. 4.12 Transverse section of the spermatic cord showing its covering content.

(b) Cremasteric artery, from inferior epigastric artery.

(c) Artery to ductus deferens, from inferior vesical artery.

3. Veins, the pampiniform venous plexus.

4. Lymphatics, especially from testis draining into pre- and para-aortic nodes, and some from the coverings draining into external iliac nodes.

5. Nerves, genital branch of genitofemoral nerve and sympathetic fibres which accompany the arteries.
6. Remains of processus vaginalis.

Coverings (Fig. 4.12)

The spermatic cord is covered by three fascial layers from within outward, these are:

1. *Internal spermatic fascia*, derived from fascia transversalis.
2. *Cremasteric fascia* consisting of loops of skeletal muscle fibres united by areolar tissue. The muscle fibres are derived from internal oblique muscle.
3. *External spermatic fascia*, derived from aponeurosis of external oblique muscle.

MECHANISMS TO MAINTAIN THE INTEGRITY OF THE INGUINAL CANAL

The inguinal canal is a site of potential weakness in the lower part of the anterior abdominal wall, and may provide herniation of abdominal viscera. But, normally it is prevented by strength and good tone of the muscles of the anterior abdominal wall by the following mechanisms:

Flap-valve Mechanism

The canal is oblique hence its deep and superficial inguinal rings do not lie opposite to each other. As a result when intra-abdominal pressure is raised the anterior and posterior walls of the canal are approximated like a flap.

Guarding of the Inguinal Rings

The deep inguinal ring is guarded anteriorly by the internal oblique muscle, and superficial inguinal ring is guarded posteriorly by the conjoint tendon and reflected part of the inguinal ligament (Fig. 4.13).

Shutter Mechanism

The internal oblique surrounds the canal in front, above, and behind like a flexible mobile arch and thus forming its

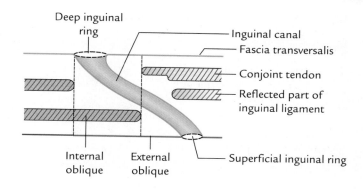

Fig. 4.13 Structures protecting the anterior and posterior walls of the inguinal canal.

anterior wall, roof, and posterior wall. Consequently, when it contracts, the roof is pulled and approximated on the floor like a shutter.

Slit-valve Mechanism

The contraction of external oblique muscle approximates the two crura medial and lateral of superficial inguinal ring like a slit valve. The intercrural fibres also help in this act.

Ball-valve Mechanism

Contraction of cremaster muscle pulls the testis up and the superficial inguinal ring is plugged by the spermatic cord.

N.B. In addition to the above mechanisms, the *interfoveolar ligament* also helps to maintain the integrity of the inguinal canal by strengthening fascia transversalis laterally. The muscle fibres arch down from the lower border of transversus abdominis to the superior ramus of pubis and constitute the interfoveolar ligament—the functional medial edge of the deep inguinal ring (Fig. 4.14).

The features of the inguinal canal are summarized in Table 4.2.

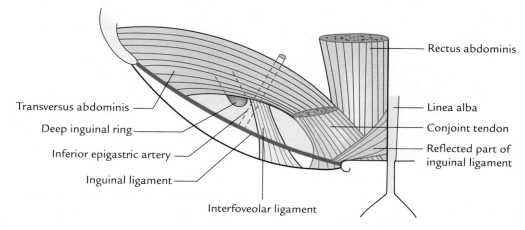

Fig. 4.14 Interfoveolar ligament.

Table 4.2 Features of the inguinal canal

Features		Formed by
Boundaries	• Anterior wall	External oblique aponeurosis (supplemented by internal oblique in the lateral 1/3rd)
	• Posterior wall	Fascia transversalis (supplemented by conjoint tendon in the medial 2/3rd)
	• Roof	Internal oblique and transversus abdominis muscles (arched fibres)
	• Floor	Inguinal ligament (supplemented by lacunar ligament medially)
Openings	• Superficial inguinal ring	Triangular aperture in external oblique aponeurosis above and lateral to the pubic crest
	• Deep inguinal ring	Oval aperture in fascia transversalis 1.25 cm above the midinguinal point

INGUINAL TRIANGLE (HESSELBACH'S TRIANGLE)

The inguinal triangle is situated deep to the posterior wall of the inguinal canal; hence, it is seen on the inner aspect of the lower part of the anterior abdominal wall.

BOUNDARIES

The boundaries of the inguinal triangle are as follows (Fig. 4.15):

Medial: Lower 5 cm of the lateral border of the rectus abdominis muscle.

Lateral: Inferior epigastric artery.

Inferior: Medial half of the inguinal ligament.

The **floor of the triangle** is covered by the *peritoneum, extraperitoneal tissue,* and *fascia transversalis.*

N.B. The medial umbilical ligament (obliterated umbilical artery) crosses the triangle and divides it into medial and lateral parts. The medial part of the floor of the triangle is strengthened by the conjoint tendon.

The lateral part of the floor of the triangle is weak, hence direct inguinal hernia usually occurs through this part.

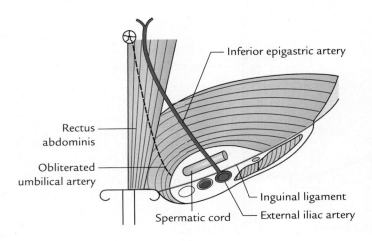

Fig. 4.15 Boundaries of the inguinal (Hesselbach's) triangle.

Labels in figure:
- Inferior epigastric artery
- Rectus abdominis
- Obliterated umbilical artery
- Spermatic cord
- Inguinal ligament
- External iliac artery

Clinical correlation

Inguinal hernias: A protrusion of abdominal viscera (e.g., loops of intestine) into the inguinal canal is termed inguinal hernia. Clinically it presents as a pear-shaped swelling above and medial to pubic tubercle, above the inguinal ligament (Fig. 4.16). There are two types of inguinal hernias, direct and indirect.

1. *Indirect inguinal hernia:* The indirect inguinal hernias occur if the hernial sac enters the inguinal canal through the deep inguinal ring, lateral to the inferior epigastric artery.

   It is common in children and young adults. The predisposing factor for this type of hernia is the complete or partial patency of the processus vaginalis.

   The indirect inguinal hernias are more common than the direct inguinal hernias and occur more often in males than females. The indirect inguinal hernia may be **congenital** or **acquired**.

   – *Congenital indirect inguinal hernia:* It occurs due to patent processus vaginalis (an outpouching of the peritoneum), connecting peritoneal cavity with the tunica vaginalis.

   – *Acquired indirect inguinal hernia:* It occurs due to increased intra-abdominal pressure as during weight lifting. When intra-abdominal pressure is increased immensely, the abdominal contents are pushed through the deep inguinal ring into the inguinal canal.

2. *Direct inguinal hernia.* The direct inguinal hernia occurs if the hernial sac enters the inguinal canal directly by pushing the posterior wall of the inguinal canal forward, medial to inferior epigastric artery through the Hesselbach's triangle. The neck of hernial sac is wide. The direct inguinal hernias are common in elderly due to weak abdominal muscles. The direct hernia leaves the triangle through its lateral part or medial part, and therefore it is of two types: (a) *lateral direct inguinal hernia,* and (b) *medial direct inguinal hernia.*

N.B.

• The term **complete inguinal hernia** is used if hernial contents reach the tunica vaginalis. If the hernial contents remain confined to inguinal canal and do

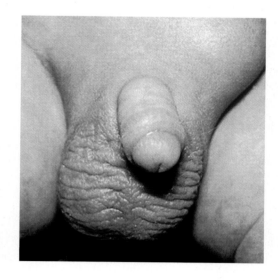
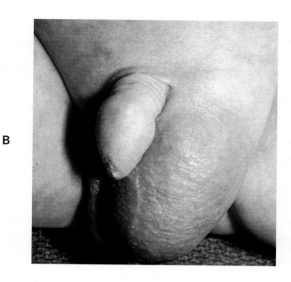

Fig. 4.16 Indirect inguinal hernia: **A**, an incomplete inguinal hernia producing a bulge in the left groin but not extending into the scrotum; **B**, a complete inguinal hernia in the left groin extending into the scrotum, obscuring the testis. (*Source:* A, Fig. 17-123 and **B**, Fig. 17-124, Pages 643–692, *Atlas of Pediatric Physical Diagnosis*, 6e, Basil J Zitelli, Sara C McIntire, and Andrew J Nowalk. Copyright 2012 Saunders. All rights reserved.)

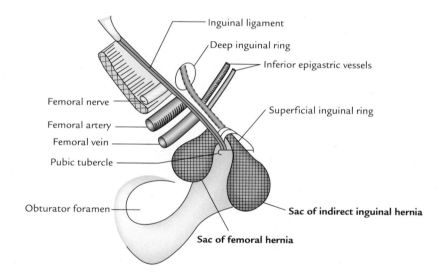

Fig. 4.17 Relationship of inguinal and femoral hernia. (*Source:* Fig. 4.7, Page 149, *Clinical and Surgical Anatomy*, 2e, Vishram Singh. Copyright Elsevier 2007, All rights reserved.)

not pass through superficial inguinal ring it is called **incomplete inguinal hernia/bubonocele.**

- The inguinal hernias occur only in men and not in other mammals. This is due to evolutionary changes which have taken place in inguinal region due to erect posture.

Differences between femoral and inguinal hernias are given in Table 4.3 and shown in Figure 4.17.

Difference between indirect and direct inguinal hernias are given in Table 4.4.

Table 4.3 Differences between inguinal and femoral hernias

	Inguinal hernia	Femoral hernia
Sex	More common in males	More common in females
Protrusion of hernial sac	Into inguinal canal	Into femoral canal
Neck of protrusion of hernia	Lies above and medial to pubic tubercle	Lies below and lateral to the pubic tubercle

Source: Modified from Table 4.2, Page 150, *Clinical and Surgical Anatomy* 2e, Vishram Singh. Copyright Elsevier 2007, All rights reserved.

Table 4.4 Differences between the indirect and direct inguinal hernia

	Indirect inguinal hernia	Direct inguinal hernia
Site of protrusion of hernial sac	Deep inguinal ring	Posterior wall of inguinal canal
Shape	Pear shaped	Globular
Extent	Generally scrotal	Rarely scrotal
Direction	Oblique (directed downward, forward, and medially)	Straight (directed forward)
Neck of hernial sac	Narrow and lies lateral to the inferior epigastric vessels	Wide and lies medial to the inferior epigastric vessels
Reducibility	Sometimes irreducible	Generally always reducible
Age group	Occurs in young age	Occurs in middle and old age
Internal ring occlusion test*	Positive	Negative

*After reducing the hernia, the pressure is applied over deep inguinal ring and patient is asked to cough. If hernia does not appear, it is indirect (because herniation occurs through the deep inguinal ring), and if hernia appears, it is direct (because herniation occurs through the Hesselbach's triangle). (*Source:* Table 4.1, Page 147, *Clinical and Surgical Anatomy*, 2e, Vishram Singh. Copyright Elsevier 2007, All rights reserved.)

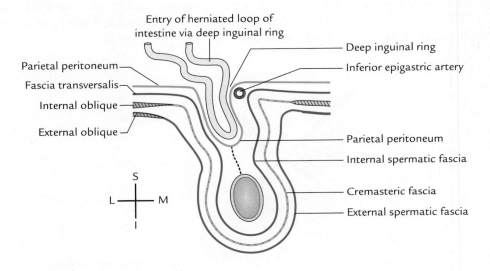

Fig. 4.18 Coverings of the indirect inguinal hernia.

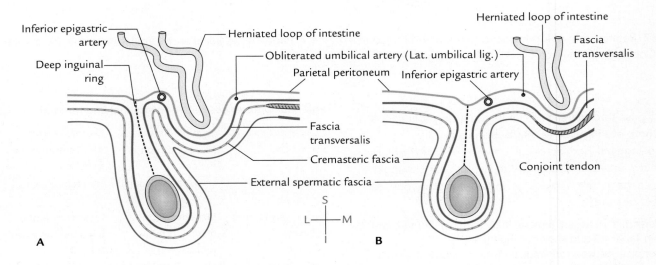

Fig. 4.19 Coverings of the direct inguinal hernia: A, lateral direct inguinal hernia; B, medial direct inguinal hernia.

Table 4.5 Coverings of the indirect and direct inguinal hernias (Figs 4.17 and 4.18)

Indirect inguinal hernia	Direct inguinal hernia
• Extraperitoneal tissue • Internal spermatic fascia • Cremasteric fascia • External spermatic fascia • Skin	• Extraperitoneal tissue • Fascia transversalis • Conjoint tendon (in medial direct hernia) • Cremaster fascia (in lateral direct hernia) • External spermatic fascia • Skin

COVERINGS OF THE INDIRECT AND DIRECT INGUINAL HERNIAS

The coverings of the hernia are the structures separating the hernial sac/peritoneal sac from the surface of the body. The coverings of indirect and direct inguinal hernias are shown in Figures 4.18 and 4.19, and are summarized in Table 4.5.

Table 4.5 clearly shows that coverings of both indirect and direct inguinal hernias are more or less same. The only difference is that in direct inguinal hernia (medial direct) internal spermatic fascia is replaced by fascia transversalis and cremasteric muscle and fascia is replaced by conjoint tendon hernia.

The differences between the indirect and direct inguinal hernias are given in Table 4.5.

Golden Facts to Remember

▸ Groin	Area of junction between the anterior abdominal wall and front of thigh
▸ Most common hernia in the inguinal region	Indirect inguinal hernia
▸ All the contents of inguinal canal lie within the spermatic cord *except*	Ilioinguinal nerve
▸ Commonest symptoms of an inguinal hernia	Presence of lump, and dragging and aching sensation in the groin
▸ Inguinal hernia	Peritoneal sac enters into the inguinal canal
▸ Femoral hernia	Peritoneal sac enters into femoral canal
▸ Most lumps in the groin move with coughing (a transmitted impulse) *except*	Hernia and vascular tumor, which expand with coughing
▸ Canal of Nuck	Peritoneal pouch in the female inguinal canal is due to persistence of processus vaginalis. It may extend into labium majus
▸ Incisional hernias	Occurs through a defect in scar of a previous abdominal operation
▸ Spigelian hernia	Passes upward through arcuate line into the lateral border of posterior rectus sheath
▸ Groin hernias	Direct and indirect inguinal and femoral hernias

Clinical Case Study

A 70-year-old patient with history of chronic bronchitis and constipation complained that he noticed a gradually increasing swelling in his right groin and often feels dragging and aching sensation at that site. On physical examination the doctor noticed a globular lump above the right pubic tubercle which expands on coughing.

After manually reducing the swelling/lump, occluded the deep inguinal ring with his thumb and asked the patient to cough. The swelling reappeared medial to the thumb. A diagnosis of *direct inguinal hernia* was made.

Questions

1. What is inguinal hernia?
2. What are the types of inguinal hernias and how they differ from each other?
3. Give the surface marking of deep inguinal canal.

Answers

1. Protrusion of abdominal viscus into the inguinal canal.
2. (a) Indirect inguinal hernia
    (b) Direct inguinal hernia
    In indirect inguinal hernia abdominal viscus (e.g., loop of intestine) protrudes into inguinal canal through deep inguinal ring, whereas in direct inguinal hernia abdominal viscus protrudes into inguinal canal by pushing its posterior wall (also see page 54).
3. It is marked 1.25 cm above the midinguinal point as an oval opening.

Male External Genital Organs

The male genital organs are classified into two types—external and internal (Table 5.1).

From surgical and clinical point of view, the male external genital organs include the following structures:

1. Penis.
2. Scrotum.
3. Testes.
2. Epididymis.
5. Spermatic cords.

The surgeons and physicians routinely examine these structures during clinical practice to diagnose a number of ailments associated with them, namely, phimosis, cancer glans penis, hydrocele, varicocele, hernias, testicular tumor, etc. The surgical procedures related to these structures (e.g., circumcision, herniorrhaphy, etc.) are also routinely performed by the surgeons.

N.B. *Axiom:* In males, the physical examination of the abdomen is not complete without the examination of external genitalia.

PENIS

The penis is the male organ of copulation and is traversed by the urethra, which provides passage for both urine and semen. It is capable of becoming hard and erect due to its engorgement with blood, a requirement for its intromission into the vagina (Fig. 5.1).

PARTS

The penis consists of the following two parts (Fig. 5.2):

1. **Root** or **radix,** an attached portion.
2. **Body** or **corpus,** a free pendulous portion.

Table 5.1 External and internal male genital organs

	Organs	Functions
External genital organs	• Penis	• Copulation • Passage for semen and urine
	• Scrotum	• Maintenance of testicular temperature for proper spermatogenesis
Internal genital organs	• Testis	• Production of sperms and male hormones
	• Epididymis	• Reservoir and maturation of sperms
	• Vas deferens	• Transportation of sperms
	• Prostate and seminal vesicles	• Production of secretions to form the bulk of semen and provide nutrition to sperms
	• Bulbourethral glands	• Produce oily secretion for lubrication of urethra

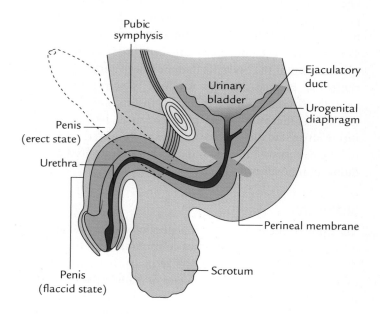

Fig. 5.1 Penis as seen in sagittal section.

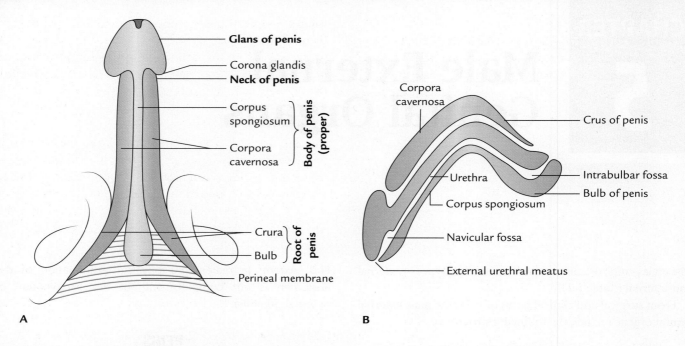

Fig. 5.2 Parts of the penis: **A**, as seen from ventral (urethral) aspect; **B**, as seen in sagittal section.

Root (Radix)

The **root of the penis** is situated in the superficial perineal pouch and is attached to the inferior aspect of the urogenital diaphragm. It comprises three masses of erectile tissue, viz. two crura (right and left) and the bulb of the penis. Each crus is firmly attached to the everted margin of the pubic arch on the corresponding side. Anteriorly, it converges toward its fellow of the opposite side, and near the inferior border of the pubic symphysis the two crura come together and continue as the corpora cavernosa of the body of the penis. The bulb is firmly attached on the inferior aspect of the perineal membrane stretching between the two crura. The bulb narrows anteriorly and continues as the corpus spongiosum of the body. Its flattened deep surface above its centre is pierced by the urethra, which traverses its substance to reach the corpus spongiosum. This part of the urethra in the bulb shows a dilatation in its floor called **intrabulbar fossa**. Each crus is covered by the ischiocavernosus muscle, and the bulb is covered by the bulbospongiosus muscle.

Body (Corpus)

The body of the penis is the free pendulous portion and lies in front of scrotum. It becomes continuous with the root of the penis. In general usage, the term penis stands for the body of penis. In the flaccid state, it hangs free below the pubic symphysis, anterior to the scrotum, and terminates in an acorn-like enlargement called glans penis. For convenience

of study and proper understanding the body of penis is further divided into three parts: body proper, neck, and glans penis (Fig. 5.3).

Body Proper

Shape

In the flaccid state, it is a long (cylindrical) pendulous structure, and directed downwards and forwards. *In erect state*, it is directed upwards and forward and assumes a triangular prism-like shape on cross section with rounded angles. The surfaces of penis are described in this state.

Surfaces

There are two surfaces — ventral and dorsal.
- The ventral surface faces backward and downward.
- The dorsal surface faces forward and upward.

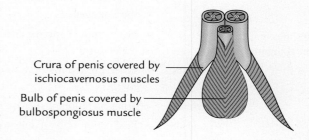

Fig. 5.3 Muscles covering the parts of the root of penis as seen from the ventral (urethral) aspect of the penis.

Glans Penis (Fig. 5.4)

It is an enlarged, conical structure at the distal end of the penis, with sagittal slit-like aperture on its summit called **external urethral meatus**. The projecting margin of the base of glans is called **corona glandis** which overhangs the neck of the penis.

Neck of Penis

It is an obliquely grooved constriction just behind the base of the glans.

STRUCTURE

It is composed of three elongated masses of erectile tissue, which are capable of considerable enlargement when engorged with blood during an erection. The three erectile tissue masses include two corpora cavernosa and one corpus spongiosum (Fig. 5.2).

Corpora Cavernosa (Figs 5.2, 5.3, and 5.4)

The two corpora cavernosa form the greater part of the body of penis. They are the forward continuation of the crura. The two corpora cavernosa, throughout their length, lay in close apposition with one another and are surrounded by a common fibrous envelope called the *tunica albuginea*. Tunica albuginea consists of superficial and deep layers. The longitudinally arranged superficial fibres form a tube to enclose both corpora, while the circular deep fibres surround each corpus separately and form at their junction in the midline the *septum of penis*. This septum is complete proximally but replaced distally by fibrous bands like the teeth of a comb called *pectiniform septum*.

The wide groove between the two corpora cavernosa on the ventral (urethral) surface lodges the corpus spongiosum. A similar but narrower groove on the dorsal surface lodges the deep dorsal vein of the penis being flanked on each side by the dorsal artery and dorsal nerve of the penis. The corpora cavernosa do not reach the end of the penis but terminate as conical extremities within the hollow on the internal aspect of glans penis.

Corpus Spongiosum

The corpus spongiosum is the forward continuation of the bulb. It is cylindrical and tapers slightly toward the distal end where it suddenly expands to form a conical enlargement – the **glans penis**. Throughout its length, it is traversed by the spongy part of the urethra. It is also surrounded by a thin fibrous sheath of tunica albuginea.

COVERINGS

Skin of Penis (Fig. 5.5)

It is remarkably thin, delicate, dark, and hairless. It envelops the body of penis completely. It is loosely attached to the fascial sheath of the penis and hence is freely mobile. At the neck of the penis, it is folded upon itself to form the **prepuce** or **foreskin**, which covers the glans for a variable distance. The prepuce is retracted during coitus or manually. The internal layer of prepuce is continuous with the thin skin covering the glans firmly. The skin covering the glans is continuous with the mucous membrane of the urethra at the external urethral orifice. On the urethral aspect of the glans, a small median fold passes from the inner aspect of prepuce to the glans immediately proximal to the external urethral meatus. The sensitivity of the **frenulum of prepuce** plays an important role in orgasm.

Prepuce of the skin

It is a fold of skin, which covers the glans for a variable extent and is attached to the neck of the penis.

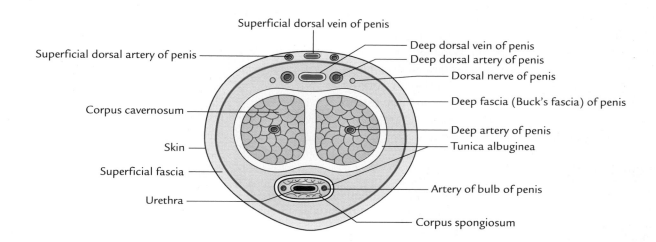

Fig. 5.4 Transverse section through the body of the penis.

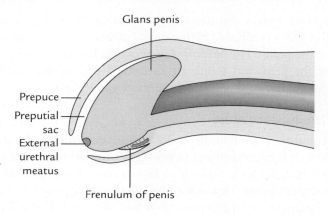

Fig. 5.5 Schematic diagram to show glans penis, prepuce, preputial sac, and frenulum of the penis.

Frenulum of the prepuce

It is a median fold of skin on the ventral surface of glans, which passes from the inner surface of prepuce to the external urethral meatus. It is highly sensitive.

Preputial sac

It is a potential space/cleft between the glans and the prepuce.

Superficial Fascia of the Penis

It consists of two layers—superficial and deep. The superficial layer is devoid of fat and consists of loose areolar tissue. It may contain few muscle fibres—the *peripenic muscle*. The deep layer in the lower part of the anterior abdominal wall is condensed and forms the fascia of penis termed **deep fascia of the penis** or **Buck's fascia**. It surrounds both corpora cavernosa and corpus spongiosum, but does not extend beyond the neck of penis. Buck's fascia separates the superficial and deep dorsal veins of the penis.

SUPPORTS OF PENIS

The ligaments support the weight of the free pendulous part (body) of the penis. They are two in number (Fig. 5.6).

1. **Fundiform ligament:** It springs from the lower part of the linea alba and splits into two lamellae, which enclose the proximal part of the body of penis and then unite on its urethral aspect with the septum of scrotum.

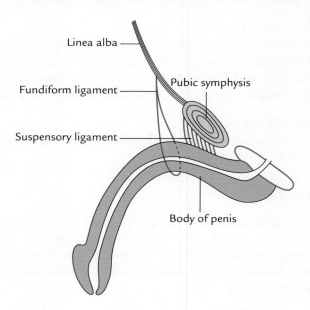

Fig. 5.6 Ligaments of the penis.

2. **Suspensory ligament:** It is deep to the fundiform ligament and triangular in shape. Its narrow upper end is attached in front of the pubic symphysis and broad lower part blends with Buck's fascia (fascia of penis) on either side of the body of penis.

ARTERIAL SUPPLY

The penis is supplied by the following four pairs of arteries (Figs 5.7 and 5.8):

1. Deep arteries of the penis.

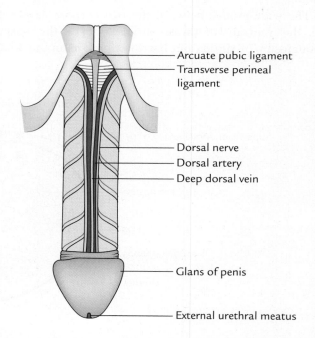

Fig. 5.7 Dorsal nerve and vessels of the penis after removal of deep fascia of the penis (Buck's fascia).

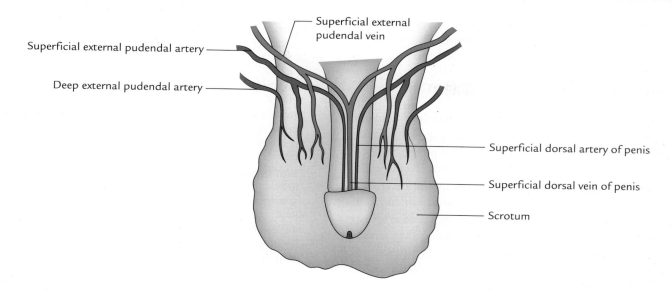

Fig. 5.8 Superficial vessels of the penis.

2. Dorsal arteries of the penis.
3. Arteries of the bulb.
4. Superficial dorsal arteries of penis.

Out of these, the first three pairs of arteries arise from *internal pudendal arteries*, branches of anterior divisions of internal iliac arteries, while the last pair arises from *superficial external pudendal arteries*, branches of femoral arteries.

N.B. The penis is supplied chiefly by deep arteries and dorsal arteries. Deep arteries are the principal vessels for filling the lacunae of erectile tissue during erection of the penis. Each deep artery of the penis runs lengthwise in corpus cavernosum and gives off numerous branches. These arteries give rise to minute arteries which directly open into the cavernous spaces. In the flaccid state of the penis, these vessels project in the lacunae as looped or spiral vessels and hence termed "helicine arteries." The dorsal arteries run on the dorsum beneath the deep fascia and supply the glans penis and distal part of corpus spongiosum, prepuce, and frenulum of prepuce. The arteries of bulb supply the bulb and proximal half of the corpus spongiosum. The superficial external pudendal arteries supply the skin and fascia of the penis.

VENOUS DRAINAGE

The following two veins mainly drain the venous blood from the penis (Figs 5.7 and 5.8):

1. Superficial dorsal vein of the penis.
2. Deep dorsal vein of the penis.

N.B. The main veins contrary to the arteries lie in the midline separated from each other by the deep (Buck's) fascia of penis.

- **Superficial dorsal vein of the penis:** It lies in the superficial fascia on the dorsal aspect of the penis in the midline and is usually visible through the skin. Proximally, it divides into right and left branches, which drain into the superficial external pudendal veins.
- **Deep dorsal vein of the penis:** It lies deep to the deep fascia of penis in the median plane dorsally in the narrow groove between the two corpora cavernosa.

Deep vein drains most of the venous blood from the cavernous tissue. Proximally it passes through the gap between the perineal membrane and the lower border of the pubic symphysis to drain into the prostatic venous plexus. The other veins correspond to the arteries.

LYMPHATIC DRAINAGE

The lymphatic drainage is important because of its role in metastasis of penis cancer, which occurs frequently. Lymph vessels from the glans penis drain into the deep inguinal lymph nodes, especially into the lymph node of **Cloquet**. The lymph vessels from the rest of penis drain into superficial inguinal lymph nodes.

NERVE SUPPLY

1. **Sensory innervation:** Sensory supply to the penis is derived from the following:
   - Dorsal nerve of penis.
   - Ilioinguinal nerve.
2. **Motor innervation:** The muscles of penis are supplied by the perineal branch of pudendal nerve.
3. **Autonomic innervation:** The autonomic nerves of the penis are derived from the pelvic (inferior hypogastric) plexus via the prostatic plexus. The sympathetic nerves are vasoconstrictor while parasympathetic fibres are

vasodilator. The parasympathetic fibres (*nervi erigentes*) are derived from S2, S3, and S4 spinal segments. The autonomic fibres are distributed through the pudendal nerve.

MECHANISM OF ERECTION AND EJACULATION

The mechanism of erection of penis is purely a vascular phenomenon and occurs in response to the parasympathetic stimulation. The sexual arousal leads to rapid inflow of blood from **helicine arteries** in the cavernous spaces of erectile tissue of the penis. The filling of blood in the cavernous spaces leads to the compression of the veins, which drain erectile tissues. (This is associated with simultaneous spasm of venous smooth muscle sphincters.) Since the venous outflow is occluded, the blood pressure in the cavernous spaces causes inflation and rigidity of the erectile tissue called **erection**. The pressure within the corpora cavernosa is 100 mmHg at the time of penile erection.

N.B.
- The strong fibrous envelope (tunica albuginea) greatly contributes to the stiffness of the engorged corpora.
- Erection is controlled by nervi erigentes (S2–S4).

The **ejaculation** consists of two processes—emission and ejaculation. The emission is the transmission of seminal fluid from vasa deferentia, seminal vesicles, and prostate into the prostatic urethra. The ejaculation is the onward transmission of seminal fluid from the prostatic urethra to the exterior.

The sympathetic outflow from T11 to L2 spinal segments leads to emission of semen by causing constriction of smooth muscle of vasa deferentia, seminal vesicles, and prostate. It also constricts the internal urethral opening to prevent the retrograde flow of semen into the bladder.

The rhythmic contraction of bulbospongiosus, supplied by the perineal nerve (somatic), compresses the penile urethra and expels the fluid to the exterior—**ejaculation**.

N.B. The neural controls of erection and ejaculation are different; erection is mediated by **parasympathetic nerve fibres** whereas ejaculation is mediated by **sympathetic** and **somatic nerve fibres**.

Clinical correlation

- **Impotence:** The failure to achieve tumescence erection is called impotence. The commonest causes of erectile dysfunction are: (a) psychogenic disturbance with failure to relax the smooth muscle in the corpora, (b) arterial insufficiency because of atheromatous disease, and (c) involvement of nervi erigentes (parasympathetic outflow) secondary to diabetes.
- **Priapism:** The persistant erection is termed **priapism**. It occurs due to persistant spasm of venous smooth muscle sphincters.
- **Peyronie's disease/chordee:** It occurs due to a localized thickening or plaque of the corpora cavernosa, which prevents expansion of a segment of erectile tissue during erection.
  As a result penis becomes curved especially during erection.
- **Phimosis:** It is a narrowing of the distal end of the prepuce (foreskin), which prevents its retraction over the glans penis and may interfere with the micturition (passage of urine).
- **Paraphimosis:** It is an uncommon condition in which narrowing of the prepuce is insufficient to interfere with the micturition, but the prepuce is just sufficiently tight to get stuck on the glans posteriorly on erection and thus interfere with copulation.
- **Circumcision:** It is the surgical removal of the prepuce (foreskin of the penis). In children and adults, the circumcision is sometimes required to relieve the patient from a tightly constricting prepuce (phimosis). The ritual of circumcision for religious reasons is one of the oldest operative procedures in the world (for details, see *Clinical and Surgical Anatomy*, 2nd Edition by Vishram Singh).

SCROTUM

The scrotum (L. scrotum = bag) is a large pendulous sac of skin located below and behind the penis. It is considered as an out-pouching of the lower part of the anterior abdominal wall. It contains the following structures:

1. Testes.
2. Epididymis.
3. Lower parts of the spermatic cords.

EXTERNAL FEATURES

The scrotum presents the following external features:

1. The scrotum is divided into right and left halves by a median ridge or raphe, which indicates the line of fusion of the two halves of the scrotum. This ridge is continued forward in the midline to the undersurface of the penis and backward in the midline of the perineum to the anus (Fig. 5.9).
2. The skin is rugose (corrugated) and dark in colour. The rugosity of the skin occurs due to the presence of subcutaneous dartos muscle.
3. The left half of the scrotum hangs lower than the right half, because the left spermatic cord is longer than the right spermatic cord.

LAYERS OF THE SCROTUM (Fig. 5.10)

The scrotal wall from without inward is made up of the following five layers:

1. Skin.
2. Dartos muscle (which replaces the superficial fascia).

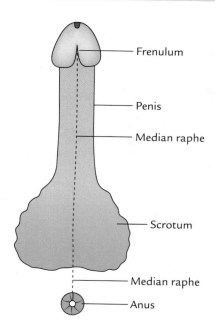

Fig. 5.9 Inferior aspects of the scrotum and penis showing median raphe.

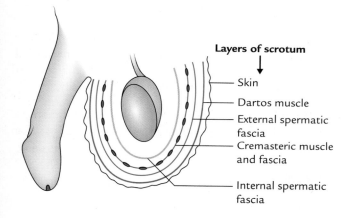

Fig. 5.10 Layers of the scrotum.

3. External spermatic fascia.
4. Cremasteric muscle and fascia.
5. Internal spermatic fascia.

The comparison between the layers of the anterior abdominal wall and the scrotum is given in Table 5.2.

The cavity of the scrotum is partly divided into two halves, right and left, by a septum; the dartos muscle extends into this septum. Each half of the scrotal cavity contains the testis, epididymis, and lower part of the spermatic cord of the corresponding side.

N.B. The subcutaneous dartos muscle helps in the regulation of temperature within the scrotal cavity. Remember the testis needs proper temperature for proper

Table 5.2 Comparison between the layers of the anterior abdominal wall and the scrotum

Layer of anterior abdominal wall	Layer of scrotum
Skin	Skin
Superficial fascia	Dartos muscle
External oblique muscle	External spermatic fascia
Internal oblique muscle	Cremasteric muscle and fascia
Transversus abdominis muscle	No corresponding layer (*Note:* The transversus abdominis muscle does not continue into the scrotum)
Fascia transversalis	Internal spermatic fascia

spermatogenesis. Hence, during the summer under the influence of warmth, the relaxed scrotum becomes flaccid and elongated. Contrary to this, in the winter season under the influence of cold, dartos muscle contracts and scrotum becomes rounded and small with enhanced skin rugosity.

BLOOD SUPPLY

The following arteries supply the scrotum:
1. Superficial external pudendal artery.
2. Deep external pudendal artery.
3. Scrotal branches of the internal pudendal artery.
4. Cremasteric artery, a branch of the inferior epigastric artery.

NERVE SUPPLY (Fig. 5.11A)

1. Anterior one-third of the scrotum is supplied by ilioinguinal nerve (L1) and genital branch of genitofemoral nerve (L1).
2. Posterior two-third of the scrotum is supplied by posterior scrotal branches of the perineal nerve (S3) and perineal branch of the posterior cutaneous nerve of the thigh (S3).
3. The involuntary dartos muscle is supplied by the sympathetic fibres through genital branch of the genitofemoral nerve.

N.B. The areas supplied by L1 and S3 spinal segments are separated by the ventral axial line (Fig. 5.11B).

LYMPHATIC DRAINAGE

The lymph vessels from the scrotum drain into the superficial inguinal lymph nodes.

DEVELOPMENT

The scrotum develops from labioscrotal swellings and urogenital folds, which fuse in the midline to form the

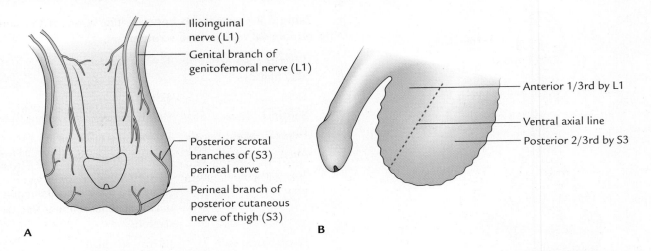

Fig. 5.11 Nerve supply of the scrotum: A, cutaneous nerves of the scrotum anterior view; B, lateral view showing segmental innervation.

scrotum. The site of fusion of urogenital folds is marked by midline fibrous ridge/raphe on the scrotum. The labioscrotal folds in the female form the labia majora and urogenital folds remain separate and form the labia minora.

Clinical correlation

- **Scrotal edema:** The scrotum is a common site of edema due to laxity of the skin and its dependent position.
- **Sebaceous cysts:** These often occur in the scrotum due to the presence of a large number of hair and sebaceous glands in the scrotum.
- **Scrotal elephantiasis:** It is a clinical condition characterized by a massive swelling and enlargement of the scrotum due to accumulation of interstitial fluid in the scrotal wall following blockage of lymph vessels by slender worms of filariasis (*Wuchereria bancrofti*).

TESTIS

The testis is a male gonad. It is homologous with the ovary in the female. It is a mobile organ and lies in each half of the scrotal sac. The functions of the testis include production of spermatozoa and secretion of **testosterone** (or dihydrotestosterone), a male hormone, responsible for the development and maintenance of the secondary sex characteristics of the maleness.

SHAPE AND MEASUREMENTS

Shape
- It is oval/ellipsoid in shape (compressed from side to side).

Measurement
It measures approximately 4 × 3 × 2.5 cm (length = 4 cm, breadth = 2.5 cm, anteroposterior diameter = 3 cm) and weight = 10–15 g.

POSITION IN THE SCROTUM

The testis is suspended in the scrotum by the spermatic cord. It lies obliquely, so that its upper pole is tilted slightly forward and laterally, and lower pole backward and medially.

N.B. The left testis lies slightly at the lower level than the right because the left spermatic cord is slightly longer than the right. This is because descent of left testis begins early.

EXTERNAL FEATURES

The testis presents the following external features:

- Two poles—upper and lower.
- Two borders—anterior and posterior.
- Two surfaces—medial and lateral.

Both the upper and lower poles are convex and smooth. The upper pole provides attachment to the spermatic cord. The anterior border is rounded and completely covered by the tunica vaginalis. The posterior border is straight and covered only partly by the tunica vaginalis. It provides attachment to the epididymis. On the lateral aspect the epididymis is separated from the testis by the extension of the cavity of tunica vaginalis called **sinus of the epididymis** (Fig. 5.12).

Both the medial and lateral surfaces are smooth and slightly convex.

N.B. A small oval body is often found attached to the upper pole of the testis. It is called **appendix of the testis** and represents the remnant of the paramesonephric duct.

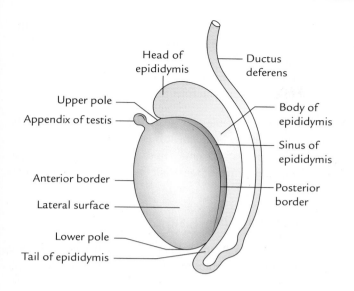

Fig. 5.12 External features of the testis (left testis as seen from the lateral aspect).

COVERINGS

Three coats cover the testis (Fig. 5.13). From superficial to deep these are:

1. Tunica vaginalis.
2. Tunica albuginea.
3. Tunica vasculosa.

Tunica Vaginalis

It is a serous sac representing the persistent lower portion of the processus vaginalis. It is invaginated by the testis from behind. As a result, it presents parietal and visceral layers with a potential cavity between them.

Thus, the tunica vaginalis completely encloses the testes on the front and sides.

Clinical correlation

Hydrocele (Fig. 5.14): It is the accumulation of the fluid within the tunica vaginalis. The fluid may collect following inflammation of the testis because tunica vaginalis is closely related to the front and side of the testis but most hydroceles are idiopathic. The fluid from tunica vaginalis can be removed by inserting a fine trocar and canula through the scrotal skin.

The canula traverses the following structures: (a) skin, (b) dartos muscle, (c) external spermatic fascia, (d) cremasteric muscle and fascia, (e) internal spermatic fascia, and (f) parietal layer of the tunica vaginalis.

For types of hydrocele see the book *Clinical and Surgical Anatomy* by Vishram Singh.

N.B. The collection of blood and pus in the tunica vaginalis is called **hematocele** and **pyocele**, respectively.

Tunica Albuginea

It is a thick, dense layer of fibrous tissue enclosing the testis. It is covered by the visceral layer of tunica vaginalis except where it is in direct contact with the epididymis (i.e., superiorly and posteriorly).

Tunica Vasculosa

It is the innermost vascular layer of the testis, lining the lobules of the testis.

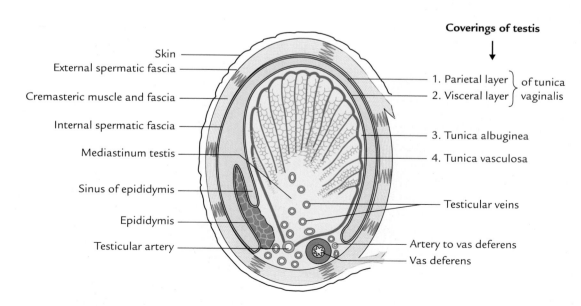

Fig. 5.13 Transverse section of the left testis and its surrounding structures to show the coverings of the testis.

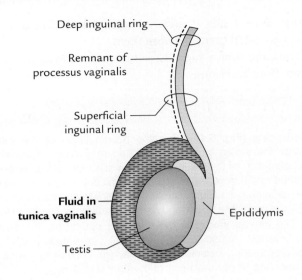

Fig. 5.14 Hydrocele.

STRUCTURE (Figs 5.13 and 5.15)

The testis is enclosed in a fibrous capsule, the *tunica albuginea*. Posteriorly, the tunica albuginea is thickened to form an incomplete vertical septum/ridge, the *mediastinum testis*. Numerous incomplete fibrous septa extend from the mediastinum to the inner aspect of the tunica albuginea and divide the interior of the testis into 200–300 lobules. Each lobule contains two to four coiled seminiferous tubules, lined by thick multilayered germinal epithelium that produces spermatozoa. The thin, thread-like loops of seminiferous tubules join each other and become straighter as they pass toward the mediastinum forming straight *tubules*. The straight seminiferous tubules do not produce spermatozoa

but discharge them into the network of channels called the *rete testis*. The small *efferent ductules* connect the channels of rete testis to the upper end of the epididymis. The interstitial cells, which produce male sex hormones, lie in the areolar tissue between the seminiferous tubules.

N.B. *Number of lobules in testis:* 200–300. Number of seminiferous tubules in each lobule: 2–4. Length of each seminiferous tubule: 60 cm. Thus, if all the seminiferous tubules are joined together, their overall length becomes 500 m.

ARTERIAL SUPPLY (Fig. 5.16)

The testicular artery supplies the testis, which arises from the abdominal aorta in the abdomen at the level of L2 vertebra. Then it passes downward and laterally to enter the deep inguinal ring, traverses through the inguinal canal within the spermatic cord to reach the testis. At the posterior border of testis, it is divided into a number of small branches and two large (medial and lateral) branches. The medial and lateral branches pierce the tunica albuginea, and ramify on the surface of lobules of the testis to form the tunica vasculosa.

VENOUS DRAINAGE (Fig. 5.17)

The *pampiniform plexus of veins* (the veins emerging from the testis form a plexus of veins called pampiniform plexus) drains the venous blood from the testis. This plexus ascends up and at the superficial inguinal ring condenses to form four veins, which pass through the inguinal canal within the spermatic cord. At the level of deep inguinal ring, they join to form a two testicular veins which accompany the testicular

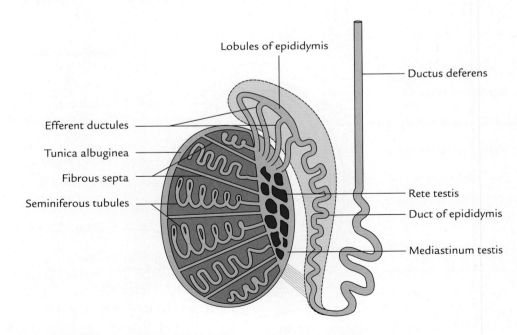

Fig. 5.15 Longitudinal section of the testis and epididymis showing their structures.

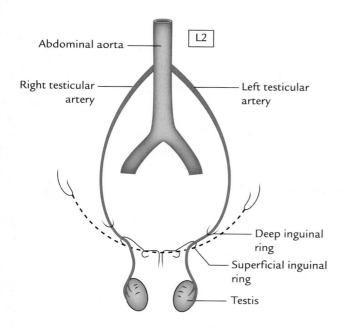

Fig. 5.16 Arterial supply of the testis.

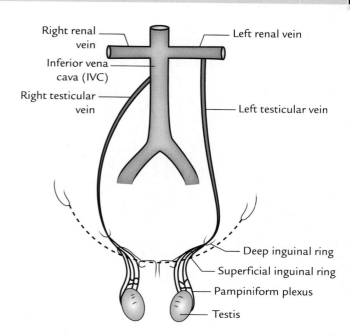

Fig. 5.17 Venous drainage of the testis.

artery. On the right side, the testicular vein drains into the inferior vena cava at an oblique angle while on the left side it drains into the left renal vein at a right angle.

Varicocele: It is a clinical condition in which veins of the pampiniform plexus become dilated, tortuous, and elongated. It commonly affects the adolescents and young adults. It mostly occurs on the left side due to the following reasons: (a) left testicular vein drains at a right angle in the left renal vein hence venous pressure is high in the left testicular vein, (b) compression of the left testicular vein by loaded constipated sigmoid colon, and (c) blockage of entry of the left testicular vein in the left renal vein sometimes may occur by growing malignant tumor of the left kidney.

Clinically varicocele presents as:
(a) Vague, dragging sensations and aching pain in the scrotum.
(b) On palpation, the veins of pampiniform plexus feel like **'bag of worms'.**

N.B. It is must for clinicians to investigate the left kidney in rapidly developing left-sided **varicocele**.

LYMPHATIC DRAINAGE (Fig. 5.18)

The lymph vessels from the testis ascend along the testicular vessels in the spermatic cord and drain into pre-aortic and para-aortic group of lymph nodes at the level of the second lumbar vertebra.

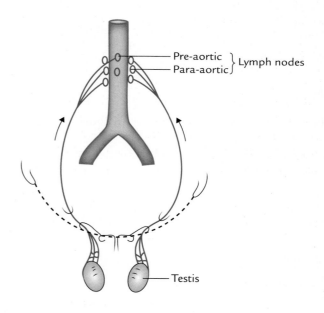

Fig. 5.18 Lymphatic drainage of the testis.

N.B.
• The testicular arteries arise in the abdomen, the testicular veins drain in the abdomen, and testicular lymph vessels drain in the abdominal lymph nodes. This is because during development the testis has migrated from high up on the posterior abdominal wall, down through the inguinal canal into the scrotum, dragging its blood supply and lymph vessels along it.
• The blood vessels and lymph vessels of the testis are shown in Figure 5.19.

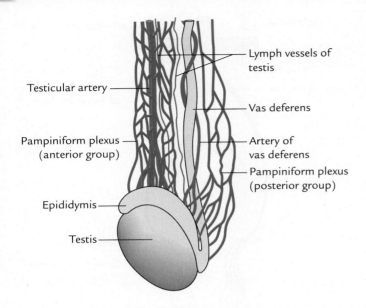

Fig. 5.19 Blood vessels and lymph vessels of the testis.

EPIDIDYMIS

The epididymis is a comma-shaped structure, which lies on to the superior and posterolateral surface of the testis. It is made up of highly coiled tubes.

PARTS

The epididymis from above downward is divided into three parts: *head*, *body*, and *tail*.

The head (the upper expanded part) is connected to the upper pole of testis by *efferent ductules* and consists of highly coiled efferent ductules. The body (middle part) and tail (lower period part) are made up of a single highly coiled duct of epididymis, which emerges from the tail as the vas deferens.

FUNCTIONS

The functions of epididymis are:

1. Storage and maturation of spermatozoa.
2. Absorption of the fluid.
3. Addition of substances to the seminal fluid to nourish the maturating spermatozoa.

N.B. Laterally, a distinct groove exists between the testis and the epididymis. A fold of visceral layer of tunica vaginalis invaginates it to form the *sinus of epididymis*.

Clinical correlation

- **Tumors of the testis:** The two main varieties of testicular tumors are seminoma (carcinoma of the seminiferous tubules) and teratoma (malignant change in the totipotent cells). The cancer cells from testis spread upward via the lymph vessels to the lumbar (pre- and para-aortic) lymph nodes at the level of L1/L2 vertebra and produce secondary tumor in the abdomen.
- **Torsion of the testis:** It is a clinical condition in which rotation of the scrotum occurs around the spermatic cord within the scrotum. It commonly affects the active young people and children, and is accompanied by severe pain.

DEVELOPMENT OF TESTIS AND EPIDIDYMIS

The testis develops in the abdominal cavity on its posterior wall from the genital ridge on the medial side of the developing mesonephros at the level of T10 segment. All the components of the testis (tunica albuginea, fibrous septa, seminiferous tubules, straight tubules, rete testis, and Sertoli cells) develop from the genital ridge except primordial germ cells (spermatogonia), which develop from the wall of yolk sac and migrate secondarily into the genital ridge.

Most of the mesonephric tubules atrophy, but about 10–15 tubules persist and form the efferent ductules of the testis.

The mesonephric duct forms the duct of epididymis, vas deferens, seminal vesicles, and ejaculatory duct.

EMBRYOLOGICAL REMNANTS IN RELATION TO TESTIS AND EPIDIDYMIS (Fig. 5.20)

These are as follows:

1. *Appendix of testis:* It is a oval body attached to the upper pole of testis (for details see page 67).

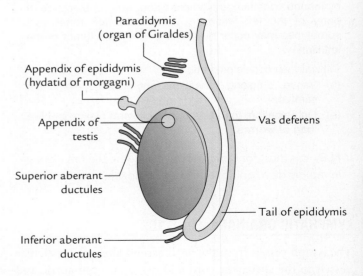

Fig. 5.20 Embryological remnants in relation to testis and epididymis.

2. *Appendix of epididymis (hydatid of Morgagni):* It is a small pedunculated rounded body attached to the head of epididymis. It is remnant of cranial end of mesonephric (Wolffian) duct.
3. *Paradidymis (organ of Giraldes):* It consists of 3 or 4 small free tubules which are found in the spermatic cord, just above the head of epididymis. They are remnants of caudal mesonephric tubules.
4. *Superior aberrant ductules:* They are 2 or 3 in number and attached to the upper end of testis above the afferent ductules of testis. They are remnants of the upper mesonephric tubules.
5. *Inferior aberrant ductules:* They are 1 or 2 in number and attached to the tail of epididymis. They are remnants of the intermediate mesonephric tubules.

N.B. The embryological remnants (vide supra) may sometime form cysts in relation to the testis and epididymis.

DESCENT OF THE TESTIS (Fig. 5.21)

The testis develops in the abdominal cavity where the temperature is high and not suitable for proper spermatogenesis. Hence, it migrates out of the abdominal cavity into the scrotum.

At an early stage of intrauterine life, the developing testis lies in the upper abdomen on the medial side of the mesonephros. A fold of the peritoneum called *processus vaginalis* extends in front of the testis and reaches the scrotum. Just after the formation of processus vaginalis, a cord-like fibromuscular band, the *gubernaculum testis*, develops and connects the mesonephric duct, and the lower pole of the testis to the base of the scrotum. Differential body growth in the embryo and fetus results in the descent of the testis from the abdominal cavity to the scrotum.

Each testis begins to descend during the 2nd month of the intrauterine life (IUL).

- It reaches the iliac fossa by the 3rd month of IUL.
- It rests at the deep inguinal ring from 4th to 6th month of IUL.
- It traverses the inguinal canal during the 7th month and reaches the superficial inguinal ring by the 8th month of IUL.
- It enters the scrotum at the 9th month of IUL.
- It reaches the base of the scrotum at or just after birth.

Factors Responsible for Descent of the Testis

These factors are as follows:

1. Differential growth of the body wall.
2. Increased intra-abdominal pressure and temperature.
3. Hormones (male sex hormones produced by the testis, and maternal gonadotrophins).

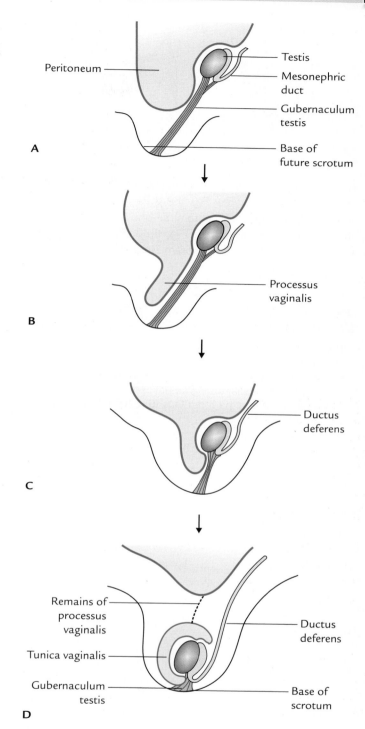

Fig. 5.21 Descent of the testis (stages **A**, **B**, **C**, and **D** in sequence) note the fate of processus vaginalis.

4. Contraction of the gubernaculum (a band of loose fibromuscular tissue extending from the lower pole of the testis to the base of the scrotum).
5. Calcitonin gene-related peptide (CGRP), a neurotransmitter secreted by the genitofemoral nerve.

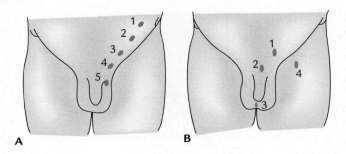

A   B

Fig. 5.22 A, Five sites of incomplete descent; **B,** four sites of ectopic testis. (*Source:* Fig. 4.8A, Page 152, *Clinical and Surgical Anatomy*, 2e, Vishram Singh. Copyright Elsevier 2007, All rights reserved. B. Fig. 4.8B, Page 152, *Clinical and Surgical Anatomy*, 2e, Vishram Singh. Copyright Elsevier 2007, All rights reserved.)

Clinical correlation

The testis may be subject to the following congenital anomalies:

- **Cryptorchidism (incomplete descent of testis):** In this condition, the testis, during its descent, although it travels through its normal path but fails to reach the base of the scrotum. Thus, it may be found (a) within the abdomen, (b) at the deep inguinal ring, (c) within the inguinal canal, (d) at the superficial inguinal ring, or (e) high up in the scrotum (Fig. 5.22A).

  The **complications of cryptorchidism** are:
  - It may fail to produce spermatozoa.
  - It is prone to undergo malignant change.
- **Ectopic testis (maldescent of the testis):** In this condition, the testis travels down along an abnormal path, and therefore fails to reach the scrotum. Thus, it may be found (a) in the superficial fascia of the lower part of the anterior abdominal wall, (b) in front of the pubis, (c) in the perineum, or (d) in the thigh (Fig. 5.22B).

  In the past the ectopic testis was attributed to the gonad following a subsidiary tail of gubernaculum. But now it is felt that it occurs because processus vaginalis reaches an abnormal site and testis follows it.

N.B. It is necessary for the testis to be in the scrotum for proper spermatogenesis. Therefore, it is necessary that the undescended testis is brought down in the scrotum (by a surgical procedure) before puberty.

An ectopic testis usually develops normally, but it is susceptible to trauma. Therefore, it should also be placed in the scrotum by a surgical procedure.

Golden Facts to Remember

- Most important difference between penis and clitoris | Penis is traversed by the urethra whereas clitoris is not
- Lymph node involved in the cancer (carcinoma) of penis | Lymph node of Cloquet (deep inguinal lymph node present in the femoral canal)
- Carcinoma penis is the most common in those races | That do not practice ritual circumcision
- Common sites of carcinoma penis | Neck (coronary sinus) and frenulum
- Phimosis | Narrowing of the distal end of the prepuce (foreskin)
- Paraphimosis | Tight prepuce which gets stuck to glans penis at erection
- Commonest cause of scrotal swelling | Hydrocele
- Lymph nodes involved in cancer testis | Pre-aortic and para-aortic lymph nodes
- Nervi erigentes | Pelvic splanchnic nerves carrying parasympathetic fibres from S2, S3, and S4 spinal segments
- Varicocele mostly occurs on | Left side

Clinical Case Study

An educated mother brought her 6-month-old son to the hospital and complained that the right scrotum of her son was empty. On physical examination, the doctors found the presence of the testis only in the left half of the scrotum and a small swelling about 1.5 cm in diameter in the inguinal region on the right side. A clinical diagnosis of "**cryptorchidism**" was made.

Questions

1. What is cryptorchidism?
2. What are the disadvantages of cryptorchidism?
3. Enumerate the factors responsible for descent of testis.
4. What is ectopic testis?

Answers

1. It is a condition in which the descent of the testis is arrested in its course and fails to reach the scrotum.
2. (a) It fails to develop properly and produce spermatozoa that may cause infertility.
   (b) It is more prone to malignancy.
3. See page 71.
4. It is a condition in which the testis descends along an abnormal path and hence fails to reach the scrotum. Also, see clinical correlation on page 72.

Abdominal Cavity and Peritoneum

ABDOMINAL CAVITY

BOUNDARIES

The abdomen is defined as a part of trunk that lies between the diaphragm above and the pelvic inlet below.

The boundaries of the abdominal cavity are as follows:

Roof: It is formed by the *diaphragm*, which also forms the upper parts of the lateral and posterior walls.

- **Anterior wall:** It is formed by three pairs of flat muscles (external oblique, internal oblique, and transversus abdominis) and their aponeuroses, and a pair of vertical muscles (rectus abdominis). The vertical muscles lie in the anterior median region, one on each side of the anterior midline, and are enclosed in the aponeuroses of the flat muscles.

- **Lateral wall:** The upper part of each lateral wall between the ribs and the iliac crest (also called *flank*) is formed by three flat muscles. The lower part of each lateral wall is formed by the ilium of hip bone covered internally by the iliacus muscle.

- **Posterior wall:** It is formed by the vertebral column, muscles attached to it (diaphragm, psoas major, and quadratus lumborum), and thoraco-lumbar fascia. Below this, it is formed by the posterior part of ilium and iliacus muscle covering it.

Floor: It is absent inferiorly as the abdominal cavity communicates with the pelvic cavity at the pelvic brim.

N.B. The abdomen and pelvic cavities are lined by a thin serous membrane called peritoneum.

SHAPE

In transverse section, the abdominal cavity is kidney shaped because the vertebral column protrudes into it posteriorly in the midline. Thus, there is a deep paravertebral gutter on each side of the vertebral column. In median section the abdominal cavity is oblong longitudinally, and its posteroinferior part is continuous with the pelvic cavity.

CONTENTS

There are three distinct layers of structures posterior to the peritoneal cavity. From behind forward these are:

1. **Kidneys, ureters,** and **suprarenal glands:** They lie on each side of vertebral column in the paravertebral gutter, enclosed in the fascial lining of the abdominal cavity.
2. **Abdominal aorta** and **inferior vena cava:** They lie on the anterior surface of the vertebral column and are enclosed in the endoabdominal fascia.
3. **Stomach, intestines, their associated glands (liver, pancreas with their ducts), and spleen:** They lie anteriorly and are surrounded to a greater or lesser extent by the peritoneal cavity.

NINE REGIONS OF THE ABDOMINAL CAVITY

The clinicians divide the abdominal cavity into nine regions to describe the location of abdominal organs and the pain associated with them during physical examination.

The abdominal cavity is divided into nine regions (Fig. 6.1) by four imaginary planes (two vertical and two horizontal) on the anterior abdominal wall.

1. **Superior horizontal plane:** It corresponds to the transpyloric plane of Addison. It is placed midway between the suprasternal notch and the pubic symphysis. This however is an awkward estimation during physical examination for a clinician, and a simpler and practical method is to locate a point midway between the umbilicus and the lower end of the body of sternum. The xiphoid process should not be used because its size is variable. The transpyloric plane lies at the level of lower border of L1 vertebra and cuts the costal margin at the 9th costal cartilages.

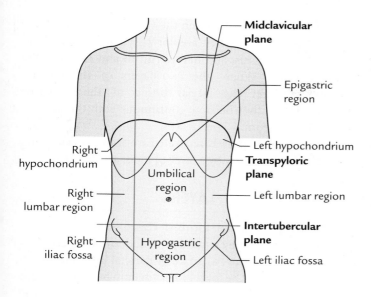

Fig. 6.1 Nine regions of the abdomen.

N.B. Occasionally the **subcostal plane** is used in preference to the transpyloric plane. This is drawn through the lowest parts of the costal margins at the 10th costal cartilages and lies at the level of the body of L3 vertebra.

2. **Inferior horizontal plane (intertubercular plane):** It is drawn at the level of tubercles of the iliac crests, which are palpable 5 cm posterior to the anterior superior iliac spine. The intertubercular plane lies at the level of upper border of L5 vertebra.

3. **Right and left vertical planes (midclavicular planes):** Each vertical plane passes vertically downward from the midpoint of the clavicle to the midinguinal point (a point midway between the anterior superior iliac spine and the pubic symphysis).

Nine regions thus marked out are arranged into three horizontal zones of abdomen: upper, middle, and lower. From right to left, in the upper abdomen they are designated as right hypochondrium, epigastric region, and left hypochondrium. In the middle abdomen they are designated as right lumbar region, umbilical region, and left lumbar region. In the lower abdomen they are designated as right iliac fossa, hypogastric (pubic) region, and left iliac fossa (Table 6.1).

Table 6.1 Regions of the abdomen

Zone	Regions (right to left)
Upper abdomen	Right hypochondrium, epigastric region, left hypochondrium
Middle abdomen	Right lumbar region, umbilical region, left lumbar region
Lower abdomen	Right iliac fossa, hypogastric region (pubic), left iliac fossa

Table 6.2 Abdominal regions and their main contents*

Region	Contents
Right hypochondrium	• Liver • Gallbladder
Epigastric region	• Stomach • Pancreas • Duodenum
Left hypochondrium	• Spleen • Left colic flexure
Right lumbar region	• Right kidney • Right ureter • Ascending colon
Umbilical region	• Loops of small intestine • Aorta • Inferior vena cava
Left lumbar region	• Left kidney • Left ureter • Descending colon
Right iliac fossa	• Caecum • Appendix
Hypogastric region	• Coils of small intestine • Urinary bladder (if distended) • Uterus (if enlarged)
Left iliac fossa	• Sigmoid colon

*This information is based on the clinical data.

The abdominal viscera/structures located in the nine regions of the abdomen are given in Table 6.2.

Clinical correlation

Clinical significance of nine regions of the abdomen: The knowledge of structures present in the nine regions helps the clinician to know the source of pain. The general guidelines are as follows:

• **Pain in the right hypochondrium** comes from the gallbladder and biliary ducts.
• **Pain in the epigastric region** comes from the stomach and duodenum.
• **Pain in the left hypochondrium** comes from the pancreas.
• **Pain in the right lumbar region** comes from the right kidney.
• **Pain in the umbilical region** comes from the small intestine.
• **Pain in the left lumbar region** comes from the left kidney.
• **Pain in the right iliac fossa** comes from the vermiform appendix.
• **Pain in the hypogastrium** comes from the urinary bladder and uterus.
• **Pain in the left iliac fossa** comes from the sigmoid colon.

It is important to note that pain in the abdomen usually occurs due to two reasons: (a) inflammation, and (b) obstruction of conducting muscular tubes such as the bowel or the ureter.

FOUR QUADRANTS OF THE ABDOMINAL CAVITY

For more general clinical descriptions, the abdominal cavity is divided into four quadrants by a horizontal **transumbilical plane** passing through the umbilicus and a vertical median plane intersecting the horizontal plane at the umbilicus (Fig. 6.2). The four quadrants thus formed are:

1. Right upper quadrant.
2. Left upper quadrant.
3. Right lower quadrant.
4. Left lower quadrant.

PERITONEUM

The **peritoneum** is a large thin serous membrane, which lines the interior of the abdominopelvic cavity. It is made up of a tough layer of elastic tissue lined with the simple squamous epithelium and forms the largest serous sac of the body. It is similar to the pleura and serous pericardium in consisting of parietal and visceral layers. These layers are separated from each other by a potential space called peritoneal cavity, which is filled with a thin capillary film of fluid. This fluid lubricates the two layers of the peritoneal cavity and facilitates the movement of those parts of the abdominal viscera, which are ensheathed by the visceral layer. The mobile parts of intra-abdominal digestive tube are completely surrounded by the visceral layer of peritoneum except for a small area where it passes from the tube to the posterior abdominal wall as a double-layered fold called **mesentery**. Between the two layers of mesentery is an extraperitoneal fatty areolar tissue in which blood vessels, lymph vessels, and nerves run to and fro from the digestive tubes. Where the two layers of the visceral peritoneum meet the fascial lining of the posterior abdominal wall, they become continuous with the parietal layer of peritoneum.

The peritoneal lining is separated from the fascial lining of the abdominal cavity by a layer of loose areolar tissue.

LAYERS

Initially the peritoneum forms a closed sac, but when it becomes invaginated by a number of abdominal viscera it is divided into two layers: (a) an outer parietal layer and (b) an inner visceral layer. The folds of peritoneum by which viscera are suspended are called **mesentery** (Fig. 6.3). Thus, the peritoneum presents two layers: parietal layer called **parietal peritoneum** and visceral layer called **visceral peritoneum**. The parietal peritoneum is a simple layer lining the internal surface of the abdominopelvic walls. The arrangement of the visceral layer is complex. It forms folds, which surround the intricately folded and tightly packed gut tube. The differences between the parietal and visceral peritoneum are given in Table 6.3.

DIFFERENCES BETWEEN MALE AND FEMALE PERITONEUM (Fig. 6.4)

- In the male, the peritoneum is a closed serous sac lined with mesothelium (squamous epithelium; Fig. 6.4A).
- In the female, the peritoneum is not a closed sac because it communicates with the exterior through uterine tubes, uterus, and vagina (Fig. 6.4B). It is also lined by mesothelium as in male.

N.B. The peritoneum covering the ovaries is lined by cuboidal epithelium.

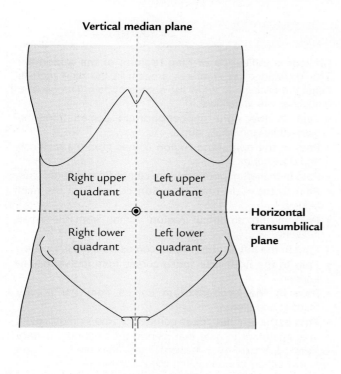

Fig. 6.2 Four quadrants of the abdomen.

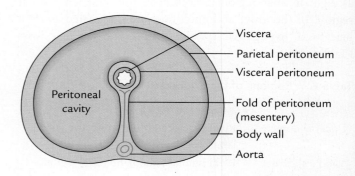

Fig. 6.3 Schematic transverse section of the abdomen showing arrangement of the peritoneum.

Table 6.3 Differences between parietal and visceral peritoneum

Parietal peritoneum	Visceral peritoneum
Arrangement of the parietal layer of the peritoneum is simple	Arrangement of the visceral layer of peritoneum is complex
It lines the inner surface of the abdominopelvic walls (parietes) from which it is separated by extraperitoneal connective tissue and therefore can be easily stripped off	It forms mesenteries, which surround the intricately folded and tightly packed gut tube, liver, and spleen. It is firmly adherent to the outer surface of the viscera and cannot be stripped off, in fact it forms part and parcel of the viscera
Embryologically it is derived from the somatopleuric layer of the lateral plate mesoderm	Embryologically it is derived from the splanchnopleuric layer of the lateral plate mesoderm
It is innervated by somatic nerves and therefore is sensitive to pain due to prick and cut	It is innervated by the autonomic nerves and therefore is insensitive to pain due to prick and cut

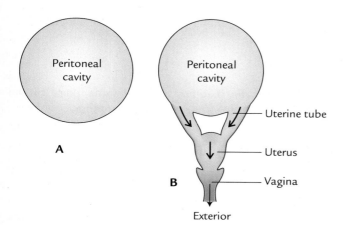

Fig. 6.4 Peritoneal cavity: **A**, in the male; **B**, in the female.

Table 6.4 Retroperitoneal organs

Classification	Organs
Primarily retroperitoneal	• Kidneys • Suprarenal glands • Ureters
Secondarily retroperitoneal (mesentery lost during development by zygosis)	• Pancreas (except tail) • Duodenum (except initial 2 cm) • Ascending colon • Descending colon • Caecum • Rectum (upper two-third)

FOLDS

These are formed by the visceral layer of the peritoneum.

1. Many organs within the abdomen are suspended by the peritoneal folds. These organs are mobile within the abdominal cavity. The degree and direction of their mobility depend on the size and direction of the folds.

   Apart from allowing mobility to organs, the peritoneal folds also provide pathways for passage to nerves, vessels, and lymphatics.
2. The organs that lie outside the peritoneal cavity (**retroperitoneal organs**) are fixed and immobile.
3. Some organs are initially suspended by the peritoneal folds, i.e., they possess mesenteries but later on lose their mesenteries by a process called **zygosis** and become retroperitoneal.

   The retroperitoneal organs are given in Table 6.4.

N.B. The **zygosis** is a process of absorption of the mesentery. One layer of the mesentery fuses with the parietal peritoneum and then fused portions of visceral and

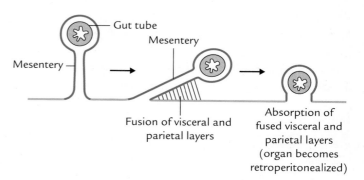

Fig. 6.5 Process of zygosis.

parietal peritoneum are absorbed and organ become retroperitonealized (Fig. 6.5).

Functions

The **functions of peritoneal folds** are as follows:

1. To provide mobility to the viscera.
2. To provide passage to vessels and nerves.

CLASSIFICATION OF THE PERITONEAL FOLDS

The peritoneal folds are classified into three types: mesentery/mesocolon, omenta, and ligaments.

1. **Mesentery/mesocolon:** The fold suspending the small intestine is called mesentery and the fold suspending the colon is called mesocolon.
2. **Omenta (singular omentum):** These are the peritoneal folds that connect the stomach with other viscera. The examples are:
   (a) *Greater omentum*, a fold connecting the stomach with the transverse colon.
   (b) *Lesser omentum*, a fold connecting the stomach with the liver.
   (c) *Gastrosplenic omentum*, a fold connecting the stomach with the spleen (in general usage it is termed gastrosplenic ligament).
3. **Ligaments:** They are the folds that connect organs to the abdominal wall or to each other. The examples are *gastrosplenic ligament* (between stomach and spleen), *lienorenal ligamentum* (between kidney and spleen), and *coronary ligaments* (between liver and diaphragm).

EMBRYOLOGICAL BASIS OF UNDERSTANDING THE PERITONEAL FOLDS

A little description of the *development* of gut makes it easier to understand the various peritoneal folds. The developing gut is divided from above downward into three parts: foregut, midgut, and hindgut. Each part has its own artery—a ventral branch of the abdominal aorta. The *coeliac artery* is the artery of foregut, *superior mesenteric artery* is the artery of midgut, and *inferior mesenteric artery* is the artery of hindgut (Fig. 6.6). The derivatives of the foregut, midgut, and hindgut are given in Table 6.5.

The abdominal part of foregut possesses both ventral and dorsal mesenteries, which are termed **ventral mesogastrium**

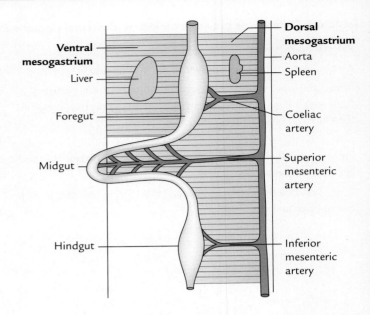

Fig. 6.6 Schematic diagram showing three parts of the primitive gut with their arteries and mesenteries.

and **dorsal mesogastrium**, respectively (Fig. 6.6). The developing liver divides the ventral mesogastrium into two parts: ventral and dorsal.

The fate of ventral mesogastrium is as under (Fig. 6.7). The ventral part forms the **falciform** and **coronary ligaments** between the body wall and the liver; and dorsal part forms the **lesser omentum** between the liver and the curvature of the stomach.

The fate of dorsal mesogastrium is as under:

1. The larger caudal part becomes greatly elongated to form the **greater omentum.** The smaller cranial part becomes divided into dorsal and ventral parts by the development of spleen within it. The ventral part forms the **gastrosplenic ligament** whereas the dorsal part forms the **lienorenal** and **gastrophrenic ligaments.**
2. The cross-sectional views of ventral and dorsal mesogastria of the foregut and their derivatives are shown in Figure 6.8.

The midgut and hindgut possess only the dorsal mesentery. The fate of dorsal mesentery is as follows (Fig. 6.9):

1. It forms the **mesentery of jejunum and ileum.**
2. It forms the mesentery of appendix—**mesoappendix.**
3. It forms the mesentery of transverse colon—**transverse mesocolon.**
4. It forms the mesentery of sigmoid colon—**sigmoid mesocolon.**

N.B. The mesenteries of the duodenum, ascending colon, descending colon, and rectum are lost by zygosis as a result they become retroperitonealized.

Table 6.5 Derivatives of the developing gut in the abdomen

Part	Derivatives
Foregut	• Esophagus • Stomach • Upper half of the duodenum (up to the opening of common bile duct)
Midgut	• Lower half of the duodenum (distal to the opening of common bile duct) • Jejunum • Ileum • Appendix • Caecum • Ascending colon • Right two-third of the transverse colon
Hindgut	• Left one-third of the transverse colon • Descending colon • Sigmoid colon • Rectum • Upper part of the anal canal

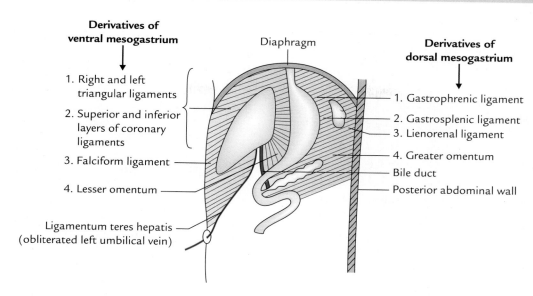

Fig. 6.7 Derivatives of ventral and dorsal mesogastria.

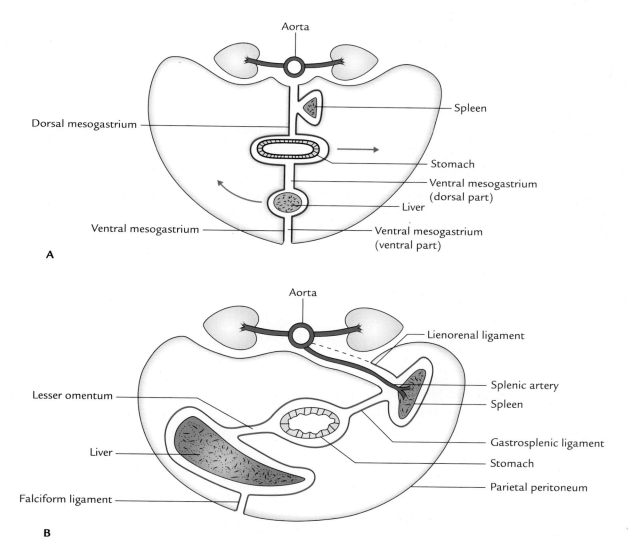

Fig. 6.8 Transverse sections of developing foregut showing ventral and dorsal mesogastria and their derivatives: A, early stage; B, later stage.

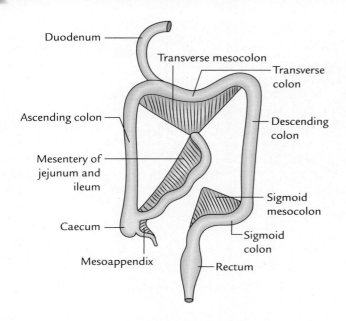

Fig. 6.9 Fate of dorsal mesentery of midgut and hindgut.

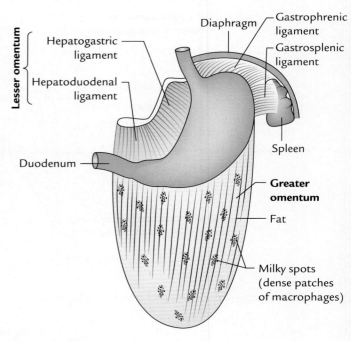

Fig. 6.10 Greater omentum.

Some of the peritoneal folds are discussed in detail in the following text.

Greater Omentum (L. Omentum = Apron)

The greater omentum is a large thick fold of peritoneum, which hangs from the greater curvature of stomach and the adjacent part of the duodenum like an apron and covers the loops of intestine to a variable extent (Fig. 6.10).

The greater omentum is made up of four layers of peritoneum, which are fused together to form a thin fenestrated membrane containing variable amount of fat.

Attachments

The anterior two layers descend from the greater curvature of the stomach (where they are continuous with the peritoneum covering the anterior and posterior surfaces of the stomach) to a variable extent and then folds on itself to form the posterior two layers. The mode of folding is such that the first layer becomes the fourth layer and the second layer becomes the third layer. The posterior two layers ascend up to the transverse mesocolon where the fourth layer loosely blends with the peritoneum on the anterior surfaces of the

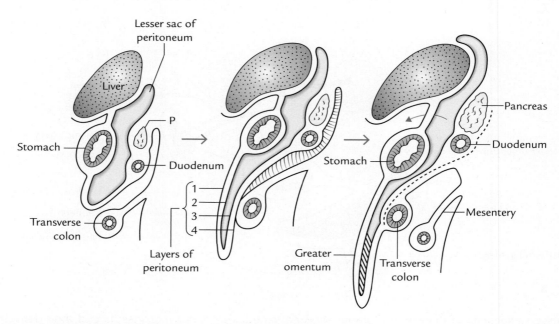

Fig. 6.11 Stages of development of greater omentum (P = pancreas).

transverse colon and transverse mesocolon above it. The part of lesser sac between the second and third layers gets obliterated except for about 1 inch (2.5 cm) below the greater curvature of the stomach (Fig. 6.11).

Contents

1. *Adipose tissue (fat)* of variable amount depending upon the nutritional status of an individual.
2. *Aggregation of macrophages,* which form dense patches called **milky spots.**
3. *Right and left gastroepiploic vessels* run between the anterior and posterior layers of the greater omentum close to the greater curvature of the stomach.

Functions

The functions of greater omentum are as follows:

1. *It is a storehouse of adipose tissue (fat).*
2. *It protects the peritoneal cavity* from infection due to the presence of a large number of macrophages.
3. *It limits the spread of infection.* The greater omentum moves to the site of infection and seals it off from the surrounding areas. It also moves to the site of perforation of gut to plug the gap to prevent the leakage of contents of gut in the peritoneal cavity. For this reason greater omentum is often termed the "**policeman of abdomen.**"
4. It is sometimes used as grafting material by the surgeons.
5. It protects the abdominal viscera from blow on the anterior abdominal wall.
6. It forms a partition between the supracolic and the infracolic compartments of the greater sac.

Lesser Omentum (Figs 6.10 and 6.12)

The lesser omentum is a double-layered fold of peritoneum between the lesser curvature of stomach and the inferior surface of the liver.

Attachments

1. **Inferiorly** it is attached to the right side of the *abdominal esophagus, lesser curvature of the stomach,* and first 2 cm of the duodenum.
2. **Superiorly** it is attached in the inverted 'L'-shaped manner to the margins of *fissure for ligamentum venosum* and *porta hepatis.*

Parts

The part of lesser omentum between stomach and liver is called *hepatogastric ligament,* and the part between duodenum and liver is called *hepatoduodenal ligament.*

N.B. The *right free margin of lesser omentum* where the anterior and posterior layers of peritoneum become continuous forms the anterior boundary of the *foramen epiploicum.*

Contents

1. *Along the lesser curvature of the stomach* the lesser omentum contains:
   (a) Right and left gastric vessels and associated gastric lymph nodes.
   (b) Branches of the left gastric nerve.
2. The *right free* margin of the lesser omentum contains:
   (a) Portal vein.

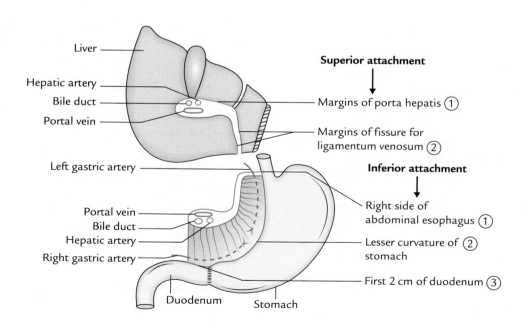

Fig. 6.12 Attachments and contents of the lesser omentum.

(b) Hepatic artery and bile duct anterior to the portal vein, with duct to the right of the artery.

(c) Autonomic nerves.

(d) Lymphatic and lymph nodes.

Mesentery (Mesentery of Small Intestine)

It is a broad fan-shaped fold of the peritoneum, which suspends the coils of the small intestine (jejunum and ileum) from the posterior abdominal wall.

The width of mesentery on an average is about 6 inches (15 cm). The maximum width is 8 inches (20 cm) in the central part and gradually diminishes toward the proximal and distal ends.

General Features

The mesentery presents two borders:

1. Attached border (or root).
2. Free border (or intestinal border).

Root of mesentery (attached border): It is attached to an oblique line across the posterior abdominal wall, extending from the duodenojejunal flexure to the ileocecal junction. The duodenojejunal flexure lies to the left side of L2 vertebra, whereas the ileocaecal junction lies at the upper part of the right sacroiliac joint.

(a) The root of mesentery from above downward crosses in front of (Fig. 6.13):

(i) Horizontal (third) part of duodenum.

(ii) Abdominal aorta.

(iii) Inferior vena cava.

(iv) Right gonadal vessels.

(v) Right ureter.

(vi) Right psoas major muscle.

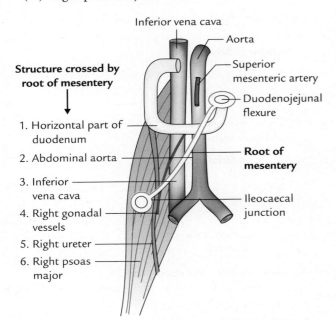

Fig. 6.13 Structures crossed by the root of the mesentery.

(b) The root of mesentery divides the infracolic compartment into two parts: right and left.

*   The right one is small and terminates in the right iliac fossa.
*   The left one is larger and passes without interruption into true pelvis.

Free border (intestinal border): It is about 6 m (20 feet) long and encloses the jejunum and ileum.

The root of mesentery is 6 inches (15 cm) long whereas its periphery (free border) is 6 m long. This accounts for the formation of folds (pleats) in it (a frill-like arrangement).

*   Its length permits the free mobility of the loops of jejunum and ileum in the abdominal cavity.
*   It has fat deposition along its root, which diminishes toward the intestinal border. Near the intestinal border it presents fat-free oval/circular windows (translucent area) of peritoneum. The amount of fat is greater in the distal part of the mesentery.

Contents

The contents of the mesentery are:

1. Superior mesenteric artery and vein (in the root)—with vein being to the right of the artery.
2. Jejunal and ileal branches of superior mesenteric artery and accompanying veins.
3. Lymphatics (lacteals).
4. Lymph nodes (100–200 in number).
5. Autonomic nerve plexuses.
6. Fat and connective tissues.
7. Jejunum and ileum (enclosed in the free border).

Clinical correlation

*   The great length of the mesentery permits the descent and protrusion of the loops of the small intestine into the hernial sacs of inguinal and femoral hernias.
*   A group of lymph nodes when infected may become adherent to an adjoining loop of the small intestine and may result in the mechanical *intestinal obstruction*.
*   An acute terminal *mesenteric lymphadenitis* is often indistinguishable from *acute appendicitis*.
*   The failure of the root of mesentery to fuse over its entire length with the posterior abdominal wall allows a peritoneal pocket to be formed which may form a sac of an intraperitoneal hernia called *mesenteric parietal hernia of Waldeyer*.

Transverse Mesocolon

The transverse mesocolon is a broad horizontal fold of peritoneum, which suspends the transverse colon from the posterior abdominal wall.

The line of attachment of the root of transverse mesocolon on the posterior abdominal wall (or rather to the organs that lie on the posterior abdominal wall at that level) is horizontal with an upward inclination toward the left. From right to left, it is attached to the anterior aspect of the head and anterior border of the body of pancreas (Fig. 6.14).

Sigmoid Mesocolon

The sigmoid mesocolon is a triangular fold of peritoneum, which suspends the sigmoid colon from the pelvic wall. The attachment of the root of sigmoid mesocolon on to the pelvic wall takes the form of an inverted 'V', the apex of which lies at the division of the left common iliac artery. The intersigmoid recess of peritoneum is found at the apex of the V-shaped attachment and the left ureter lies behind the peritoneum of this recess.

The left limb of V is attached along the upper half of the left external iliac artery and the right limb to the posterior pelvic wall extending downward and medially from the apex to the median plane of sacrum up to the level of S3 vertebra (Fig. 6.15).

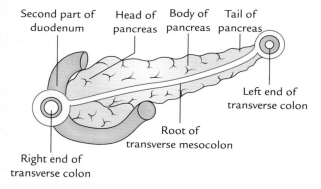

Fig. 6.14 Attachments of the root of transverse mesocolon.

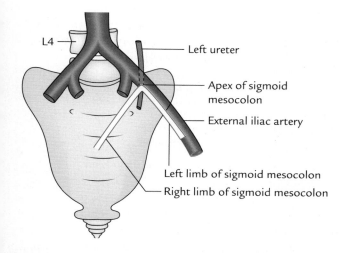

Fig. 6.15 Attachments of the root of sigmoid mesocolon.

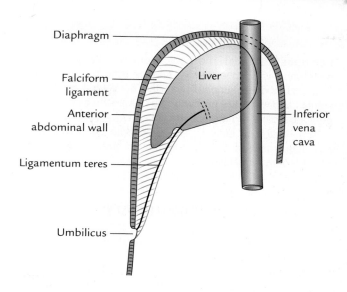

Fig. 6.16 Attachments of the falciform ligament.

Falciform Ligament

The falciform ligament is a sickle-shaped fold of peritoneum, which connects the anterosuperior surface of the liver to the supraumbilical part of the anterior abdominal wall and the inferior surface of the diaphragm.

Its concave inferior margin contains the ligamentum teres (the obliterated left umbilical vein). The ligamentum teres extends from the umbilicus to the notch for this ligament on the inferior border of the liver and joins the left branch of the portal vein at the left end of the porta hepatis (Fig. 6.16).

The contents of falciform ligament contain the following structures:

1. Ligamentum teres.
2. Paraumbilical veins, tributaries of portal vein.
3. Numerous small veins which connect paraumbilical vein with the diaphragmatic veins.

FUNCTIONS

1. Provides a slippery surface for the free movement of the abdominal viscera.
2. Provides a moist surface to prevent friction between the adjacent viscera.
3. Guards the viscera against infection by phagocytic cells within its mesothelial lining.
4. Prevents the spread of infection by wrapping around the inflamed site and sealing the site of perforation by its fold, e.g., greater omentum.
5. Provides a large surface area for absorption of fluids.
6. Provides healing power for its mesothelial cells, which can transform into fibroblasts.
7. Provides storage of fat in its folds, e.g., greater omentum, particularly in obese persons.

Peritoneal dialysis: The peritoneum is a semipermeable membrane with an extensive surface area much of which overlies blood and lymphatic capillary beds. Hence, diffusible solutes and water are exchanged between the blood and the peritoneal cavity as a result of concentration gradient.

The peritoneal dialysis is a procedure by which waste products such as urea are removed from the blood in patients with renal failure.

PERITONEAL CAVITY

1. The peritoneal cavity is the largest and most complex serous sac in the body.
2. It is a potential space between the parietal and visceral layers of the peritoneum.
3. In the male it is a closed cavity, but in the female it communicates with the exterior through ostia of uterine tubes, uterus, and vagina; therefore, pelvic infections are common in the females.

• Normally, the peritoneal cavity is only a potential space and contains only a thin film of serous fluid, which lubricates the adjacent surfaces of peritoneum so that they can glide over one another but the peritoneal cavity is capable of great distension following the collection of fluid (ascitis), blood (**hemoperitoneum**), and air (**pneumoperitoneum**).

• **Paracentesis abdominis:** It is a procedure by which excessive collection of intraperitoneal fluid is evacuated by canula inserted through the abdominal wall. After emptying the urinary bladder with catheter, the canula is introduced on a trocar either through the anterior midline, where linea alba is relatively bloodless, or through the flank (lateral to McBurney's point, where there is no danger of injuring—*inferior epigastric vessels*). The canula inserted in the flank will pass through the skin, superficial fascia, aponeurosis of external oblique muscle, internal oblique muscle, transversus abdominis muscle, fascia transversalis, extraperitoneal fat, and parietal peritoneum.

SUBDIVISIONS OF THE PERITONEAL CAVITY

The peritoneal cavity may be broadly divided into two parts:

1. Greater sac.
2. Lesser sac (or omental bursa).

The *greater sac* is the larger (main) compartment of the peritoneal cavity and extends across the whole breadth and length of the abdomen.

The *lesser sac* is the smaller compartment of the peritoneal cavity, which lies behind the stomach, liver, and lesser omentum as a diverticulum from the greater sac.

The *two sacs* communicate with each other through the foramen epiploicum (Figs 6.17, 6.18, and 6.19).

N.B. The small pockets of peritoneum (**fossae** and **recesses**) may be separated from the main peritoneal cavity by small

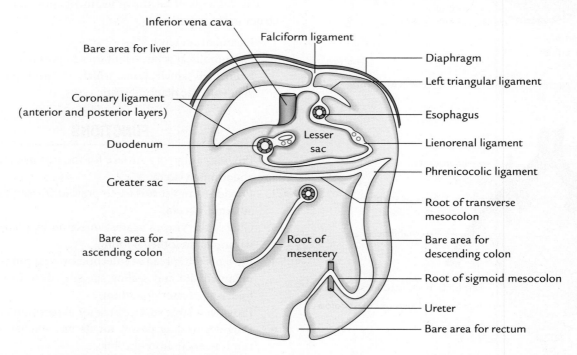

Fig. 6.17 Attachments of the peritoneum on the posterior abdominal wall. Note the division of peritoneal cavity into greater sac (orange colour) and lesser sac (light blue colour).

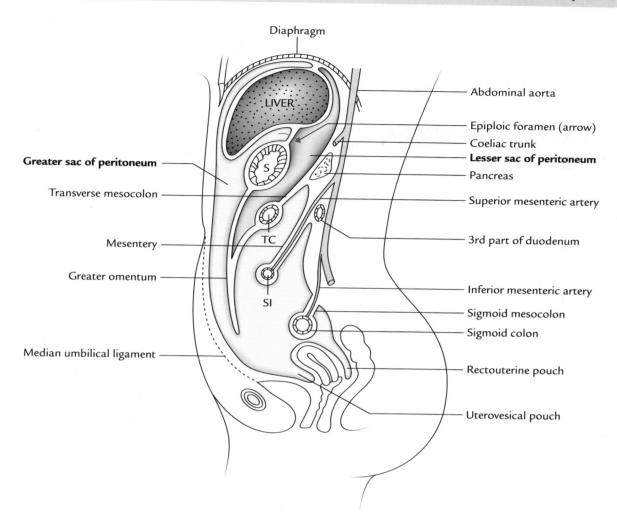

Fig. 6.18 Sagittal section of the abdominopelvic cavity (female) to show the vertical disposition of peritoneum (S = stomach, TC = transverse colon, SI = small intestine).

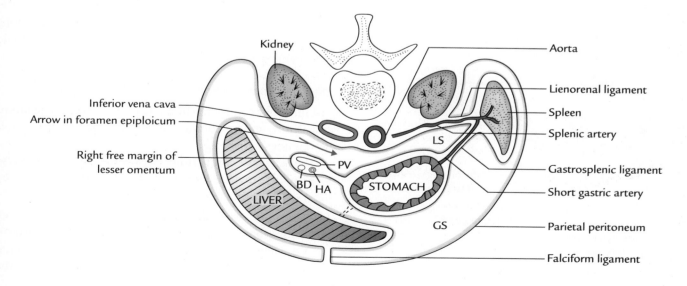

Fig. 6.19 Horizontal section through supracolic compartment of the abdomen showing horizontal disposition of peritoneum (PV = portal vein, BD = bile duct, HA = hepatic artery, LS = lesser sac, GS = greater sac).

inconstant peritoneal folds. They are more frequently found in infants but soon obliterate, but some of them may persist in adult life and then may at times be the site of an internal hernia and strangulation of the extraperitoneal tissue of the abdominal walls.

TRACING OF THE PERITONEUM

The peritoneum is a large serous membrane, which lines the interior of the abdomino-pelvic walls, roof, and floor. It is reflected along certain lines from these parietes to be continuous with a layer of peritoneum over certain viscera. Thus, although the peritoneum is usually divided descriptively into parietal and visceral layers, they are really parts of the same membrane (Fig. 6.17).

The vertical disposition of the peritoneum is shown in Figure 6.18. The horizontal disposition of the peritoneum is shown in Figures 6.19 and 6.20.

GREATER SAC

As discussed earlier, it is the main part of the peritoneal cavity and into this sac protrudes all the peritoneal organs.

SUPRACOLIC AND INFRACOLIC COMPARTMENTS OF THE PERITONEAL CAVITY

The abdominal part of the peritoneal cavity is divided into anterosuperior supracolic and posteroinferior infracolic compartments by transverse colon and its mesentery—the transverse mesocolon (Fig. 6.21).

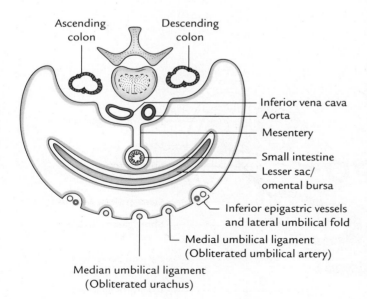

Fig. 6.20 Horizontal section through infracolic compartment of the abdomen showing horizontal disposition of peritoneum.

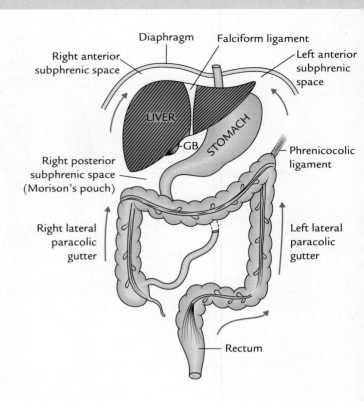

Fig. 6.21 Schematic diagram showing subphrenic spaces and paracolic gutters (GB = gallbladder).

Supracolic Compartment

The supracolic compartment is largely under the cover of costal margin and diaphragm.

The supracolic compartment of peritoneal cavity surrounds the liver, stomach, spleen, and the superior part of the duodenum. It lies anterior to the pancreas, duodenum, kidney, and suprarenal glands. The attachments of the liver to the diaphragm and anterior abdominal wall define the subdivisions of the supracolic compartment. The subdivisions of supracolic compartment are described under the topic subphrenic spaces on p. 87.

Infracolic Compartment

The infracolic compartment is filled with the coils of jejunum and ileum, and surrounded by ascending, transverse, and descending colons.

The infracolic compartment below the level of transverse mesocolon is divided into **right** and **left infracolic** spaces by the root of the mesentery of the small intestine.

1. The **right infracolic space** is triangular with its apex lying below at the ileocaecal junction. It is bounded on the right side by the ascending colon, above by the transverse mesocolon, and on the left side by the mesentery of the small intestine.

2. The **left infracolic space** is larger than the right infracolic space and is quadrangular in shape. It is bounded above by

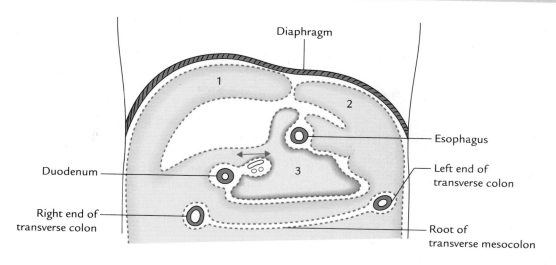

Fig. 6.22 Anatomy of the subphrenic spaces, the viscera having been removed: 1 = right anterior intraperitoneal compartment, 2 = left anterior intraperitoneal compartment, 3 = left posterior intraperitoneal compartment/lesser sac.

the transverse mesocolon, on the right by the root of mesentery, and on the left by the descending colon. Below it is continuous across the pelvic brim into the pelvic cavity.

N.B. *Right and left paracolic gutters*

- Lateral to the ascending colon is the **right paracolic gutter**. It is continuous above with the **hepatorenal pouch** and below with the pelvic cavity. Therefore, it may be infected by downward spread of infection from hepatorenal (Morison's) pouch and lesser sac or by an upward spread of infection from appendix.
- Lateral to the descending colon is the **left paracolic gutter**. It is limited above by the phrenicocolic ligament (a small transverse fold of peritoneum stretching between the left colic flexure and the diaphragm), below it is continuous with the pelvic cavity. Therefore, it may be infected by an upward spread of infection from the pelvis.

INTRAPERITONEAL FOSSAE

The peritoneal cavity presents a number of small pockets/recesses called fossae into which loops of bowel may become caught and get strangulated. The important ones are:

1. **Lesser sac:** A diverticulum of the peritoneal cavity behind the stomach (see page 88).
2. **Paraduodenal fossa:** A peritoneal recess between the duodenojejunal flexure and the inferior mesenteric vein. Its orifice looks to the right.
3. **Retrocaecal fossa:** A recess of the peritoneum behind caecum, in which the appendix frequently lies.

4. **Intersigmoid fossa:** A triangular recess formed by the inverted V-shaped attachment of the sigmoid mesocolon. This recess is open inferomedially.

SUBPHRENIC SPACES

Below the diaphragm, six spaces are defined in relation to the periphery of the liver called subphrenic spaces. These spaces are of great importance to surgeons because pus often collects in these spaces forming subphrenic abscesses. The ligaments of the liver play a major role in delimiting these spaces.

Of these six spaces, three are on the right side and three on the left side. Out of the three spaces on each side, two are intraperitoneal and one is extraperitoneal. They are named as follows (Fig. 6.22):

1. Right posterior intraperitoneal compartment.
2. Right anterior intraperitoneal compartment.
3. Right extraperitoneal compartment.
4. Left posterior intraperitoneal compartment.
5. Left anterior intraperitoneal compartment.
6. Left extraperitoneal compartment.

RIGHT POSTERIOR INTRAPERITONEAL COMPARTMENT (HEPATORENAL POUCH OR MORISON'S POUCH)

It is situated between the posteroinferior surface of the liver and front of the right kidney (Fig. 6.23).

Boundaries

Anterior: Posteroinferior (visceral) surface of the liver.
Posterior: Peritoneum covering the front of the upper pole of the right kidney and the diaphragm.

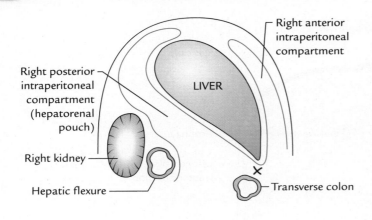

Fig. 6.23 Hepatorenal pouch as seen in the sagittal section.

Above: Posterior (inferior) layer of the coronary ligament.
Below: Transverse colon and mesocolon.

Communications

On the left: It communicates through foramen epiploicum with the lesser sac of peritoneum (omental bursa).

   Along the sharp inferior border of liver: It communicates with the right anterior intraperitoneal compartment.

Clinical correlation

Clinical significance of hepatorenal pouch: In supine position, hepatorenal pouch of Morison is the most dependant part of the peritoneal cavity above the pelvic brim. Hence, fluid from various locations will tend to collect here. It is important to note that the right posterior intraperitoneal and right anterior intraperitoneal compartments communicate with each other along the sharp anterior border of the liver. But if abscess forms in one of these compartments, the pus is prevented from extending around the sharp inferior border of the liver to enter other compartment due to the formation of adhesions between transverse colon and greater omentum and inferior border of the liver.

RIGHT ANTERIOR INTRAPERITONEAL COMPARTMENT

It is situated between the anterior surface of the right lobe of the liver and diaphragm in front of the superior layer of coronary ligament and right triangular ligament (Fig. 6.22).

Boundaries

Anterior: Diaphragm and anterior abdominal wall.
Posterior: Anterior surface of the liver.
Superior: Superior layer of the coronary ligament.
Left: Right side of the falciform ligament.
Right: Fossa communicates with the right posterior intraperitoneal compartment.
Below: Open.

RIGHT EXTRAPERITONEAL COMPARTMENT

It is the space between the bare area of the liver and the diaphragm.

Boundaries

Anterior: Superior layer of the coronary ligament.
Posterior: Inferior layer of the coronary ligament.
Left: Inferior vena cava.
Right: Fusion of the two layers of coronary ligament to form the *right triangular ligament.*
Above: Diaphragm.
Below: Posterior surface of the liver.

N.B. The right extraperitoneal compartment is completely shut off and if it is distended by fluid or pus, the liver may be pushed down and the diaphragm may be pushed up.

LEFT POSTERIOR INTRAPERITONEAL COMPARTMENT (LESSER SAC)

The lesser sac (also called omental bursa) is a diverticulum of the peritoneal cavity behind the stomach. It communicates with the greater sac through a slit-like aperture called epiploic foramen (or foramen of Winslow).

Boundaries (Fig. 6.24)

Anterior wall: From above downward, it is formed by:
   (a) caudate lobe of the liver,
   (b) lesser omentum,
   (c) posteroinferior surface of the stomach, and
   (d) anterior two layers of the greater omentum.
Posterior wall: From below upward, it is formed by:
   (a) posterior two layers of the greater omentum, and
   (b) structures forming the stomach bed except spleen are:
      – Transverse colon.
      – Transverse mesocolon.
      – Pancreas.
      – Upper part of the left kidney and left suprarenal gland.
      – Diaphragm.

N.B. All the structures forming the stomach bed are separated from the stomach by the lesser sac except spleen, which is separated from the stomach by the greater sac.

Recesses of Lesser Sac

The lesser sac (omental bursa) presents the following three recesses:

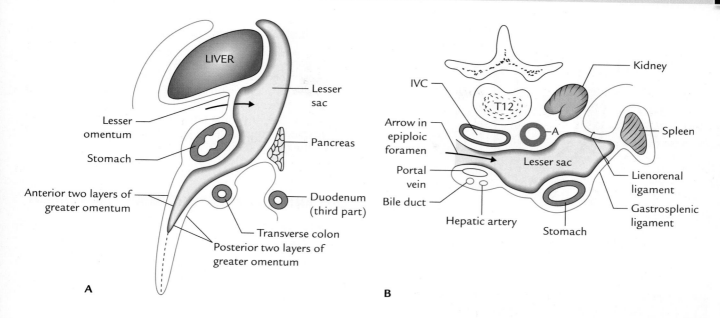

Fig. 6.24 Lesser sac: **A**, as seen in the sagittal section; **B**, as seen in the transverse section (IVC = inferior vena cava, A = aorta).

1. **Superior recess:** It lies behind the lesser omentum and the liver. The portion behind the lesser omentum is termed *vestibule of the lesser sac.*
2. **Inferior recess:** It lies between the anterior two layers and the posterior two layers of the greater omentum.
3. **Splenic recess:** It lies between the gastrosplenic and lienorenal ligaments.

N.B. The lesser sac is somewhat akin to an empty hot water bottle with its neck facing towards the right (Fig. 6.25).

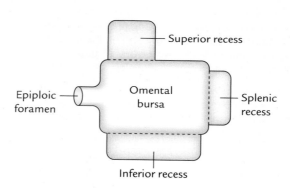

Fig. 6.25 Schematic diagram to show the recesses of lesser sac (omental bursa).

Clinical correlation

Pseudocyst of pancreas: The collection of fluid in the lesser sac occurs most frequently, as a result of *acute pancreatitis* or sometimes after pancreatic injury forming *"pseudocyst of pancreas."* The pseudocyst of pancreas projects forward either between the stomach and liver or between the stomach and transverse colon.

The perforation of posterior wall of stomach also results in the passage of its fluid contents in the lesser sac.

Foramen Epiploicum (Foramen of Winslow)

The foramen epiploicum is a vertical slit through which lesser sac of peritoneum (omental bursa) communicates with the greater sac of peritoneum. It is situated behind the right free margin of lesser omentum at the level of T12 vertebra.

Boundaries (Fig. 6.26)

Anterior:	Right free border of the lesser omentum containing bile duct, vertical part of the hepatic artery, and portal vein. Remember duct and artery are anterior to the vein with the duct being to the right of the artery. (The duct is dexter, which means to the right.)
Posterior:	Inferior vena cava and right suprarenal gland.
Superior:	Caudate process of the caudate lobe of the liver.
Inferior:	First part of the duodenum and horizontal part of the hepatic artery.

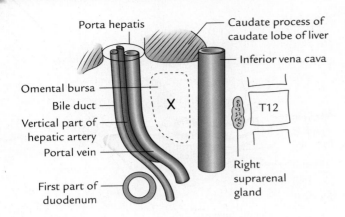

Fig. 6.26 Boundaries of the foramen epiploicum.

• Control of hemorrhage during cholecystectomy: If the cystic artery is torn during cholecystectomy, the surgeon can stop hemorrhage by compressing the hepatic pedicle (formed by the right free margin of lesser omentum), containing portal vein, hepatic artery and bile duct, between the index finger and thumb. This is achieved by inserting the index finger in the foramen of Winslow and compressing the hepatic pedicle against it by the thumb (Fig. 6.27).

LEFT ANTERIOR INTRAPERITONEAL COMPARTMENT

It lies between the *left lobe of the liver* and the diaphragm in front of the *left triangular ligament*.

Boundaries

Anterior: Abdominal wall.
Posterior: Liver.
Above: Left triangular ligament.
Right: Falciform ligament.
Left: Open.
Below: Open.

Communications

1. Below it is continuous in front of the lesser omentum and stomach.
2. To the left, it is continuous around the spleen.

Clinical correlation

• **Internal hernia:** Sometime the loop of the small intestine may herniate into the lesser sac through foramen epiploicum, producing an internal hernia.

This hernia if strangulated cannot be reduced by cutting any of the important boundaries of the foramen of Winslow (for details, see *Clinical and Surgical Anatomy*, 2nd Edition by Vishram Singh). However, it can be reduced by aspirating the gut contents and pushing the herniated loop out from the lesser sac by inserting the index finger into it through the anterior two layers of greater omentum or through the transverse mesocolon.

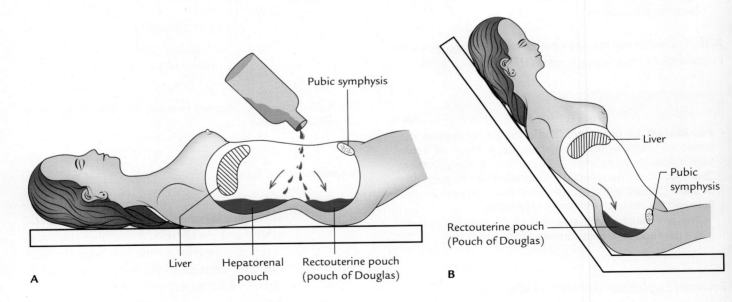

Fig. 6.27 Most dependent pouches of the peritoneal cavity where the fluid, or blood, or pus collects: **A**, when subject is in supine position; **B**, when subject is in semi-upright position.

N.B. The right and left anterior intraperitoneal compartments are separated from each other by the falciform ligament.

The abscess in this space may be formed by the following operations on the stomach, spleen, splenic flexure of colon, and tail of the pancreas.

LEFT EXTRAPERITONEAL COMPARTMENT

It is merely the loose connective tissue around the upper pole of the left kidney and left suprarenal gland.

It is hardly infected and therefore is the least important of the six subphrenic spaces.

N.B. Under the modern facilities of CT scan and ultrasound the accuracy of diagnosis of subphrenic abscess has improved tremendously. The radiologists are now able to drain subphrenic abscess by percutaneous catheters under the guidance of ultrasound.

RECTOUTERINE POUCH (OF DOUGLAS)

It is a pouch of peritoneum situated between the rectum and the uterus. It is the most dependent part of the peritoneal cavity in the upright position. In the supine position it is the most dependent part of the pelvic cavity.

Boundaries

The rectouterine pouch is bounded (Fig. 14.11):

Anteriorly: By the uterus and the upper one-third of the vagina (posterior fornix of vagina).

Posteriorly: By the rectum.

Inferiorly (floor): By the rectovaginal fold of the peritoneum. The floor of the pouch is about 5.5 cm above the perineal skin.

Clinical significance of rectouterine pouch: The rectouterine pouch is the most dependent part of the peritoneal cavity below the pelvic brim the pus tends to collect here and form the pelvic abscess (Fig. 6.27). The pus can be drained either through the rectum or through the posterior fornix of the vagina (**posterior colpotomy**).

N.B. The hepatorenal pouch is the *most dependent* part of the abdominal cavity in supine position (Fig. 6.27B) above the pelvic brim. As a result, pus tends to collect in it following an upper abdominal surgery, *viz.,* cholecystectomy. Therefore as a routine, surgeons insert a tube in this pouch to facilitate gravitational drainage. The hepatorenal and rectouterine pouches communicate with each other through the right paracolic gutter, which serve as a route of infection from the abdomen to the pelvis.

Golden Facts to Remember

- Largest and most complicated serous sac in the body — Peritoneal cavity
- Primordium of the peritoneal cavity — Intraembryonic celom
- Largest serous cavity in the body — Peritoneal cavity
- Policeman of the abdomen — Greater omentum
- Largest fold of the peritoneum — Mesentery
- Most dependent part of the peritoneal cavity in the abdomen in supine position — Hepatorenal pouch (of James Rutherford Morison)
- Clinically the term "abdominal wall" stands for — Anterior abdominal wall
- Situs inversus — Lateral transposition of the abdominal viscera

Clinical Case Study

A 45-year-old patient was admitted in the hospital with severe pain in the abdomen associated with fever and tachycardia. On palpation, the doctor found tenderness and guarding of the abdominal wall, and on auscultation, he noted the absence of bowel sounds. His pulse rate increased gradually during 1–2 hours of observation. He was diagnosed as a case of "acute peritonitis."

Questions

1. What is peritonitis?
2. Enumerate the means by which infection may gain access to the peritoneal cavity.
3. What is the anatomical basis of tenderness and guarding of the anterior abdominal wall?
4. What will be the nature of pain if visceral peritoneum is inflamed?

Answers

1. Peritonitis is the inflammation of the peritoneum.
2. (a) Traumatic and surgical penetration of the abdominal wall; (b) perforation of the gastrointestinal tract; (c) hematogenous or lymphatic spread; and (d) rupture of the uterine tube.
3. The parietal peritoneum is innervated by the somatic nerves of the anterior abdominal wall. An inflamed parietal peritoneum is extremely sensitive to palpation and leads to tenderness. The muscles of the abdominal wall become tense, guarding to produce a rigid abdomen and thereby minimize the pain.
4. The visceral peritoneum is innervated by autonomic nerves. Therefore, the inflamed visceral peritoneum results in diffuse, crampy, or colicky abdominal pain, which may be referred to specific dermatomes on the abdominal wall.

Abdominal Part of Esophagus, Stomach, and Spleen

ABDOMINAL PART OF THE ESOPHAGUS

The abdominal part of the esophagus is only 1.25 cm long. It enters the abdomen through the esophageal opening of the diaphragm, runs downward and to the left in front of the left crus of the diaphragm, and behind the left lobe of the liver to end by opening into the cardiac end of the stomach.

The esophageal opening of the diaphragm is situated at the level of T10 vertebra slightly to the left of the median plane. The cardiac end of the stomach is situated at the level of T11 vertebra about 2.5 cm to the left of the median plane. Thus, the abdominal part of the esophagus extends only from T10 to T11 vertebra.

Its right border becomes continuous with the lesser curvature of the stomach, whereas it's left border is separated from the fundus of the stomach by a notch called **cardiac notch**.

The **relations of abdominal part of the esophagus** are as follows:

1. It is covered by the peritoneum only anteriorly and to the left.
2. Posteriorly it is related to the posterior vagal trunk and the diaphragm.
3. Anteriorly it is related to the anterior vagal trunk and the left lobe of the liver.
4. The esophageal branches of the left gastric artery and accompanying veins run along its left side.

N.B. The veins from the abdominal part of the esophagus drain partly into the portal and partly into the systemic circulation. The veins drain into the portal circulation through the left gastric vein and into the systemic circulation through the hemiazygos vein. Thus, it is one of the important sites of **portocaval anastomosis**.

Clinical correlation

- **Esophageal varices:** The lower end of the esophagus is one of the important sites of *portocaval anastomosis*. In portal hypertension (e.g., due to cirrhosis of the liver), the portocaval anastomotic channels open and become dilated and tortuous forming *esophageal varices*. Their rupture may cause severe and fatal hematemesis (vomiting of blood).
- **Achalasia cardia:** Due to neuromuscular incoordination sometimes the lower end of the esophagus fails to open and does not allow smooth passage of food leading to *dysphagia* called *achalasia cardia.* Marked dilatation of the esophagus may occur due to accumulation of food within it.
- The lower end of the esophagus is prone for inflammation and ulceration due to acidic regurgitation from the stomach.
- The lower end of the esophagus is the commonest site of carcinoma.

STOMACH

Synonyms: *Gaster* (in Greek); *venter* (in Latin).

The stomach is the widest and most distensible part of the alimentary canal between the esophagus and the duodenum.

The main functions of stomach are:

1. Forms a reservoir of food.
2. Mixes food with gastric secretions to form a semifluid substance called **chyme**.
3. Controls the rate of delivery of chyme into the small intestine to allow proper digestion and absorption in the small intestine.
4. Hydrochloric acid secreted by the gastric glands destroys bacteria present in the food and drink.
5. Castle's intrinsic factor present in the gastric juice helps in the absorption of vitamin B_{12} in the small intestine.

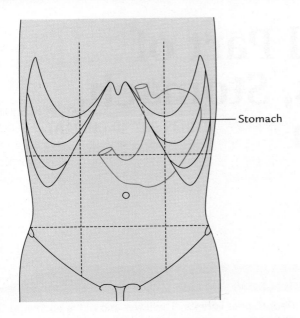

Fig. 7.1 Location of the stomach (demarcated by red line).

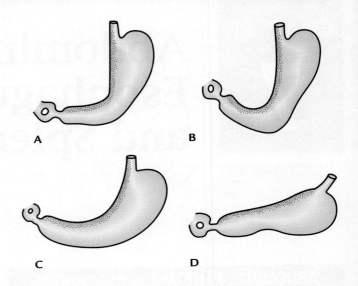

Fig. 7.2 "Types" of shape of the stomach as seen in barium meal X-ray of abdomen: A, reversed L-shaped; B, J-shaped; C, semilunar shaped; D, steer-horn shaped.

LOCATION

The stomach is situated in the upper left part of the abdomen occupying left hypochondriac, umbilical, and epigastric regions. It extends obliquely from the left hypochondriac region into the epigastric region (Fig. 7.1).

Most of the stomach lies under cover of the left costal margin and lower ribs.

Shape

The stomach is mostly "J" shaped. Its long axis passes downward, forward, and to the right and finally backward and slightly upward. It tapers from the fundus on the left of the median plane to the narrow pylorus slightly to the right of the median plane.

N.B.

- Both the shape and position of the stomach vary greatly according to the build of an individual. It is:
  1. High and transverse (steer-horn type) in short obese persons.
  2. Low and elongated in tall and weak persons.
- Even in the same individual the shape of the stomach depends upon the:
  1. Volume of fluid or food it contains.
  2. Position of body (erect or supine position).
  3. Phase of respiration.
- The shape of the stomach is studied by radiographic examination using barium meal. Generally, four types of shape of the stomach are seen in barium meal X-ray (Fig. 7.2): (A) reversed "L" shaped, (B) "J" shaped, (C) semilunar shaped, and (D) steer-horn shaped.

Size and Capacity

Length: 10 inches.
Capacity: The capacity of the stomach is variable as the stomach is highly distensible:

1. At birth the capacity is only 30 ml (1 ounce).
2. At puberty the capacity is 1000 ml (1 L).
3. In adults the capacity is 1500 to 2000 ml.

EXTERNAL FEATURES

The stomach presents the following external features (Fig. 7.3):

1. **Two ends:** Cardiac and pyloric.
2. **Two curvatures:** Greater and lesser.
3. **Two surfaces:** Anterior (anterosuperior) and posterior (posteroinferior).

Ends

Cardiac End (Upper End)

It joins the lower end of the esophagus and presents an orifice called *cardiac orifice.*

Pyloric End (Lower End)

It joins the proximal end of the duodenum and presents an orifice called *pyloric orifice.*

The stomach is relatively fixed at upper and lower ends but mobile in between.

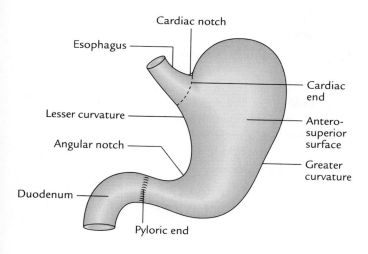

Fig. 7.3 External features of the stomach.

Table 7.1 Cardiac and pyloric orifices of the stomach

Cardiac orifice	Pyloric orifice
It is at the junction between the lower end of the esophagus and stomach, and marks the level at which curvatures begin	It is at the junction between the pyloric end of the stomach and first part of the duodenum
It is situated to the left of the median plane behind the left 7th costal cartilage, 2.5 cm from its junction with the sternum at the level of lower border of T11	It is about 1.5 cm to the right of median plane at the lower border of L1 (i.e., transpyloric plane)
It does not have an anatomical sphincter but is guarded by the physiological sphincter	It has anatomical *pyloric sphincter* formed by the thickening of a circular coat of muscle assisted by a deep set of longitudinal fibres of the stomach

The details of cardiac and pyloric orifices are given in Table 7.1.

N.B.

- The *cardiac end of the stomach* is less mobile and less likely to vary in position whereas the *pyloric end of the stomach* is more mobile and more likely to vary in position.

Curvatures

The stomach presents two curvatures—lesser and greater.

Lesser Curvature

It is concave and forms the shorter right border of the stomach. The most dependent part of this curvature—the

angular notch/incisura angularis, indicates the junction of the body and pyloric part. The lesser curvature provides attachment to the lesser omentum.

Greater Curvature

It is convex and forms the longer left border of the stomach. At its upper end this curvature presents a *cardiac notch* which separates it from the left aspect of the esophagus. The greater curvature provides attachment to the greater omentum, gastrosplenic, and gastrophrenic ligaments.

Surfaces

Anterosuperior (Anterior) Surface

It faces forward and upward.

Posteroinferior (Posterior) Surface

It faces backward and downward.

PARTS

The stomach has four parts (Fig. 7.4):

1. Cardiac part (or cardia).
2. Fundus.
3. Body.
4. Pyloric part.

Cardiac Part

It is the part around the cardiac orifice.

Fundus

The fundus is the upper dome-shaped part of the stomach situated above the horizontal plane drawn at the level of cardiac notch. Superiorly, the fundus *usually* reaches the level of the left 5th intercostal space just below the nipple, hence gastric pain sometimes imitates the pain of angina pectoris. The cardiac notch lies between the fundus and the esophagus.

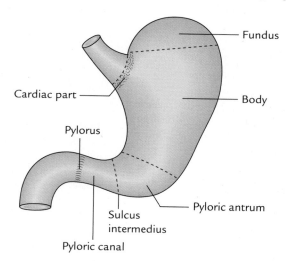

Fig. 7.4 Parts of the stomach.

N.B.

- The fundus is generally distended with gas/air, which is clearly seen as a radiolucent shadow under the left dome of the diaphragm in a skiagram.
- **Traube space:** It is a topographic area overlying the fundus of the stomach which is tympanic on percussion. It is bounded *superiorly* by the lower border of the left lung, *inferiorly* by the left costal margin, *on the left side* by the lateral end of the spleen, and *on the right side* by the lower border of the left lobe of the liver.

Body

The body is the major part of the stomach between the fundus and the pyloric antrum. It can be distended enormously along the greater curvature.

Pyloric Part

The pyloric part is the funnel-shaped outflow region of the stomach. A line drawn downward and to the left from an angular notch to the greater curvature separates it from the body. It extends from the angular notch to the gastroduodenal junction. It is divided into three parts: **pyloric antrum, pyloric canal,** and **pylorus.**

1. **Pyloric antrum** is the proximal wide part which is separated from the pyloric canal by an inconstant sulcus, sulcus intermedius present on the greater curvature. It is about 3 inches (7.5 cm) long and leads into the pyloric canal.
2. **Pyloric canal** is a distal narrow and tubular part measuring 1 inch (2.5 cm) in length. It lies on the head and neck of the pancreas.
3. **Pylorus** (Greek *gatekeeper*) is the distal most and sphincteric region of the pyloric canal. The circular

muscle fibres are markedly thickened in this region, which control the discharge of stomach contents through the pyloric orifice into the duodenum.

N.B.

- The position of the pyloric orifice is indicated on the surface by (a) a **circular sulcus**—*pyloric constriction produced by the underlying pyloric sphincter or pylorus;* and (b) the **prepyloric vein of Mayo** on the anterior surface of the pylorus.

RELATIONS

Peritoneal Relations

The stomach is covered by the peritoneum except where blood vessels run along its curvatures and a small area (called **bare area of the stomach**) posteriorly near the cardiac orifice. The **bare area of the stomach** is directly related to the left crus of the diaphragm.

The peritoneal folds extending from the lesser and greater curvatures of the stomach to other structures are as follows (Fig. 7.5):

1. *Lesser omentum,* extends from the lesser curvature of the stomach to the liver.
2. *Greater omentum,* extends from the lower two-third of the greater curvature to the transverse colon (for details see page 80).
3. *Gastrosplenic ligament,* extends from the upper one-third of the greater curvature (i.e., fundus) to the spleen (near the hilum).
4. *Gastrophrenic ligament,* extends from the uppermost part of the fundus to the diaphragm.

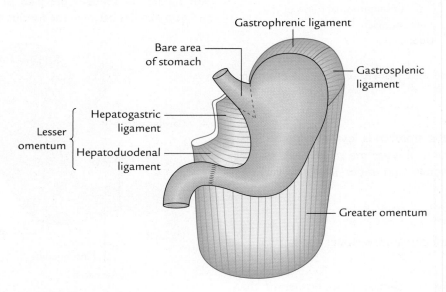

Fig. 7.5 Peritoneal relations of the stomach.

Visceral Relations

1. **Relations of the anterior (anterosuperior) surface (Fig. 7.6):**
   (a) On the right side this surface is related to the gastric impression of the left lobe of the liver and near the pylorus to the quadrate lobe of the liver.
   (b) The left half of this surface is related to the diaphragm and rib cage.
   (c) The lower part of this surface is related to the anterior abdominal wall.

N.B. *Gastric triangle:* It is a triangular area of the stomach in contact with the anterior abdominal wall. It is bounded on the left side by the left costal margin, on the right side by the lower border of the liver, and inferiorly by the transverse colon. In complete esophageal obstruction, **gastrostomy** is performed in this area to feed the patient.

2. **Relations of the posterior (posteroinferior) surface:** This surface is related to a number of structures on the posterior abdominal wall, which collectively form the **stomach bed** (Fig. 7.7). These structures are:
   (a) Diaphragm.
   (b) Left kidney.
   (c) Left suprarenal gland.
   (d) Pancreas.
   (e) Transverse mesocolon.
   (f) Left colic flexure (splenic flexure of colon).
   (g) Splenic artery.
   (h) Spleen.

Mnemonic: "Dr S3 Kills Patients Mercilessly"
D = diaphragm, S3 = splenic artery, suprarenal gland (left), and splenic flexure, K = kidney (left), P = pancreas, M = mesocolon (transverse).

N.B. All the structures forming the stomach bed are separated from the stomach by the lesser sac except spleen, which is separated from the stomach by the greater sac of peritoneum.

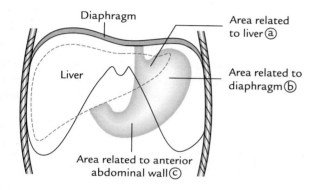

Fig. 7.6 Anterior relations of the stomach.

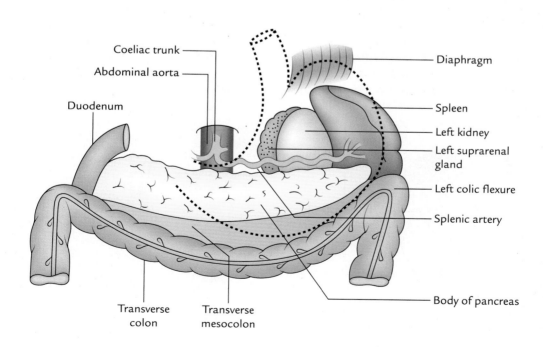

Fig. 7.7 The "stomach bed."

MICROSCOPIC STRUCTURE

The wall of the stomach consists of four coats. From outside inward, these are serous, muscular, submucous, and mucous coats.

- The **serous coat** is formed by the peritoneum.
- The **muscular coat** consists of three layers of unstriped muscles—outer longitudinal, middle circular, and inner oblique (Fig. 7.8).

Close to the pyloric end the longitudinal muscle coat separates into superficial and deep fibres. The deep fibres turn inward at the pylorus and join with circular muscle coat to help form the pyloric sphincter.

The circular muscle coat thickens at the pylorus to form a ring of muscle called pyloric sphincter.

The major sphincteric component of the pyloric sphincter is derived from the circular muscle coat and its minor dilator component is derived from the longitudinal muscle coat (Fig. 7.9).

- The submucous coat consists of loose areolar tissue.
- The mucous membrane is thick, soft, and velvety. It presents a number of temporary folds (rugae) which disappear when the stomach is distended.
- The mucous membrane of the stomach is lined by simple columnar epithelium which form simple tubular glands.
  - Glands in the cardiac region secrete mucus.
  - Glands in the fundus and body contain mucus neck cells which secrete mucus, parietal/oxyntic cells which secrete hydrochloric acid and gastric intrinsic factor, and chief cells which secrete pepsinogen.
  - Glands in the pyloric region secrete mucus.

N.B. Anatomically, the stomach is divided into 4 parts, viz. cardia, fundus, body, and pylorus (Fig. 7.4). However, histologically the stomach is divided into 3 parts, viz. cardia, body, and pylorus, because fundus and body share the common histological features.

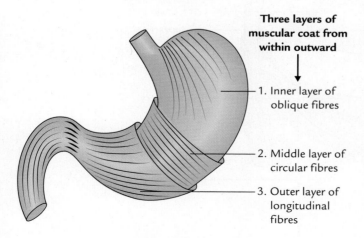

Three layers of muscular coat from within outward
↓

1. Inner layer of oblique fibres

2. Middle layer of circular fibres

3. Outer layer of longitudinal fibres

Fig. 7.8 Three layers of the muscular coat of the stomach.

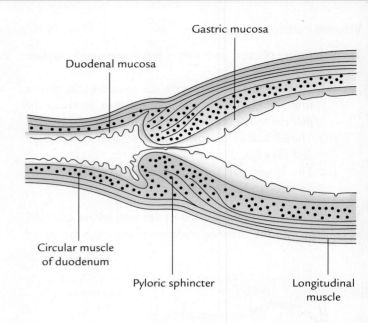

Gastric mucosa

Duodenal mucosa

Circular muscle of duodenum

Pyloric sphincter

Longitudinal muscle

Fig. 7.9 A longitudinal section through pyloroduodenal junction showing the thickening of circular muscle coat in the pylorus forming pyloric sphincter and merging of deep fibres of longitudinal muscle coat in the sphincter.

INTERIOR OF THE STOMACH

When the stomach is cut open, the interior of the stomach presents the following features (Fig. 7.10):

1. **Gastric folds/gastric rugae:** The mucosa of an empty stomach is thrown into numerous folds called *gastric rugae*. They are longitudinal along the lesser curvature

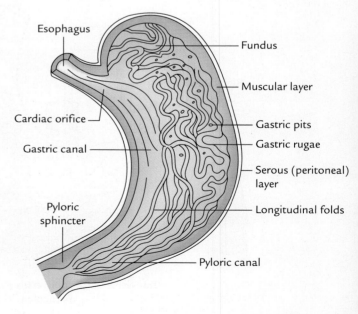

Esophagus

Fundus

Muscular layer

Cardiac orifice

Gastric pits

Gastric canal

Gastric rugae

Serous (peritoneal) layer

Longitudinal folds

Pyloric sphincter

Pyloric canal

Fig. 7.10 Interior of the stomach showing folds in mucous lining.

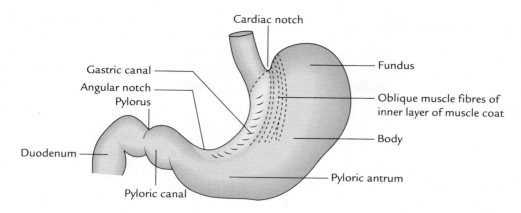

Fig. 7.11 Gastric canal.

and irregular in the remaining part. The rugae are flattened when the stomach is distended.

2. **Gastric pits:** These are small depressions on the mucosal surface in which open the gastric glands.

3. **Gastric canal (or Magenstrasse):** A longitudinal furrow that forms temporarily during swallowing between the longitudinal folds of the mucosa along the lesser curvature (Fig. 7.11). The gastric canal forms due to firm attachment of the gastric mucosa to the underlying muscular layer, which does not have an oblique layer at this site. This canal allows a rapid passage of swallowed liquids along the lesser curvature to the lower part before it spreads to the other parts of the stomach.

Thus, the lesser curvature is subject to maximum insult of the swallowed spicy food and irritable liquids (e.g., alcohol), which makes it vulnerable to the gastric ulceration.

N.B. The interior of the stomach can be directly examined in the living person by an endoscope. The gastric mucosa is reddish brown during life except in the pyloric part, where it is pink.

ARTERIAL SUPPLY

The stomach has rich arterial supply derived from the coeliac trunk and its branches. The arteries supplying the stomach are (Fig. 7.12):

1. *Left gastric artery*, a direct branch from the coeliac trunk.
2. *Right gastric artery*, a branch of the common hepatic artery.
3. *Left gastroepiploic artery*, a branch of the splenic artery.
4. *Right gastroepiploic artery*, a branch of the gastroduodenal artery.
5. *Short gastric arteries* (five to seven in number), branches of the splenic artery.

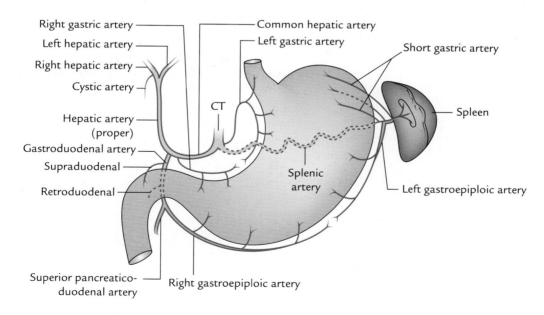

Fig. 7.12 Arteries of the stomach (CT = coeliac trunk).

VENOUS DRAINAGE

The veins of the stomach correspond to the arteries and drain directly or indirectly into the portal vein. The veins of the stomach are (Fig. 7.13):

1. Left gastric vein.
2. Right gastric vein.
3. Left gastroepiploic vein.
4. Right gastroepiploic vein.
5. Short gastric veins.

The left and right gastric veins drain directly into the portal vein. The left gastroepiploic and short gastric veins drain into the splenic vein. The right gastroepiploic vein drains into the superior mesenteric vein.

LYMPHATIC DRAINAGE

The knowledge of lymphatic drainage of the stomach is clinically very important because gastric cancer (carcinoma of stomach) spreads through the lymph vessels.

For descriptive purposes, the stomach is divided into four lymphatic territories as follows:

First, divide the stomach into right two-third and left one-third by a line along its long axis. Now divide the right two-third into upper two-third (area 1) and lower one-third (area 4), and left one-third into upper one-third (area 3) and lower two-third (area 2). In this way, four lymphatic territories are marked out and numbered 1 to 4 (Fig. 7.14A).

Mode of lymphatic drainage from four lymphatic territories into different groups of lymph nodes is as follows (Fig. 7.14B):

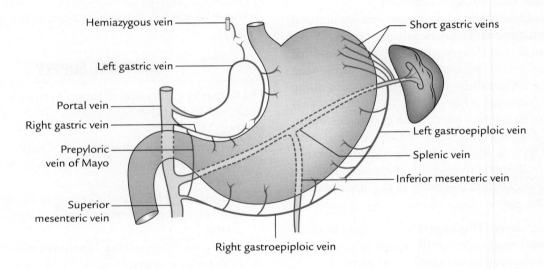

Fig. 7.13 Venous drainage of the stomach.

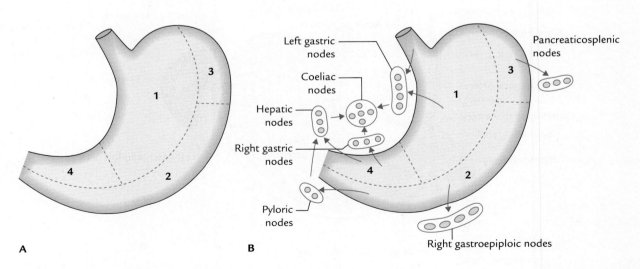

Fig. 7.14 Lymphatic drainage of the stomach: A, lymphatic territories; B, lymph node groups draining the lymphatic territories of the stomach.

1. *Area 1* is the largest area along the lesser curvature. The lymph from this area is drained into **left gastric lymph nodes** along the left gastric artery. These lymph nodes also drain the abdominal part of the esophagus.
2. *Area 2* includes the pyloric antrum and pyloric canal along the greater curvature of the stomach. (The carcinoma of the stomach most frequently occurs in this area.) The lymph from this area is drained into **right gastroepiploic lymph nodes** along the right gastroepiploic artery and **pyloric nodes**, which lie in the angle between the first and second parts of the duodenum.
3. *Area 3* (also called pancreaticosplenic area) drains into pancreaticosplenic (pancreaticolienal) nodes along the splenic artery.
4. *Area 4* includes the pyloric antrum and pyloric canal along the lesser curvature of the stomach. The lymph from this area is drained into **right gastric nodes** along the right gastric artery and **hepatic nodes** along the hepatic artery.

The efferents from all these lymph node groups pass to the *coeliac nodes*. Efferents from coeliac nodes enter the *cysterna chyli* through *intestinal lymph trunk*.

Clinical correlation

Gastric carcinoma (gastric cancer): It commonly occurs in the region of pyloric antrum along the greater curvature of the stomach. The gastric cancer spreads by lymph vessels to the left supraclavicular lymph nodes. The enlarged and palpable left supraclavicular node (**Virchow's node**) may be the first sign of gastric cancer (**Troisier's sign**). The cancer cells reach the left supraclavicular lymph node through the thoracic duct.

NERVE SUPPLY

The stomach has both sympathetic and parasympathetic innervation.

Sympathetic Innervation

The sympathetic fibres are derived from T6 to T10 spinal segments via greater splanchnic nerves, and coeliac and hepatic plexuses. They reach the stomach by running along its arteries.

The sympathetic supply to the stomach is (a) vasomotor, (b) motor to pyloric sphincter, and inhibitory to the remaining gastric musculature, and (c) serves as the chief pathway for pain sensations from the stomach.

Parasympathetic Innervation

The parasympathetic fibres are derived directly from the vagus nerves (Fig. 7.15).

The anterior vagal trunk derived largely from the left vagus nerve and partly from the right vagus nerve enters the abdomen on the anterior surface of the esophagus. Soon after entering the abdomen it gives off three branches in the vicinity of the lesser curvature.

1. *Hepatic branch* (or branches), which runs in the upper part of the lesser omentum to the porta hepatis to supply the liver and gallbladder. It also gives a branch to the pyloric antrum.
2. *Coeliac branch,* which follows the left gastric artery to the celiac plexus.
3. *Gastric branch/nerve of Latarjet* (largest of the three branches), which follows the lesser curvature and distributes anterior gastric branches to the stomach as far as the pylorus.

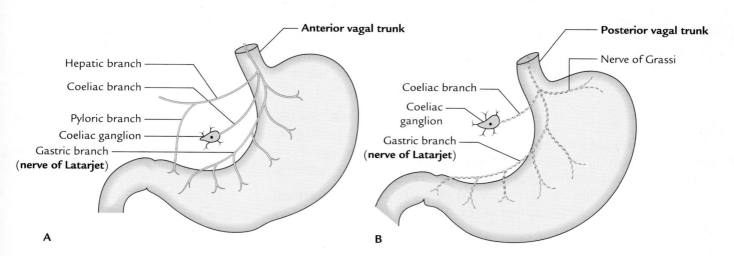

Fig. 7.15 Parasympathetic innervation of the stomach: A, distribution of the anterior vagal trunk; B, distribution of the posterior vagal trunk.

The **posterior vagal trunk** derived largely from the right vagus nerve and partly from the left vagus nerve enters the abdomen on the posterior surface of the esophagus; soon after entering the abdomen it also gives rise to three types of branches.

1. *Coeliac branch* to the coeliac ganglion.
2. *Nerve of Grassi* is the name given to one or more branches of the posterior vagal trunk which arises at the level of the gastroesophageal junction and supplies the gastric fundus.
3. *Gastric branch* (nerve of Latarjet) which runs along the lesser curvature and gives branches to the posterior surface of the stomach.

N.B. The nerves of Latarjet supply the acid and pepsin secreting areas of the stomach.

Clinical correlation

- **Vagotomy (a surgical procedure of cutting the vagus nerves):** It is done to cure the chronic duodenal ulcers. There are three different types of vagotomies:
(a) *Truncal vagotomy:* In this procedure the trunks of both gastric nerves are divided at the lower end of esophagus.
(b) *Selective vagotomy:* In this procedure the hepatic and coeliac branches are preserved but the main trunks of gastric nerves along with nerve of Laterjet are cut.

N.B. The above two procedures cause denervation of pyloric antrum with subsequent defect in gastric emptying.

(c) *Highly selective vagotomy:* In this procedure only parietal cells of the stomach are denervated. The nerve of Laterjet is dissected out and cut. In this procedure gastric emptying is not affected, hence it is regarded by many as the procedure of choice in surgical treatment of duodenal ulcer.
- **Gastric pain:** It is usually referred to the epigastric region because the stomach is supplied by T6–T10 spinal segments.

Vagotomy

The vagus nerves largely control the secretion of acid by the parietal cells of the stomach. Since excess acid secretion is the main cause of peptic ulcers, the section of vagal trunks (vagotomy) as they enter the abdomen is carried out to reduce the production of acid. Vagotomy is of three types:

1. **Truncal vagotomy:** In this both the vagal trunks (anterior and posterior) are sectioned at the lower end of the esophagus.

2. **Selective vagotomy:** In this, the nerves of Latarjet are selectively cut to denervate the acid and pepsin secreting area of the stomach.

The disadvantage of both truncal and selective vagotomy is that pyloric antrum is denervated. Consequently the gastric emptying is affected.

3. **Highly selective vagotomy:** In this only parietal cells of the stomach are denervated by cutting the anterior and posterior gastric branches, particularly the nerve of Grassi. The advantage of high selective vagotomy is that nerves of Latarjet and their antral branches are preserved. As a result, the gastric emptying remains normal.

SPLEEN

Synonym: *Splen* (in Greek); *Lien* (in Latin).

The spleen is the largest lymphoid organ in the body (strictly speaking a hemolymphoid organ). The main functions of the spleen are:

1. To filter blood by removing worn-out RBCs and microbial agents from the circulation.
2. To manufacture RBCs in fetal life and lymphocytes after birth.
3. To provide immunity to the body by producing immunoglobulin M (IgM) by plasma cells.
4. To store RBCs and release them in circulation when required.

LOCATION

The spleen is located in the left hypochondrium between the fundus of the stomach and the diaphragm, behind the midaxillary line opposite the 9th, 10th, and 11th ribs. Its long axis lies parallel to the long axis of the 10th rib. It moves a bit in living during respiration.

Size, Shape, and Colour

The spleen is a wedge-shaped soft organ with purple colour. The size of the spleen roughly corresponds to the fist of the subject.

N.B. *Classification of the spleen according to its shape (Fig. 7.16):* According to the shape or form, the spleen is classified into three types: (a) wedge-shaped (44%), (b) tetrahedral (42%), and (c) triangular (14%).

Measurement

Measurements of the spleen are:
Thickness: 1 inch.
Breadth: 3 inches.
Length: 5 inches.
Weight: 7 oz.

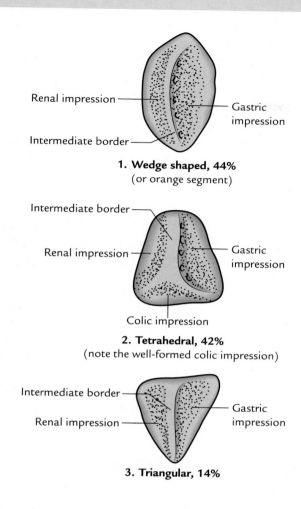

Renal impression

Gastric impression

Intermediate border

1. Wedge shaped, 44%
(or orange segment)

Intermediate border

Renal impression

Gastric impression

Colic impression

2. Tetrahedral, 42%
(note the well-formed colic impression)

Intermediate border

Gastric impression

Renal impression

3. Triangular, 14%

Fig. 7.16 Types of the spleen according to its shape.

N.B. *The Harris' dictum of odd numbers* 1, 3, 5, 7, 9, 11 summarizes some splenic statistics, *viz.,* it measures 1 inch in thickness, 3 inches in breadth, 5 inches in length, weighs 7 oz, and lies deep to 9, 10, and 11 ribs.

Surface Projection

The spleen is marked on the surface on the left side of the back of the trunk. Its long axis corresponds to that of the 10th rib. Its upper border corresponds to the upper border of the 9th rib, and its lower border corresponds to the lower border of the 11th rib. Its medial end lies about 5 cm from the posterior midline of the body at the level of spine of T10 vertebra and lateral end at the midaxillary line (Fig. 7.17).

EXTERNAL FEATURES

The spleen presents the following external features (Fig. 7.18):

1. Two ends (anterior and posterior).
2. Three borders (superior, inferior, and intermediate).
3. Two surfaces (diaphragmatic and visceral).

N.B. Some authorities also describe **two angles**: (a) **anterobasal angle** at the junction of superior border with anterior end and (b) **posterobasal angle**, at the junction of inferior border with the anterior end. The anterobasal angle is called **clinical angle of spleen** because it is felt first when the spleen is enlarged.

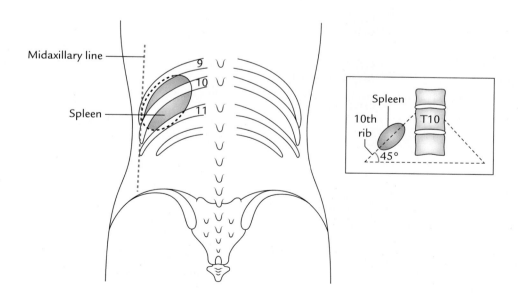

Midaxillary line

9

10

11

Spleen

Spleen

10th rib

T10

45°

Fig. 7.17 Location of the spleen as seen from the posterior aspect. Figure in the inset shows that the axis of spleen corresponds to the long axis of the 10th rib of the left side which makes an angle of about 45° with the horizontal plane.

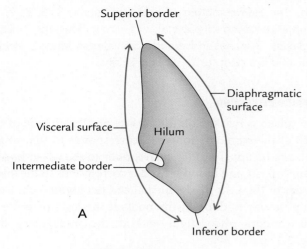

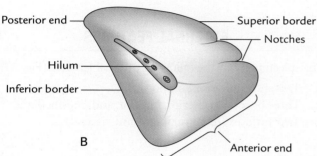

Fig. 7.18 A, External features of the spleen: A, as seen in the transverse section; B, as seen from the visceral surface. Note the characteristic notches on the superior border of the spleen.

Ends

The **anterior end** (lateral end/lower pole) is broad and is more like a border. It is directed downward, forward, and to the left. It is related to the left colic flexure in front and phrenicocolic ligament below.

The **posterior end** (medial end/upper pole) is blunt and rounded. It is directed upward, backward, and medially towards the vertebral column. It is related to the upper pole of the left kidney.

Borders

Superior Border

The superior border is thin and convex. It separates the visceral surface (gastric impression) from the diaphragmatic surface. **It characteristically presents one or two notches** near its anterior end. These notches indicate that the spleen develops by the fusion of separate masses of lymphoid tissue (lobulated development).

Inferior Border

The **inferior border** separates the visceral surface (renal impression) from the diaphragmatic surface. It is rounded and corresponds to the lower border of the 11th rib.

Intermediate Order

The **intermediate border** is rounded and separates the gastric impression from the renal impression on the visceral surface.

Surfaces

Diaphragmatic Surface

The **diaphragmatic surface** is smooth, convex, and directed upward, backward, and to the left.

Visceral Surface

The **visceral surface** is concave and irregular. It presents four impressions: gastric, renal, colic, and pancreatic.

- The *gastric impression* is produced by the fundus of the stomach. It is the largest impression and lies between the superior and intermediate borders. The *hilum of spleen* is located in the lower part of this impression.
- The *renal impression* is produced by the left kidney and lies below and behind the gastric impression between the intermediate and inferior borders.
- The *colic impression* is produced by the left colic flexure. It is triangular in shape and situated in front of the lateral end.
- The *pancreatic impression* (occasional) is produced by the tail of the pancreas. It is located between the hilum and the colic impression.

RELATIONS

Peritoneal Relations

The spleen is completely enclosed in the peritoneum except at its hilum, from where two peritoneal folds extend — one to the stomach and one to the left kidney, called gastrosplenic and lienorenal ligaments, respectively (Fig. 7.19).

1. *Gastrosplenic ligament* extends from the hilum of the spleen to the upper one-third of the greater curvature of the stomach. It contains short gastric vessels.

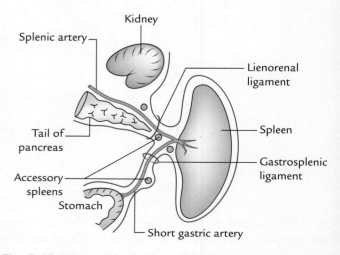

Fig. 7.19 Peritoneal relations of the spleen.

2. *Lienorenal ligament* extends from the hilum of the spleen to the anterior surface of the left kidney. It contains (a) tail of the pancreas, (b) splenic vessels, and (c) pancreaticosplenic lymph nodes.

N.B. *Phrenicocolic ligament*: It is a triangular fold of the peritoneum which extends from the left colic flexure to the diaphragm opposite to the 10th rib. It passes below the lateral end of the spleen, which it supports; hence, it is also termed *sustentaculum lienis*.

Visceral Relations

The **visceral surface of the spleen** is related to the following viscera (Fig. 7.20):

1. Fundus of the stomach.
2. Anterior surface of the left kidney.
3. Left colic flexure.
4. Tail of pancreas.

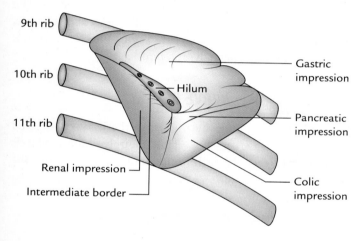

Fig. 7.20 Visceral surface of the spleen showing different impressions.

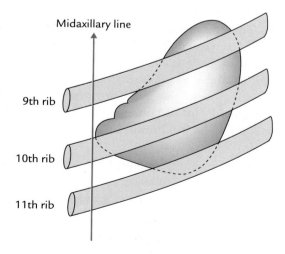

Fig. 7.21 Diaphragmatic surface of the spleen showing relation to 9th, 10th, and 11th ribs.

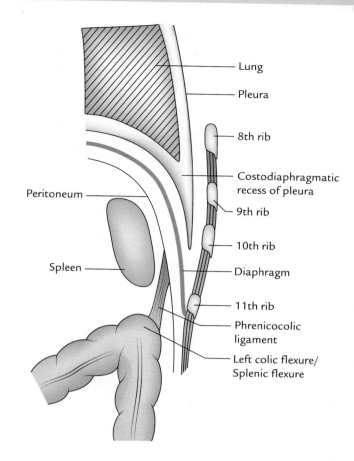

Fig. 7.22 Longitudinal section through the midaxillary line to show the relations of diaphragmatic surface of the spleen.

These viscera produce impressions on this surface (for details see visceral surface on page 104).

The **diaphragmatic surface of the spleen** is related to the diaphragm, which separates it from the costophrenic recess of the pleura, lung, and 9 to 11 ribs (Figs 7.21 and 7.22).

ARTERIAL SUPPLY (Fig. 7.23)

The spleen is supplied by the splenic artery, the largest branch of the coeliac trunk (Fig. 7.23). It traverses through the lienorenal ligament to reach near the hilum of the spleen, where it divides into five or more branches, which enter the spleen through its hilum to supply it.

The splenic artery is remarkably tortuous to allow movements of the spleen following distension of the stomach and movements of diaphragm, without obstruction to the blood flow.

N.B. The spleen is classified into two types, diffuse and compact, depending upon the branching pattern of the terminal branches of the splenic artery, which enter the hilum.

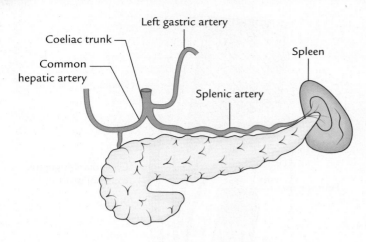

Fig. 7.23 Arterial supply of the spleen.

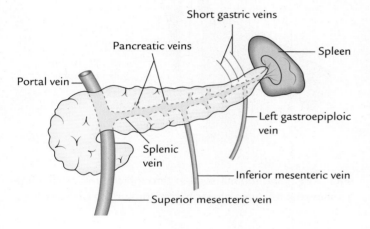

Fig. 7.24 Venous drainage of the spleen.

(a) *Diffuse type of spleen*, if the terminal branches are long and arise far away from the hilum.

(b) *Compact type of spleen*, if the terminal branches are small and arise close to the hilum.

VENOUS DRAINAGE

The venous blood from the spleen is drained by the splenic vein, which is formed at the hilum by the union of five or more tributaries which emerge from the splenic substance. The splenic vein runs a straight course from left to right behind the body of pancreas. Behind the neck of pancreas it joins the *superior mesenteric vein* to form the *portal vein*. Its *tributaries* are (Fig. 7.24):

1. Short gastric veins.
2. Left gastroepiploic vein.
3. Pancreatic veins.
4. Inferior mesenteric vein.

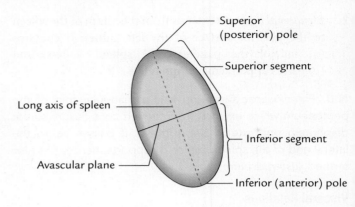

Fig. 7.25 Vascular segments of the spleen.

LYMPHATIC DRAINAGE

The splenic tissue proper has no lymphatics. The tissue fluid formed in the spleen freely enters the venous sinusoids. The splenic lymphatics are confined to its trabeculae, capsule, and visceral peritoneum. They drain along the splenic vessels into the pancreaticolienal lymph nodes.

NERVE SUPPLY

The spleen is supplied by the sympathetic fibres derived from the coeliac plexus. They supply blood vessels (vasomotor) and smooth muscle fibres present in the trabeculae and capsule.

SEGMENTS OF THE SPLEEN

The splenic artery within the spleen usually gives two branches—superior and inferior. These branches usually do not anastomose and each branch supplies its own territory (segment). Thus, an avascular zone exists between these two territories. Thus, the spleen presents two segments, superior and inferior, separated by an avascular plane passing perpendicular to the long axis of the spleen (Fig. 7.25). The knowledge of these vascular segments is essential for segmental resection of the spleen to preserve the splenic tissue if required (for details, see *Clinical and Surgical Anatomy*, 2nd Edition by Vishram Singh).

N.B. The branches of the splenic artery within the spleen are segmental in distribution whereas the tributaries of the splenic vein within the spleen are intersegmental.

DEVELOPMENT

The spleen develops between the two layers of the upper part of the dorsal mesogastrium from a number of condensations of mesenchymal cells. These separate masses of mesenchymal cells (called splenunculi) fuse together to form the lobulated spleen. The notches on the superior border of the adult spleen indicate the lobulated development of the organ.

Accessory Spleens

The failure of fusion of splenunculi results in the formation of accessory spleens (splenunculi). These are usually found in the derivatives of the dorsal mesogastrium, *viz.* (Fig. 7.19): (a) in the gastrosplenic ligament, (b) in the lienorenal ligament, and (c) in the greater omentum. Rarely they are formed in the left spermatic cord and in the broad ligament of the uterus (left side).

Clinical correlation

- **Palpation of the spleen:** The normal spleen is not palpable; however, it can be mapped out by percussion. When it is enlarged more than double of its size, it becomes palpable at the left costal margin during deep inspiration.
- **Splenomegaly:** The enlargement of the spleen (splenomegaly) occurs in number of diseases. The spleen may increase in size by as much as tenfold (massive splenomegaly). The common causes of massive splenomegaly are: (a) malaria, (b) cirrhosis of liver, (c) chronic myeloid leukemia, and (d) kala-azar.

  The very large (massive) spleen projects downward and medially toward the right iliac fossa in the direction of the axis of the 10th rib. The enlarged spleen may be differentiated from the enlarged kidney by the presence of one or more notches on its superior border (for details, see *Clinical and Surgical Anatomy*, 2nd Edition by Vishram Singh).
- **Splenectomy:** The splenectomy (surgical removal of the spleen) is sometimes performed when the spleen is ruptured or inadvertently nicked at operation. It is also performed in the treatment of certain blood diseases. If the accessory spleens are located in the splenic pedicle they should also be removed. The removal of spleen does not impair the immune response seriously.

N.B.

Rupture of spleen: Although well protected by 9th, 10th, and 11th ribs, the spleen is the most frequently ruptured organ in the abdomen following severe external blow. The pain is referred to the left shoulder due to irritation of the left dome of diaphragm by the splenic blood. It is called '**Kehr's sign**'.

Golden Facts to Remember

➤ Most dilated and distensible part of the digestive tube	Stomach
➤ Most fixed part of the stomach	Cardiac end (gastroesophageal junction)
➤ Angle of His	Cardiac notch
➤ Bare area of the stomach	Triangular non-peritoneal area on the posterior surface of the cardiac end
➤ Commonest site of gastric ulcer	Along the lesser curvature
➤ Commonest site of gastric cancer	Pyloric antrum along the lesser curvature
➤ Virchow's node	Left supraclavicular lymph node
➤ Troisier's sign	Enlarged and palpable left supraclavicular lymph node in gastric cancer
➤ Most commonly ruptured organ in abdomen	Spleen
➤ Commonest site of accessory spleens (splenunculi)	Gastrosplenic or lienorenal ligament
➤ Largest lymphoid organ in the body	Spleen
➤ Clinically the most important surface feature of the spleen	Presence of notches on its superior border

Clinical Case Study

A 65-year-old man was admitted in the hospital with a history of loss of appetite, indigestion, and epigastric pain. Pain was not relieved by taking antacids, food, or vomiting. He had lost 10–20 kg weight in 1–2 months. He also gave the history of vomiting of large quantities of indigested food. On examination the doctors made the following observations: (a) wasting and pallor, (b) a palpable left supraclavicular node (often called Virchow's node), (c) epigastric tenderness, and (d) epigastric mass (on deep palpation at full respiration). He was diagnosed as a case of "gastric cancer" (carcinoma of the stomach).

Questions

1. What is the commonest site of carcinoma of the stomach?
2. What are premalignant conditions of gastric cancer?
3. Which age group and sex are commonly affected by gastric cancer?
4. Give anatomical basis of vomiting of large quantities of undigested food.
5. How do the cancer cells reach the left supraclavicular node?

Answers

1. Pyloric antrum along the greater curvature of the stomach.
2. (a) Chronic gastric ulcer, (b) pernicious anemia, and (c) gastric polyps.
3. Individuals between the ages of 50 and 70 years. The males are affected two or three times more than females.
4. Cancer of pylorus often obstructs the outflow tract of the stomach, which leads to vomiting.
5. Stomach → lymph vessels → lymph nodes → intestinal lymph trunk → thoracic duct → left supraclavicular lymph node.

Liver and Extrahepatic Biliary Apparatus

LIVER

The liver (Greek *hepar:* liver) is the largest gland of the body, occupying much of the right upper part of the abdominal cavity. It consists of both exocrine and endocrine parts. The liver performs a wide range of metabolic activities necessary for homeostasis, nutrition, and immune response. Its main functions are:

1. It secretes bile and stores glycogen.
2. It synthesizes the serum proteins and lipids.
3. It detoxifies blood from endogenous and exogenous substances (e.g., toxins, drugs, alcohol, etc.) that enter the circulation.
4. It produces hemopoietic cells of all types during fetal life.

LOCATION

The liver almost fully occupies the right hypochondrium, upper part of the epigastrium, and part of the left hypochondrium up to the left lateral (midclavicular) line. It lies mostly under cover of the ribs and costal cartilages immediately below the diaphragm. It extends upward under the rib cage as far as the 5th rib anteriorly on the right side (below the right nipple) and left 5th intercostal space anteriorly on the left side (below and medial to the left nipple).

In the midline, the upper border lies at the level of the xiphisternal joint. The sharp inferior border crosses the midline at the level of transpyloric plane (at the level of L1 vertebra; Fig. 8.1).

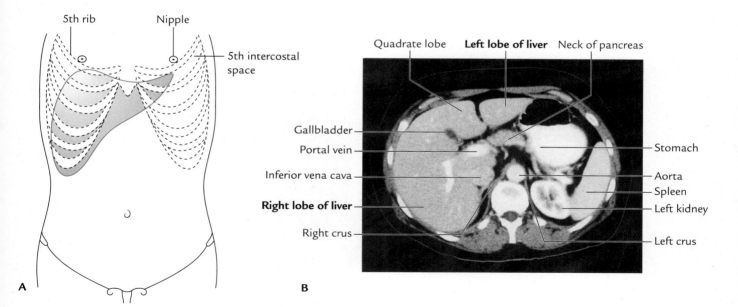

Fig. 8.1 Location of the liver: A, surface projection of the liver as seen from the front; B, CT scan of the abdomen showing the location of the liver. (*Source:* Fig. 4.85B, Page 286, *Gray's Anatomy for Students*, Richard L Drake, Wayne Vogl, Adam WM Mitchell. Copyright Elsevier Inc. 2005, All rights reserved.)

N.B. The liver is much larger in newborn and young children due to its hemopoietic function in fetal life, and occupies 2/5th of the abdomen.

SHAPE, SIZE, AND COLOUR

Shape
The liver is wedge shaped and resembles a four-sided pyramid laid on one side with its base directed towards the right and apex directed towards the left.

Weight
- *In males:* 1.4 to 1.8 kg.
- *In females:* 1.2 to 1.4 kg.
- *In newborn:* 1/18th of the body weight.
- *At birth:* 150 g.
- *Proportional weight:* In adult 1/40th of the body weight.

Colour
It is red-brown in colour.

EXTERNAL FEATURES (Figs 8.2–8.5)

The wedge-shaped liver presents two well-defined surfaces, diaphragmatic and visceral and one well-defined border, inferior border. The **diaphragmatic surface** is convex and extensive. It faces upwards, forward, to the right and backwards. The **visceral surface** is relatively flat and faces inferiorly. These two surfaces meet in front at the sharp **inferior border**. Conventionally the diaphragmatic surface is further subdivided into superior, anterior, right lateral, and posterior surfaces, but there is no distinct demarcation between these surfaces (Fig. 8.2).

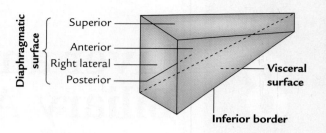

Fig. 8.2 Schematic diagram to show shape (wedge shaped) and surfaces of the liver.

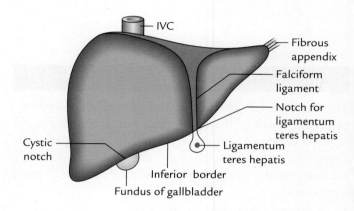

Fig. 8.3 Liver—viewed from the front.

Diaphragmatic Surface

The dome-shaped diaphragmatic surface includes smooth peritoneal areas which face superiorly, anteriorly and to the right and a rough bare area (devoid of the peritoneum) which faces posteriorly.

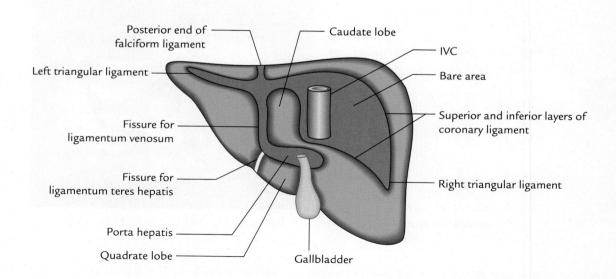

Fig. 8.4 Liver—viewed from behind.

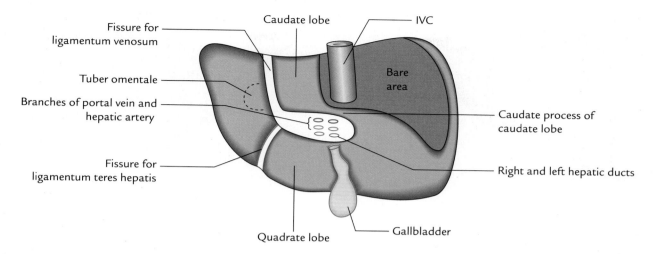

Fig. 8.5 Liver—viewed from below.

- The inferior vena cava (IVC) is embedded in the *deep sulcus* in the left part of the bare area. In most cases, this sulcus is roofed by the fibrous tissue termed *ligament of IVC* which may contain hepatic tissue converting the sulcus into the tunnel.
- The peritoneal ligaments are coronary, left and right triangular and falciform ligaments.

Visceral Surface (Inferior Surface)

The visceral surface is relatively flat or concave. It is directed downward, backward, and to the left. It is separated in front from the diaphragmatic surface by the sharp inferior border and behind from the diaphragm by the posterior layer of coronary ligament. The *notable features* on the visceral surface are:

- Fossa for the gallbladder.
- Fissure for the ligamentum teres hepatis.
- Porta hepatis.

The visceral surface is covered by the peritoneum except at the *fossa for gallbladder* and the porta hepatis.

The notable features of diaphragmatic and visceral surfaces of the liver are summarized in detail in Table 8.1.

Table 8.1 Notable features on diaphragmatic and visceral surfaces of the liver

Surface	Features
Diaphragmatic surface	• Bare area of the liver • Groove for inferior vena cava • Fissure for ligamentum venosum • Attachment of coronary, right, and left triangular and falciform ligaments
Visceral surface	• Fissure for ligamentum teres hepatis • Porta hepatis • Fossa for gallbladder

Inferior Border

The features of the inferior border are as follows:

1. It separates the diaphragmatic surface from the visceral surface.
2. It is rounded laterally where it separates the right lateral surface from the inferior surface.
3. It is thin and sharp medially where it separates the anterior surface from the inferior surface.
4. It presents two notches:
    (a) *Notch for ligamentum teres* or *interlobar notch:* It is located just to the right of the median plane.
    (b) *Cystic notch:* It is located about 5 cm to the right of the median plane and often corresponds to the fundus of the gallbladder.
5. In the epigastrium, it extends from the right 9th costal cartilage to the 8th left costal cartilage, thus it ascends sharply to the left.
6. In the median plane, it lies in the transpyloric plane.

LOBES OF THE LIVER

The lobes of the liver are classified into two types: (a) anatomical lobes and (b) physiological (functional) lobes.

Anatomical Lobes (Fig. 8.6)

- On the *diaphragmatic surface,* the liver is divided into two lobes, right and left, by the attachment of the falciform ligament (Fig. 8.6A). The right lobe which forms the base of the wedge-shaped liver is approximately six times larger than the **left lobe**.
- On the *visceral surface,* the liver is divided into four lobes: (a) right lobe, (b) left lobe, (c) quadrate lobe, and (d) caudate lobe by fissures and fossae present on this

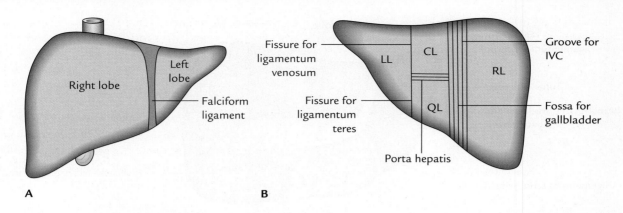

Fig. 8.6 Anatomical lobes of the liver: **A**, on the diaphragmatic surface of the liver; **B**, on the visceral surface of the liver (RL = right lobe, LL = left lobe, CL = caudate lobe, QL = quadrate lobe).

surface (Viz. fissures for ligamentum teres and ligamentum venosum, porta hepatis, groove of the IVC and fossa for the gallbladder). These fissures and fossae form an H-shaped figure (Fig. 8.6B).

(a) **Right lobe** to right of the fossa for gallbladder.

(b) Left lobe to the left of the fissures for ligamentum teres and ligamentum venosum.

(c) **Quadrate lobe,** between the fossa for gallbladder and the fissure for ligamentum teres below the porta hepatis.

(d) **Caudate lobe,** between the groove for IVC and the fissure for ligamentum venosum above the porta hepatis.

N.B. The anatomical lobes demarcated by surface features only serve as useful landmarks but they are not true lobes as they do not correspond to the internal architecture of the liver.

Physiological Lobes/Functional Lobes/True Lobes (Fig. 8.7)

The division of the liver into lobes is based on the intrahepatic distribution of branches of the bile ducts, hepatic artery, and portal vein.

The liver is divided into right and left physiological lobes by an imaginary sagittal plane/line (**Cantlie's plane/line**). **On the posteroinferior surface** this plane passes through the fossa for gallbladder, to the groove for IVC. (*Note:* Caudate lobe is equally shared between the right and left lobes.) **On the anterosuperior surface** of the liver, this plane passes from the IVC to the cystic notch present a little to the right of the falciform ligament.

The physiological right and left lobes are approximately equal in size.

Each true lobe of the liver has its own *primary branch* of the hepatic artery and portal vein and is drained by its own hepatic duct.

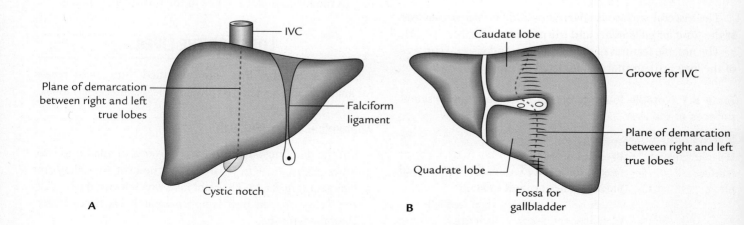

Fig. 8.7 True/physiological lobes of the liver: **A**, plane of demarcation on anterosuperior surface; **B**, visceral surface is shown by the interrupted redline.

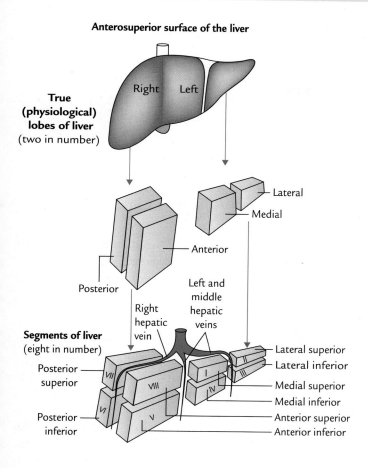

Anterosuperior surface of the liver

True (physiological) lobes of liver (two in number)

Segments of liver (eight in number)

Fig. 8.8 Segments of the liver.

HEPATIC SEGMENTS (SEGMENTS OF THE LIVER)

These are structural units of the liver (Fig. 8.8). There are eight hepatic segments. They are deduced as follows (Fig. 8.8).

The right physiological lobe is divided into anterior and posterior parts, and the left physiological lobe into medial and lateral parts.

Each of these parts is further divided into upper and lower parts and form eight surgically resectable hepatic segments. The veins draining the hepatic segments are intersegmental, i.e., they drain more than one segment.

On the surface of the liver, there is no identifiable demarcation between anterior and posterior segments of the right lobe. The fissures for ligamentum teres and ligamentum venosum mark the junction between the medial and lateral segments of the left lobe. The caudate and *quadrate lobes* are incorporated into the upper and lower areas of the medial segment of left lobe.

N.B. The caudate lobe is regarded as a separate special segment by many authorities because it is drained by both right and left hepatic ducts and supplied by both right and left branches of the hepatic artery and portal vein.

Couinaud's segments: According to nomenclature of Couinaud, the hepatic segments are numbered I to VIII (Fig. 8.8), I to IV in the left hemiliver and V to VIII in the right hemiliver. According to this nomenclature, the segment I corresponds to the caudate lobe and segment IV corresponds to the quadrate lobe.

Segment I to IV of the left lobe are supplied by the left branch of hepatic artery, left branch of portal vein and drained by left hepatic duct. The segments V to VIII of right lobe are supplied by right hepatic artery, right branch of portal vein and drained by right hepatic duct.

Clinical correlation

Segmental resection of liver: The hepatic segments are not well defined as the bronchopulmonary segments. The anatomy of hepatic segments is still of controversial usefulness in partial resection of the liver. Therefore, a true lobe rather than a segment should be resected in most instances of partial hepatectomy.

A large volume of liver (80%) can be removed safely because healthy hepatocytes have great capacity of regeneration.

The liver can regrow to its original size within 6–12 months.

PERITONEAL RELATIONS

Most of the liver is covered by the peritoneum. The areas which are not covered by the peritoneum are:

1. *Bare area of the liver:* It is a triangular area on the posterior aspect of the right lobe (details on p. 115).
2. *Fossa for gallbladder,* on the inferior surface of the liver between right and quadrate lobes.
3. *Groove for IVC,* on the posterior surface of the right lobe of the liver.
4. *Groove for ligamentum venosum.*
5. *Porta hepatis.*

LIGAMENTS

Ligaments of the liver are of two types: (a) false and (b) true.

False Ligaments

The false ligaments are actually peritoneal folds and include:

1. Falciform ligament.
2. Coronary ligament.
3. Right triangular ligament.
4. Left triangular ligament.
5. Lesser omentum.

Falciform Ligament

It is a sickle-shaped fold of the peritoneum connecting the liver to the undersurface of the diaphragm and the anterior abdominal wall up to the umbilicus (see details on page 83).

Coronary Ligament

It is a triangular fold of the peritoneum connecting the bare area of the liver to the diaphragm. It consists of two layers—upper and lower. The upper layer is reflected from the diaphragm to the liver whereas the lower layer is reflected from the liver to the upper end of the kidney.

1. *When traced on the right side*, the layers are continuous with the right triangular ligament.
2. *When traced on the left side*, the upper layer is continuous with the right layer of the falciform ligament and the lower layer is continuous with the peritoneal reflection along the right border of the caudate lobe.

Right Triangular Ligament

It is a small triangular fold of the peritoneum which connects the right lateral surface of the liver to the diaphragm. It encloses the apex of the bare area of liver.

Left Triangular Ligament

It is a very-very small triangular fold of the peritoneum which connects the upper surface of the left lobe to the diaphragm.

1. *When traced to the left side*, both layers come close to each other to form a free margin.
2. *When traced to the right side*, the upper layer is continuous with the left layer of the falciform ligament and the lower layer becomes continuous with the anterior layer of the lesser omentum along the left margin of the fissure for ligamentum venosum.

Lesser Omentum

It is the fold of peritoneum connecting the lesser curvature of the stomach and proximal 1 inch (2.5 cm) of duodenum to the visceral surface of the liver. The hepatic attachment is J-shaped with vertical limb being attached to the margins of fissure for ligamentum venosum and horizontal limb being attached to the margins/lips of porta hepatis (see details on page 81).

True Ligaments

The true ligaments are actually the remnants of fetal structures and include:

1. Ligamentum teres hepatis.
2. Ligamentum venosum.

Ligamentum Teres Hepatis

It is the remnant of the obliterated left umbilical vein and extends from the umbilicus to the left branch of the portal vein.

Ligamentum Venosum

It is the remnant of the obliterated ductus venosus which in fetal life connects the left branch of the portal vein with the IVC.

RELATIONS

Diaphragmatic Surface

Superior Surface

1. The convex right and left parts of this surface fit into the corresponding domes of the diaphragm, which separate them from the corresponding lung and pleura.
2. The central depressed area of this surface is related to the central tendon of the diaphragm, which separates it from the pericardium of the heart. Hence, this area is often termed *cardiac impression.*

Anterior Surface

It is related to the xiphoid process and anterior abdominal wall in the median plane and diaphragm on each side. The falciform ligament is attached to this surface a little to the right of the median plane.

Right Lateral Surface

It is related to the diaphragm opposite 7th to 11th ribs in the midaxillary line. Through the diaphragm:

1. **Upper one-third** of this surface is related to both the lung and the pleura (remember the lung extends up to the 8th rib).
2. **Middle one-third** of this surface is related to the costodiaphragmatic recess of pleura (remember the pleura extends up to the 10th rib).
3. **Lower one-third** of this surface is related to 10th and 11th ribs (i.e., it is related neither to the lung nor to the pleura).

N.B. For taking biopsy of the liver, the needle is inserted in the midaxillary line in 9th or 10th intercostal space to avoid injury to the lung (for details, see *Clinical and Surgical Anatomy,* 2nd Edition by Vishram Singh).

Posterior Surface (Fig. 8.9)

This surface presents: bare area of the liver, groove for IVC, caudate lobe, fissure for ligamentum venosum, and posterior surface of the left lobe.

1. The **bare area of the liver** is a triangular area to the right of groove for the IVC between the two layers of coronary and right triangular ligaments. It is in direct contact with the diaphragm. The right suprarenal gland is related to the inferomedial part of this area, i.e., near the groove for IVC.
2. The **groove for IVC** as the name indicates lodges the IVC. Its floor is pierced by the hepatic veins.
3. The **caudate lobe** is related to the superior recess of the lesser sac.

N.B. The caudate lobe presents two processes: a **papillary process**, which arises from its left side, and a **caudate process** above the porta hepatis, which connects it to the rest of the liver.

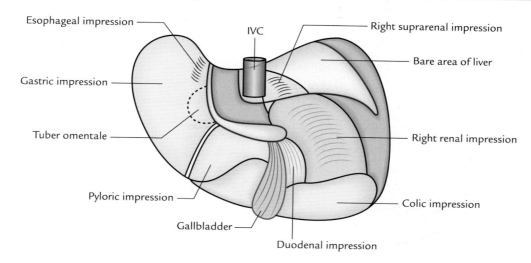

Fig. 8.9 Visceral relations of the liver (relations of the inferior/visceral surface of the liver).

4. The fissure for ligamentum venosum is a deep cleft to the left of the caudate lobe. The ligamentum venosum lies in its floor.
5. The posterior surface of the left lobe is related to the abdominal part of the esophagus, just to the left of the upper part of fissure for ligamentum venosum and causes esophageal impression. The fundus of the stomach is related just to the left of the esophageal impression.

Visceral Surface (Inferior Surface; Fig. 8.9)

1. The *inferior surface of the left lobe* is related to the anterosuperior surface of the stomach, which produces a *gastric impression*. Near the left side of the fissure for ligamentum venosum, this surface presents a slight elevation that comes in contact with the lesser omentum. Hence, it is called *tuber omentale/omental tuberosity.*
2. The *fissure for ligamentum teres* is a deep cleft to the left of the quadrate lobe. The ligamentum teres lies in its floor.
3. The *inferior surface of the right lobe* presents three prominent features: quadrate lobe, fossa for gallbladder, and porta hepatis. The relations of the inferior surface are:
   (a) The *quadrate lobe* is related to the pyloric end of the stomach and the first part of the duodenum.
   (b) The *fossa for gallbladder* lies to the right of the quadrate lobe, occupied by the gallbladder with its cystic duct close to the right end of the porta hepatis.
   (c) The *right colic flexure* is related to the inferior surface to the right of the gallbladder near the inferior margin and produces colic impression.
   (d) The *junction of first and second parts of the duodenum* is related to the right upper part of the fossa for gallbladder and adjoining part of the right lobe and produces the duodenal impression.
   (e) The *right kidney* is related to the inferior surface posterior to the colic impression and to the right

of the duodenal impression and causes renal impression.

N.B. *Porta hepatis* (gateway of the liver) is a horizontal fissure on the inferior surface of the liver between the quadrate lobe and the caudate lobe. The main structures entering the porta hepatis are right and left branches of the hepatic artery and portal vein, and the main structures leaving the porta hepatis are right and left hepatic ducts. They lie in the order from posterior to anterior as vein, artery, and duct (VAD). Also present in the porta hepatis are lymph nodes and nerves of the liver.

The relations of diaphragmatic and visceral surfaces of the liver are summarized in Table 8.2.

Clinical correlation

- **Surgical importance of the bare area of the liver:** The bare area of the liver is indirect contact with the diaphragm, which separates it from the right pleural cavity. Surgically, it is important because it encloses the **right extraperitoneal subphrenic space**. In amoebic hepatitis, the pus may collect in this space and form a subphrenic abscess which may burst into the right pleural cavity through the diaphragm.
  A potential anastomosis of venous capillaries exists in the region of bare area between the liver and the diaphragm. It becomes functional under certain pathological conditions (e.g., portal hypertension).
- **Needle biopsy of the liver (Fig. 8.10):** In needle biopsy of the liver, the needle is inserted in the midaxillary line through 9th or 10th intercostal space. The needle passes through the chest wall, costodiaphragmatic recess of the pleura, diaphragm, and right anterior intraperitoneal space to enter the liver. Needle inserted above the 8th intercostal space will injure the lung.

Table 8.2 Relations of diaphragmatic and visceral surfaces of the liver

Surface		Relations
Diaphragmatic surface (parietal surface)	**Superior surface** with diaphragm intervening	• Corresponding lung and pleura on either side • Pericardium and heart in the centre
	Anterior surface	• Xiphoid process • Anterior abdominal wall
	Right lateral surface with diaphragm intervening	• Lung and pleura in the upper one-third • Costodiaphragmatic recess in the middle one-third • 10th and 11th ribs in the lower one-third
	Posterior surface: (a) with peritoneum intervening (b) with peritoneum not intervening	• Abdominal part of the esophagus • Right suprarenal gland • Inferior vena cava
Visceral surface (inferior surface)	(a) with peritoneum intervening (b) with peritoneum not intervening	• Stomach • Duodenum • Right colic flexure • Right kidney • Gallbladder

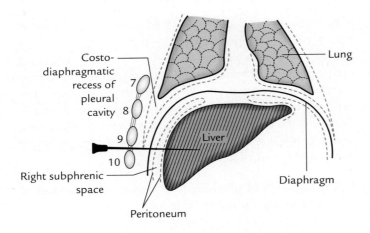

Fig. 8.10 Needle biopsy of the liver.

BLOOD SUPPLY

The liver is a highly vascular organ. It receives blood from two sources. The arterial blood (oxygenated) is supplied by the hepatic artery and venous blood (rich in nutrients) is supplied by the portal vein. In a normal adult (in the recumbent position), nearly one-third of the cardiac output passes through the liver. About 80% of this is delivered through the portal vein and 20% is delivered through the hepatic artery.

VENOUS DRAINAGE

Most of the venous blood from liver is drained by three large hepatic veins: (a) **left hepatic vein** between medial and lateral segments of the left true lobe, (b) **middle hepatic** vein between true right and left true lobes, and (c) **right hepatic**

vein between anterior and posterior segments of the right true lobe. These veins do not have the extrahepatic course. They emerge in the upper part of the groove for IVC and open directly in the IVC, just below the central tendon of the diaphragm. The three veins may enter the IVC independently but the left and middle veins usually join, so that only two major veins join the IVC.

N.B.

• The middle hepatic vein lies in the sagittal plane that divides the liver into true right and left lobes. Therefore, it is a useful landmark in radiological and ultrasonographic investigations.

• In addition to three large hepatic veins, several small accessory veins including a separate vein from the caudate lobe emerge in the lower part of the groove for IVC and open into the IVC.

• The hepatic veins are intersegmental (vide supra).

LYMPHATIC DRAINAGE

A network of **superficial lymphatics** exists in the capsule of the liver underneath the peritoneum. The **superficial lymphatics** from the **posterior aspect of the liver** converge toward the bare area of the liver and communicate with the extraperitoneal lymphatics which perforate the diaphragm and drain into the **posterior mediastinal lymph nodes**. The **superficial lymphatics from the anterior aspect of the liver** drain into three or four nodes that lie in the porta hepatis (**hepatic nodes**). The nodes also receive the lymphatics from the gallbladder. Efferents from these nodes run downward along the hepatic artery to coeliac nodes.

The lymphatics accompanying the portal triads constitute the **deep lymphatics**. The deep lymphatics form two trunks. The ascending trunk enters the thorax through the vena caval opening and terminates in the nodes around the IVC. The descending trunk empties in hepatic nodes located in the porta hepatis.

NERVE SUPPLY

The liver is supplied by both sympathetic and parasympathetic fibres. The sympathetic fibres are derived from the coeliac plexus. They run along the vessels in the free margin of the lesser omentum and enter the porta hepatis.

The parasympathetic fibres are derived from the hepatic branch of the anterior vagal trunk, which reaches the porta hepatis through the lesser omentum.

Pain occurring due to distension of the hepatic capsule and hepatic peritoneum due to inflammation and swelling of the liver (hepatitis) run along the sympathetic fibres. The pain is often referred to the epigastrium and sometimes to the shoulder.

FACTORS KEEPING THE LIVER IN POSITION

These are as follows:

1. **Hepatic veins** connecting the liver to the IVC.
2. **Intra-abdominal pressure** maintained by the tone of abdominal muscles.
3. **Peritoneal ligaments** connecting the liver to the abdominal walls.

MICROSCOPIC STRUCTURE

In a classical description, the liver consists of hexagonal lobules (classical liver lobules) made up of anastomosing cords of hepatocytes radiating away from the central vein, a radicle of hepatic vein. At the periphery of the lobules in the corners of hexagon are portal triads/tracts. Each triad contains three structures viz. radicle of bile duct (hepatic ductal), hepatic artery (hepatic arteriole), and portal vein (portal venule) (Fig. 8.11A). The plates/cords of hepatocytes are separated by vascular spaces called **sinusoids** which connect the portal vein of the triad to the central vein of the lobule. The blood flow in the sinusoids is from the periphery of the lobule toward the central vein.

The sinusoids intervening between the cords of hepatocytes are lined by endothelial cells, which present frequent intercellular spaces/fenestrations. The fenestrations allow plasma (but not the blood cells) to leave the sinusoids and enter the perisinusoidal spaces (spaces of Disse) between the endothelial lining and hepatocytes. Many of the cells of endothelial lining are capable of phagocytic activities (**Kupffer cells**).

The bile produced by hepatocytes first enters the bile canaliculi situated between the opposite sides of adjacent hepatocytes. The bile canaliculi drain into the *bile ductules* of the portal triads which in turn unite to form the larger intrahepatic ducts.

The portal triads are embedded in the perilobular connective tissue which pervades the liver and is continuous with the capsule of the organ.

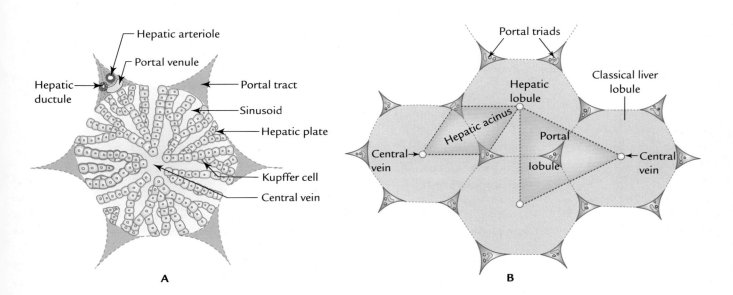

A

B

Fig. 8.11 A, classical liver lobule; B, functional units of liver, viz. portal lobule and hepatic acinus. (*Source*: A. Fig. 12.14, Page 239, *Textbook of Histology and a Practical Guide*, JP Gunasegaran. Copyright Elsevier 2010, All rights reserved. B. Fig. 12.17, Page 241, *Textbook of Histology and a Practical Guide*, JP Gunasegaran. Copyright Elsevier 2010, All rights reserved.)

N.B. To study certain pathological conditions, it is useful to divide liver into functional units called portal lobules and hepatic acini.

- The **portal lobule** is a triangular unit/area of liver parenchyma bounded by three adjacent central veins. It includes the portions of three classical lobules with portal triad in the centre (Fig. 8.11B).
- The **liver acinus/hepatic acinus** is a diamond-shaped unit/area of liver parenchyma. It includes portions of two classical liver lobules with portal triad at each side of elliptical area and central vein on each end (Fig. 8.11B).

Clinical correlation

Cirrhosis of the liver: The hepatocytes sometimes may undergo necrosis following their injury and death caused by infection, toxins, alcohol, and poisons. The dead hepatocytes are replaced by fibrous tissue by the proliferation of the perilobular connective tissue. The resultant hepatic fibrosis is clinically termed *cirrhosis of the liver*. The patient develops jaundice due to obstruction of bile flow. Resistance to blood flow through cirrhotic liver is increased which leads to increase of pressure in the radicles of portal vein in the triads. Since portal vein and its tributaries are devoid of valves, the increased venous pressure in the portal vein causes engorgement and distension of all its tributaries, as well as of spleen. This clinical condition is called **portal hypertension**.

DEVELOPMENT

The liver develops from a diverticulum (**hepatic bud**) from the distal end of the foregut. The hepatic bud elongates cranially and gives rise to a small accessory bud on its right side called **pars cystica** which forms cystic duct and gallbladder. The main bud called **pars hepatica** grows into the septum transversum. It bifurcates and gives rise to right and left hepatic ducts and liver parenchyma. The septum transversum contains the vitelline veins and umbilical veins before the hepatic bud invades it. These vessels subdivide to form sinusoids which invade the liver parenchyma breaking it up into hepatic cords. The bile canaliculi and ductules are formed in the liver parenchyma and establish connections with the extrahepatic bile ducts at a later stage.

EXTRAHEPATIC BILIARY APPARATUS

The **extrahepatic biliary apparatus** receives the bile from liver, stores and concentrates it in the gallbladder, and transmits it to the second part of the duodenum when required.

It consists of five components (Fig. 8.12):

1. Right and left hepatic ducts.
2. Common hepatic duct.
3. Gallbladder.
4. Cystic duct.
5. Bile duct (formerly, common bile duct).

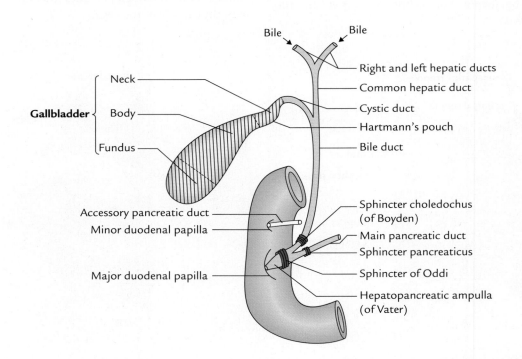

Fig. 8.12 Components of the extrahepatic biliary apparatus. *Note:* the sphincters around hepatopancreatic ampulla and terminal parts of the bile, and main pancreatic ducts.

The anatomical knowledge of the extrahepatic biliary apparatus is extremely important clinically because it is often affected in various disease processes such as cholecystitis (inflammation of gallbladder), cholelithiasis (formation of stones in the gallbladder), obstruction of common bile duct (CBD), etc. Further, it is frequently visualized by various imaging techniques.

HEPATIC DUCTS

The right and left hepatic ducts from the right and left lobes of the liver emerge through porta hepatis and unite near its right end to form the **common hepatic duct**, which passes downward for about 2.5 cm (1 inch) and then joined on its right side by the cystic duct to form the CBD. The angle between the cystic duct and the common hepatic duct is acute and is **called cystohepatic angle**. In the right free margin of the lesser omentum, the common hepatic duct lies on the right side of the hepatic artery proper, in front of the portal vein.

N.B. The accessory hepatic ducts are seen in about 15% of cases. They usually emerge from right lobe of the liver and may open in one of the following sites: (a) common hepatic duct, (b) cystic duct, (c) bile duct, and (d) gallbladder (Fig. 8.13).

GALLBLADDER

The gallbladder is an elongated pear-shaped sac of about 30–50 ml capacity. It stores and concentrates the bile and discharges it into the duodenum by its muscular contraction. Radiopaque substances, which are excreted in the bile, are also concentrated in it. Therefore, they are used to demonstrate radiographically (cholecystography) the cavity of gallbladder and its ability to concentrate and contract.

N.B. *Hormonal control of gallbladder emptying:* When the food rich in fat enters the duodenum, the duodenal cells

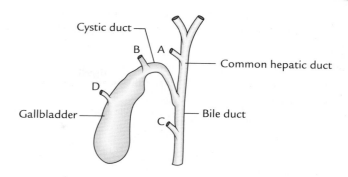

Fig. 8.13 Sites of termination of the accessory hepatic ducts.

liberate a hormone called cholecystokinin (CCK). This hormone is carried to the gallbladder and causes its contraction. There is a reflex mediation, when the gallbladder contracts, the sphincter of Oddi relax. Thus concentrated bile is emptied into the gallbladder.

Location (Fig. 8.14)

The gallbladder lies in the fossa for gallbladder on the inferior surface of the right lobe of the liver along the right edge of the quadrate lobe. It extends from the right extremity of porta hepatis to the inferior border of the liver. It is usually attached to the liver substance by connective tissue and has venous communications with it. But it may be suspended from the liver by a short mesentery, or partly buried in it.

Dimensions

Length: 10 cm.
Width: 3 cm (at its widest part).

Parts and Relations (Fig. 8.15)

The gallbladder is divided into the following three parts: fundus, body, and neck.

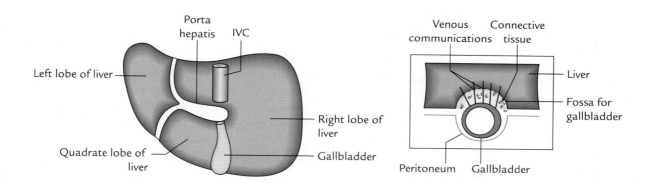

Fig. 8.14 Location of the gallbladder on the inferior surface of the right lobe of the liver. Figure in the inset on the right side shows connective tissue and venous communication between gallbladder and liver.

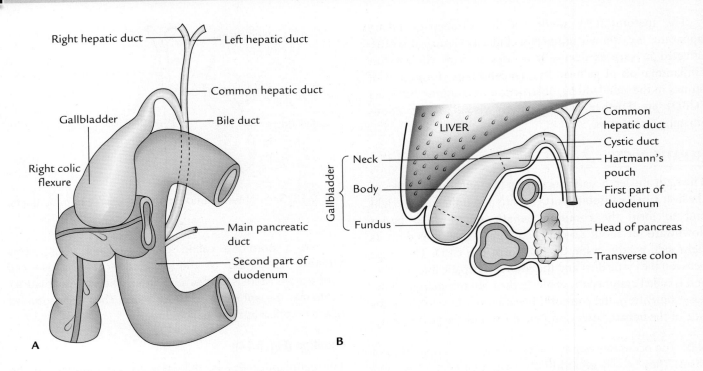

Fig. 8.15 Relations of the gallbladder: **A**, as seen from the front after removal of the liver; **B**, as seen in sagittal section through the gallbladder fossa.

Fundus

1. It is the expanded blind end of the organ. It projects from the inferior border of the liver and touches the anterior abdominal wall at the tip of the right 9th costal cartilage, deep to the point where the right linea semilunaris meets the costal margin.
2. It is completely surrounded by peritoneum.
3. It is related anteriorly to the anterior abdominal wall and posteriorly to the transverse colon.
4. It is continuous through the body of the gallbladder with the narrow neck.

Body

1. It is directed upward, backward, and to the left to join the neck at the right end of the porta hepatis.
2. Its upper surface is related directly to the liver and is devoid of the peritoneum.
3. Its undersurface is covered by the peritoneum and is related to the second part of the duodenum.

Neck

1. It is the narrow upper end of the gallbladder lying near the right end of the porta hepatis.
2. It joins the cystic duct and its junction with this duct is marked by a constriction.
3. It is attached to the liver by loose areolar tissue in which cystic artery is embedded.

4. It is related inferiorly to the first part of the duodenum.
5. Its posteromedial wall shows a pouch-like dilatation (**Hartmann's pouch**) directed downward and backward.
6. The gall stones lodged in this pouch may cause adhesion with the first part of the duodenum and may perforate it.
7. The neck turns sharply downward to become continuous with the cystic duct.

Structure of the Gallbladder

The wall of the gallbladder consists of the following layers:

1. Serous layer of the peritoneum.
2. Subserous layer of the loose areolar tissue.
3. Fibromuscular layer of the fibrous tissue mixed with smooth muscle fibres, which are arranged in loose bundles disposed in longitudinal, circular, and oblique directions.
4. Mucous membrane is loosely connected with the fibrous layer and is elevated into minute rugae which give it a **honeycomb** appearance. The epithelium lining consists of a single layer of tall columnar cells.

Arterial Supply (Fig. 8.16)

The gallbladder is supplied by the cystic artery (a branch of right hepatic artery). It may arise from the main trunk of the hepatic artery, from the left hepatic artery, or from the gastroduodenal artery.

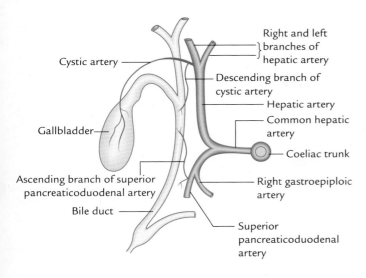

Fig. 8.16 Blood supply of the gallbladder and bile duct.

Venous Drainage

The venous drainage of the gallbladder is twofold (a) by the cystic vein, which drains into the portal vein and (b) by a number of small veins, which pass from the superior surface of the gallbladder to the liver through the gallbladder bed to drain into the hepatic veins.

Lymphatic Drainage

1. The majority of lymph vessels from the gallbladder drain into (a) the **cystic lymph node** of Lund, located in the **Calot's triangle** and (b) the node alongside the upper part of the bile duct (node at the anterior border of epiploic foramen), which finally drains into the coeliac group of lymph nodes.
2. Few lymph vessels from the upper surface of gallbladder directly communicate with subscapular lymph vessels of the liver.

N.B. Cystic node is constantly enlarged in cholecystitis.

Nerve Supply

The gallbladder receives its nerve supply via cystic plexus formed by the sympathetic fibres (T7–T9), parasympathetic fibres (right and left vagus nerve), and fibres of the right phrenic nerve.

Clinically, gallbladder pain is referred to (i) the inferior angle of the right scapula by sympathetic fibres, (ii) the tip of the right shoulder via the right phrenic nerve, and (iii) the stomach by vagus.

CYSTIC DUCT

1. The cystic duct is about 3–5 cm long and runs backward and downward from the neck of the gallbladder to run

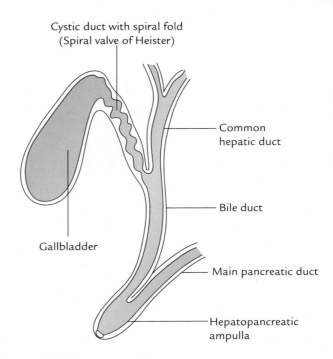

Fig. 8.17 Spiral valve of Heister.

in the lesser omentum with common hepatic duct and joins it at an acute angle to form the bile duct.
2. Its junction with common hepatic duct is usually situated immediately below the porta hepatis.
3. The mucous membrane lining the interior of the cystic duct is thrown into a series of crescentic folds (5–10 in number). They project into the lumen in a spiral fashion forming a **spiral fold called "spiral valve (of Heister; Fig. 8.17)."**

The valve of Heister keeps the duct open so that bile can pass through it both in and out of the gallbladder.

When the CBD is closed at its inferior end, the bile secreted by the liver fills the duct and passes through the cystic duct into the gallbladder.

When the CBD is open, the bile flows into it from the common hepatic and cystic ducts.

The flow of bile is augmented by the contraction of the gallbladder. It is coordinated by the relaxation of sphincter of CBD under the influence of **cholecystokinin**, a hormone released by the duodenal mucosa.

BILE DUCT/COMMON BILE DUCT (CBD)

Formation

It is formed near the porta hepatis by the union of cystic and common hepatic ducts. It is usually 7.5 cm (3 inches) long and about 6 mm in diameter.

Parts

It is divided into four parts (Fig. 8.18):

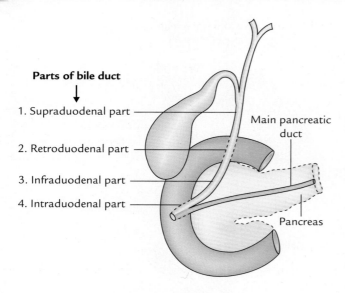

Parts of bile duct
↓

1. Supraduodenal part
2. Retroduodenal part
3. Infraduodenal part
4. Intraduodenal part

Main pancreatic duct

Pancreas

Fig. 8.18 Parts of the bile duct (dark green colour).

1. Supraduodenal part.
2. Retroduodenal part.
3. Infraduodenal (or pancreatic) part.
4. Intraduodenal part.

Supraduodenal Part

It is about 2.5 cm long and descends in the right free margin of the lesser omentum to the right of the hepatic artery proper and anterior to the portal vein.

Retroduodenal Part

It descends behind the first part of the duodenum with the gastroduodenal artery on its left and IVC on its posterior aspect.

Infraduodenal (Pancreatic) Part

It runs in the groove on the upper and lateral parts of the posterior surface of the pancreas and is sometimes completely embedded in the pancreatic tissue. Here it lies in front of the IVC from which it is separated by a thin layer of pancreatic tissue.

It is accompanied on its left side by the gastroduodenal artery, which gives origin to the superior pancreaticoduodenal artery.

The superior pancreaticoduodenal artery crosses the bile duct either anteriorly or posteriorly. Clinically it is a source of hemorrhage in the exposure of infraduodenal part of the bile duct. Near the middle second part of the duodenum, it comes in contact with the pancreatic duct.

Intraduodenal (or Intramural) Part

It enters the posteromedial surface of the descending (second) part of the duodenum a little below to its middle. The main pancreatic duct also enters the wall of the duodenum at the same site. The two ducts run obliquely in the wall of the duodenum and unite to form an expansion, the *hepatopancreatic ampulla* (or **ampulla of Vater**), which bulges the mucous membrane of duodenum inward forming the **major duodenal papilla**. The distal constricted end of this ampulla opens on the summit of the major duodenal papilla 8–10 cm distal to the pylorus.

Sphincters Around the Terminal Parts of Bile and Pancreatic Ducts and Ampulla

The intramural parts (terminal parts) of bile and pancreatic ducts as well as ampulla are surrounded by **smooth muscle** sphincters (Fig. 8.12). The sphincter around the bile duct is called **sphincter choledochus** (of Boyden), the sphincter around the pancreatic duct is called **sphincter pancreaticus**, and the sphincter around the ampulla is known as **sphincter ampullae** (of Oddi). The three sphincters are independent of duodenal musculature. The sphincters remain closed until the gastric contents enter the duodenum, stimulating its mucosa to release a hormone called cholecystokinin. This hormone in addition to causing contraction of the gallbladder relaxes these sphincters allowing bile and pancreatic secretions to enter the duodenum.

Arterial Supply of the Bile Duct/Common Bile Duct (Fig. 8.16)

The upper part of bile duct is supplied by a twig from the descending branch of cystic artery while its lower part is supplied by the ascending branch of the superior pancreaticoduodenal artery.

> **Clinical correlation**
>
> Arterial supply of the common bile duct (CBD) is clinically important because if the anastomosis between the superior and inferior pancreaticoduodenal arteries is poor, the ligation of superior pancreaticoduodenal artery during surgery can lead to gangrene of the common bile duct.

CYSTOHEPATIC TRIANGLE OF CALOT

The **cystohepatic triangle** (Fig. 8.19) is bounded on the right side by the cystic duct, on the left side by common hepatic duct, and above by inferior surface of the liver. The apex of triangle faces downward between the cystic and common hepatic ducts. The *contents of the triangle* are right hepatic artery, cystic artery, and cystic lymph node of Lund. It is in this triangle that most of aberrant segmental right hepatic ducts and arteries are usually encountered. The accessory hepatic ducts terminate either into the gallbladder or into the common hepatic duct or even into the bile duct, and are

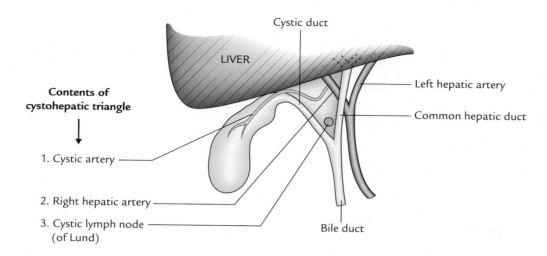

Cystic duct

LIVER

Left hepatic artery

Common hepatic duct

Contents of cystohepatic triangle

↓

1. Cystic artery

2. Right hepatic artery

3. Cystic lymph node (of Lund)

Bile duct

Fig. 8.19 Boundaries and contents of the cystohepatic triangle (yellow-coloured area).

responsible for oozing of bile from the wound after cholecystectomy.

The identification of cystohepatic triangle and its contents helps the surgeon to locate the pedicle of gallbladder and its ligation in **cholecystectomy.** The errors in gallbladder surgery often occur from failure to appreciate the common variations of the extrahepatic biliary system. This occurs especially when the right hepatic artery in this triangle presents a caterpillar-like loop called **Moynihan's hump (Fig. 8.20)**, which may be inadvertently clamped, ligated along with cystic pedicle, and cut leading to profuse bleeding.

N.B. The **cystic node of Lund** (a solitary node) present in the apical part of this triangle receives most of the lymph from gallbladder and is constantly found enlarged in **cholecystitis.**

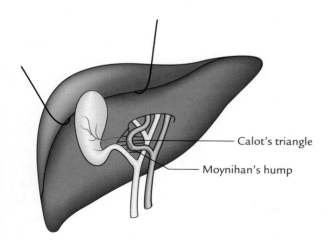

Calot's triangle

Moynihan's hump

Fig. 8.20 Moynihan's hump.

- **Cholecystitis:** The cholecystitis is the inflammation of the gallbladder. It may be acute or chronic.
  (a) Acute cholecystitis: It occurs usually in adult women and is characterized by (i) sudden pain in the hypochondrium referred to the inferior angle of the right scapula or to the tip of right shoulder, (ii) vomiting, and (iii) positive Murphy's sign—if the finger is pressed under the right costal margin at the tip of the 9th costal cartilage when the patient is asked to take a deep breath, she/he feels sharp *pain* and winces with a "catch" in the breath as the diseased gallbladder meets the examining finger.

    The symptoms of cholecystitis are aggravated on taking fatty meals because the gallbladder contracts to pour the bile into the duodenum when fat reaches the duodenum. Fat in the duodenum induces liberation of a local hormone cholecystokinin–pancreozymin (CCK-PZ), which reaches the gallbladder through the blood stream and stimulates its contraction.
  (b) **Chronic cholecystitis usually leads to formation of stones in the gallbladder (cholelithiasis):** It usually occurs typically in fat, fertile, flatulous female of forty (5F).
- **Referred pain of gallbladder:** In acute cholecystitis, the inflammation of the gallbladder may cause irritation of the subdiaphragmatic parietal peritoneum, which is supplied in part by the phrenic nerve (C3, C4, and C5 spinal segments). This may lead to referred pain over the tip of the right shoulder for being supplied by the supraclavicular nerves (C3 and C4 spinal segments).
- **Biliary colic:** It is usually caused by the spasm of smooth muscle of the gallbladder wall in an attempt to expel the gallstone. It is intermittent and is most intense when stone (calculus) is impacted either at the terminal end of cystic duct or at the lower end of the bile duct because the smooth muscle everywhere in the biliary duct system is

sparse except at the terminal portions of the cystic and bile ducts. The afferent fibres from the gallbladder enter the thoracic segments of spinal cord (T7–T9), hence referred pain is felt in the right upper quadrant or epigastrium (T7–T9) dermatomes.

- **Obstruction of CBD:** The obstruction of CBD usually occurs due to gallstones, pancreatic carcinoma, or enlarged neoplastic hepatic lymph nodes. It causes obstruction to bile flow, which leads to jaundice.
- **Courvoisier's law:** This law states that the *obstructive jaundice* with *distended* and *palpable gallbladder* is most likely due to extrinsic obstruction of CBD (e.g., carcinoma of head of pancreas). On the contrary, *obstructive jaundice with non-distended, non-palpable gallbladder* is due to an intrinsic obstruction of CBD (e.g., impaction by gallstones) because in this case previous cholecystitis makes the gallbladder fibrotic and contracted.

IMAGING OF THE BILIARY TRACT

CHOLECYSTOGRAPHY

Gallbladder is not opaque to X-ray, but when certain radiopaque dyes are given by either mouth or intravenous injection they are excreted by the liver from blood into bile and reach the gallbladder. In the gallbladder, the dye is concentrated and thus the gallbladder becomes opaque to X-rays.

ULTRASOUND

The ultrasonography is a noninvasive imaging technique to visualize the gallbladder and other components of the biliary apparatus. This technique has largely replaced the cholecystography.

ENDOSCOPIC RETROGRADE CHOLANGIOPANCREATOGRAPHY (ERCP)

In this technique, under direct vision through a fibre-optic endoscope, a catheter is inserted into the hepatopancreatic ampulla and radiopaque contrast medium is injected, and bile and pancreatic ducts are visualized.

N.B. The bile and pancreatic ducts can now also be visualized by the noninvasive magnetic resonance imaging (MRI) technique.

Golden Facts to Remember

► Largest gland in the body	Liver
► Most obvious features on the diaphragmatic surface of the liver	Inferior vena cava and bare area of the liver
► Only part of the liver that is covered by the peritoneum of	Caudate lobe, the lesser sac
► Gateway of the liver	Porta hepatis
► Cantlie line/plane	Line/plane of demarcation between right and left true (physiological) lobes of the liver
► Most obvious feature on the visceral surface of the liver	Porta hepatis
► Fibrous appendix of the liver	Fibrous band at the left extremity of the liver representing the degenerate part of the left lobe
► Riedel's lobe	Tongue-like process projecting from the inferior border of the liver just to the right of the gallbladder

Clinical Case Study

A 55-year-old man, a chronic alcoholic, was admitted in the hospital with complaints of weakness, repeated episodes of vomiting blood, and pain in the right upper part of the abdomen. On physical examination, the doctor found jaundice, enlarged liver and spleen, and dilated tortuous veins radiating from the umbilicus. An ultrasound of the upper abdomen revealed fatty degeneration of the liver. He was diagnosed as a case of **cirrhosis of the liver.**

Questions

1. What is the cirrhosis of the liver and give its cause?
2. Give the reason of vomiting blood and mention its sources.
3. What is portal hypertension?
4. Name the term used by clinicians for dilated radiating veins around the umbilicus.

Answers

1. Following injury and death of hepatocytes (caused by alcohol, toxins, etc.), the liver parenchyma undergoes fatty degeneration and is replaced by fibrous tissue called **hepatic fibrosis/cirrhosis of liver.**
2. Rupture of esophageal varices formed due to portal hypertension.
3. Normal portal pressure is about 5–15 mmHg. The portal pressure of about 40 mmHg is called portal hypertension.
4. Caput medusae.

CHAPTER

9

Duodenum, Pancreas, and Portal Vein

DUODENUM

The duodenum is the first, shortest, widest, and the most fixed part of the small intestine. It extends from the pylorus to the duodenojejunal flexure. It was so named by Herophilus in 300 BC because its length was approximately equal to the combined width of 12 fingers.

The term "duodenum" is the Latin corruption of Greek word "do-deka-daktulos" meaning 12 fingers.

The duodenum is 10 inches (25 cm) long. It begins at the pylorus which lies on the transpyloric plane about 2.5 cm to the right of the median plane and ends at the duodenojejunal junction which lies about 2.5 cm to the left of the median plane and little below the transpyloric plane.

The duodenum is retroperitoneal except the proximal 2.5 cm, which is suspended above by the lesser omentum and below by the greater omentum.

The **main function** of the duodenum is digestion. It receives chyme from the stomach which is mixed with bile and pancreatic enzymes here.

SHAPE AND LOCATION (Fig. 9.1)

The duodenum is a "C"-shaped loop of the small intestine. The concavity of the duodenal loop encloses the head of pancreas.

The duodenum is located in the abdominal cavity above the level of the umbilicus opposite to the L1, L2, L3 vertebrae.

N.B. The duodenum along with the pancreas, which is closely related to it, is the most deeply located portion of the alimentary tract and the least accessible to physical examination.

PARTS AND RELATIONS

For descriptive purposes, the 25 cm long duodenum is divided into four parts (Fig. 9.2):
1. Superior (first) part, 5 cm (2 inches) long.

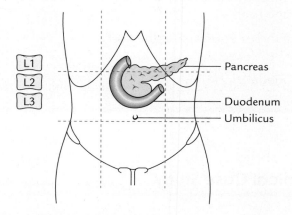

Fig. 9.1 Location of the duodenum.

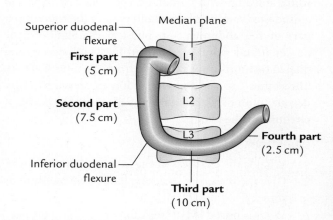

Fig. 9.2 Parts of the duodenum.

2. Descending (second) part, 7.5 cm (3 inches) long.
3. Horizontal (third) part, 10 cm (4 inches) long.
4. Ascending (fourth) part, 2.5 cm (1 inch) long.

FIRST PART

Course

It begins at the pylorus, passes upward, backward, and laterally to the right side of the vertebral column to reach the neck of the gallbladder, where it curves downward (**superior**

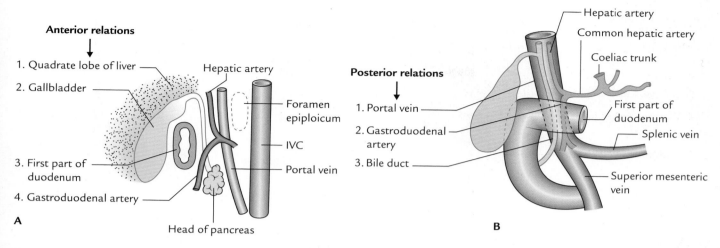

Fig. 9.3 Relations of the first part of the duodenum: **A,** anterior relations as seen in sectional view; **B,** posterior relations as seen from anterior aspect (IVC = inferior vena cava).

duodenal flexure) to become continuous with the second part of the duodenum.

Features

1. It develops from the foregut.
2. It is only partly retroperitoneal.
3. It is freely mobile and distensible.
4. It has no circular folds in the mucous membrane of its initial 2.5 cm—seen as the **duodenal cap** in barium meal radiographs.
5. It is the site for duodenal ulcer.
6. It is supplied by the branches of coeliac trunk/artery.

Relations (Fig. 9.3)

Anteriorly: Quadrate lobe of the liver and gallbladder.
Posteriorly: Portal vein, gastroduodenal artery, and common bile duct (CBD).
Superiorly: Epiploic foramen being separated from it by the portal vein and bile duct.
Inferiorly: Head and neck of the pancreas.

N.B. Peculiar features of the first part of the duodenum are:
- Only part (first inch of the first part) which is intraperitoneal hence freely movable.
- Only part supplied by end arteries.
- Only part which is devoid of circular mucus folds.

SECOND PART

Course

It begins at the superior duodenal flexure, passes downward, in front of the medial part of the right kidney, till the lower border of the L3 vertebra where it curves toward the left (**inferior duodenal flexure**) to become continuous with the third part.

Features

1. Its upper half develops from the foregut and lower half from the midgut.
2. It lies behind the transverse mesocolon.
3. It receives the bile duct, the chief and accessory pancreatic ducts.
4. It is the only part of the intestine supplied by double rows of vasa recta, arising from anterior and posterior pancreaticoduodenal arterial arcades.

Relations (Fig. 9.4)

Anteriorly: Gallbladder and right lobe of the liver, transverse colon, transverse mesocolon (commencement), and coils of the small intestine.
Posteriorly: Right kidney and right renal vessels, right edge of the inferior vena cava (IVC), and right psoas major muscle.
Medially: Head of the pancreas.
Laterally: From below upward, ascending colon, right colic flexure, and right lobe of the liver.

THIRD PART

Course

It runs horizontally to the left, across the lower part of the body of L3 vertebra, crosses in front of IVC, and then takes a smooth curve upward to become continuous with the ascending part of the duodenum.

Relations (Fig. 9.5)

Anteriorly: Root of the mesentery, superior mesenteric vessels, and coils of the jejunum.
Posteriorly: Right psoas major, right ureter, IVC, abdominal aorta, and right gonadal vessels.

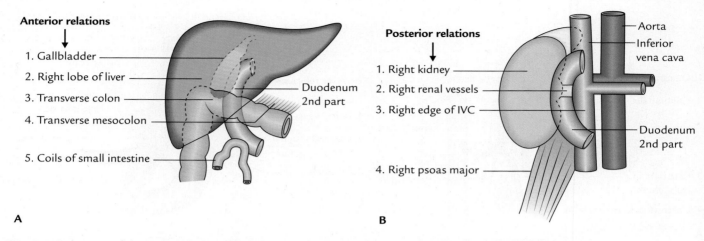

Fig. 9.4 Relations of the second part of the duodenum: A, anterior relations; B, posterior relations.

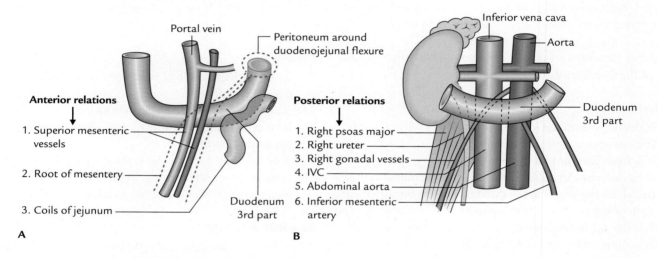

Fig. 9.5 Relations of the third part of the duodenum: A, anterior relations; B, posterior relations.

Superiorly: Head of the pancreas with its uncinate process.
Inferiorly: Coils of the jejunum.

FOURTH PART

Course

It runs upward, on or immediately to the left of the abdominal aorta, from the end of the third part to the upper border of the L2 vertebra where it turns forward (ventrally) to become continuous with the jejunum (**duodenojejunal flexure**).

Relations (Fig. 9.6)

Anteriorly: Transverse colon and transverse mesocolon.
Posteriorly: Left psoas major muscle, left sympathetic chain, left gonadal vessels, and inferior mesenteric vein.
Superiorly: Body of the pancreas.
On to the left: Left kidney and left ureter.
On to the right: Upper part of the root of mesentery.

INTERIOR OF THE DUODENUM

Being a part of the small intestine, the mucous membrane of the duodenum presents circular folds (**valves of Kerckring**), but they begin in the second part and become large and closely set below the level of the major duodenal papilla. In addition to this, the interior of the second part of the duodenum presents the following special features (Fig. 9.7):

1. **Major duodenal papilla:** It is a well-marked conical projection on the posteromedial wall and situated 8–10 cm distal to the pylorus. On its summit opens the common hepatopancreatic duct (formed by the union of bile and main pancreatic ducts).

2. **Minor duodenal papilla:** It is a small conical projection situated 2 cm proximal (and ventral) to the major duodenal papilla. The accessory pancreatic duct opens on its summit.

3. **Arch of plica semicircularis:** The plica semicircularis forms an arch above the major duodenal papilla like a hood (cf. monk's hood).

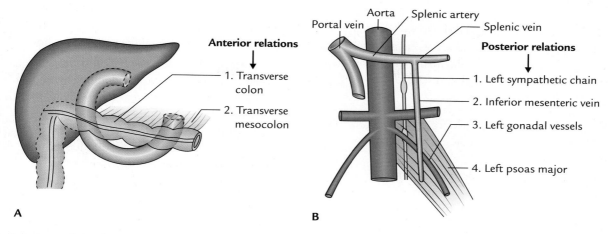

Fig. 9.6 Relations of the fourth part of the duodenum: **A**, anterior relations; **B**, posterior relations.

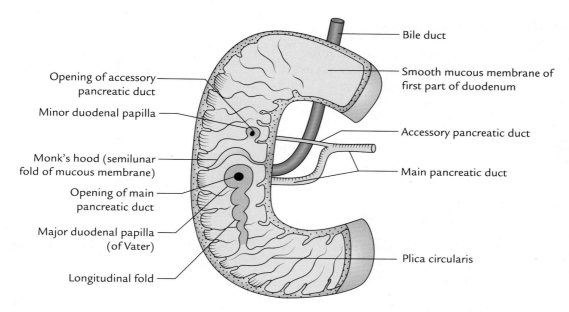

Fig. 9.7 Interior of the duodenum.

4. **Plica longitudinalis:** It is a vertical tortuous fold of the mucous membrane extending downward from the major duodenal papilla.

N.B. It is very important to recognize the major duodenal papilla because it is often catheterized under direct vision using a duodenal endoscope and a radiopaque material is filled in the bile and pancreatic ducts (for details, see page 124; endoscopic retrograde cholangiopancreatography).

SUSPENSORY MUSCLE OF DUODENUM (LIGAMENT OF TREITZ)

It is a *fibromuscular band*, which suspends the duodenojejunal flexure from the right crus of the diaphragm. Its upper end is attached on to the right crus of the diaphragm and the lower

end attached on to the posterior surface of the duodenojejunal flexure (Fig. 9.8). This band contains:

(a) Striated muscle fibres in the upper part.
(b) Elastic fibres in the middle part.
(c) Non-striated muscle fibres in the lower part.

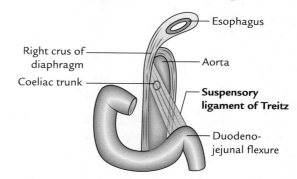

Fig. 9.8 Suspensory ligament of Treitz.

The ligament of Treitz fixes the duodenojejunal flexure and prevents it from being dragged down by the weight of loops of the small intestine. It also serves as an important landmark in the radiological diagnosis of incomplete rotation or malrotation of the small intestine.

N.B.

- Sometimes, the ligament of Treitz may kink the duodenojejunal flexure and may cause partial intestinal obstruction.
- The ligament of Treitz if short the duodenum will be O-shaped, and if long the duodenum will be reverse J-shaped. Thus, three shapes of the duodenum are recognized, viz., "C"-, "O"-, and "L"-shaped (i.e., reverse J-shaped).

DUODENAL RECESSES (FOSSAE)

In the region of duodenojejunal junction, small pocket like pouches of peritoneum called **duodenal recesses** do occur (Fig. 9.9).

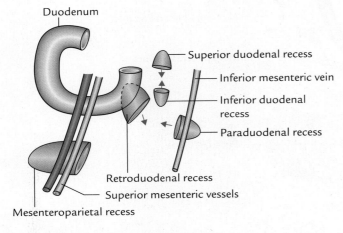

Fig. 9.9 Duodenal recesses.

These are sometimes responsible for strangulated retroperitoneal hernia. The important peritoneal recesses around the duodenojejunal flexure are as follows:

1. *Superior duodenal recess:* It lies to the left upper end of the fourth part of the duodenum, behind the superior duodenojejunal peritoneal fold with its mouth looking downward.
2. *Inferior duodenal recess:* It lies a little below the superior recess behind the inferior duodenojejunal peritoneal fold with its orifice looking upward.
3. *Paraduodenal recess:* It is the lowest when present. It lies to the left of the fourth part of the duodenum behind the paraduodenal fold of the peritoneum with its orifice facing medially. The paraduodenal fold contains **inferior mesenteric vein** in its free border edge.
4. *Retroduodenal recess:* It is the largest of duodenal recesses, but is rarely present. If present, it lies behind the third and fourth parts of the duodenum. Its orifice looks downward and to the left.

The *incidence of duodenal recesses* (vide supra) are: superior duodenal recess 50%, inferior duodenal recess 75%, paraduodenal recess 20%, and retroduodenal recess, occasional.

N.B. *Mesenteroparietal recess*: It is found only in 1% individuals. It lies below the duodenum behind the upper part of the mesentery. The superior mesenteric vessels lie in the anterior wall of its opening.

ARTERIAL SUPPLY (Fig. 9.10)

The upper half of the duodenum develops from the foregut and the lower half from the midgut. Therefore, the arterial supply of the upper half is derived from the coeliac trunk (artery of the foregut) and that of the lower half from the superior mesenteric artery (artery of the midgut). The

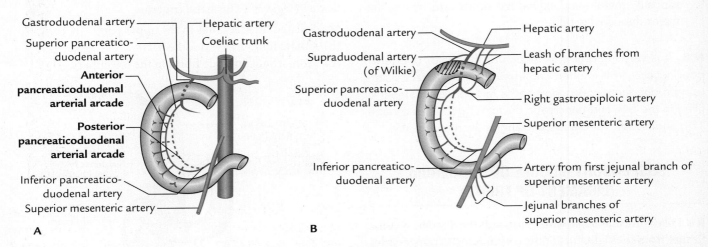

Fig. 9.10 Arterial supply of the duodenum: A, pancreaticoduodenal arterial arcades; B, various arteries supplying the duodenum.

different arteries of the duodenum derived directly or indirectly from the above two arteries are:

1. **Superior pancreaticoduodenal artery,** a branch of gastroduodenal artery (a branch of hepatic artery from the coeliac trunk).
2. **Inferior pancreaticoduodenal artery,** a branch of the superior mesenteric artery.

Each of the above two arteries divide into anterior and posterior branches. Respective branches of superior and inferior pancreaticoduodenal arteries anastomose to form **anterior** and **posterior pancreaticoduodenal arterial arcades.**

Each anastomotic arterial arcade gives off a row of vasa recta. The vasa recta of the anterior arcade supply the anterior surface and those of the posterior arcade supply the posterior surface of the duodenum. Between the two rows of vasa recta lies the head of the pancreas.

3. **Supraduodenal artery of "Wilkie":** Usually it is a branch of the gastroduodenal artery from the coeliac trunk and supplies the anterosuperior and posterosuperior surfaces of the first part.
4. **Retroduodenal branches of the gastroduodenal artery.**
5. **Leash of branches of the hepatic artery.**
6. **Branches from the right gastroepiploic artery.**
7. **Artery from the first jejunal branch of the superior mesenteric artery:** It supplies branches to the fourth part of the duodenum.

N.B. Arteries 3,4,5, and 6 exclusively supply the first part of the duodenum.

VENOUS DRAINAGE

The veins correspond to the arteries but are superficial to them. They drain into the splenic, superior mesenteric, and portal veins.

LYMPHATIC DRAINAGE

The lymph vessels follow the arteries and most of them drain into **pancreaticoduodenal nodes** lying along the inner curve of the duodenum (junction of the pancreas and duodenum). From here the efferents drain into coeliac and superior mesenteric lymph nodes and ultimately via intestinal lymph trunk into the cisterna chyli.

NERVE SUPPLY

The **sympathetic nerves** to the duodenum are derived from T6–T9 segments of the spinal cord and **parasympathetic nerves** from both the vagi through coeliac and superior

mesenteric plexuses. From these plexuses, fibres run along the arteries of the duodenum to supply it.

Clinical correlation

- **Duodenal ulcer:** The duodenal ulcers commonly occur in the first part of the duodenum because it is supplied by a series of end arteries and receives the acidic chyme from the stomach. In barium meal X-ray of abdomen, the first part of the duodenum presents a triangular shadow having a well-demarcated base and less distinct apex called **duodenal cap** or **bulb**. When duodenal ulcer is present in the first part, a small fleck of barium is found filling the ulcer crater and the duodenal cap is said to be deformed (Fig. 9.11).
- **Duodenal injuries:** The second part of the duodenum is most protected from external injury because it lies in the paravertebral gutter—a deeper plane than the forward curvature of the vertebral column. The third part of the duodenum is most vulnerable to external injury because it gets crushed between the vertebral column and the anterior abdominal wall following violence.
- **Duodenal diverticula:** They are congenital and almost always occur in the medial wall of the second part of the duodenum. They are thought to be caused by herniation of the duodenal lining through the gaps in the muscle coat where arteries and ducts pierce the wall.
- **Referred pain:** The pain arising from duodenum is poorly localized and referred to the central epigastrium.

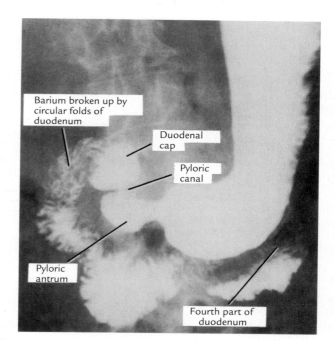

Fig. 9.11 Radiograph of the stomach and duodenum after barium meal. (*Source:* Fig. 5.25, Page 250, *Last's Anatomy: Regional and Applied,* 12th ed, Chummy S Sinnatamby. Copyright Elsevier Ltd. 2011, All rights reserved.)

PANCREAS

The pancreas is a soft, finely lobulated, elongated exo-endocrine gland. The exocrine part secretes the pancreatic juice and the endocrine part secretes the hormones, *viz.,* insulin, etc.

The pancreas (in Greek *pan*: all 1 *kreas*: flesh) is presumably so named because of its fleshy appearance.

The pancreatic juice helps in the digestion of lipids, carbohydrates, and proteins, whereas the pancreatic hormones maintain glucose homeostasis.

LOCATION (Fig. 9.12)

The pancreas lies more or less horizontally on the posterior abdominal wall in the epigastric and left hypochondriac regions. It crosses the posterior abdominal wall obliquely from concavity of the duodenum to the hilum of spleen opposite the level of T12–L3 vertebrae (Fig. 9.12A).

The greater part of the gland is retroperitoneal behind the serous floor of the lesser sac. Its left extremity—the tail, lies in the lienorenal ligament.

N.B. The pancreas is deeply located in the upper part of the abdomen, and hidden by many organs, hence not accessible for physical examination (Fig. 9.12B).

SIZE AND SHAPE

The pancreas is "J"-shaped or retort shaped being set obliquely. The bowl of retort represents its head and the stem of retort represents its neck, body, and tail. Its measurements are:

Length:	12–15 cm.
Width:	3–4 cm.
Thickness:	1.5–2 cm.
Weight:	80–90 g.

PARTS (SUBDIVISIONS) AND RELATIONS

For descriptive purposes, the pancreas is subdivided into four parts (Fig. 9.13):

1. Head (with one process—uncinate process).
2. Neck.
3. Body (with one process—tuber omentale).
4. Tail.

HEAD OF THE PANCREAS

It is the enlarged, disc-shaped right end of the pancreas, which lies in the concavity of the C-shaped duodenal loop in front of the L2 vertebra.

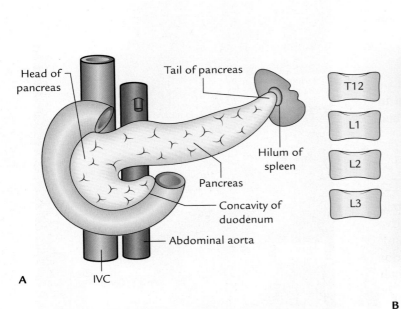

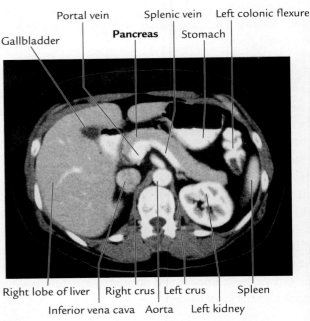

Fig. 9.12 Location of the pancreas: A, head lies opposite L1 and L3 vertebrae, body lies more or less in transpyloric plane (lower border of L1), and tail is at the level of T12 vertebra; B, CT scan of abdomen showing location of the pancreas. (*Source:* Fig. 4.88A, Page 289, *Gray's Anatomy for Students*, Richard L Drake, Wayne Vogl, Adam WM Mitchell. Copyright Elsevier Inc. 2005, All rights reserved.)

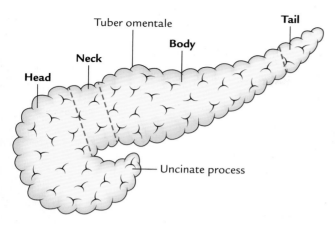

Fig. 9.13 Parts of the pancreas.

External Features

The head presents the following external features:

1. *Three borders:* Superior, inferior, and right lateral.
2. *Two surfaces:* Anterior and posterior.

3. *One process:* Uncinate process. (It is a hook-like process from the lower and left part of the head. It extends toward the left behind the superior mesenteric vessels.)

Relations (Fig. 9.14)

Superior border is related to:

(a) first part of the duodenum, and
(b) superior pancreaticoduodenal artery.

Inferior border is related to:

(a) third part of the duodenum, and
(b) inferior pancreaticoduodenal artery.

Right lateral border is related to:

(a) second part of the duodenum, and
(b) anterior and posterior pancreaticoduodenal arterial arcades.

Anterior surface is related from above downward to:

(a) gastroduodenal artery,

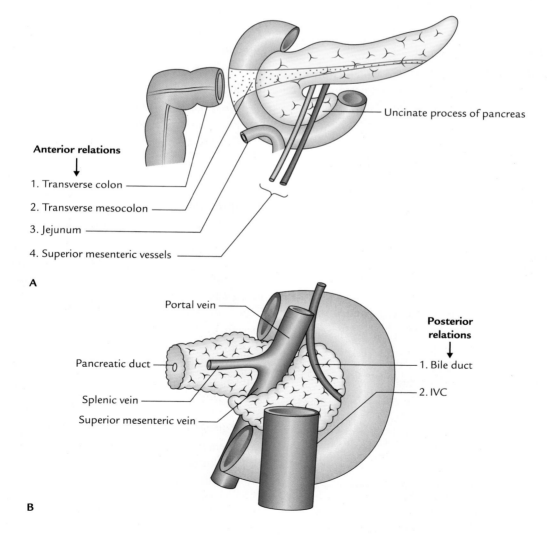

Fig. 9.14 Relations of the head of pancreas: A, anterior relations; B, posterior relations.

(b) transverse colon,

(c) root of the transverse mesocolon, and

(d) jejunum.

Posterior surface is related to:

(a) IVC,

(b) left renal vein,

(c) bile duct (lying in a groove, and may be found embedded in the pancreatic tissue), and

(d) right crus of diaphragm.

Uncinate process is related to:

(a) anteriorly to superior mesenteric vessels, and

(b) posteriorly to the abdominal aorta.

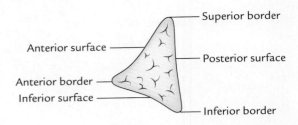

Fig. 9.16 Surfaces and borders of the body of pancreas as seen in cross section.

Lower border is related to the root of the transverse mesocolon.

BODY OF THE PANCREAS

1. It is the elongated part of the gland extending from its neck to the tail.

2. It passes toward the left of midline with a slight upward and backward inclination.

3. It lies in front of the vertebral column at or just below the transpyloric plane.

External Features

It is somewhat triangular in cross section (Fig. 9.16) and presents:

1. *Three borders:* Anterior, superior, and inferior.

2. *Three surfaces:* Anterior, posterior, and inferior.

3. *One process:* Tuber omentale (a part of the body projects above the lesser curvature of the stomach and comes in contact with the lesser omentum across the lesser sac).

Relations (Fig. 9.17)

Anterior border provides the attachment to the root of transverse mesocolon.

Superior border is related to the coeliac artery above the tuber omentale, hepatic artery to the right, and splenic artery to the left of tuber omentale.

Inferior border is related to superior mesenteric vessels (at its right end).

Anterior surface (concave and directed forward and upward) is related to:

(a) lesser sac, and

(b) stomach.

Posterior surface (devoid of peritoneum) is related to:

(a) aorta and origin of the superior mesenteric artery,

(b) left kidney and left suprarenal glands, and

(c) splenic vein usually lies in a groove below the level of splenic artery.

Inferior surface (covered by peritoneum) is related to:

(a) duodenojejunal flexure,

NECK OF THE PANCREAS

It is a slightly constricted part of the gland which connects the head with the body. It is about 2.5 cm (1 inch) long and is directed forward, upward, and to the left.

External Features

It presents the following external features:

Two surfaces: Anterior and posterior.
Two borders: Upper and lower.

Relations

Anterior surface is related to pylorus.

Posterior surface is related to (Fig. 9.15) commencement of the portal vein.

Upper border is related to the first part of the duodenum.

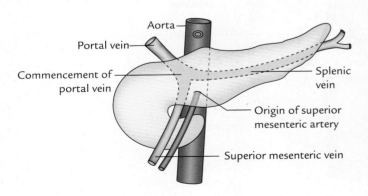

Fig. 9.15 Posterior relations of the neck of pancreas.

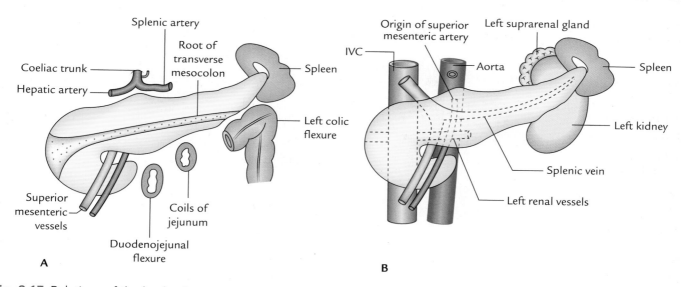

Fig. 9.17 Relations of the body of pancreas: A, anterior and inferior relations; B, posterior relations.

(b) coils of jejunum, and
(c) left colic flexure.

TAIL OF THE PANCREAS

1. It is the narrow left extremity of the pancreas.
2. It lies in the lienorenal ligament along with splenic vessels.
3. It is mobile unlike the other major retroperitoneal parts of the gland.

4. It contains the largest number of islets of Langerhans per unit of tissue as compared to other parts of the gland.

Relations

These are related to the visceral surface of spleen between gastric impression and colic impression.

The visceral relations of the different parts of pancreas together are shown in Figure 9.18.

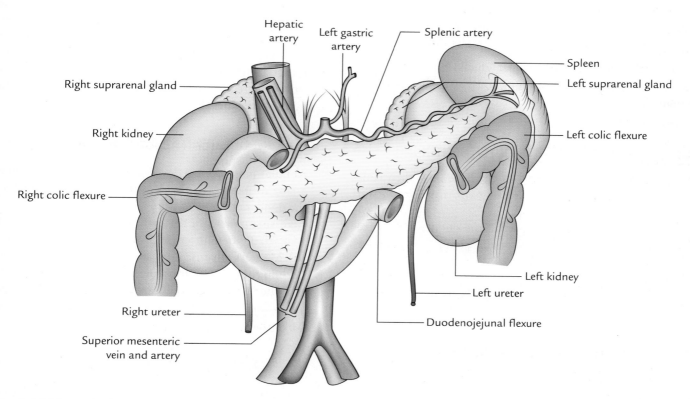

Fig. 9.18 Visceral relations of the different parts of the pancreas.

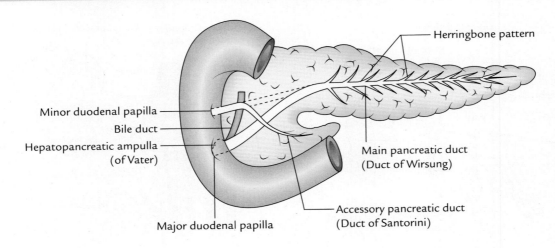

Fig. 9.19 Pancreatic ducts.

DUCTS OF THE PANCREAS (Fig. 9.19)

Usually there are two ducts: main and accessory, which drain the exocrine secretion into the duodenum.

MAIN PANCREATIC DUCT (OF WIRSUNG)

1. It begins in the tail and traverses the whole length of the gland near its posterior surface.
2. At the neck, it turns downward, and then to the right to enter into the second part of duodenum.
3. It joins the bile duct as it pierces the duodenal wall to form the **hepatopancreatic ampulla** (of **Vater**) which opens by a narrow mouth on the summit of major duodenal papilla 8–10 cm distal to the pylorus.

It receives tributaries (smaller ducts) throughout its length, at right angle to its long axis in a "herringbone pattern."

It is the only duct in 90% of cases.

ACCESSORY PANCREATIC DUCT (OF SANTORINI)

1. It begins in the lower part of the head, and then runs upward and medially, crossing in front of main pancreatic duct.
2. It opens into the second part of the duodenum on the summit of minor duodenal papilla about 2–3 cm above the opening of main pancreatic duct (6–8 cm distal to pylorus).
3. In 40% of cases, it communicates with the main duct while crossing it.

DEVELOPMENT (Fig. 9.20)

The pancreas develops from two separate buds: the **ventral pancreatic bud** and the **dorsal pancreatic bud**, hence it has two ducts.

1. The smaller ventral pancreatic bud arises in common with hepatic bud for the liver (subsequently the bile duct).
2. The larger dorsal pancreatic bud arises more proximally, directly from the duodenum.

Following rotation of the gut, the ventral pancreatic bud (which forms the posterior part of the head and uncinate process) passes along with the bile duct into the position dorsal to the dorsal pancreatic bud (which forms the remaining whole part of the gland). The two buds now fuse and their ducts anastomose with each other in such a way that the duct of ventral pancreas forms the proximal part of the main pancreatic duct while the duct of dorsal pancreas forms the remainder distal part of the pancreatic duct. The proximal part of the dorsal pancreatic duct between the anastomosis and duodenum remains narrow and forms the **accessory pancreatic duct**. It usually communicates with the main pancreatic duct (Fig. 9.20).

CONGENITAL ANOMALIES

1. **Annular pancreas** is a developmental anomaly in which a ring of pancreatic tissue encircles the second part of the duodenum.
2. **Accessory pancreatic tissue** may be found in (a) stomach wall, (b) duodenum (most common), (c) small intestine, (d) Meckel's diverticulum, (e) greater omentum, and (f) hilum of spleen. It occurs in the form of yellowish, lobulated nodules, usually single (1–6 mm) in diameter; about one-third of these nodules contain islets of Langerhans.

ARTERIAL SUPPLY (Fig. 9.21)

The pancreas is a high vascular structure and supplied by the following arteries:

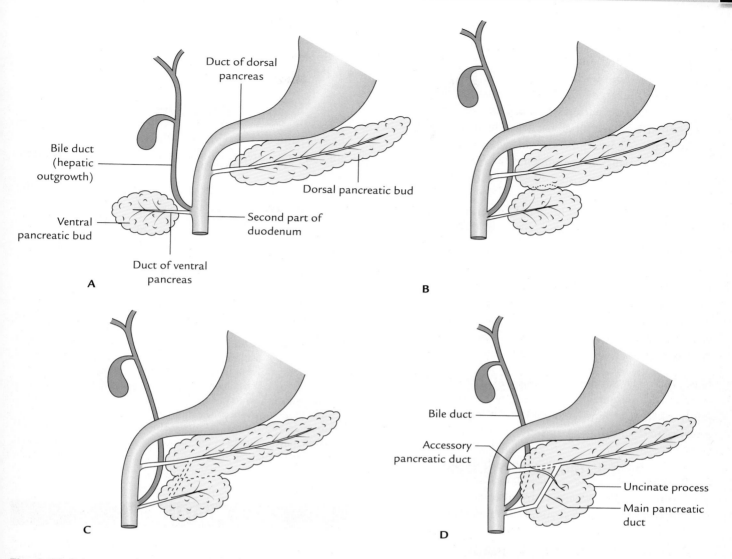

Fig. 9.20 Schematic diagrams showing stages (A, B, C, and D) of formation of the adult pancreas and its ducts (main and accessory) by the fusion of the dorsal and ventral pancreatic buds.

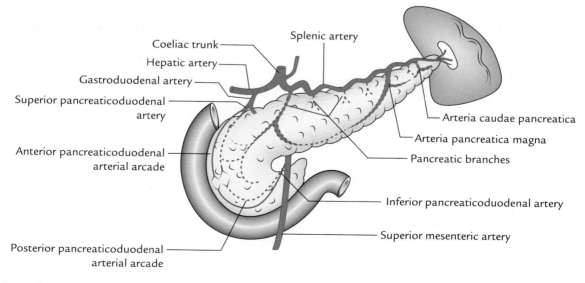

Fig. 9.21 Arterial supply of the pancreas.

1. **Splenic artery, a branch of coeliac trunk:** The splenic artery is the branch of coeliac trunk and it is the main source of blood supply to the pancreas. Its branches supply the body and tail of pancreas. Two branches are named. One large branch which arises near the tail and runs toward the neck is called *arteria pancreatica magna.* Another relatively small branch, which runs toward the tip of the tail, is termed *arteria caudae pancreatica.*
2. **Superior pancreaticoduodenal artery:** The *superior pancreaticoduodenal artery* is a branch of gastroduodenal artery.
3. **Inferior pancreaticoduodenal artery:** The *inferior pancreaticoduodenal artery* is a branch of superior mesenteric artery.

Both the superior and inferior pancreaticoduodenal arteries divide into *anterior and posterior branches,* which run between the concavity of the duodenum and the head of pancreas. *The anastomoses between anterior and posterior branches form anterior and posterior pancreaticoduodenal arterial arcades.*

N.B. Since the pancreas develops at the junction of the foregut and midgut, it is supplied by the branches of the artery of foregut (coeliac trunk) and the branches of the artery of midgut (superior mesenteric artery).

VENOUS DRAINAGE (Fig. 9.22)

The veins of the pancreas drain into (a) portal vein, (b) superior mesenteric vein, and (c) splenic vein.

LYMPHATIC DRAINAGE

The lymphatics from the pancreas follow the arteries and drain mainly into the following groups of lymph nodes:

1. Pancreaticosplenic nodes (main group).
2. Coeliac nodes.
3. Superior mesenteric nodes.
4. Pyloric nodes.

NERVE SUPPLY

The sympathetic and parasympathetic nerve fibres reach the gland along its arteries from coeliac and superior mesenteric plexuses.

The sympathetic supply is vasomotor whereas the parasympathetic supply controls the pancreatic secretion.

Clinical correlation

- **Carcinoma of the head of pancreas** is common. It compresses the bile duct leading to persistent obstructive jaundice. It may press the portal vein or may involve the stomach due to close vicinity of these structures to the head of pancreas.
- **Acute pancreatitis** is the acute inflammation of the pancreas. It occurs due to obstruction of pancreatic duct, ingestion of alcohol, viral infections (mumps), or trauma. It is serious condition because activated pancreatic enzymes leak into the substance of pancreas and initiates the autodigestion of the gland. Clinically, it presents as very severe pain in the epigastric region radiating to the back, fever, nausea, and vomiting. The serum amylase, level is raised four times.

PORTAL VEIN

The portal vein is an important venous channel [about 3 inches (7.5 cm) in length], which collects blood from (i) abdominal and pelvic parts of the alimentary tract (except lower part of the anal canal), (ii) gallbladder, (iii) pancreas,

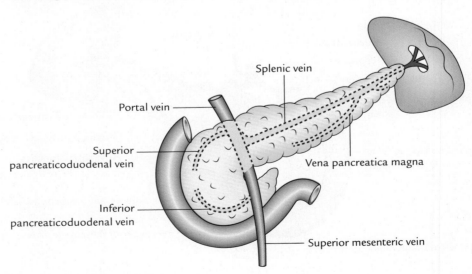

Fig. 9.22 Venous drainage of the pancreas.

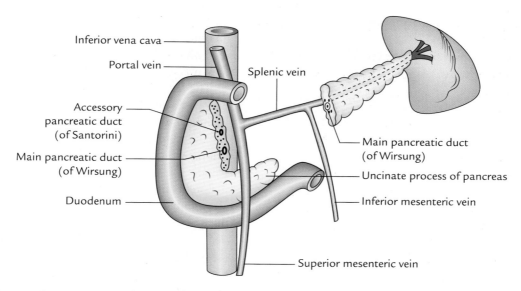

Fig. 9.23 Formation of the portal vein behind the neck of pancreas.

and (iv) spleen, and transports it to the liver. The important features of the portal vein are:

1. It provides about 80% of the blood that flows through the liver.
2. Its tributaries and branches contain up to one-third of the total volume of blood in the entire body.
3. The portal vein and its tributaries are devoid of valves.
4. It transports the products of digestion of carbohydrates, proteins, and other nutrients from the intestine and also products of red cell destruction (etc.) from the spleen to the liver.
5. It divides into branches which, like those of hepatic artery, discharge their blood into sinusoids of the liver, which are drained by hepatic veins into the IVC.
6. It begins like vein from capillary bed of the gut and terminates like an artery in the hepatic sinusoids.

FORMATION, COURSE, AND BRANCHES

The portal vein is formed behind the neck of pancreas by the union of superior mesenteric vein and splenic vein at the level of L2 (Figs 9.23 and 9.24).

It runs upward and a little to the right behind the neck of pancreas, then ascends posterior to the first part of the duodenum to enter the right free edge of the lesser omentum. It ends at the right end of porta hepatis by dividing into a right branch and a left branch.

1. **Right branch:** It is shorter and wider and enters the right lobe of liver after receiving the cystic vein.
2. **Left branch:** It is longer and narrower. It passes to the left end of porta hepatis giving branches to the caudate and quadrate lobes. Then unites with ligamentum teres and ligamentum venosum receives paraumbilical veins

(which run with ligamentum teres in the falciform ligament) before entering into the left lobe of the liver.

N.B. *Intrahepatic course (Fig. 9.25):* After entering the liver, each branch of the portal vein divides and redivides, like those of the hepatic artery to end ultimately into the hepatic sinusoids. Here the portal venous blood mixes with the hepatic arterial blood, and is separated from the liver cells by a single layer of phagocyte and fenestrated epithelium. From hepatic sinusoids the blood is drained by hepatic veins into the IVC.

PARTS AND RELATIONS (Fig. 9.24)

For the purpose of description, the portal vein is divided into three parts (Fig. 9.24):

1. *Infraduodenal part* which lies below the first part of the duodenum.

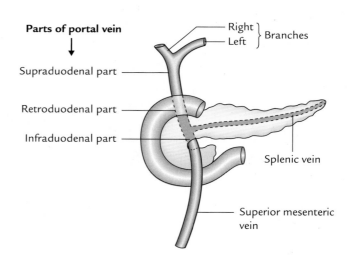

Fig. 9.24 Course and parts of the portal vein.

2. *Retroduodenal part* which lies posterior to the first part of the duodenum,

3. *Supraduodenal part* which lies above the first part of the duodenum in the right free margin of lesser omentum.

The relations of different parts of the portal vein are as follows:

Infraduodenal Part

Anterior: Neck of pancreas.
Posterior: IVC.

Retroduodenal Part

Anterior: First part of the duodenum.
              Bile duct.
              Gastroduodenal artery.
Posterior: IVC.

Supraduodenal Part

Anterior: Hepatic artery (on the left) and bile duct (on the right).
Posterior: IVC.

TRIBUTARIES

The portal vein receives the following tributaries (Fig. 9.25):

1. *Splenic vein,* a larger formative tributary.
2. *Superior mesenteric vein,* a smaller formative tributary.

3. *Superior pancreaticoduodenal vein* joins the portal vein behind the first part of duodenum.

4. *Left and right gastric veins* join the portal vein the right free margin of lesser omentum.

  The *left gastric vein* at the cardiac end of the stomach receives a few esophageal veins from the lower end of esophagus.

  The *right gastric vein* receives the prepyloric vein (of Mayo) which runs vertically in front of the pylorus.

5. *Cystic vein* joins the right branch of the portal vein before it enters the right lobe of the liver.

6. *Paraumbilical veins* are small veins that run along the ligamentum teres in the falciform ligament and join the left branch of the portal vein before it enters the left lobe of the liver.

PORTOCAVAL (PORTOSYSTEMIC) ANASTOMOSES (Fig. 9.26)

There are many sites in the abdominal cavity where anastomosis exists between the portal and systemic venous systems. These communications between the veins of the portal and caval (systemic) systems form important routes of collateral circulation in cases of portal obstruction.

The **important sites of portocaval anastomoses** are as follows (Fig. 9.27):

1. **Umbilicus:** Here the left branch of the portal vein communicates with the superficial veins of the anterior

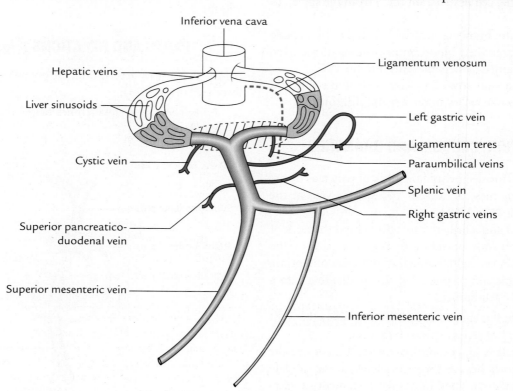

Fig. 9.25 Tributaries of the portal vein.

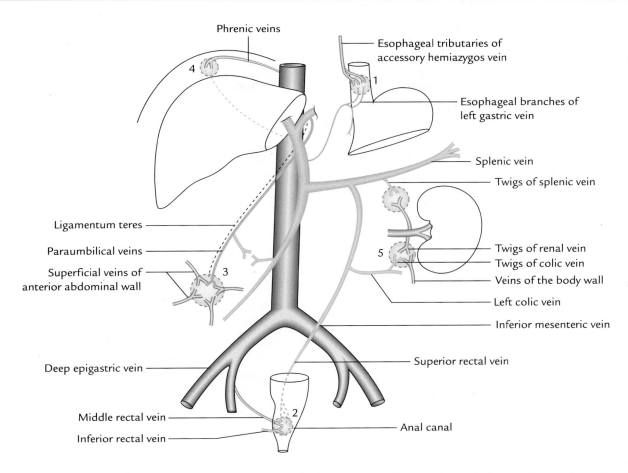

Fig. 9.26 Sites of portocaval anastomosis: 1 = lower end of esophagus; 2 = anal canal; 3 = in the region of umbilicus; 4 = at the bare area of liver; 5 = between the colic veins and the renal veins.

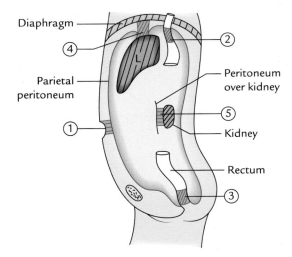

Fig. 9.27 Highly schematic diagram to show the sites of portocaval anastomosis: 1 = umbilicus; 2 = lower end of esophagus; 3 = anal canal; 4 = bare area of liver; 5 = anterior aspect of kidney.

abdominal wall around umbilicus, through paraumbilical veins (of Sappey). In portal obstruction, the superficial veins around the umbilicus become distended and tortuous (varicosity). This whorl of prominent distended tortuous (snake-like) veins around the umbilicus is known as caput medusae[1]—a sign of diagnostic value to the clinicians.

2. **Lower end of esophagus:** Here the esophageal tributaries of left gastric vein (draining into the portal vein) anastomose with esophageal tributaries of accessory hemiazygos vein (systemic).

    In portal obstruction as in *liver cirrhosis*, these collateral channels become distended and tortuous, forming esophageal varices, which may rupture causing hematemesis (vomiting of blood) and may even bleed to death.

3. **Anal canal:** Here the superior rectal (hemorrhoidal) vein which ultimately drains into the portal vein

---

[1]Caput: head of Medusa (in Greek Medusae). Medusa (a mythical lady) was the daughter of Phorcys and captivated Neptune with her golden hair and became by him the mother of Pegasus. As a punishment, Minerva changed her hair into serpents and empowered her eyes so that everything her eyes looked upon changed to stone. Perseus slew and decapitated her and from the blood that dropped serpents sprung.

Table 9.1 Anastomoses between the portal and systemic venous systems

Site of anastomosis	Veins forming portocaval anastomosis	Clinical signs
Lower third of the esophagus	Left gastric vein ↑↓ Esophageal veins draining into azygos vein	Esophageal varices
Umbilicus	Paraumbilical veins ↑↓ Superficial veins of anterior abdominal wall	Caput medusae
Mid-anal canal	Superior rectal vein ↑↓ Middle and inferior rectal veins	Hemorrhoids

anastomoses with middle and inferior rectal veins, the tributaries of internal iliac (systemic) vein. The distension and dilatation of these anastomotic channels result in the formation of **hemorrhoids** or **piles** which may be responsible for repeated bleeding per annum.

4. **Extraperitoneal surfaces of retroperitoneal organs.** Veins of retroperitoneal organs such as duodenum, ascending colon, and descending colon (portal) anastomose with the retroperitoneal veins of the posterior abdominal wall and renal capsule (systemic). The renal vein anastomosis with splenic and azygos veins.

5. **Bare area of liver:** Here the hepatic venules (portal) anastomose with phrenic and intercostal (systemic) veins.

The three very-very important sites of portocaval anastomoses are given in Table 9.1.

Clinical correlation

Portal hypertension: Obstruction of the portal vein or its branches leads to the increase in the portal venous pressure called **portal hypertension**, i.e., pressure above 40 mmHg (normal being 5–15 mmHg). This leads to enlargement of collateral channels. The most common cause of portal hypertension is *alcoholic cirrhosis* of the liver.

The effects of portal hypertension are:

1. Splenomegaly (enlargement of the spleen).
2. Ascites (accumulation of fluid in the peritoneal cavity).
3. Esophageal varices.
4. Hemorrhoids.

Golden Facts to Remember

- Most movable part of the duodenum — First part
- Duodenal cap — Triangular shadow of the first part seen in barium meal X-ray
- Most vulnerable part of the duodenum for peptic ulceration — First part
- Most common site for a diverticulum in the small intestine — Duodenum
- Most protected part of the duodenum from external injury — Second part
- Most vulnerable part of the duodenum for external injury — Third part
- Commonest sites of accessory pancreatic tissue — Duodenum
- Most of the nutrition to the liver is provided by — Portal vein
- Part of the pancreas containing maximum number of islets of Langerhans — Tail

Clinical Case Study

A 65-year-old male patient was admitted in the hospital with the following complaints: progressive jaundice, pale greasy stools, itching of skin, loss of appetite and weight, and back pain. On examination the doctors found palpable gallbladder and ascites. After thorough investigations he was diagnosed as a case of "**carcinoma of the head of pancreas.**"

Questions

1. What is the anatomical basis of jaundice in carcinoma of the head of pancreas?
2. What is Courvoisier's law?
3. What are the important posterior relations of the head of pancreas?
4. Give the source of development of common bile duct and main pancreatic duct (of Wirsung).

Answers

1. This is due to obstruction of CBD. The CBD being embedded in the head of pancreas on its posterior surface is blocked by cancer infiltration. This leads to stasis of bile in the biliary tree. The bile escapes through ruptured bile canaliculi into blood. As a result, the patient develops jaundice. This type of jaundice is called **obstructive jaundice.**
2. The obstructive jaundice with palpable gallbladder indicates carcinoma of the head of pancreas whereas obstructive jaundice without palpable gallbladder indicates obstruction of bile duct due to gallstone (also see Clinical correlation on page 124).
3. (a) Bile duct and (b) IVC.
4. (a) The CBD develops from the hepatic bud. (b) The small proximal part of the main pancreatic duct develops from the duct of ventral pancreatic and larger distal part of main pancreatic duct part develops from the duct of dorsal pancreatic bud.

Small and Large Intestines

SMALL INTESTINE

Anatomically the small intestine extends from the pylorus to the ileocaecal junction. It is about 6 m long and divided into three parts: duodenum, jejunum, and ileum (Fig. 10.1). The proximal fixed part which is about 10 inches (25 cm) long is called **duodenum**. The remaining long part which is freely mobile is divided into two parts—**jejunum** and **ileum**.

The duodenum is principally retroperitoneal and fixed. It receives chyme from the stomach, bile from the gallbladder, and pancreatic juice from the pancreas. The fixation of duodenum is essential because mobile duodenum will cause twisting and kinking of common bile duct (CBD) and pancreatic ducts which open into it. It is intimately related with pancreas and extra hepatic biliary apparatus. Hence, clinically it is considered as a separate entity. It is described in detail in Chapter 9.

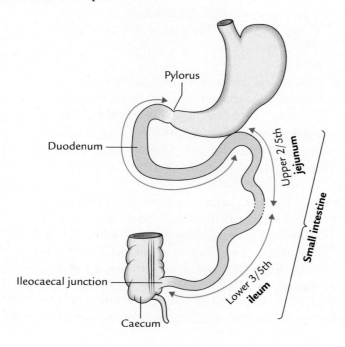

Fig. 10.1 Parts of the small intestine.

The jejunum and ileum are principally concerned with the digestion and absorption of digested food; hence these two parts together form the **small intestine proper**. The following description of the small intestine is confined only to the jejunum and ileum.

JEJUNUM AND ILEUM

The small intestine proper extends from the *duodenojejunal flexure* to the *ileocaecal junction*. Its upper two-fifth forms the *jejunum* and its lower three-fifth forms the *ileum*. However, there is no definite line of demarcation. The jejunum and ileum are suspended from the posterior abdominal wall by a large fold of peritoneum called the **mesentery of small intestine**; hence, the small intestine enjoys a considerable mobility. The structure of the small intestine corresponds to its functional requirements.

STRUCTURE

The wall of the small intestine consists of four layers. From within outward, these are: (a) mucosa, (b) submucosa, (c) muscle layer, and (d) serosa.

Mucosa

The mucosa presents the following three relevant features.

Larger Surface Area

For digestion and absorption of nutrients, the surface area of mucus membrane is enormously increased by plicae circulares, villi, and microvilli.

(a) *Plicae circulares* (or *valves of Kerckring*): These are circular folds, which are permanent and are not obliterated by distension.

(b) *Villi*: The surface of circular folds is thrown into small (0.5 mm or less in length) finger-like projections called *villi*.

(c) *Microvilli*: The surface epithelium covering the villi presents microvilli (or striated border).

N.B.
- The total surface area of mucosa of the small intestine is about 200 m^2.
- The entire epithelial lining of the small intestine is replaced in every 2 to 4 days.

Intestinal Glands (Crypts of Lieberkühn)

In between the bases of villi, the epithelium is invaginated in the lamina propria to form intestinal glands. They secrete digestive enzymes and mucous.

Lymphatic Follicles

The lamina propria of the mucous membrane contains two types of lymphatic follicles.

1. **Solitary lymph follicles:** These are 1–2 mm in diameter and are distributed throughout the length of the small intestine.
2. **Aggregated lymph follicles:** They form circular or oval patches called **Peyer's patches**. Each Peyer's patch consists of about 260 solitary lymph follicles and its length varies from 2 to 10 cm. They are present lengthwise along the antimesenteric border. Peyer's patches are small, circular, and fewer in the distal part of the jejunum, and large, oval, and numerous in the ileum particularly in its distal part (Fig. 10.2). In the distal part of the ileum where Peyer's patches are much larger and most numerous may extend in the submucosa after breaking the muscularis mucosa.

Submucosa

It is made up of loose areolar tissue and contains blood vessels, lymph vessels, and nerve plexus (**Meissner's plexus**).

Muscle Layer

It is made up of outer longitudinal and inner circular layers of smooth muscle. **Auerbach's plexus of nerves** is present between these two layers.

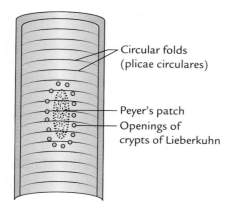

Fig. 10.2 Interior of ileum showing a Peyer's patch.
- Circular folds (plicae circulares)
- Peyer's patch
- Openings of crypts of Lieberkuhn

Serosa

It is formed by the visceral peritoneum and is lined by the simple squamous epithelium.

> **Clinical correlation**
>
> **Typhoid and tubercular ulcers: Peyer's patches** may be felt through the antimesenteric border of the ileum. They may ulcerate in *typhoid fever* forming characteristic vertically oriented, oval ulcers which may sometimes perforate. For this reason, patients suffering from typhoid fever are given nonspicy soft diets.
>
> **N.B.** After healing, the typhoid, ulcers do not cause intestinal obstruction like tubercular ulcers. Note, the tubercular ulcers are circularly placed; hence, after healing they often cause constriction of the lumen of small intestine by fibrous tissue, leading to intestinal obstruction.

ARTERIAL SUPPLY

The jejunum and ileum are supplied by the jejunal and ileal branches (12–15 in number) of the superior mesenteric artery. They arise from the left side of the superior mesenteric artery and enter the mesentery to reach the intestine. The terminal part of the ileum is supplied by the ileal branches of the ileocolic branch of the superior mesenteric artery. As soon as these enter the mesentery they break up into smaller branches which anastomose with each other to form a series of **arterial arcades** which are more complex in the ileum than in the jejunum.

From the convexities of the terminal arcades, small parallel straight vessels called "**vasa recta**" arise and pass to the mesenteric border of the gut to be distributed alternatively to the opposite surfaces of the small intestine. The anastomosis between the vasa recta is poor.

VENOUS DRAINAGE

The veins correspond to the branches of superior mesenteric artery and drain into the portal vein, which carries the products of protein and carbohydrates to the liver.

LYMPHATIC DRAINAGE

The lymph vessels from the small intestine pass through a large number of mesenteric nodes (lymph nodes present in the mesentery) and finally drain into **superior mesenteric nodes** present around the origin of superior mesenteric artery. The lymphatics of the small intestine have a circular course in its wall. The **circular tubercular ulcers** and subsequent strictures in the small intestine are due to involvement of these lymphatics in tuberculosis.

NERVE SUPPLY

The small intestine is supplied by both sympathetic and parasympathetic nerve fibres. The sympathetic supply is derived from T10–T11 spinal segments through splanchnic nerves and superior mesenteric plexus. For this reason, pain from the jejunum and ileum is referred to the umbilical region. The parasympathetic supply is derived from the vagus nerves through the coeliac and superior mesenteric plexuses.

The *sympathetic fibres* are motor to the gut-sphincters whereas the *parasympathetic fibres* stimulate the peristalsis and are inhibitory to the sphincters.

MESENTERY OF THE SMALL INTESTINE

It is a broad fan-shaped fold of the peritoneum, which suspends the small intestine (jejunum and ileum) from the posterior abdominal wall. It has the **root** (attached margin) and **free margin** (intestinal margin). The root is attached to an oblique line across the posterior abdominal wall extending from the *duodenojejunal flexure* to the *ileocaecal junction*.

The duodenojejunal flexure lies to the left side of second lumbar vertebra, whereas ileocaecal junction lies at the right sacroiliac joint.

The **root of mesentery** is about 6 inches (15 cm) long while its **free margin** (periphery of the mesentery) is about 6 m long. This accounts for the formation of folds/ pleats in it (a frill-like arrangement resembling a full skirt; Fig. 10.3).

The mesentery of small intestine is described in detail in Chapter 6, p. 82.

Surface Marking of the Root of Mesentery (Fig. 10.4)

The point representing the duodenojejunal flexure lies 1 cm below the transpyloric plane and 2.5 cm to the left of midline. The point representing the ileocaecal junction corresponds to the point of intersection between right lateral and transtubercular planes.

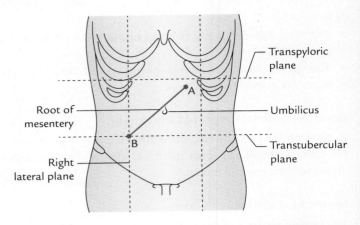

Fig. 10.4 Surface marking of the root of the mesentery: A, point representing duodenojejunal flexure; B, point representing ileocaecal junction.

Clinical correlation

- The great length of the mesentery permits the descent of the loop of small intestine into the sac of inguinal or femoral herniae.
- A group of lymph nodes when infected may become adherent to an adjoining loop of small intestine and may result in the mechanical obstruction. An acute terminal *mesenteric lymphadenitis* is often indistinguishable from an *acute appendicitis*.
- **Mesenteric cyst:** The mesentery is the site of cystic swellings which mostly arise from the mesenteric lymph nodes. Clinically, the mesenteric cyst presents as a painless, cystic fluctuant swelling in the umbilical region. On examination, the characteristic feature of the swelling is that it is more mobile in the direction at right angles to the line of the attachment of the mesentery and less mobile along the line of attachment of the mesentery.
- The *failure of root* of mesentery to fuse over its entire length with the posterior abdominal wall allows a pocket of the peritoneum to be formed which may form a sac of an intraparietal hernia called *mesenteric parietal hernia of Waldeyer*.

The differences between the duodenum and small intestine proper (jejunum and ileum) are given in the following box:

Duodenum	Small intestine proper
• Short in length (25 cm)	• Long in length (<6 m)
• Supplied by two rows of vasa recta	• Supplied by single row of vasa recta
• Presence of Brunner glands in submucus coat	• Absence of glands in submucus coat

DIFFERENCES BETWEEN THE JEJUNUM AND ILEUM (Fig. 10.5)

Both jejunum and ileum have characteristic features which make them recognizable during operation by the surgeons.

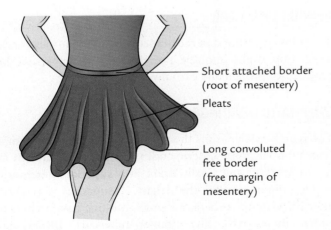

Fig. 10.3 Mesentery of the small intestine resembling a full skirt.

Labels: Short attached border (root of mesentery); Pleats; Long convoluted free border (free margin of mesentery)

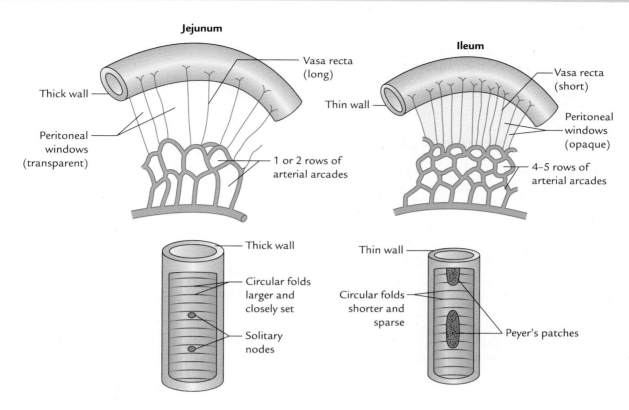

Fig. 10.5 Differences between the jejunum and ileum.

The jejunum is more vascular than the ileum and is slightly wider in diameter than the ileum. It feels thicker between the finger and thumb than the ileum, because its mucous membrane is thrown into more and closely set circular folds (plicae circulares). The ileum, on the other hand, possesses many more aggregated lymph follicles (Peyer's patches) in its wall than jejunum.

The differences between jejunum and ileum are given in detail in Table 10.1.

DEVELOPMENT

The jejunum and ileum develop from the U-shaped midgut loop having cephalic and caudal limbs. The cephalic limb gives rise to the jejunum and upper part of the ileum, and the caudal limb gives rise to the lower part of the ileum. In the embryonic life, the apex of the midgut loop communicates with the yolk sac through the **vitello-intestinal duct**. The vitelline duct is generally obliterated by the sixth week of intrauterine life.

Table 10.1 Differences between the jejunum and ileum

Features	Jejunum	Ileum
Walls	Thicker and more vascular	Thinner and less vascular
Lumen	Wider and often found empty (diameter = 4 cm)	Narrower and often found full (diameter = 3.5 cm)
Circular folds/plicae circulares (valves of Kerckring)	Longer and closely set	Smaller and sparsely set
Villi	More, larger, thicker, and leaf-like	Less, shorter, thinner, and finger-like
Aggregated lymph follicles (Peyer's patches)	Small, circular, and few in number, and found only in the distal part of the jejunum	Large oval and more in number (± 10 cm × 1.5 cm), and found throughout the extent of ileum being maximum in the distal part
Mesentery	Contains less fat and becomes semitranslucent between the vasa recta called peritoneal windows	Contains more fat and there are no peritoneal windows between the vasa recta
Arterial arcades	One or two rows with long vasa recta	Four or five rows with short vasa recta

Clinical correlation

Meckel's diverticulum (or ileal diverticulum; Fig. 10.6): It is the persistent proximal part of the *embryonic vitello-intestinal duct.* It presents the following characteristic features:

1. It occurs in 2 percent of the subjects.
2. It is usually 2 inches (5 cm) long.
3. It is situated about 2 feet (60 cm) proximal to the ileocaecal junction.
4. It is more common in men.
5. The calibre and structure of its wall are similar to that of the ileum.
6. Its apex may be free or attached to the umbilicus by a fibrous band.
7. It is attached to the antimesenteric border of the ileum.
8. It may contain ectopic gastric mucosa and pancreatic tissue.

Normally, it is symptomless but may cause the following *clinical problems:*

1. It may cause intestinal obstruction.
2. When it contains ectopic gastric mucosa or pancreatic tissue, its thin wall may ulcerate, perforate, and bleed to mimic the *acute abdomen.*
3. When inflamed, its symptoms are similar to that of "*acute appendicitis.*"

N.B. *Dictum:* In a clinically diagnosed case of acute appendicitis, if a healthy appendix is found during operation the surgeon should look for Meckel's diverticulum.

LARGE INTESTINE

The large intestine is about 1.5 m long and extends from the caecum in the right iliac fossa to the anus in the perineum. Apart from the transverse colon and sigmoid colon, it is more fixed in position than the small intestine.

The *functions of the large intestine* are:

1. Absorption of water from fluid contents in it to help form the feces.
2. Storage, lubrication, and expulsion of feces.
3. Synthesis of vitamin B complex by normal bacterial flora present its lumen.
4. Protection from invasion by microorganisms by its mucoid secretion which is rich in IgA group of antibodies.

PARTS

For descriptive purposes, the large intestine is divided into the following four parts:

1. Caecum and appendix.
2. Colon.
3. Rectum.
4. Anal canal.

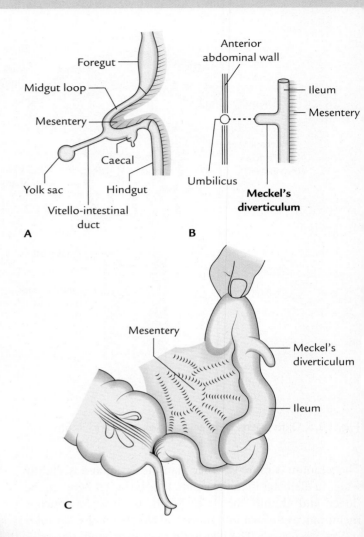

Fig. 10.6 Meckel's diverticulum: **A,** vitello-intestinal duct connecting midgut loop with yolk sac; **B,** Meckel's diverticulum (schematic representation); **C,** Meckel's diverticulum as seen during surgery.

The colon is further divided into four parts: ascending colon, transverse colon, descending colon, and sigmoid colon (Fig. 10.7).

N.B. All the parts of the large intestine are retroperitoneal and fixed except appendix, transverse colon, and sigmoid colon which are intraperitoneal and possess mesenteries. The mesenteries of these parts are termed mesoappendix, transverse mesocolon, and sigmoid mesocolon, respectively.

STRUCTURE

The structure of the large intestine differs in different parts. Hence, the following account deals only with the structure of colon—the longest part, as a representative of the large intestine. Similar to the small intestine, the colon also consists of four layers. From within outward these are mucosa, submucosa, muscle layer, and serosa.

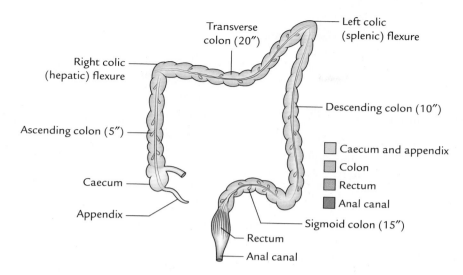

Fig. 10.7 Parts of the large intestine.

Mucosa

The mucosa does not present transverse circular folds (plicae circulares) and villi. However, temporary folds involving mucosa and submucosa are present in the undescended colon. The surface epithelium is absorptive in nature and consists of columnar cells bearing microvilli.

Intestinal glands (crypts of Lieberkühn) are long and tubular and possess a large number of goblet cells. The lamina propria of the mucous membrane contains abundant diffuse lymphatic tissue but is devoid of Peyer's patches.

Submucosa

It is made up of loose areolar tissue and contains blood vessels, lymph vessels, and nerve plexus (Meissner's plexus).

Muscle Layer

It consists of outer longitudinal and inner circular layers of smooth muscle. The outer longitudinal layer is not continuous, rather, it is arranged into three thick longitudinal bands called **teniae coli**. The inner circular layer of smooth muscle is thin as compared to the small intestine.

Serosa

It covers the transverse colon and the sigmoid colon but the parts of ascending and descending colons are covered by tunica adventitia.

CARDINAL (DISTINGUISHING) FEATURES

The three cardinal features of the large intestine are the presence of (a) teniae coli, (b) appendices epiploicae, and (c) sacculations (or haustrations) (Fig. 10.8).

Teniae Coli

These are three ribbon-like bands of the longitudinal muscle coat. These bands converge proximally at the base of the

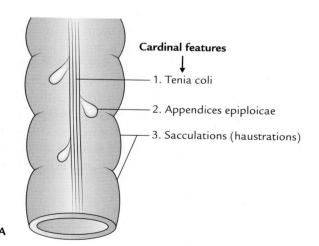

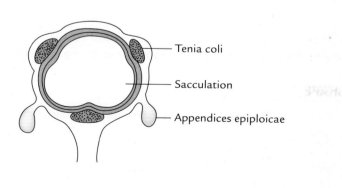

Fig. 10.8 Cardinal features of the large intestine: **A,** surface view; **B,** in cross-sectional view.

appendix and spread out distally to become continuous with the longitudinal muscle coat of the rectum. Thus, teniae coli are present on all the parts of colon and caecum.

Location

In the caecum, ascending colon, and descending colon, the positions of teniae are anterior (*Teniae libera*), posteromedial (*Teniae mesocolica*), and posterolateral (*Teniae omentalis*), but in the transverse colon the corresponding positions are inferior, posterior, and superior, respectively.

Appendices Epiploicae

These are small bags of visceral peritoneum filled with fat attached to the teniae of large intestine. Thus, they are absent in the appendix, rectum, and anal canal. The appendices epiploicae are most numerous on the sides of sigmoid colon and posterior surface of the transverse colon.

Sacculation (or Haustrations)

These are a series of pouches/dilatations in the wall of caecum and colon between the teniae. They are produced because length of teniae fall short of the length of circular muscle coat. The sacculations are responsible for the characteristic puckered appearance of the large intestine.

The differences between the small and large intestines are given in Table 10.2.

CAECUM

The caecum (L. caecum = blind) is the large dilated blind sac at the commencement (proximal end) of the large intestine. It is situated in the right iliac fossa above the lateral half of the inguinal ligament. Its surface projection occupies the triangular region limited by the right lateral plane, the transtubercular plane, and the inguinal ligament.

It communicates:

(a) Superiorly with the ascending colon.
(b) Medially at the ileocaecal junction with ileum, and posteromedially with appendix.

N.B. The caecum is so named because it forms the blind end of the large intestine below the level of ileal opening.

SHAPE

Generally the caecum appears as a dilated pendulous sac inferior to the ileocaecal junction.

The growth of caecum from birth leads to a change in its shape and in the position of the attachment of appendix. At birth, the caecum is conical in shape and the vermiform appendix is attached at its apex. Later the caecal growth results in the formation of two saccules, one on either side of anterior teniae coli. The growth of right saccule is greater

Table 10.2 Differences between the small and large intestines*

Features	Small intestine	Large intestine
Length	6 m	1.5 m
Lumen	Narrower	Wider
Mobility	More	Less
Transverse mucous folds	Permanent and not obliterated by distension of the gut	Temporary and obliterated by distension of the gut
Villi	Present	Absent
Peyer's patches	Present	Absent
Appendices epiploicae	Absent	Present
Teniae coli	Absent	Present
Sacculation	Absent	Present

*Clinically, it is important for the students to know that (a) the small intestine is a common site for worm infestation, typhoid, and tubercular ulcers whereas the large intestine a common site for amebiasis and carcinoma. (b) The infection and irritation of the small intestine lead to diarrhea, whereas the infection and irritation of the large intestine lead to dysentery.

than the left so that the apex of caecum and the base of appendix are pushed toward the left and nearer to the ileocaecal junction. As a result the base of appendix is attached at the posteromedial wall of the caecum.

Types of Caecum (Fig. 10.9)

The caecum and vermiform appendix develop from the caecal bud arising from the caudal limb of the primitive intestinal loop. The proximal part of the bud dilates to form caecum and the distal part remains narrow and forms the vermiform appendix. On the basis of growth of the caecum later on, four types of caecum may be found in adults (Fig. 10.9).

1. *Conical type/fetal type (2%):* The caecum is conical and the appendix is attached at its apex.
2. *Infantile type (3%):* The caecum is quadrate in shape (due to equal size of right and left saccules) and the appendix is attached at the depressed bottom.
3. *Normal type (80–90%):* The right saccule is larger than the left and the appendix is attached on the posteromedial aspect about 2 cm below the ileocaecal junction.
4. *Exaggerated type (4–5%):* The right saccule is immensely large (due to its exaggerated growth) and the left saccule is absent. The appendix is attached just below the ileocaecal junction.

DIMENSIONS

Length: 6 cm (2½ inches).
Width: 7.5 cm (3 inches).

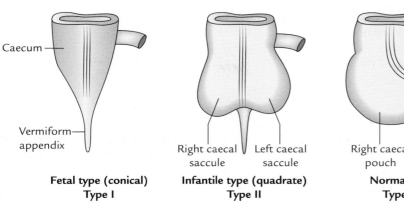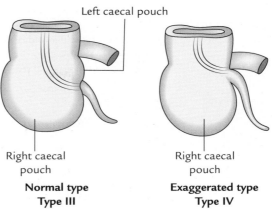

Fig. 10.9 Types of caecum.

N.B. Caecum is one of those organs of the body which have greater width than length (viz. prostate, pituitary gland, isthmus of thyroid gland, and coeliac trunk).

RELATIONS

Visceral Relations

Anterior:

1. Coils of the small intestine.
2. Greater omentum.
3. Anterior abdominal wall (in the right iliac region).

Posterior (Fig. 10.10):

1. Right psoas major and iliacus muscles.
2. Femoral nerve, lateral cutaneous nerve of the thigh, and genitofemoral nerve of the right side.
3. Right gonadal vessels.

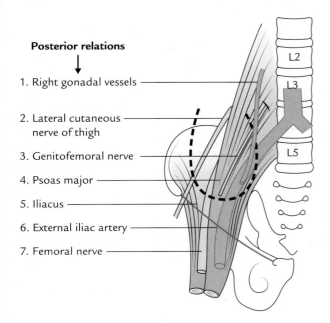

Fig. 10.10 Posterior relations of the caecum. The position of caecum is outlined by a thick broken black line.

4. Right external iliac artery (sometimes).
5. Retrocaecal recess (often contains the vermiform appendix).

Peritoneal Relations (Fig. 10.11)

In about 90% individuals, the caecum is almost completely surrounded by the peritoneum and has wide *retrocaecal recess* which may ascend up posterior to the lower part of the ascending colon and then called *retrocolic recess*. The vermiform appendix frequently lies in the retrocaecal recess.

In 10% of individuals, the upper part of its posterior surface is non-peritoneal and lies directly on fascia iliaca. The other recesses in the ileocaecal region are superior ileocaecal recess underneath the superior ileocaecal fold, and inferior ileocaecal recess underneath the inferior ileocaecal fold.

N.B. The caecum may have mesentery. It is mobile in 20% subjects, more often in females than in males.

The **peritoneal folds in relation to the caecum and the terminal part of the ileum** are discussed as follows:

1. **Superior ileocaecal fold:** It lies between the ileum and the ascending colon.
   (a) It is a fold of the peritoneum from the posterior abdominal wall raised by the anterior caecal artery. Therefore, it is also called vascular fold of caecum.
   (b) It guards the superior ileocaecal recess and opens downward and to the left.
2. **Inferior ileocaecal fold:** It extends from the anteroinferior aspect of the terminal part of the ileum to the caecum or appendix.
   (a) It does not contain any blood vessels, hence also called "**bloodless fold of Treves.**"
   (b) It lies in front of the ileocaecal recess which looks downward and to the left.
3. **Caecal fold:** It lies on the posterior surface and forms the right boundary of the posterior ileocaecal recess.

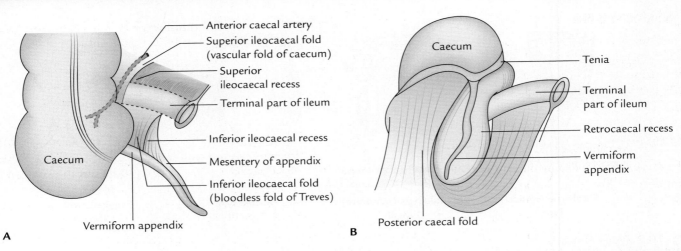

Fig. 10.11 Peritoneal relations of caecum: **A**, anterior view of ileocaecal region; **B**, inferior view of ileocaecal region. Note retrocaecal recess containing vermiform appendix (caecum has been pulled forward and upward).

INTERIOR OF THE CAECUM (Fig. 10.12)

The interior of the caecum presents two orifices—ileocaecal orifice and appendicular orifice.

The ileocaecal orifice is the prominent feature of the interior of the caecum.

Ileocaecal Orifice (Fig. 10.12)

It is present on the posteromedial aspect of the cecocolic junction where the ileum opens into the large intestine. The orifice measures about 2.5 cm transversely. This orifice is guarded by a valve called **ileocaecal valve**. The valve has two lips: upper and lower. The **upper lip** is smaller and horizontal. It lies at the level of ileocolic junction. The lower lip is longer and concave upwards. It lies at the level of ileocaecal junction. The two lips meet at the ends and are continued as the mucous folds called **caecal frenula**, which may act as

caecocolic sphincter. Each lip is made up of thickening of circular muscle coat covered by the submucosa and mucosa.

The *ileocaecal valve regulates the flow of contents from the ileum to the caecum and prevents regurgitation of contents of the caecum into the ileum.*

Clinical correlation

- A **barium enema** that fills the colon completely always enters in the terminal part of the ileum to a variable extent.
- Failure of relaxation of ileocaecal sphincter in longstanding large bowel obstruction may cause distension and rupture of caecum, if the obstruction is not relieved.

  The caecum acts as a guide to surgeon during operation for intestinal obstruction. The *dictum* is that if caecum is distended, the obstruction is in the large intestine and if it is empty the obstruction is in the small intestine.

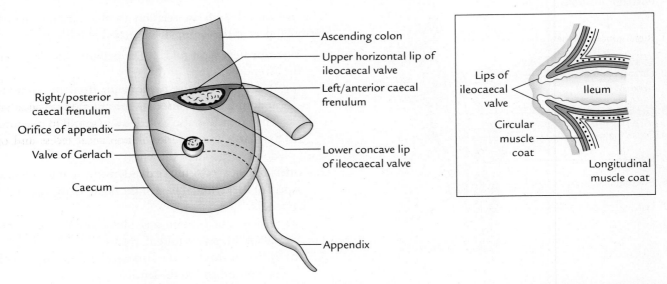

Fig. 10.12 Interior of caecum showing ileocaecal and appendicular orifices and associated ileocaecal valve and valve of appendicular orifice, respectively. Figure in the inset shows the projection of ileum into the lumen of the caecum.

Appendicular Orifice

It is a small circular orifice situated about 2 cm below and slightly behind the ileocaecal orifice. The orifice is guarded by insignificant semicircular fold of mucous membrane called **valve of Gerlach** attached to the lower margin of the opening (Fig. 10.12).

BLOOD SUPPLY AND LYMPHATIC DRAINAGE

The caecum is supplied by the **anterior and posterior caecal branches of the ileocolic artery**, a branch of superior mesenteric artery (Fig. 10.13).

The veins of the caecum follow the arteries and drain into the superior mesenteric vein, which finally drains into the portal system.

The lymph vessels from the caecum drain into the ileocolic lymph nodes, which in turn drain into the superior mesenteric group of pre-aortic lymph nodes.

NERVE SUPPLY

The sympathetic nerve supply is derived from T11 and L1 spinal segments through superior mesenteric plexus. The *parasympathetic nerve supply* is derived from both vagus nerves.

VERMIFORM APPENDIX

The vermiform appendix is a narrow worm-like diverticulum, which arise from the posteromedial wall of the caecum about 2 cm below the ileocaecal junction.

DIMENSIONS

The appendix varies in length from 2 to 20 cm (average 9 cm). The average width is about 5 mm. The diameter of lumen varies with age. It is more in children than adult and often obliterated after mid-adult life. The length also varies with age. It is longer in children than in adults.

PARTS

The appendix presents three parts—base, body, and tip.

1. The **base** is attached to the posteromedial wall of the caecum about 2 cm below the ileocaecal junction. All the three teniae of caecum converge to the base of the appendix. This anatomical fact serves as guide to the surgeon to search for the appendix during appendicectomy.
2. The **body** is a narrow tubular part between the base and the tip.
3. The **tip** is the least vascular distal blind end. It may be directed in various directions.

SURFACE ANATOMY (Fig. 10.14)

The base of the appendix is marked on the surface by a point 2 cm below the intersection between the transtubercular plane and the right midclavicular line (right lateral plane).

N.B. The point representing the base on the surface (vide supra) and McBurney's point do not exactly correspond anatomically but they are in close approximation topographically. For this reason, clinicians equate the surface marking of the appendix to McBurney's point.

POSITIONS (Fig. 10.15)

The appendix usually lies in the right iliac fossa. The base of appendix is fixed but the remaining part may occupy any of

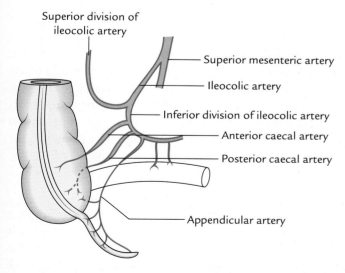

Fig. 10.13 Arterial supply of the caecum and appendix.

Superior division of ileocolic artery
Superior mesenteric artery
Ileocolic artery
Inferior division of ileocolic artery
Anterior caecal artery
Posterior caecal artery
Appendicular artery

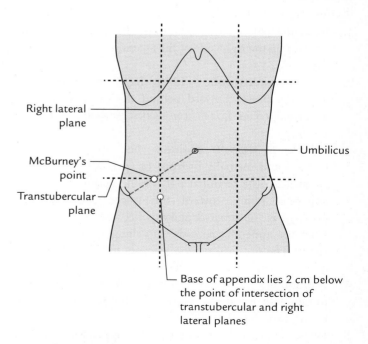

Fig. 10.14 Surface marking of the appendix.

Right lateral plane
McBurney's point
Transtubercular plane
Umbilicus
Base of appendix lies 2 cm below the point of intersection of transtubercular and right lateral planes

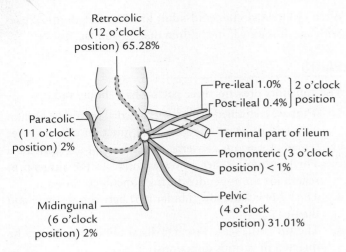

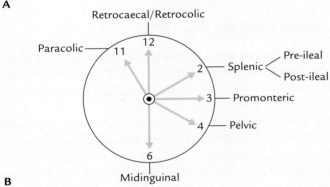

Fig. 10.15 Positions of vermiform appendix (after Treves): A, actual positions; B, positions according to the needle of clock.

the following positions, which are often indicated with an hour hand of a clock.

1. **Paracolic (11 o'clock) position:** The appendix passes upward on the right side of the ascending colon in 2% of the cases.

2. **Retrocaecal/retrocolic (12 o'clock) position:** The appendix passes upward behind the caecum and the ascending colon. *It is the commonest position (65.28%) of the appendix.*

3. **Splenic (2 o'clock) position:** The appendix passes upward and medially in front of (**pre-ileal**) or behind (**post-ileal**) the terminal part of the ileum. The tip of appendix points toward the spleen. The pre-ileal position is the most dangerous because inflammation from the appendix spreads into the general peritoneal cavity. The pre-ileal position occurs in 1% of the cases and post-ileal in 0.4% of the cases.

4. **Promonteric (3 o'clock) position:** The appendix passes horizontally toward the sacral promontory. The position is very rare (less than 1%).

5. **Pelvic (4 o'clock) position:** The appendix descends downward and medially, and crosses the pelvic brim to

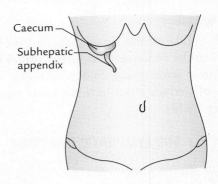

Fig. 10.16 Subhepatic appendix.

enter the true pelvis. In females, it may be related to the right uterine tube. It is the *second commonest position* (31.01%).

6. **Midinguinal/subcaecal (6 o'clock) position:** The appendix passes vertically downward below the caecum (subcaecal) and points toward the inguinal ligament. It occurs in 2% of the cases.

N.B. *Subhepatic appendix (Fig. 10.16):* It is an abnormal position of the appendix in which it lies underneath the liver in the right hypochondrium. It is a development anomaly, which occurs due to failure in the descent of caecal bud. The caecum and appendix develop from **caecal bud** that arises from postarterial segment of midgut loop (near its apex).

After the return of herniated midgut loop in the abdominal cavity, the caecal bud occupies the subhepatic position. When the postarterial segment of midgut loop elongates to form ascending colon, the caecal bud gradually descends to reach the right iliac fossa. The arrest of its descent leads to subhepatic position of caecum and appendix. The inflammation of subhepatic appendix causes pain and tenderness in the right hypochondrium and may mimic *acute cholecystis* (inflammation of the gall bladder).

PERITONEAL RELATIONS

The vermiform appendix is an intraperitoneal structure. The appendix is suspended by a small triangular fold of the peritoneum derived from the posterior/left layer of mesentery of the ileum. It is called the *mesentery of appendix or mesoappendix.* The appendicular artery runs within the free margin of mesoappendix. Occasionally the mesoappendix fails to reach the apex of appendix.

ARTERIAL SUPPLY

The appendix is supplied by a single appendicular artery, a branch of inferior division of ileocolic artery (Fig. 10.13). It passes behind the terminal part of the ileum to enter the mesoappendix and runs in its free margin to reach the tip of appendix which is the least vascular part. The appendicular artery is an end artery. When the mesoappendix is short, the appendicular artery rests directly on the appendicular wall near the tip of appendix. In appendicitis, this part of the artery is affected and thrombosed, leading to gangrenous change in the tip which may perforate.

VENOUS DRAINAGE

The vein corresponds to the artery and drains into the superior mesenteric vein which in turn drains into the portal vein.

LYMPHATIC DRAINAGE

The lymph vessels of the appendix drain into **ileocolic lymph nodes** directly or through appendicular nodes in the mesoappendix.

NERVE SUPPLY

The **sympathetic nerve supply**, which carries the pain sensations from the appendix, is derived from the T10 spinal segment via lesser splanchnic nerve and superior mesenteric plexus. For this reason, the pain of appendicitis is referred to the umbilical region.

The **parasympathetic nerve supply** is derived from both vagus nerves.

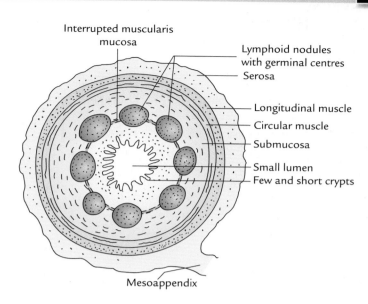

Fig. 10.17 Microscopic structure of appendix as seen in its transverse section.

Clinical correlation

- **Appendicitis:** The inflammation of the appendix is called appendicitis. Acute appendicitis is a common occurrence and is a surgical emergency. It commonly occurs due to obstruction of its lumen by fecaliths or edema.

  The initial pain of appendicitis is the referred pain and is felt in the umbilical region because both have same segmental nerve supply (i.e., T10 spinal segment). Gradually the pain is localized in the right iliac fossa. It is due to involvement of local parietal peritoneum (i.e., parietal peritoneum in the region of right iliac fossa). The overlying musculature undergoes spasm causing guarding of anterior abdominal wall. On palpation maximum tenderness is elicited at **McBurney's point** which is marked on the surface by a point at the junction of medial two-third and lateral one-third of a line extending from the umbilicus to the right anterior superior iliac spine.
- **Psoas test in appendicitis:** When the appendix is retrocaecal in position it lies on and irritates the right psoas major when inflamed (appendicitis). The forced extension of the right thigh in such patients causes increase in pain in the right iliac fossa.
- **Obturator test in appendicitis:** When the appendix is pelvic in position, it may irritate the obturator internus muscle. The flexion and medial rotation of the right thigh on the abdomen causes pain in the lower abdomen.
- **Appendectomy:** The incision for appendectomy is purely based on the anatomy of the anterior abdominal wall. A gridiron (5 shape of a cross beam) incision is given (i.e.,

incision is given at right angle to the spino-umbilical line) in the right iliac fossa. The three flat muscles are split along the direction of their fibres. The fascia transversalis and parietal peritoneum are incised together. The appendix is delivered through the wound and cut at its base and removed.

MICROSCOPIC STRUCTURE (Fig. 10.17)

The appendix has relatively small angulated circular lumen as compared to its thick wall. The wall of the appendix consists of four layers from within outwards, these are: mucosa, submucosa, muscular layer, and serosa.

1. **Mucosa:** The surface of the mucous membrane is lined by the simple columnar cells and numerous goblet cells. It is devoid of villi. The intestinal glands (crypts of Lieberkuhn) are few and short.
2. **Submucosa:** It contains a **ring of large lymphoid follicles** with germinal centres. Hence, the appendix is commonly considered as an **abdominal tonsil.**
3. **Muscle layer:** It consists of outer longitudinal and inner circular layers of smooth muscle.
4. **Serosa:** It is made up of visceral peritoneum.

N.B. Muscularis mucosa is disrupted by lymphatic nodules.

COLON

For descriptive purposes, the colon is divided into four parts (Fig. 10.18): (a) ascending colon, (b) transverse colon, (c) descending colon, and (d) sigmoid colon.

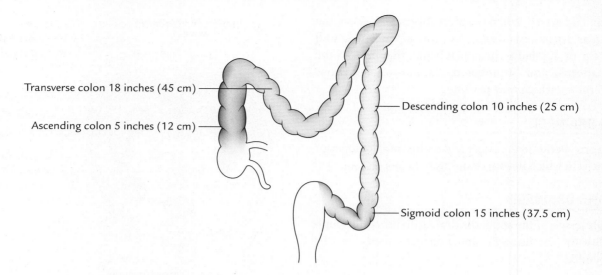

Fig. 10.18 Subdivisions of the colon and their length.

Ascending Colon

1. The ascending colon is an upward continuation of the caecum. It is about 5 inch (12.5 cm) in length and extends from the caecum, at the level of ileocaecal orifice, to the inferior surface of the right lobe of the liver where it bends to the left to form the **hepatic (right colic) flexure.**
2. It lies in the right paracolic gutter and covered by the peritoneum on the front and sides, which binds it to the posterior abdominal wall.
3. Its posterior surface lies on three muscles: iliacus, quadratus lumborum, and transversus abdominis.
4. During its course from the caecum to the undersurface of the liver, it crosses three nerves. From below upward these are: lateral cutaneous nerve of thigh, ilioinguinal nerve, and iliohypogastric nerve.
5. Anteriorly it is related to the coils of the small bowel and right edge of the greater omentum.

N.B.
- Sometimes ascending colon possesses a mesentery called **ascending mesocolon.**

- Right margin of the greater omentum is sometimes fused with its peritoneal covering. In that case, the right half of the transverse colon is often closely related to the ascending colon, forming the so-called *"double-barreled gun."*

Transverse Colon

1. It is the longest (20 inch/50 cm in length) and most mobile part of the large intestine.
2. It extends from the right colic flexure (in right lumbar region) to the left colic flexure (in the left hypochondriac region).
3. Strictly speaking transverse colon is not transverse but forms a dependent loop in front of loops of small intestine between the right and left colic flexures. The lowest point of loop usually extends up to the level of umbilicus but may sometimes extend into the pelvis. Thus, the transverse colon is usually 'U'-shaped.

The differences between the right and left colic flexures are given in Table 10.3.

Table 10.3 Differences between the right (hepatic) and left (splenic) flexures

Features	Right colic flexure	Left colic flexure
Location	Right lumbar region (where it is related to the inferior surface of right lobe of the liver)	Left hypochondrium (immediately below the spleen)
Level	1 inch (2.5 cm) below the transpyloric plane, at the level of L2 vertebra	1 inch (2.5 cm) above the transpyloric plane, at the level of T12 vertebra
Angulation	Wider	Acute
Attachment to diaphragm	No attachment	Attached to diaphragm at the level of 10th and 11th ribs by phrenicocolic ligament

Relations

Anterior: Greater omentum and anterior abdominal wall.
Posterior: Second part of the duodenum, head of the pancreas, and coils of the jejunum and ileum.

Clinical correlation

- The anterior surface of the transverse colon is closely related to the anterior abdominal wall. This makes exposure of transverse colon easy for surgeons to perform colostomy (making a hole in it).
- If the loops of the jejunum and ileum are distended, the transverse colon may be pushed up. Occasionally it passes anterior to the stomach and if distended with gas it may mask the dullness of the liver to percussion and mimic the presence of gas in the peritoneal cavity.

Transverse Mesocolon

The transverse colon is suspended from the posterior abdominal wall by a large double-layered fold of the peritoneum called *transverse mesocolon.*

It is fused with the posterior surface of the greater omentum and divides the peritoneal cavity into supra- and infracolic compartments.

Thus, it forms a natural barrier against the spread of the infection between the supra- and infracolic compartments.

1. On the posterior abdominal wall, it is attached to the second part of the duodenum, head, and body (lower margin) of the pancreas and anterior surface of the left kidney.
2. The contents of the transverse mesocolon are middle colic vessels, ascending branches of the right and left colic vessels, lymph nodes, lymphatics, and nerve plexuses embedded in the loose areolar tissue containing variable amount of the fat.

Development

The proximal two-third of transverse colon develops from the midgut and the distal one-third from the hindgut. The differences between the right two-third and the left one-third of the transverse colon are given in Table 10.4.

Descending Colon

1. The descending colon is longer (25 cm), narrower, and more deeply located than the ascending colon.

2. It extends from the left colic flexure to the front of the left external iliac artery at the level of pelvic brim where it becomes continuous with the pelvic colon (sigmoid colon).

It is covered by the peritoneum on the front and sides which fixes it in the left paracolic gutter and iliac fossa.

Course and Relations

1. Its proximal part descends vertically downward from the left colic flexure to the left iliac fossa. During this course it passes in front of three muscles and three nerves. The muscles are quadratus lumborum, transversus abdominis, and iliacus. The nerves are iliohypogastric, ilioinguinal, and lateral cutaneous nerve of the thigh.
2. Its distal part turns medially from the left iliac fossa to the front of the left external iliac vessels. During this course it passes in front of the femoral nerve, psoas major muscle, testicular vessels, genitofemoral nerve, and left external iliac vein.

Clinical correlation

The loaded (with feces) descending colon may compress the left testicular and common iliac veins. This is one of the predisposing factors for greater frequency of varicosity of veins forming pampiniform plexus in the left spermatic cord (*varicocele*) and veins draining the left lower limb (*varicose vein in the left lower limb*).

Sigmoid Colon (Pelvic Colon)

The sigmoid colon is about 15 inches (37.5 cm) long and connects the descending colon with the rectum. It is S-shaped and hence its name, sigmoid colon (G. Sigma = S-shaped alphabet).

It extends from the lower end of descending colon at the left pelvic inlet to the pelvic surface of the third piece of sacrum, where it becomes continuous with the rectum.

During its course it forms a sinuous loop which hangs free in the lesser pelvis. In the pelvis it lies in front of the bladder and uterus, below the loops of ileum.

The loop of sigmoid colon consists of three parts: (a) first part runs downward in contact with the left pelvic wall; (b) second part transverses the pelvic cavity horizontally

Table 10.4 Differences between the right two-third and left one-third of the transverse colon

Features	Right two-third of transverse colon	Left one-third of transverse colon
Development	From midgut	From hindgut
Arterial supply	Middle colic artery, a branch of superior mesenteric artery (artery of midgut)	Left colic artery, a branch of inferior mesenteric artery (artery of hindgut)
Nerve supply	By vagus nerves	By pelvic splanchnic nerves

between the bladder and the rectum in male (uterus and rectum in female); and (c) third part runs backward to reach the midline in front of third sacral vertebra.

Sigmoid (Pelvic) Mesocolon

The sigmoid colon is suspended from the pelvic wall by a large peritoneal fold called sigmoid mesocolon. The sigmoid mesocolon has an inverted V-shaped attachment/root.

The left limb: The left limb of the root is attached on the external iliac artery. It extends from the end of the descending colon to the middle of the common iliac artery. Here it turns sharply downward and to the right across the lesser pelvis to the third piece of the sacrum, forming the right limb. The right limb is attached on the pelvic surface of the sacrum. The meeting point of two limbs is called apex. The students must remember the following facts in relation to the apex of "Λ."

1. Just lateral to the apex of the Λ, a pocket-like extension of the peritoneal cavity passes upward posterior to the root of the mesocolon. It is called **intersigmoid recess**. The left ureter lies behind this recess.
2. The inferior mesenteric artery divides near the apex of Λ.
3. The *superior rectal artery* enters the right limb and sigmoidal arteries enter the left limb.

ARTERIAL SUPPLY

The colon is supplied by the following arteries (Fig. 10.19):

1. Ileocolic artery.
2. Right colic artery.
3. Middle colic artery.
4. Left colic artery.
5. Sigmoidal arteries.
6. Superior rectal artery.

The first three arteries are the branches of the superior mesenteric artery and the last three are the branches of the inferior mesenteric artery.

The supply of different parts of the colon by these arteries is as under:

(a) The lower smaller part of the ascending colon is supplied by the ileocolic artery and its larger upper part is supplied by the right colic artery.
(b) The right two-third of the transverse colon is supplied by the middle colic artery and the left one-third by the left colic artery.
(c) The descending colon is supplied by the left colic artery.
(d) The sigmoid colon is supplied by the sigmoidal branches of the inferior mesenteric artery and superior rectal artery. The sigmoidal arteries are usually two to three in number.

Marginal Artery of Drummond (Fig. 10.19)

1. It is a circumferential anastomotic arterial channel extending from the ileocaecal junction to the rectosigmoid junction. It is located close (about 3 cm) to the inner margin of the colon.
2. It is formed by the anastomoses between the branches of colic branches of the superior mesenteric artery (i.e., ileocolic, right colic, and middle colic) and colic branches of the inferior mesenteric artery (left colic and sigmoidal). The vasa recta arise from the marginal artery and supply the colon.

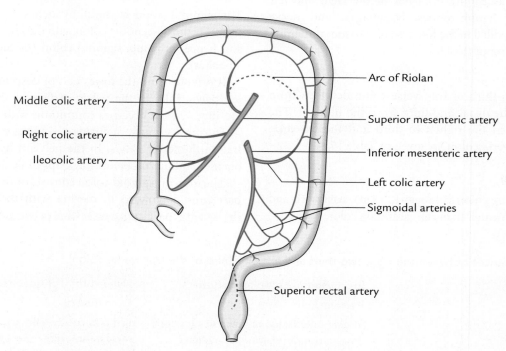

Fig. 10.19 Arterial supply of the colon. Note the formation of marginal artery of Drummond.

N.B. *Critical point of colon:* It lies at the level of splenic flexure. At this level, the ascending branch of the left colic artery often fails to anastomose with the left branch of the middle colic artery. However, there is anastomotic channel between the main trunk of the middle colic and the ascending branch of the left colic called *"arc of Riolan."* If this anastomosis is not well developed, the arterial supply of splenic flexure is jeopardized and splenic flexure undergoes ischemic changes.

Earlier it was thought that the critical point of the colon is on the sigmoid colon (**critical point of Sudeck**) where the anastomosis between the sigmoidal branches of inferior mesenteric and superior rectal arteries was thought to be insufficient.

VENOUS DRAINAGE

1. The veins draining the colon accompany the arteries.
2. The veins accompanying the ileocolic, right colic, and middle colic arteries join the *superior mesenteric vein*, while the veins, accompanying the branches of inferior mesenteric artery, join the inferior mesenteric vein. The superior and inferior mesenteric veins finally drain into the portal circulation.

LYMPHATIC DRAINAGE (Fig. 10.20)

The lymphatic drainage of the colon is clinically very important because carcinoma of the colon spreads through lymphatic route.

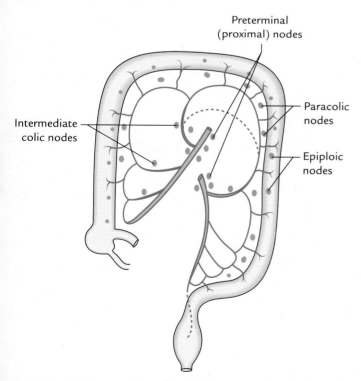

Fig. 10.20 Lymphatic drainage of the colon.

There are numerous colic lymph nodes, which drain the lymph from the colon. These nodes have common pattern of distribution. They are arranged in following four groups:

1. *Epiploic nodes,* are small nodules and lie on the wall of the colon.
2. *Paracolic nodes,* lie very close to the marginal artery (of Drummond), i.e., along the medial borders of the ascending and descending colons and along the mesenteric borders of transverse and sigmoid colons.
3. *Intermediate colic nodes,* lie along the ileocolic, right colic, middle colic and left colic, arteries, and drain into terminal nodes.
4. *Preterminal nodes,* lie along trunks of superior and inferior mesenteric arteries.

The rectum and anal canal are described in detail in Chapter 19.

Clinical correlation

- **Examination of the interior of colon:** Barium enema is used for visualizing the interior of the colon. The typical pattern of the colon due to the presence of sacculations is clearly seen. Nowadays, endoscopic examination of the interior of the colon is extensively done.
- **Congenital megacolon/Hirschsprung disease:** It occurs when neural crest cells fail to migrate and form the **myenteric plexus** (parasympathetic ganglia) in the sigmoid colon and rectum during embryonic development. This condition results in absence of peristalsis. As a result the normal proximal colon becomes grossly dilated due to the fecal retention causing abdominal distension. The constricted segment usually corresponds to rectosigmoid junction (for details, see *Clinical and Surgical Anatomy*, 2nd Edition by Vishram Singh).
- **Cancer (carcinoma) of colon:** Cancer of colon (actually large intestine) is a leading cause of death in the Western world. It is relatively common in people who are above 50 years of age and nonvegetarian. It is slow growing tumor and causes constriction of the colon. The growth is restricted to the wall of colon for a considerable time before it spreads by lymphatics. In advanced cases, it spreads to the liver via portal circulation. If diagnosed early, hemicolectomy (partial resection of the colon) is done to treat the patient.
- **Surgical resection for cancer:** While planning resection of the colon affected by carcinoma, the surgeon should remember the following anatomical facts:
  - (a) Lymph from gut may miss the epiploic and paracolic nodes and go directly to the intermediate and preterminal nodes.
  - (b) The territory of lymphatic drainage is divided fairly accurately into areas corresponding to the areas supplied by the main arteries.
  - (c) Removal of lymph nodes is possible only after ligating the main arteries.

  Thus, the whole segment of colon being supplied by the ligated artery should be removed to avoid gangrene.

  The sites of carcinoma in colon and segment of bowel of colon to be removed is given in Table 10.5.

Table 10.5 Sites of the carcinoma in colon

Sites of carcinoma	Vessels to be ligated	Segments of colon to be removed
Caecum and ascending colon	Ileocolic, right colic, and right branch of middle colic	Terminal part of the ileum, caecum, ascending colon, hepatic flexure, proximal one-third of transverse colon
Hepatic flexure and right two-third of transverse colon	Ileocolic, right colic, and middle colic	Terminal part of the ileum, caecum, ascending colon, and right two-third of transverse colon
Left one-third of transverse colon and splenic flexure	Middle colic and left colic	From middle of the ascending colon to the beginning of sigmoid colon
Descending and sigmoid colons	Inferior mesenteric artery	Descending and pelvic colon

- **Diverticulosis:** The diverticulosis is a common clinical condition of the colon and mostly involves the sigmoid colon. It consists of the herniation of the lining mucosa through the circular muscle between the teniae coli.

  The herniation occurs where the circular muscle coat is the weakest, i.e., where it is pierced by the blood vessels.

  The inflammation of diverticula is termed *diverticulitis*.

- **Volvulus:** It is a clinical condition, in which a portion of gut rotates (clockwise/anticlockwise) on the axis of its mesentery. It usually occurs due to adhesion of antimesenteric border of the gut to the parietes or any other viscera. It may correct itself spontaneously or the rotation may continue until the blood supply of the gut is cut off leading to ischemia. The sigmoid colon is susceptible to volvulus because of extreme mobility of its mesentery—the pelvic mesocolon.

- **Intussusception:** It is a clinical condition in which a proximal segment of the bowel invaginates into the lumen of an adjoining distal segment. This may cut off the blood supply to the bowel and cause gangrene. The various forms of intussusception are *ileoileal, ileocaecal,* and *colocolic.* The ileocaecal intussusception is the most common form (for details, see *Clinical and Surgical Anatomy,* 2nd Edition by Vishram Singh).

SUPERIOR AND INFERIOR MESENTERIC VESSELS

These vessels include superior and inferior mesenteric arteries and veins.

SUPERIOR MESENTERIC ARTERY (Fig. 10.21)

Origin

It arises from the front of the abdominal aorta behind the body of pancreas near its neck at the level of L1 vertebra about ½ inch (1.25 cm) below the origin of coeliac trunk.

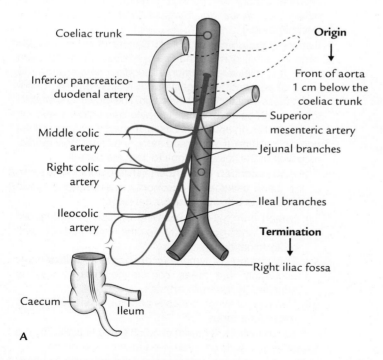

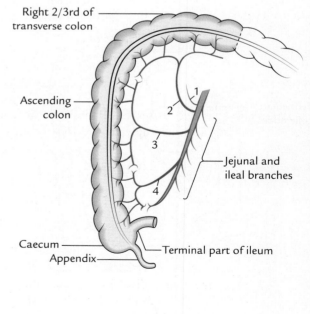

Fig. 10.21 Superior mesenteric artery: A, course and branches; B, a part of gut supplied by the superior mesenteric artery (1 = inferior pancreaticoduodenal artery; 2 = middle colic artery; 3 = right colic artery; 4 = ileocolic artery).

Course

From its origin, it runs downward and to the right passing first in front of the uncinate process of the pancreas, and then in front of the third part of the duodenum to enter the root of mesentery where it runs between its two layers.

It terminates in the right iliac fossa by anastomosing with a branch of ileocolic artery—one of its own branches.

Throughout its course, the *superior mesenteric artery* is accompanied by the *superior mesenteric vein* on its right side.

Relations

Anteriorly from above downward it is related to the body of pancreas and splenic vein.

Posteriorly from above downward it is related to the left renal vein, uncinate process of the pancreas, third part of the duodenum, IVC, right ureter, and right psoas major.

Branches

The superior mesenteric artery gives off five sets of branches as follows:

1. Inferior pancreaticoduodenal artery.
2. Middle colic artery.
3. Right colic artery.
4. Ileocolic artery.
5. Jejunal and ileal branches.

All the branches arise from its right side except jejunal and ileal branches which arise from its left side.

Inferior pancreaticoduodenal artery: It arises from the right side at the upper border of the horizontal part of the duodenum and soon divides into anterior and posterior branches which run in the pancreaticoduodenal groove and end by anastomosing with the anterior and posterior branches of the superior pancreaticoduodenal artery. Inferior pancreaticoduodenal artery is the first branch of superior mesenteric artery.

Middle colic artery: It arises from the right side, just below the pancreas, and runs upward and forward to pass between the two layers of transverse mesocolon, where it divides into right and left branches. The right branch anastomoses with the ascending branch of the right colic artery and the left branch anastomoses with the ascending branch of the left colic artery, a branch of the inferior mesenteric artery.

Right colic artery: It arises from the right side near the middle of the superior mesenteric artery, runs to the right behind the peritoneum and divides into ascending and descending branches. The ascending branch anastomoses with the right branch of the middle colic artery and the descending branch anastomoses with the ascending branch of the ileocolic artery to form the beginning of the marginal artery of Drummond (p. 158).

Ileocolic artery: It is the lowest branch arising from the right side. It runs downward and to the right, and divides into the ascending and descending branches. The ascending branch anastomoses with the descending branch of the right colic artery and the descending (inferior) branch anastomoses with the terminal end of the superior mesenteric artery. The descending/inferior branch of the ileocolic artery also gives rise to:

(a) Anterior and posterior caecal arteries to the caecum.
(b) Appendicular artery to the appendix.
(c) Ileal branch to the terminal part of the ileum.

Jejunal and ileal branches: These branches, about 12–15 in number arise from the convex left side of the superior mesenteric artery. They pass between the two layers of the mesentery of small intestine. They branch and anastomose with each other to form a series of **arterial arcades** from which further branches arise and form the second, third, and even fifth tiers of arterial arcades.

The number of these arcades increases from the jejunum to ileum. Finally the straight branches called **vasa recta** arise from these arcades which pass on either side of the small intestine to supply it. The vasa recta are longer and less numerous in the jejunum than in the ileum.

N.B. The whole of the small intestine proper (i.e., jejunum and ileum) is supplied by the jejunal and ileal branches of the superior mesenteric artery except the terminal part of the ileum which is supplied by the ileocolic branch of the superior mesenteric artery.

Distribution

The superior mesenteric artery is the artery of the midgut, hence it supplies all the derivatives of the midgut, *viz.*, lower half of the duodenum (below the opening of hepatopancreatic duct), jejunum and ileum, caecum and appendix, ascending colon and right two-third of the transverse colon, and lower half of the head of pancreas.

SUPERIOR MESENTERIC VEIN (Fig. 10.22)

The superior mesenteric vein is the major tributary of the portal vein. It is formed in the right iliac fossa by the union of small veins emerging from the ileocaecal region. It runs upward accompanying the superior mesenteric artery (the vein being right to the artery) and terminates behind the neck of pancreas by joining the splenic vein to form the portal vein.

The tributaries of superior mesenteric vein are as follows:

1. Veins corresponding to the branches of superior mesenteric artery.
2. Right gastroepiploic vein.
3. Inferior pancreaticoduodenal vein.

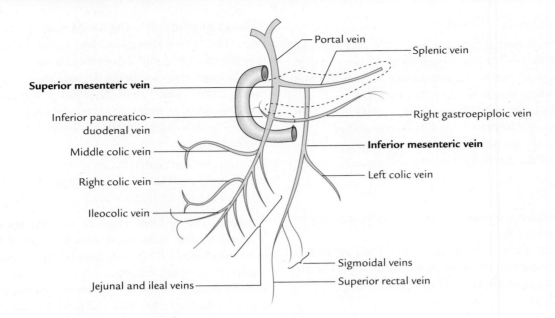

Fig. 10.22 Superior and inferior mesenteric veins and their tributaries.

The superior mesenteric vein drains venous blood from the small intestine which is rich in nutrients, large intestine up to the junction of proximal two-third and distal one-third of the transverse colon, stomach, and pancreas.

INFERIOR MESENTERIC ARTERY (Fig. 10.23)

Origin

The inferior mesenteric artery arises from the front of the abdominal aorta behind the third (horizontal) part of the duodenum at the level of L3 vertebra, about 3–4 cm above the termination (bifurcation) of the abdominal aorta.

Course and Branches

After arising from the aorta, it runs downward and to the left behind the peritoneum to cross the termination of the left common iliac artery (medial to ureter) at which point it becomes the **superior rectal artery**. The superior mesenteric artery gives rise to the following branches:

1. Left colic artery.
2. Sigmoidal arteries (two to three in number).
3. Superior rectal artery (continuation).

Distribution

The inferior mesenteric artery is the artery of hindgut, hence it supplies all the parts of gut derived from hindgut, viz., left one-third of the transverse colon, descending colon, rectum, and upper part of the anal canal.

N.B. The lowest sigmoidal artery anastomoses with the colic branch (first branch) of the superior rectal artery and this anastomosis is insufficient (weak point) in the marginal artery of

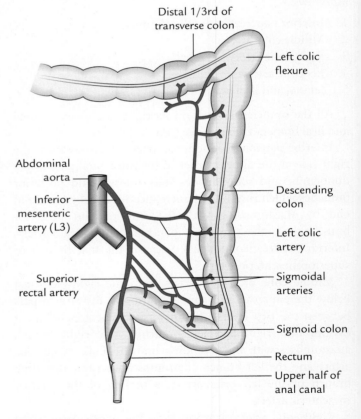

Fig. 10.23 Inferior mesenteric artery, its branches, and distribution.

the colon. Hence, the point of origin of the last sigmoidal artery from the inferior mesenteric artery is called **critical point of Sudeck**. Therefore, while ligating the inferior mesenteric artery it should be done proximal to Sudeck's point to avoid ischemia and necrosis of the sigmoid colon and rectum.

INFERIOR MESENTERIC VEIN

The inferior mesenteric vein is an upward continuation of the superior rectal vein. It ascends behind the peritoneum lateral to the inferior mesenteric artery. Then it passes lateral to the duodenojejunal flexure and anterior to the left renal vein to terminate by joining the splenic vein behind the pancreas. It may deviate to the right and join the superior mesenteric vein or its junction with the splenic vein.

The tributaries of the inferior mesenteric vein correspond to the branches of the inferior mesenteric artery.

Golden Facts to Remember

➤ Most fixed part of small intestine	Duodenum
➤ Longest and most mobile part of large intestine	Transverse colon
➤ Most common type of intussusception	Ileocolic
➤ Most common true diverticulum of gastrointestinal tract	Meckel's diverticulum (remnant of vitello-intestinal duct)
➤ Commonest site of intestinal diverticulosis	Sigmoid colon
➤ Most common site for intestinal tuberculosis	Ileocaecal junction
➤ Most common site for carcinoma colon	Rectosigmoid junction
➤ Narrowest part of the small intestine	2 feet (60 cm) proximal to ileocecal junction
➤ Most common site for ischemia of colon	Splenic flexure
➤ Commonest position of appendix	Retrocaecal/Retrocolic

Clinical Case Study

A 25-year-old medical student came to the surgical OPD of a hospital with the history of acute colicky pain around the umbilicus, fever, and vomiting a day before and now he was feeling pain in the region of right iliac fossa. On examination, the surgeon found the area of maximum tenderness at McBurney's point and guarding of the anterior abdominal wall in the region of right iliac fossa. The "*psoas test*" was positive. He was diagnosed as a case of *acute appendicitis*.

Questions

1. What is McBurney's point and what is its clinical significance?
2. Give the anatomical basis of initial pain in umbilical region and later in the region of right iliac fossa in this case.
3. Name the various positions of the appendix and mention the most common position.
4. What is the common incision given by surgeons to perform appendicectomy?

Answers

1. McBurney's point is located at the junction of the medial two-third and lateral one-third of the line joining the anterior superior iliac spine and umbilicus. Clinically, it corresponds to the base of appendix. It is the site of maximum tenderness in acute appendicitis.
2. Since the appendix is innervated by T10 spinal segment through the lesser splanchnic nerve, the initial pain is visceral and referred to the skin around the umbilicus because it is also innervated by T10 spinal segment. When the parietal peritoneum in right iliac fossa becomes involved by inflamed appendix, the pain becomes somatic in nature and localized to the right iliac fossa.
3. The various positions of the appendix are paracolic, retrocaecal, splenic, promonteric, pelvic, and midinguinal. The most common position is retrocaecal (60%).
4. Gridiron muscle splitting incision at McBurney's point.

Kidneys, Ureters, and Suprarenal Glands

KIDNEYS

Synonyms: *Ren*: kidney (in Latin); *Nephros*: kidney (in Greek).

The kidneys are two bean-shaped, reddish-brown organs within the abdomen situated on the posterior abdominal wall.

They are the major excretory organs and remove the waste products of protein metabolism and excess of water and salts from the blood and are thus essential for maintaining the electrolyte and water balance in the tissue fluids of the body, necessary for survival.

LOCATION

The kidneys lie on the posterior abdominal wall, one on each side of the vertebral column, behind the peritoneum, opposite 12th thoracic and upper three lumbar (T12–L3)

vertebrae. They occupy epigastric, hypochondriac, lumbar and umbilical regions (Fig. 11.1).

1. The right kidney lies at a slightly lower level than the left one due to the presence of liver on the right side.
2. The left kidney is little nearer to the median plane than the right.
3. Their long axes are slightly oblique (being directed downward and laterally) so that their upper ends or poles are nearer to each other than the lower poles (Fig. 11.1A inset). The upper poles are 2.5 cm away from the midline, the hilum are 5 cm away from the midline, and the lower poles are 7.5 cm away from the midline (Fig. 11.2).
4. Both kidneys move downward in vertical direction for 2.5 cm during respiration.
5. Transpyloric plane passes through the upper part of the hilum of the right kidney and through the lower part of the hilum of the left kidney.

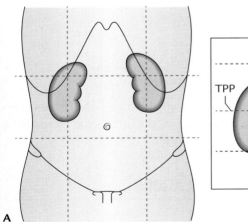
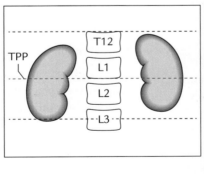
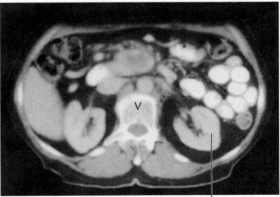

Fig. 11.1 Location of the kidneys: **A**, surface projection in relation to the anterior abdominal wall. The figure in the inset on the right shows the vertebral levels of the kidneys. Note the transpyloric plane (TPP) passes through the upper part of the hilum of the right kidney and the lower part of the hilum of the left kidney; **B**, CT scan in the axial plane showing location of the kidneys in relation to the vertebral column (V). (*Source*: B. Fig. 4.158, Page 360, *Gray's Anatomy for Students*, Richard L Drake, Wayne Vogl, Adam WM Mitchell. Copyright Elsevier Inc. 2005, All rights reserved.)

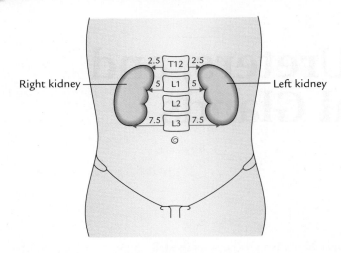

Fig. 11.2 Distances of the upper poles, hila, and lower poles of kidneys from the midline.

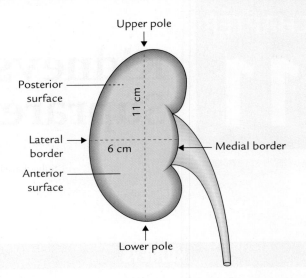

Fig. 11.3 External features and measurements of the kidney.

Shape and Measurements

Shape: Bean shaped.

Measurements:
Length: 11 cm. (left kidney is slightly longer and narrower).
Width: 6 cm.
Thickness: (anteroposterior) 3 cm.
Weight: 150 g in males; 135 g in females.

EXTERNAL FEATURES (Fig. 11.3)

Each kidney presents the following external features:

1. Two poles (superior and inferior).
2. Two surfaces (anterior and posterior).
3. Two borders (medial and lateral).
4. A hilum.

POLES

1. The *superior (upper) pole* is thick and round and lies nearer to the median plane than the inferior pole. It is related to the suprarenal gland.
2. The *inferior (lower) pole* is thin and pointed and lies 2.5 cm above the iliac crest.

SURFACES

1. The *anterior surface* is convex and faces anterolaterally.
2. The *posterior surface* is flat and faces posteromedially. However, in practice it is difficult to recognize anterior and posterior surfaces. This however is done easily by seeing the relationship of structures present at the hilum (vide infra).

BORDERS

1. The *medial border* of each kidney is convex above and below near the poles and concave in the middle. It slopes downward and laterally, and presents a vertical fissure in its middle part called **hilum/hilus** which has anterior and posterior lips.
2. The *lateral border* of each kidney is convex.

HILUM

The medial border (central part) of the kidney presents a deep vertical slit called **hilum**. It transmits, from before backward, the following structures (Fig. 11.4):

1. Renal vein.
2. Renal artery.
3. Renal pelvis.
4. Subsidiary branch of renal artery.

In addition to the above structures the hilum also transmits lymphatics and nerves, the latter being sympathetic and mainly vasomotor in nature.

RELATIONS

ANTERIOR RELATIONS (Fig. 11.5)

The anterior relations of two kidneys are different.
   Anterior surface of the right kidney:

1. Right suprarenal gland.
2. Right lobe of the liver.
3. Second part of the duodenum.

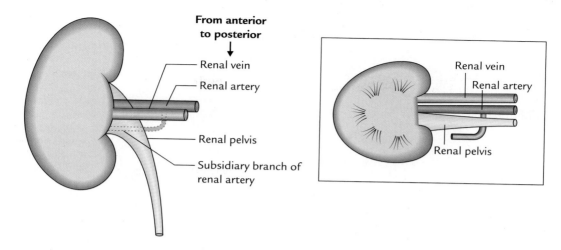

Fig. 11.4 Relationship of structures passing through the hilum of kidney. Figure in the inset is the schematic transverse section of the kidney showing this relationship.

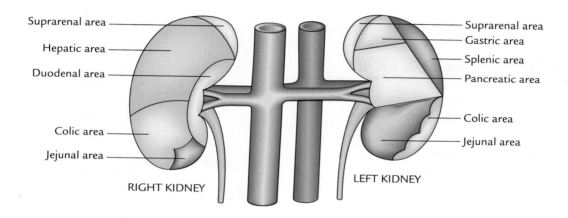

Fig. 11.5 Anterior relations of the kidneys.

4.   Hepatic (right colic) flexure.
5.   Jejunum.

Out of these, liver and jejunum are separated from the kidney by peritoneum.

Anterior surface of the left kidney:
1.   Left suprarenal gland.
2.   Spleen.
3.   Stomach.
4.   Pancreas and splenic vessels.
5.   Left colic flexure.
6.   Jejunum.

Out of these, stomach, spleen, and jejunum are separated from the kidney by peritoneum.

POSTERIOR RELATIONS (Fig. 11.6)

The posterior relations of two kidneys are the same except that right kidney is related to one rib while left kidney is related to two ribs:

1.   **Four muscles:** Diaphragm, quadratus lumborum, psoas major, and transversus abdominis.

2.   **Three nerves:** Subcostal (T12), iliohypogastric (L1), and ilioinguinal (L1). The subcostal nerve is accompanied by the subcostal vessels.

3.   **One or two ribs:** The right kidney is related to the 12th rib whereas the left kidney is related to the 11th and 12th ribs.

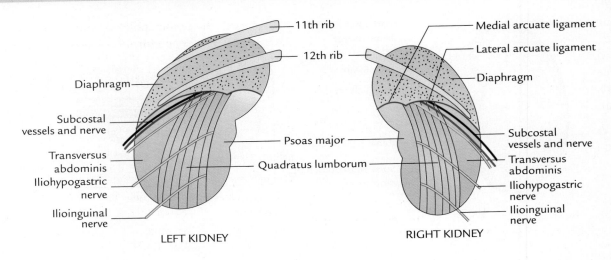

Fig. 11.6 Posterior relations of the kidneys.

N.B. The posterior relations of both the kidneys are same except that the right kidney is related only to the 12th rib and the left kidney to the 11th and 12th ribs.

CAPSULES (COVERINGS) OF KIDNEY

From within outwards, the kidney is surrounded by four capsules/coverings as follows (Fig. 11.7):

1. Fibrous capsule (true capsule).
2. Perirenal (perinephric) fat.
3. Renal fascia (false capsule).
4. Pararenal (paranephric) fat.

FIBROUS CAPSULE (TRUE CAPSULE)

It is a thin membrane which closely invests the kidney. It is formed by the condensation of fibrous connective tissue in the peripheral part of the organ. It is readily stripped off from the surface of the normal kidney. The capsule passes through the hilum to line the renal sinus and becomes continuous with the walls of calyces where they are attached with the kidney. If the kidney is inflamed, this capsule becomes firmly adherent to the organ and cannot be stripped off.

PERIRENAL (PERINEPHRIC) FAT

It is a layer of adipose tissue, surrounding the fibrous capsule of the kidney. It fills the space inside the loosely fitting sheath of the renal fascia enclosing the kidney and suprarenal gland. This fatty capsule is thickest at the borders of kidney and is prolonged through hilum into the renal sinus. In chronic debilitating diseases, the depletion of perinephric fat can

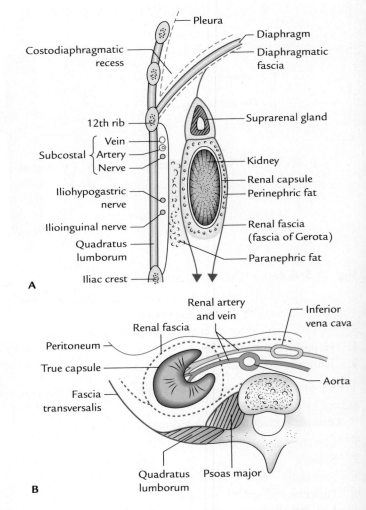

Fig. 11.7 Capsules (coverings) of the kidney: **A**, as seen in vertical section through posterior abdominal wall in the lumbar region; **B**, as seen in cross section through posterior abdominal wall in the lumbar region.

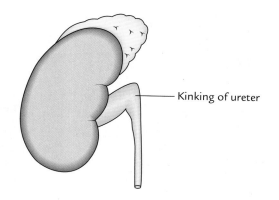

Fig. 11.8 Kinking of the ureter due to depletion of perinephric fat.

cause downward displacement of the kidney, which may lead to the kinking of the ureter (Fig. 11.8).

RENAL FASCIA (FALSE CAPSULE/ FASCIA OF GEROTA)

It is a fibroareolar sheath, which surrounds the kidney and perirenal fat.

It consists of the following two layers:

1. An ill-defined anterior layer (fascia of Toldt).
2. A well-defined posterior layer (fascia of Zuckerkandl).

Extensions

1. **Superiorly,** the two layers first enclose the suprarenal gland in a separate compartment and then fuse with each other and become continuous with the diaphragmatic fascia.
2. **Inferiorly,** the two layers remain separate and enclose the ureter. The anterior layer is gradually lost in the extraperitoneal tissue of iliac fossa while the posterior layer blends with the fascia iliaca.
3. **Laterally,** the two layers unite firmly and become continuous with the fascia transversalis.
4. **Medially,** the anterior layer passes in front of the kidney and renal vessels and merges with the connective tissue surrounding the aorta and inferior vena cava (IVC). The posterior layer passes behind the kidney and is attached to fascia covering the quadratus lumborum and psoas major.

At the medial border of the kidney, the two layers are attached by a connective tissue septum being pierced by the renal vessels. Because of this attachment (septum), perirenal effusion of the fluid does not usually extend across into the opposite perirenal space.

PARARENAL (PARANEPHRIC) FAT

It is a layer of fat lying outside the renal fascia. It consists of considerable quantity of fat being more abundant posteriorly

and toward the lower pole of the kidney. It fills the paravertebral gutter and forms a cushion for the kidney.

MACROSCOPIC STRUCTURE

When the kidney is split longitudinally, it presents the kidney proper and the renal sinus.

Kidney Proper (Fig. 11.9)

The naked eye examination of the kidney proper presents an outer cortex and an inner medulla.

The **cortex** is located just below the renal capsule and extends between the renal pyramids (vide infra) as **renal columns (columns of Bertini)**. The cortex appears pale yellow with granular texture.

The **medulla** is composed of 5–11 dark conical masses called **renal pyramids (pyramids of Malpighi)**. The apices of renal pyramids form nipple-like projections—the **renal papillae** which invaginate the minor calyces.

N.B. A renal pyramid along with its covering cortical tissue forms a lobe of the kidney.

Renal Sinus (Fig. 11.10)

It is a cavity of considerable size present within the kidney. It takes up a large part of the interior of the kidney and opens at the medial border of the kidney as hilus.

It contains:

1. Greater part of the renal pelvis, major and minor calyces.
2. Renal vessels, lymphatics, and nerves.
3. Fat.

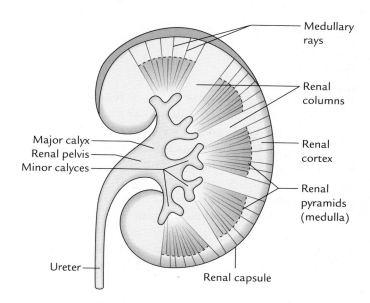

Fig. 11.9 Macroscopic structure of the kidney as seen in the longitudinal section.

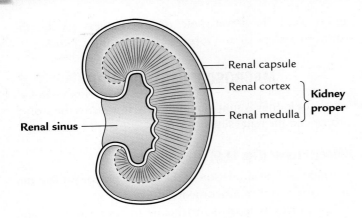

Fig. 11.10 Highly schematic diagram to show the renal sinus and kidney proper.

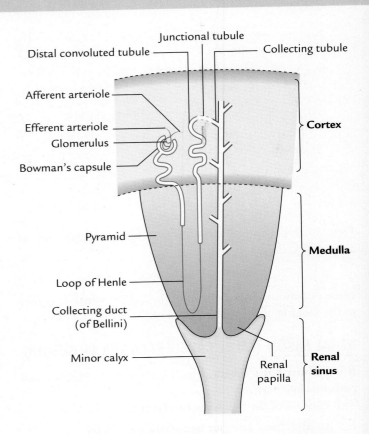

Fig. 11.11 Location of the uriniferous tubule within the kidney.

The sinus is lined by the continuation of the true capsule of the kidney. Numerous nipple-like elevations (*renal papillae*) indent the wall of the sinus. The renal pelvis within the sinus is divided into two or three large branches, called *major calyces*, which further divides to form 5–11 short branches called *minor calyces*. Each minor calyx expands as it approaches the wall of renal sinus, and its expanded end is indented and moulded around the renal papilla. The collecting tubules within the renal papilla open into the minor calyx by perforating its wall and capsule lining the sinus. Thus, the pelvis of ureter (upper funnel-shaped part of the ureter) is connected with the kidney tissue through calyces.

MICROSCOPIC STRUCTURE

Histologically, each kidney consists of 1 to 3 millions of uriniferous tubules. Each uriniferous tubule consists of two components: nephron and collecting tubule (Fig. 11.11).

1. The **nephron** is the structural and functional unit of kidney. The number of nephrons in each kidney is about 1–3 million. Each nephron consists of a glomerulus and a tubule system. The glomerulus is a tuft of capillaries surrounded by Bowman's capsule. The tubular system consists of the proximal convoluted tubule, loop of Henle, and distal convoluted tubule.

2. Each **collecting tubule** begins as a **junctional (connecting) tubule** from the distal convoluted tubule. Many collecting tubules unite together to form **collecting duct (duct of Bellini)** which opens on the apex of renal papilla.

   The collecting tubules radiate from the renal pyramid into the cortical region to form radial striations called **medullary rays**.

Clinical correlation

The total capacity of renal pelvis and major and minor calyces is about 8 ml. This fact is to be kept in mind while injecting radiopaque substance through ureter to outline these spaces because excess of substance may tear the sites of continuity between the minor calyces and renal papillae.

ARTERIAL SUPPLY

The kidneys are supplied by the renal arteries. Usually there is one renal artery for each kidney, but in about 30% individuals accessory renal arteries are also found. They commonly arise from the aorta and enter the kidney at the hilus or at one of its poles, usually the lower pole. The renal arteries have a blood flow in excess of 1 L/minute.

RENAL ARTERIES (Fig. 11.12)

The renal arteries arise directly from the abdominal aorta just below the origin of the superior mesenteric artery (i.e., at the level of intervertebral disc between L1 and L2).

1. The right renal artery passes to the right behind the inferior vena cava and right renal vein, while the left renal artery passes to the left behind the left renal vein.

2. At or near the hilum of the kidney, each renal artery divides into anterior and posterior divisions. The anterior division supplies apical, upper, middle, and lower segments, while posterior division supplies only posterior segment. The branches supplying the sgements are called *segmental arteries*. The anterior segmental arteries are usually larger than the posterior.

3. Each of these segmental arteries after supplying renal sinus divides into lobar branches (Fig. 11.13).

4. The **lobar arteries** break up into two or three **interlobar arteries** which pass through renal columns between the pyramids.

5. When an interlobar artery reaches the base of the associated pyramids, it divides dichotomously into the *arcuate arteries*.

6. The arcuate arteries run parallel to the surface of the kidney between the pyramids and the overlying cortex.

7. The renal arteries do not anastomose with adjacent arcuate arteries but give branches which pass radially

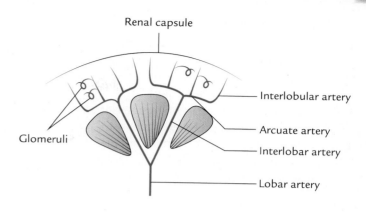

Fig. 11.13 Arrangement of arteries within the kidney.

toward the surface of the kidney which are called **interlobular arteries**.

8. The afferent arterioles from interlobular arteries pass to the capillaries of glomeruli, which then reunite to form efferent arterioles.

9. The efferent arterioles divide to form peritubular capillary plexus around the convoluted tubules.

10. The capillaries drain into the interlobular veins and then into interlobar veins, which run along the corresponding arteries.

11. The interlobular veins drain into the arcuate veins which in turn drain into interlobar veins which pass through the kidney tissue to the sinus where they join to form the renal vein.

Vascular Segments

According to Graves (1954), on the basis of distribution of major branches of the renal artery each kidney is anatomically divided into five vascular segments (Fig. 11.14). Each segment has its own artery and between the segments there is no anastomosis.

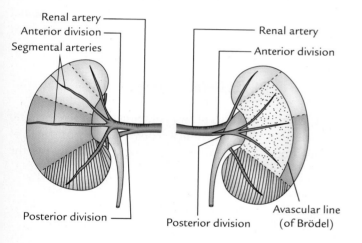

Fig. 11.12 Renal arteries.

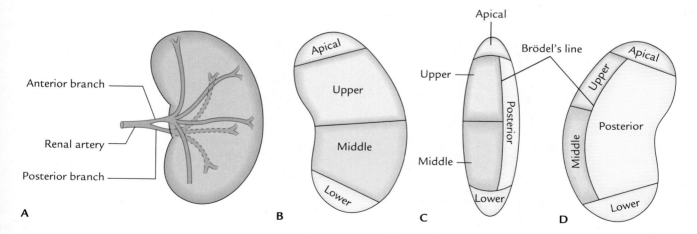

Fig. 11.14 Arterial segments of the kidney (left kidney in this figure): **A**, shows branches of the renal artery; **B, C,** and **D** show the segments as seen from anterior, lateral, and posterior aspects of the kidney, respectively.

These segments are as follows:

1. *Apical* consists of the medial side and the anterior part of the superior pole.
2. *Upper* includes the remainder of the upper pole and the upper part of the anterior aspect.
3. *Middle* includes lower part of the anterior aspect and lies between the upper and lower segments.
4. *Lower* consists of the whole of lower pole.
5. *Posterior* consists of the whole of posterior aspect of the kidney between the apical and lower segments.

For these segments, the Nomina Anatomica adopted a slightly more descriptive terms, *viz.*,

1. Superior.
2. Anterosuperior.
3. Anteroinferior.
4. Interior.
5. Posterior.

In the hilum/hilar area, the main renal artery divides into anterior and posterior divisions. The anterior division supplies the apical, upper, middle, and lower segments, while the posterior division supplies the posterior segment of the kidney.

The junction between the areas supplied by the anterior and posterior divisions of the renal artery is called **Brödel's line** (an important anatomical landmark). It is on the posterior aspect of the kidney at the junction of medial two-third and lateral one-third (Fig. 11.15). It is a functional avascular plane between the posterior segment medially and the upper and middle segments, hence suitable site for surgical incision to remove the renal stones (**nephrolithotomy**).

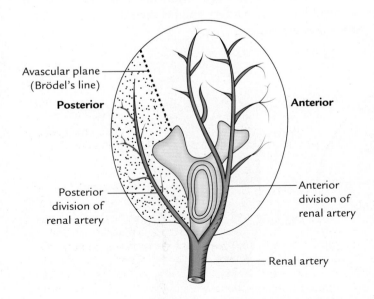

Fig. 11.15 Schematic diagram showing avascular plane of the kidney (Brödel's line).

N.B. The segmental resection of kidney is possible if the disease is localized to one or more segments.

VENOUS DRAINAGE

The venous blood from the kidneys is drained by the renal veins (right and left). The left renal vein passes in front of the aorta immediately below the origin of the inferior mesenteric artery.

LYMPHATIC DRAINAGE

The lymphatics from the kidney drain into the para-aortic lymph nodes at the level of origin of the renal arteries (L2).

NERVE SUPPLY

Each kidney is supplied by the renal plexus of nerves which reach the kidney along the renal artery. The renal plexus consists of both sympathetic and parasympathetic fibres. The sympathetic fibres are derived from T10–L1 spinal segments, and the parasympathetic fibres are derived from both vagus nerves.

DEVELOPMENT (Fig. 11.16)

1. The kidney consists of two components—excretory and collecting. The excretory component consisting of nephrons develop from the metanephros whereas the

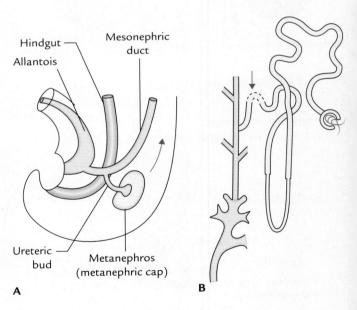

Fig. 11.16 Development of the kidney: **A**, origin of the ureteric bud from mesonephric duct; **B**, point of union between the derivatives of the ureteric bud and metanephros (metanephric cap) indicated by an arrow.

collecting system consisting of collecting tubules, collecting ducts, minor and major calyces, renal pelvis, and the ureter develops from the ureteric bud. The metanephros is derived from intermediate cell mass of the intraembryonic mesoderm while the ureteric bud is derived from the mesonephric duct.

2. Initially, the kidney develops in the pelvis and is supplied by the internal iliac artery. Subsequently it ascends up to its adult position gaining successively new arteries of supply from the common iliac and then from the abdominal aorta. The older arteries degenerate as the new ones appear until the definitive renal artery forms.

3. The hilum of the kidney is at first anterior but the kidney rotates 90° medially causing the hilum to orient medially. The fetal kidney is lobulated.

The adult derivatives of the embryonic structure forming the kidney are given in Table 11.1.

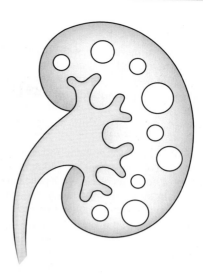

Fig. 11.17 Polycystic kidney. (*Source:* Fig. 20.9, Page 238, *Textbook of Clinical Embryology,* Vishram Singh. Copyright Elsevier 2012, All rights reserved.)

Table 11.1 Development of the kidney

Embryonic structures	Adult derivatives
Ureteric bud	• Collecting tubules • Collecting ducts • Minor calyces • Major calyces • Renal pelvis • Ureter
Metanephros	• Renal glomeruli • Bowman's capsules • Proximal convoluted tubules • Loop of Henle • Distal convoluted tubules • Connecting tubules

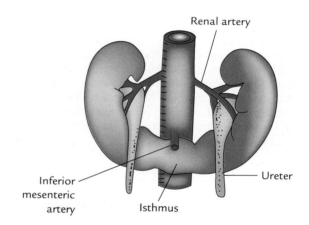

Fig. 11.18 Horseshoe kidney.

Clinical correlation

- **Congenital anomalies:**
  (a) *Lobulated kidney:* The persistence of fetal lobulation in the adult kidney: It is of no clinical significance.
  (b) *Aberrant artery:* The persistence of one of the fetal arteries is common (30% individuals), especially an artery from the aorta to the lower pole of the kidney.
  (c) *Congenital polycystic kidney:* It is is formed if the luminal continuity between the nephrons and collecting tubules fail to establish. The glomeruli continue to excrete urine which accumulates in the tubules due to lack of outlet. As a result tubules undergo cystic enlargements (retention cysts; Fig. 11.17).
  (d) *Horseshoe kidney (1 in 800;* Fig. 11.18)*:* It occurs due to fusion of the lower poles of the kidneys. The ureters pass anterior to the isthmus. The inferior mesenteric artery also passes anterior to the isthmus which limits the ascent of the horseshoe kidney.
  (e) *Renal agenesis (1 in 500):* It occurs when ureteric bud fails to develop. Unilateral renal agenesis is relatively common. A physician should never assume that a patient has two kidneys. A surgeon must confirm this fact before considering *nephrectomy.*

- **Renal pain:** The renal pain is felt in the loin and often radiates downward and forward into the groin. The nature of pain varies from dull ache to severe spasmodic pain. The renal pain occur either due to stretching of the renal capsule or due to spasm of the smooth muscle in the renal pelvis. The afferent fibres pass successively through the renal plexus, lowest splanchnic nerve, sympathetic trunk, and enter the T12 spinal segment. The pain is commonly referred along the subcostal nerve to the flank and anterior abdominal wall and along the ilioinguinal nerve (L1) into the groin.

Note: Tenderness in the kidney is elicited by applying pressure in the renal angle with the thumb during inspiration. The renal angle lies between the lower border of 12th rib and the outer border of erector spinae.

- **Floating kidney (hypermobility of the kidney):** The kidney is kept in position by the perirenal fat and renal fascia. However, each kidney moves up and down with respiration.

   If the amount of perinephric fat is reduced, the mobility of the kidney becomes excessive (floating kidney) and may reduce the symptoms of the renal colic caused by the kinking of the ureter. A floating kidney can move up and down but not from the side to side within the renal fascia.

- **Renal trauma:** Although the kidneys are well protected by the lower ribs, lumbar muscles and vertebral column, still a severe blunt injury of the abdomen may crush the kidney against the last 11th and/or 12th ribs, and the vertebral column. The penetrating injuries are usually caused by stab or gunshot wounds. Since about 25% of the cardiac output passes through the kidneys, the severe renal injury can lead to rapid blood loss.

   Blood from the ruptured kidney or pus in a perirenal abscess first distends the renal fascia, then trickles downward within the fascial compartment and may reach the pelvis.

- **Transplantation of kidney:** It is done in chronic renal failure in selected cases. The donor kidney is placed retroperitoneally in the iliac fossa with hilum parallel to the external iliac vessels. The renal artery is anastomosed end to end to the internal iliac artery and renal vein is anastomosed end to side to the external iliac vein. The ureter is implanted into the urinary bladder (*ureterocystostomy*).

EXPOSURE OF THE KIDNEY FROM BEHIND

For posterior surgical approaches to the contents of the abdominal cavity, viz., kidney and ureter or the sympathetic trunk, one should know the composition of the posterior abdominal wall in the lumbar region. This is well appreciated by the anatomical exposure of the kidney from behind.

N.B. *Loin:* It is the region on the back of the trunk, bounded above by the 12th rib, below by the iliac crest, medially by the posterior median line, and laterally by flank.

Surface Marking of Kidney on the Back (Fig. 11.19)

It is done within **parallelogram of Morris** which is drawn in the following way:

1. First two horizontal lines are drawn one at the level of spine of T11 and other at the level of spine of L3.
2. Then two vertical lines are drawn, one 2.5 cm away and other 9 cm away from the posteromedian plane.
3. The centre of hilum of the each kidney lies approximately at the lower border of L1.

Incisions

1. Give median vertical incision extending from the spine of T11 to the spine of L2.
2. Then make horizontal incisions extending from the upper and lower ends of the vertical incision.

Layers to be Reflected to Reach the Kidney

The following layers can be reflected one by one in order to expose the kidney (Fig. 11.20):

1. Skin.
2. Superficial fascia.
3. Posterior layer of the thoraco-lumbar fascia with attached latissimus dorsi and serratus posterior inferior muscles.
4. Erector spinae (sacrospinalis) muscles.

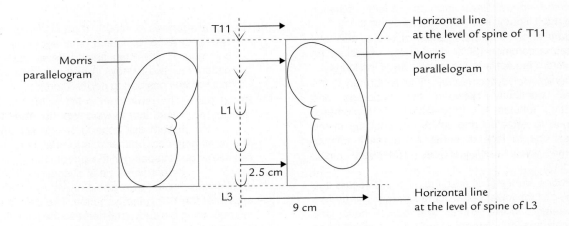

Fig. 11.19 Surface marking of the kidneys on the back.

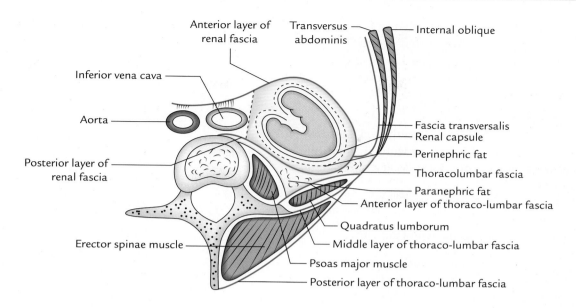

Fig. 11.20 Transverse section through lumbar region showing transverse disposition of thoracolumbar fascia and coverings of the kidney.

5. Middle layer of the thoraco-lumbar fascia.
6. Quadratus lumborum muscle.
7. Anterior layer of the thoraco-lumbar fascia.

N.B.

Renal angle:
- It is an angle between the lower border of the 12th rib and the lateral border of erector spinae muscle.
- This angle becomes full following kidney enlargements and formation of perinephric abscess.
- It is the site of tenderness in case of perinephric abscess. Renal pain is usually felt in this angle as a dull ache.

For details of the renal angle and its clinical importance, see *Clinical and Surgical Anatomy*, 2nd Edition, by Vishram Singh.

For better understanding of structures that are encountered during exposure of kidney, the students must know about the *thoraco-lumbar fascia*.

THORACOLUMBAR FASCIA (Fig. 11.20)

It is the name given to the deep fascia on the back of trunk. It binds the long extensor muscle of the vertebral column (erector spinae) to the posterolateral surfaces of the vertebral bodies.

For descriptive purposes the thoracolumbar fascia is divided into two parts: lumbar and thoracic.

Lumbar Part of Thoracolumbar Fascia

In the lumbar region, thoraco-lumbar fascia is very strong and should be called **lumbar fascia**.

Features

1. It consists of three strong layers, namely, anterior, middle, and posterior, and fills in the gap between the 12th rib and the iliac crest.
2. The posterior and middle layers are thick, dense, and strong, but the anterior layer is thin and not so strong.
3. Between the posterior and middle layers lie the erector spinae and transversus spinalis muscles.
4. Between the middle and anterior layers lies the quadratus lumborum muscle.
5. The three layers fuse laterally to form a dense aponeurotic sheet which gives origin to the internal oblique and transversus abdominis muscles.

Attachments of the anterior layer

Above: It is attached *medially* to the transverse process of the first lumbar vertebra; laterally to the 12th rib, in front of quadratus lumborum forming a thick tendinous strip called *lateral lumbocostal arch* (or *lateral arcuate ligament*).

Below: To the iliolumbar ligament and iliac crest.

Medially: To the vertical ridges on the anterior surfaces of the transverse processes of lumbar vertebrae.

N.B. The kidney lies in front of thoracolumbar fascia, which blends with the renal fascia. The subcostal nerve and vessels, iliohypogastric nerve and ilioinguinal nerve lie between the fascia and the quadratus lumborum, much exactly in the same way as the phrenic nerve in the neck lies between the scalenus anterior and the prevertebral layer of deep cervical fascia covering it.

Attachments of the middle layer

Above: It is attached to the 12th rib laterally and transverse process of first lumbar vertebra, behind the quadratus lumborum forming the *lumbocostal ligament.*

Medially: To the tips of the transverse processes of lumbar vertebrae.

Below: To the iliolumbar ligament and iliac crest.

N.B. The upper part of the quadratus lumborum is therefore embraced by the lateral *lumbocostal arch in front* and the *lumbocostal ligament behind.*

Attachments of the posterior layer

Medially: To the spines of lumbar vertebrae.

Below: To the iliac crest.

Above: Extends as the thoracic part of thoraco-lumbar fascia.

Thoracic Part of the Thoracolumbar Fascia

Attachments

Medially: To the spines of thoracic vertebrae.

Laterally: To the angles of the ribs.

Above: Extends into the cervical region deep to the serratus posterior superior to fuse with fascia of the neck.

URETER

The ureter is a narrow, thick-walled, expansile muscular tube which conveys urine from the kidney to the urinary bladder. The urine is propelled from the kidney to the urinary bladder by the peristaltic contractions of the smooth muscle of the wall of the ureter (Fig. 11.21).

Measurements

Length: 25 cm (10 inches).

Diameter: 3 mm.

COURSE (Figs 11.22 and 11.23)

The ureter begins as a downward continuation of a funnel-shaped **renal pelvis** at the medial margin of the lower end of the kidney.

The ureter passes downward and slight medially on the psoas major, which separates it from the transverse processes

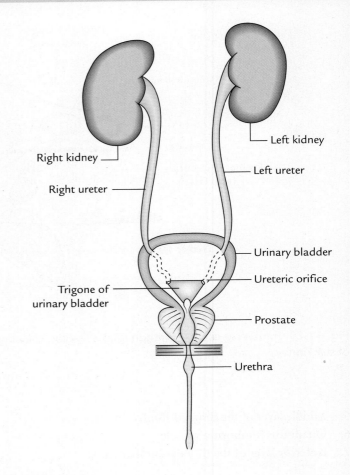

Fig. 11.21 Ureters.

of the lumbar vertebrae and enters the pelvic cavity by crossing in front of the bifurcation of the common iliac artery at the pelvic brim in front of the sacroiliac joint (Fig. 11.22).

In the pelvis, the ureter first runs downward, backward, and laterally along the anterior margin of the greater sciatic notch. Opposite to the ischial spine, it turns forward and medially to reach the base of the urinary bladder, where it enters the bladder wall obliquely (Fig. 11.23). Within the bladder wall, it narrows down, takes a sinuous course, and opens into the cavity of the bladder at the lateral angle of its trigone as ureteric orifice (Fig. 11.23).

During its course from the kidney to the urinary bladder, it runs behind the parietal peritoneum to which it is closely applied.

N.B. The **renal pelvis** is an upward funnel-shaped continuation of the ureter and therefore also named **pelvis of the ureter**. It lies partly outside and partly within the kidney.

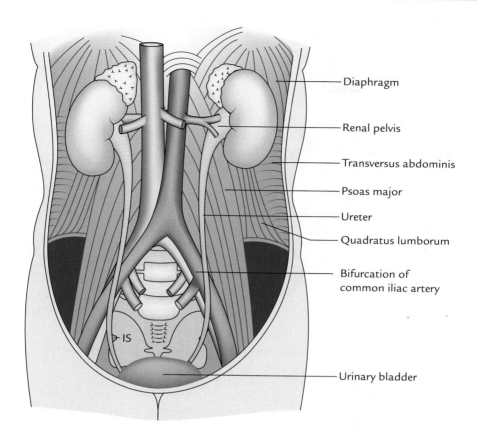

Fig. 11.22 Course of the ureters (IS = ischial spine).

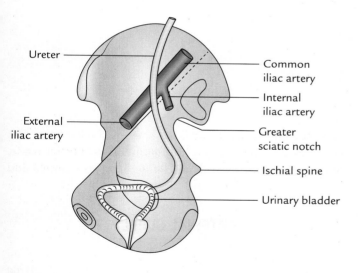

Fig. 11.23 Course of the pelvic part of the ureter.

PARTS AND RELATIONS

The ureter is generally divided into two parts: abdominal and pelvic. Each part is about the same length, i.e., 12.5 cm (5 inches).

The **abdominal part** of ureter extends from the renal pelvis to the bifurcation of the common iliac artery.

The **pelvic part** of the ureter extends from the pelvic brim (at the level of bifurcation of the common iliac artery) to the base of the urinary bladder.

Abdominal Part

The anterior and posterior relations of the abdominal part of the ureter are given in Table 11.2 and shown in Figure 11.24.

N.B. Medially the right ureter is related to inferior vena cava and left ureter is related to left gonadal vein and inferior mesenteric vein.

Pelvic Part

The pelvic part of the ureter crosses in front of all the nerves and vessels on the lateral pelvic wall except vas deferens, which crosses in front of it. Near the uterine cervix, the uterine artery lies above and in front of it, a highly important surgical relationship.

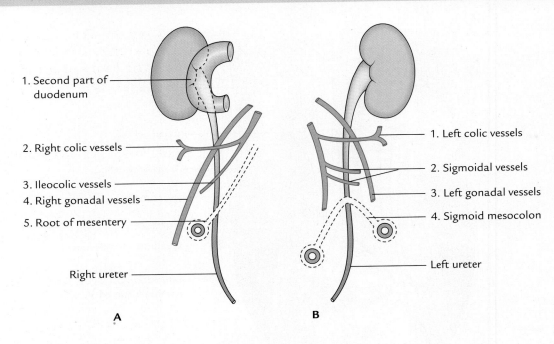

1. Second part of duodenum

2. Right colic vessels

3. Ileocolic vessels
4. Right gonadal vessels
5. Root of mesentery

Right ureter

1. Left colic vessels

2. Sigmoidal vessels

3. Left gonadal vessels

4. Sigmoid mesocolon

Left ureter

A   B

Fig. 11.24 Anterior relations of the abdominal parts of the ureters: A, right ureter; B, left ureter.

Table 11.2 Relations of the abdominal part of the ureter

	Anterior relations (Fig. 11.22)	Posterior relations
Right ureter	• Second part of the duodenum • Right colic vessels • Ileocolic vessels • Right testicular or ovarian vessels • Root of mesentery	• Right psoas major • Bifurcation of right common iliac artery
Left ureter	• Left colic vessels • Sigmoidal vessels • Left testicular or ovarian vessels • Sigmoid mesocolon	• Left psoas major • Bifurcation of left common iliac artery

SITES OF ANATOMICAL NARROWINGS/CONSTRICTIONS

The lumen of the ureter is not uniform throughout and presents three constrictions at the following sites (Fig. 11.25):

1. At the **pelviureteric junction** where the renal pelvis joins the upper end of ureter.
    It is the upper most constriction, found approximately 5 cm away from the hilum of kidney.
2. At the **pelvic brim** where it crosses the common iliac artery.
3. At the **uretero-vesical junction** (i.e., where ureter enters into the bladder).

Portions of the ureter between these constrictions show spindle-shaped dilatations. These constricted segments of the ureter are the sites of arrest of ureteric calculi.

N.B. In addition to above three sites of constrictions, two more sites of constrictions are described by the surgeons, one at juxtaposition of the vas deferens/broad ligament and other at the ureteric orifice.

ARTERIAL SUPPLY

The ureter derives its arterial supply from the branches of all the arteries related to it. The important arteries supplying ureter from above downward are (Fig. 11.26):

1. Renal.
2. Testicular or ovarian.
3. Direct branches from aorta.
4. Internal iliac.
5. Vesical (superior and inferior).
6. Middle rectal.
7. Uterine.

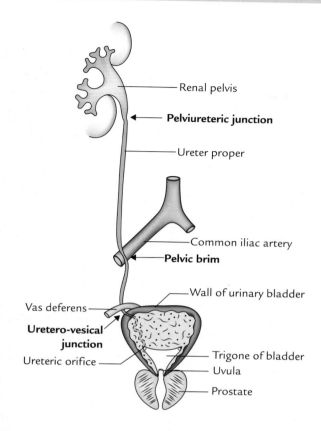

Fig. 11.25 Normal sites of anatomical constrictions in the ureter (arrows).

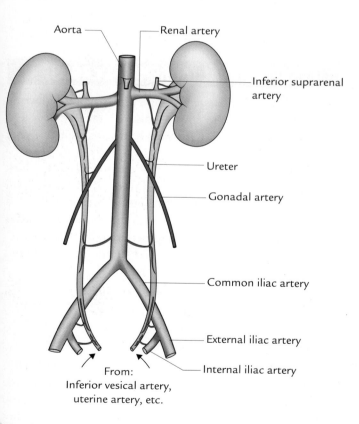

Fig. 11.26 Arterial supply of the ureter.

N.B. Arteries supplying the ureter divide into ascending and descending branches to first form a plexus in the connective tissue sheath on the surface of the ureter and then supply it.

VENOUS DRAINAGE

The venous blood from the ureter is drained into the veins corresponding to the arteries.

LYMPHATIC DRAINAGE

The lymph from the ureter is drained into lateral aortic and iliac nodes.

NERVE SUPPLY

1. The **sympathetic supply** of the ureter is derived from T12–L1 spinal segments through renal, aortic, and hypogastric plexuses.
2. The **parasympathetic supply** of ureter is derived from S2–S4 spinal segments through pelvic splanchnic nerves.

The afferent fibres travel with both sympathetic and parasympathetic nerves.

Clinical correlation

- **Mobilization of ureter:** Branches of the arteries supplying the ureter form an anastomosis in the fat and fascia around the ureter. Therefore, surgeons should bear in their mind that stripping off this fascia, while mobilizing the ureter for transplantation, will hamper the blood supply of the ureter and may cause its necrosis.
- **Identification of ureter:** Ureter is a muscular structure, and in life waves of muscular contractions produce a worm-like rhythmic movement (peristalsis) thus milking urine toward the bladder. The ureter is readily identified in life by its thick muscular wall which is seen to undergo worm-like writhing movements, especially when it is gently stroked or squeezed. Violent muscular contractions precipitated by the presence of stone in the lumen of the ureter (**ureteric calculus**) produce such a severe spasmodic pain called **renal colic** that immediate treatment is required.
- **Ureteric colic:** It occurs due to obstruction of ureteric lumen by a stone. The referred pain of ureteric colic is related to the cutaneous areas innervated by the same spinal segments as that of the ureter, i.e., T12–L2. Pain of ureteric colic commences in the loin, shoots downward and forward to the groin and then into the scrotum or labium majus.
  (a) *Pain from upper ureteral obstruction* is referred to the lumbar region (T12 and L1).
  (b) *Pain from middle ureteral obstruction* is referred to the inguinal, scrotal or mons pubis, and upper medial aspect of the thigh (L1, L2).

(c) *Pain from lower ureteral obstruction* is referred to the perineum (S2–S4).

- **Localization of a ureteric stone on the plain radiograph of the abdomen (Fig. 11.27):** To localize the stone in the ureter in plane X-ray abdomen, one must know the course of ureter in relation to the bony skeleton. Ureter lies in front of the tips of the transverse processes of the lower four lumbar vertebrae, crosses in front of the sacroiliac joint, swings out to the spine of the ischium, and then runs medially to the urinary bladder. In plane X-ray of abdomen, therefore the radiopaque shadow of ureteric calculus is usually seen at the following sites:
  (a) Near the tips of the transverse processes of lumbar vertebrae.
  (b) Overlying the sacroiliac joint.
  (c) Overlying or slightly medial to the ischial spine.
- **Injury to ureters:** According to Kenson and Hinman, the ureter may be injured at one of the following four dangerous sites:
  (a) Point where the ureter crosses the iliac vessels.
  (b) In the ovarian fossa.
  (c) Where the ureter is crossed by the uterine artery (**most dangerous site**) as damage is likely at this site during hysterectomy.
  (d) At the base of the bladder.
- **Ureteric calculus** is likely to lodge at one of the sites of anatomical narrowings of the ureter particularly:
  (a) At the pelvic ureteric junction.
  (b) Where it crosses the pelvic brim.
  (c) In the intramural part—the narrowest part.

- **Approach to ureter:** Throughout its abdominal and upper parts of the pelvic course, the ureter runs deep to the peritoneum and adheres with it closely. During surgery when the ureter is mobilized, the ureter is in danger of injury for it moves with the peritoneum. Deep to the peritoneum in the abdominal part the ureter is crossed by various blood vessels. Due to these vascular relations an extraperitoneal approach of the ureter is preferred to that of a transperitoneal approach.

DEVELOPMENT

The ureter develops from the ureteric bud arising as an outgrowth from the mesonephric duct (see page 172).

Clinical correlation

Congenital anomalies: The common congenital anomalies of ureter are: **(a) double pelvis, (b) bifid ureter,** and **(c) double ureters** (upper ureter enters below the lower ureter). Rarely the extra ureter may open ectopically into the urethra or vagina and cause urinary incontinence.

The cause of double pelvis is premature division of the ureteric bud near its termination, whereas the cause of bifid or double ureter is the too premature division of the ureteric bud.

Sometimes during the ascent of kidney, the ureter may ascend posterior to the inferior vena cava leading to post-caval ureter.

SUPRARENAL (ADRENAL) GLANDS

The suprarenal glands are an important pair of endocrine glands situated on the upper poles of the kidneys and enclosed in the same fascial sheath as that of kidneys (renal fascia).

Each gland consists of two parts: (a) a relatively thick outer cortex which develops from the mesoderm (mesodermal lining of the peritoneal cavity) and (b) a central medulla which develops from the neural crest and is equivalent to a group of sympathetic ganglion cells.

The cortex secretes a considerable number of steroid hormones which are responsible for:

1. Controlling electrolyte and water balance.
2. Maintaining blood sugar concentration.
3. Maintaining liver and muscle glycogen stores.
4. Controlling inflammatory reactions.

The medulla is composed of large granular chromaffin cells which secrete adrenaline and noradrenaline (catecholamines). These catecholamines are similar to those released by the postganglionic sympathetic fibres and are stored in good quantity in the medulla. They are readily

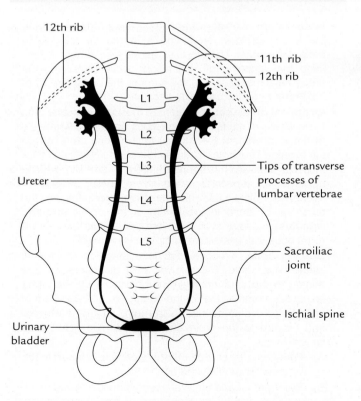

Fig. 11.27 Drawing from an intravenous pyelogram to show the relationship of the ureters to the bony landmarks.

oxidized to a dark brown colour by certain salts of chromic acid (e.g., potassium dichromate), a feature which makes the renal medulla a part of the chromaffin system of the body.

Ontogenetically, phylogenetically, structurally, and functionally the cortex and the medulla (of suprarenal gland) are distinct from each other but topographically they are similar.

As a whole each adrenal gland is yellowish in colour, otherwise in section the cortex is yellow and the medulla is dark brown in colour.

N.B. *Accessory suprarenal glands:* Small accessory suprarenal glands which may consist of adrenal cortical tissue only are usually found in loose areolar tissue around the principal gland but may be found in the spermatic cord, epididymis, or broad ligament of the uterus.

LOCATION (Fig. 11.28)

1. The suprarenal glands are located in the epigastric region of abdomen, anterosuperior to the upper part of each kidney.
2. The right suprarenal gland is wedge shaped between the diaphragm posteromedially, the inferior vena cava anteromedially, the right lobe of the liver anteriorly, and the kidney inferolaterally. *Superiorly it is related to the bare area of liver.*
3. The left suprarenal gland lies between the diaphragm posteromedially, the stomach anteriorly (with lesser sac and pancreas and splenic artery intervening), and the kidney inferolaterally.

Shape and Measurements

Shape: Each gland is flattened anteroposteriorly.

1. Right gland is triangular or pyramidal in shape bearing a resemblance to a *"top hat."*

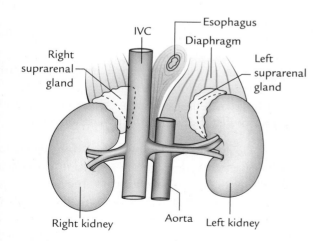

Fig. 11.28 Location of the suprarenal glands (IVC = inferior vena cava).

2. Left gland is crescentic or semilunar in shape like a *"cocked hat."*

Measurements:
Length: 50 mm.
Breadth: 30 mm.
Thickness: 10 mm.
Weight = About 5 g.

At birth the gland is about one-third of the size of kidney, whereas in adults it is only 1/30th of the size of kidney.

EXTERNAL FEATURES

1. *Right suprarenal gland:* It has base, apex, two surfaces (anterior and posterior), and three borders (medial and lateral).
2. *Left suprarenal gland:* It has two ends (narrow upper end and rounded lower end), two borders (medial and lateral), and two surfaces (anterior and posterior).
   (a) *Posterior surface of the right gland* is divided into upper convex and lower concave parts by a curved ridge.
   (b) *Posterior surface of the left gland* is divided into medial and lateral areas by a ridge.
   (c) *Anterior surface of the right gland* has narrow vertical medial area and triangular lateral area.
   (d) *Anterior surface of the left gland* has superior and inferior areas.

N.B. *Hilum:* The hilum of suprarenal gland provides emergence of the suprarenal vein. Its location differs on the two sides.
   (a) *In the right suprarenal gland,* it is short sulcus a little inferior to the apex and near the anterior border. From it the right suprarenal vein emerges to join the inferior vena cava.
   (b) *In the left supra renal gland,* it is located near the lower part of anterior surface and faces anteroinferiorly. From it the left suprarenal vein emerges to join the left renal vein.

The **relations of the suprarenal glands** are given in Table 11.3 and shown in Figure 11.29.

SHEATHS

Each suprarenal gland is surrounded by two sheaths as follows (Fig. 11.30):

1. Immediate covering of loose areolar tissue containing a considerable amount of perirenal fat.
2. Outer to this renal fascia encloses the suprarenal gland together with the kidney but the gland is separated from the kidney by a septum.

Table 11.3 Relations of the suprarenal glands (Fig. 11.27)

	Right gland	Left gland
Anterior surface	• *Medial*: Inferior vena cava • *Lateral*: Right lobe of the liver including bare area	• *Superior*: Stomach • *Inferior*: Splenic artery and pancreas
Posterior surface	• *Inferior*: Kidney • *Superior*: Crus (right) of diaphragm	• *Medial*: Crus (left) of diaphragm • *Lateral*: Kidney
Medial border	• Right coeliac ganglion • Right inferior phrenic artery	• Left coeliac ganglion • Left inferior phrenic artery • Left gastric vessels
Hilum	Near the upper end	Near the lower end
Peritoneal relations	Not related to peritoneum except a tiny area below	Related to peritoneum of omental bursa which separates it from stomach

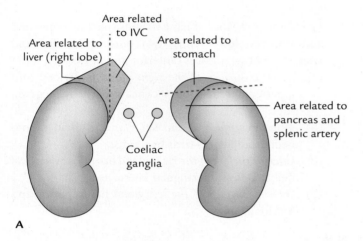

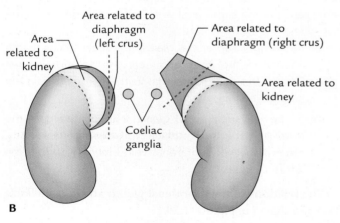

Fig. 11.29 Relation of the suprarenal glands: **A**, anterior relations; **B**, posterior relations.

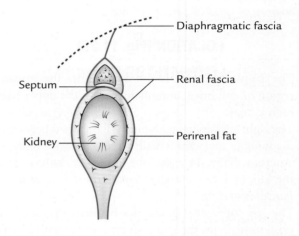

Fig. 11.30 Sheaths of the suprarenal gland.

about one-tenth of the whole gland. The histological features of the cortex and medulla are as follows:

1. The **cortex** consists of three layers/zones from superficial to deep. These are:
   (a) Outer **zona glomerulosa** is composed of nests or clumps of small polyhedral cells.
   (b) Middle **zona fasciculata** is formed of parallel straight columns of large polyhedral cells.
   (c) Inner **zona reticularis** is a mesh of interlacing cords of rounded cells.
2. The **medulla** consists of strands or clumps of chromaffin cells interspersed with sympathetic ganglion cells.

N.B. *Chromaffin cells:* These are cells which have affinity for certain salts of chromic acid, hence the name chromaffin cells. They develop from neural crest cells. They are located on posterior abdominal wall near the sympathetic ganglion. Apart from adrenal medulla, the other examples of chromaffin tissue are: paraganglia, para-aortic bodies, and glomus coccygeum (coccygeal body).

STRUCTURE OF THE SUPRARENAL GLAND

As already discussed, the suprarenal gland consists of an outer cortex and inner medulla. The medulla forms only

ARTERIAL SUPPLY

Each gland is supplied by three arteries from three different sources (Fig. 11.31):

1. *Superior suprarenal artery:* A branch of the inferior phrenic artery.
2. *Middle suprarenal artery:* A branch of the abdominal aorta.
3. *Inferior suprarenal artery:* A branch of the renal artery.

VENOUS DRAINAGE

Each gland is drained only by a single vein which emerges from the hilus of the gland (Fig. 11.32):

1. *Right suprarenal vein* drains into the inferior vena cava.
2. *Left suprarenal vein* drains into the left renal vein.

LYMPHATIC DRAINAGE

The lymph drains into lateral aortic nodes.

NERVE SUPPLY

The nerves are exceedingly numerous. They are predominantly myelinated preganglionic sympathetic fibres derived from splanchnic nerves and are distributed mainly to the chromaffin cells of the medulla which are homologous to postganglionic sympathetic neurons.

The activity of the cortex is largely controlled by adrenocorticotrophic hormone secreted by the anterior lobe of the pituitary gland.

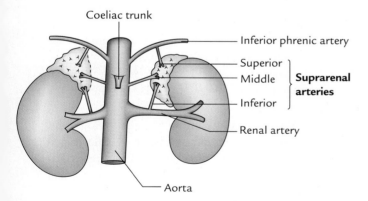

Fig. 11.31 Arterial supply of the suprarenal gland.

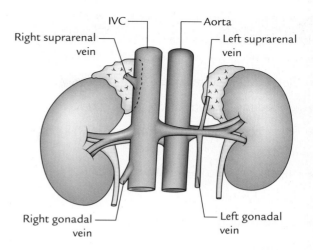

Fig. 11.32 Venous drainage of the suprarenal gland.

Clinical correlation

- A number of clinical conditions may occur following lesions affecting the cortex or medulla of the suprarenal gland. They are attributable to either excess or deficiency of secretions from respective parts of the gland.
- **Addison's disease:** It occurs due to chronic insufficiency of cortical secretion. Clinically, it presents as (a) muscle weakness and wasting, (b) increased pigmentation of skin, (c) low blood pressure, and (d) restlessness and tiredness, etc.
- **Cushing syndrome:** It occurs due to hypersecretion of the adrenal cortex. Clinically, it presents as (a) obesity involving the face (*moon face*), neck, and abdomen, (b) hypertension, (c) hirsutism, and (d) masculization (virilism) in female and feminization in male, and (e) adrenogenital syndrome in children.
- **Adrenalectomy** (bilateral removal of the adrenal glands) is sometimes done in advanced and inoperable cases of carcinoma breast and prostate. Great care must be taken during adrenalectomy. The suprarenal vein must be ligated before manipulating the gland so that catecholamines do not escape in the circulation. The right adrenal gland is more difficult to approach than the left because part of it lies posterior to the inferior vena cava.
- **Pheochromocytoma** is a tumor of the adrenal medulla. The signs and symptoms are produced due to bursts of epinephrine and norepinephrine. Clinically, it presents as (a) paroxysms of hypertension, (b) palpitation, (c) headache, and (d) excessive sweating, and pallor of the skin.

Golden Facts to Remember

▶ Number of nephrons in each kidney	1–3 million
▶ Secretory system of the kidney develops from	Metanephric cap (metanephros)
▶ Collecting system of the kidney develops from	Ureteric bud from the mesonephric duct
▶ Most common congenital anomaly of the upper urinary tract	Duplication of the renal pelvis
▶ Most common fusion anomaly of the kidney	Horseshoe kidney
▶ 90% of renal stones are	Radiopaque
▶ Ureteric stone arises in	Kidney
▶ Narrowest part of the ureter	Ureteric orifice in the urinary bladder
▶ Most common abdominal malignancy in children above 1 year	Nephroblastoma (Wilms' tumor, arising from embryonic nephrogenic tissue)
▶ Commonest cause of the renal injury	Penetrating (stab) wounds
▶ Most common tumor of the pelvicalyceal system and ureter	Transitional cell carcinoma

Clinical Case Study

A 37-year-old patient came to the emergency with excruciating abdominal pain in the left flank (loin) and inguinal region. A urine sample was positive for blood. The plane X-ray of abdomen (KUB film) revealed a possible calculus in the lower left quadrant of the abdomen. While the patient was waiting for treatment he complained that pain was worse and had moved into the upper anteromedial aspect of the thigh and scrotum. A diagnosis of "**renal colic**" was made.

Questions

1. What is renal colic?
2. Why the patient first complained of pain in the loin and inguinal region and later into the thigh and scrotum?
3. What is KUB film?
4. Name the radiological technique used to visualize the lumen of the ureter and calyces.

Answers

1. *Renal colic* occurs due to impaction of stone in the ureter and classically begins in the loin and radiates to the groin.

2. This is because first the stone was obstructing the upper part of the ureter and then moved down to obstruct the middle part of the ureter. The upper part of the ureter receives afferent innervation from the T12 spinal segment, hence pain is felt in the lumbar and inguinal regions. The middle part of the abdominal ureter receives afferent innervation from L1–L2 spinal segment, hence pain is felt in the thigh and scrotum.

3. The plane X-ray of abdomen is usually done to examine kidney, ureter, and bladder, hence the name KUB film.

4. These are intravenous and retrograde pyelography. Intravenous pyelography consists of injecting a contrast medium (iodine containing compound) into the subcutaneous vein of the arm (e.g., median cubital vein). It is excreted and concentrated by the kidneys, thus making the calyces and ureter radiopaque. In retrograde pyelography, the contrast medium is introduced into the ureter through the catheter. First, a cystoscope is passed in the urinary bladder and then a catheter is passed through the cystoscope in the ureter.

Posterior Abdominal Wall and Associated Structures

The posterior abdominal wall extends from the 12th rib above to the pelvic brim below. It is strong and stable (cf. the anterior abdominal wall is soft and distensible) because it is constructed by bones, muscles, and fasciae. It supports retroperitoneal organs, vessels, and nerves.

The posterior abdominal wall is constructed as follows (Fig. 12.1):

1. **Bony part:** In the median plane, it is made up of bodies, intervertebral disc, and transverse processes of the five lumbar vertebrae. Laterally it is divided

into upper and lower parts by the iliac crest. The part above the iliac crest is made of inner surfaces of the 12th rib and the part below the iliac crest is made of iliac fossa.

2. **Muscular part:** Above the iliac crest, from medial to lateral sides, it is made up of psoas major, quadratus lumborum, and transversus abdominis muscles. Below the iliac crest on either side of the lumbar vertebral column from *medial to lateral sides*, it is made up of psoas major and iliacus muscles.

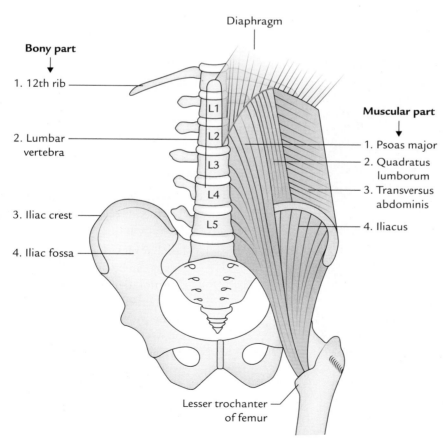

Fig. 12.1 Bones and muscles forming the posterior abdominal wall.

In addition to these muscles, the diaphragm completes the abdominal wall superiorly.

3. **Fasciae:** The psoas major and iliacus muscles are covered by fascia iliaca. The quadratus lumborum is enclosed between the anterior and posterior layers of the thoraco-lumbar fascia.

The following structures are to be studied in the posterior abdominal wall:

1. Muscles and fasciae of the posterior abdominal wall.
2. Great vessels of the abdomen (e.g., abdominal aorta and inferior vena cava [IVC]).
3. Azygos and hemiazygos veins.
4. Lymph nodes and lymphatics of the posterior abdominal wall.
5. Nerves of the posterior abdominal wall.

MUSCLES OF THE POSTERIOR ABDOMINAL WALL

Three muscles viz. psoas major, iliacus, and quadratus lumborum, on each side of the vertebral column form most of the posterior abdominal wall.

PSOAS MAJOR (Fig. 12.2)

The psoas major is a long fusiform muscle extending from the sides of lumbar vertebrae to the lesser trochanter of the femur. It is enclosed in a fascial sheath called *psoas sheath.*

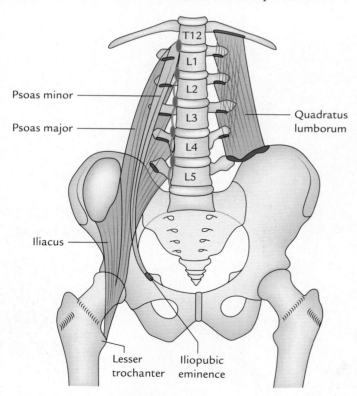

Fig. 12.2 Origin and insertion of the psoas major, psoas minor, iliacus, and quadratus lumborum muscles.

Origin

The muscle arises from 14 fleshy slips that are as follows:

1. Five slips from intervertebral discs between T12–L5 vertebrae and adjoining margins of the bodies of these vertebrae.
2. Five slips from anterior surfaces and lower borders of the transverse process of five lumbar vertebrae.
3. Four slips from tendinous arches bridging the constricted sides of the bodies of lumbar vertebrae. The lumbar vessels pass deep to these arches.

Insertion

From the site of origin, the muscle descends along the pelvic brim and enters the thigh behind the inguinal ligament. Below the ligament, the tendon forms on the lateral side of the muscle, passes in front of the hip joint, and enters the anterior surface of the tip of the lesser trochanter of the femur. A synovial bursa which may communicate with the cavity of the hip joint commonly separates this tendon from the joint capsule.

Nerve Supply

The nerve supply is by direct branches from ventral rami of L2, L3, L4 spinal nerves.

Actions

These are as follows:

1. **Acting from above,** it is the chief flexor of the thigh at the hip joint.
2. **Acting from below,** it flexes the trunk on the thigh, as in raising the trunk from recumbent to sitting position.

Relations

The psoas major is the **key muscle of the posterior abdominal wall,** because its relations provide a fair idea about the layout of structures in this region (Fig. 12.3):

1. **Lumbar plexus** forms within the substance of psoas. The plexus can be displayed only by tearing the muscle, for it does not divide the muscle into planes.
2. Five nerves emerge from underneath the lateral border of the psoas major from above downward; these are as follows:
   (a) Subcostal nerve.
   (b) Iliohypogastric nerve.
   (c) Ilioinguinal nerve.
   (d) Lateral cutaneous nerve of thigh.
   (e) Femoral nerve.
   The upper four nerves emerge above the iliac crest and runs downward and laterally across the quadratus

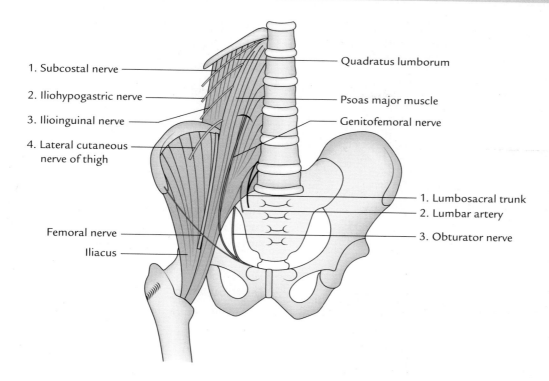

Fig. 12.3 Relations of the psoas major muscle.

lumborum muscle. The last nerve (femoral nerve) emerges below the iliac crest and runs down in the groove between the psoas and iliacus muscles.

3. One nerve (genitofemoral nerve) runs downward on the front of the psoas major and sometimes may be mistaken for the tendon of psoas minor muscle.

4. Three important structures lying on the medial side of the psoas major. From medial to lateral side these are: (a) lumbosacral trunk, (b) iliolumbar artery, and (c) obturator nerve.

N.B. *Lumbosacral triangle of Marcille (Fig. 12.4):* It is a triangular interval on each side of the body of L5 vertebra with the apex directed upward. It is bounded medially by the body of L5 vertebra, laterally by the medial border of the psoas major, and inferiorly (base) by the ala of the sacrum. The apex is formed by the junction of psoas and the body of L5 vertebra. The floor (posterior wall) is formed by the transverse process of L5 vertebra and iliolumbar ligament.

It contains four structures. From medial to lateral sides, these are:

1. Sympathetic trunk.
2. Lumbosacral trunk.
3. Iliolumbar artery.
4. Obturator nerve.

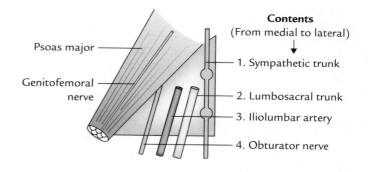

Fig. 12.4 Lumbosacral triangle (of Marcelle).

Psoas Sheath

The psoas major muscle is enclosed in a fascial sheath called (**psoas sheath**) formed by the psoas fascia. The attachments of psoas fascia are as follows:

Above: It is thickened to form *medial arcuate ligament,* which extends from the body of L1 vertebra to the tip of its transverse process.

Laterally: It blends with the anterior layer of the thoraco-lumbar fascia.

Medially: It is attached to the bodies and intervening intervertebral discs of lumbar vertebrae and presents four tendinous arches.

Below: It fuses with the arcuate line of the pelvis and the fascia covering the iliacus muscle (**iliac fascia**).

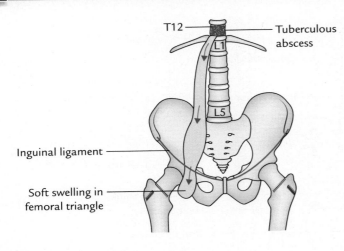

Fig. 12.5 Psoas abscess.

Clinical correlation

Psoas abscess: The psoas fascia forms a long tubular sheath (osseofibrous tunnel) called psoas sheath extending from the upper lumbar region of the posterior abdominal wall to the groin. Tubercular infection of vertebrae of the thoraco-lumbar region causes destruction of their bodies leading to the formation of an abscess. The pus cannot spread anteriorly due to anterior longitudinal ligament. Therefore, it spreads laterally into the psoas sheath forming psoas abscess. The pus can also enter the psoas sheath from the posterior mediastinum through a gap deep to *medial arcuate ligament*. Pus may then spread downward along the psoas muscle, under the inguinal ligament into the femoral triangle where it produces a soft swelling (Fig. 12.5).

PSOAS MINOR (Fig. 12.2)

This muscle is present in about 50% individuals. When present, it runs downward in front of psoas major. In form and shape, it resembles the plantaris muscle of the leg and is confined to the abdomen.

Origin

It arises from the side of the intervertebral disc between T12 and L1 vertebrae and adjoining parts of their bodies.

Insertion

From the site of origin, the muscle runs in front of the psoas major and ends in a long flat tendon, which is inserted into the iliopubic eminence.

Nerve Supply

It is by a branch of L1 spinal nerve.

Action

It is a weak flexor of the trunk.

ILIACUS (Fig. 12.2)

It is a fan-shaped muscle and forms the lateral component of the iliopsoas muscle.

Origin

It arises from the upper two thirds of the floor of iliac fossa, inner lip of iliac crest and upper surface of the lateral part of the sacrum.

Insertion

The fibres converge on and fuse with the lower part of the psoas major laterally and inserted with it on the anterior surface of lesser trochanter and an area (2.5 cm long) below it.

Nerve Supply

It is by the femoral nerve.

Actions

Along with the psoas major, it causes flexion of the thigh and the lumbar part of the vertebral column.

QUADRATUS LUMBORUM (Fig. 12.2)

It is a quadrilateral muscle which fills the medial half of the gap between the 12th rib, the iliac crest, and the tips of transverse processes of lumbar vertebrae. The quadratus lumborum muscle is enclosed between the anterior and middle layers of the thoraco-lumbar fascia.

Origin

It arises from:

(a) Posterior one-third of the inner lip of the iliac crest and iliolumbar ligament.
(b) Lower two to four transverse processes of lumbar vertebrae.

Insertion

The muscles run upward and medially pass posterior to the lateral arcuate ligament to be inserted into the medial part of the anterior surface of the 12th rib. It is also inserted into the upper lumbar transverse processes, posterior to its slips of origin.

Nerve Supply

It is by ventral rami of T12–L3/L4 lumbar spinal nerves.

Actions

These are as follows:

1.   It is a lateral flexor of the lumbar vertebral column.

2. It fixes the 12th rib during inspiration for effective contraction of the diaphragm.
3. Muscles of both sides acting together extend the lumbar vertebral column.

FASCIAE OF THE POSTERIOR ABDOMINAL WALL

The fasciae of posterior abdominal wall are:

1. Psoas fascia.
2. Fascia iliaca.
3. Thoraco-lumbar fascia.

The psoas fascia is described on p. 187, the fascia iliaca on p. 43, and thoraco-lumbar fascia on p. 175.

GREAT VESSELS OF THE ABDOMEN

The great vessels of the abdomen are abdominal aorta and inferior vena cava.

ABDOMINAL AORTA (Figs 12.6, 12.7, and 12.8)

The abdominal aorta begins as the continuation of descending thoracic aorta at the aortic orifice of the diaphragm opposite to the lower border of the T12 vertebra or intervertebral disc between vertebrae T12 and L1. It descends vertically downward and slightly to the left, in front of the vertebral column, and terminates in front of the lower part of the body of L4 vertebra (about 1.25 cm) to the left of the median plane by dividing into *right and left common iliac arteries.*

Measurements

Length: 10–11 cm.
Width: 2 cm.

Relations

Posterior:

1. Bodies of the upper four lumbar vertebrae and intervening intervertebral discs.
2. Anterior longitudinal ligament.
3. Third and fourth left lumbar veins.

Anterior: From above downward, the aorta is related to the following structures:

1. Pancreas and splenic vein.
2. Left renal vein.
3. Third part of the duodenum.
4. Root of the mesentery.
5. Coils of the small intestine separated by parietal peritoneum.

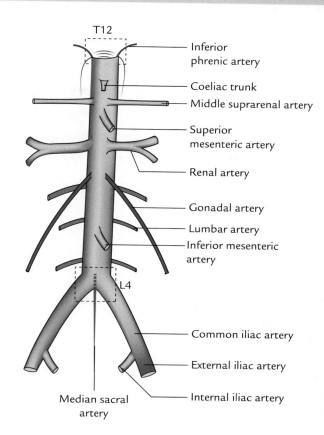

Fig. 12.6 Course and branches of the abdominal aorta.

Right side: Inferior vena cava.
Left side: Left sympathetic trunk.

Branches

The abdominal aorta gives three sets of branches:

1. Three unpaired ventral branches to the gut.
2. Three paired lateral branches to three paired glands (suprarenal glands, kidneys, and gonads).
3. Paired posterolateral branches to the abdominal wall.

In addition to the above, the aorta also gives rise to paired inferior phrenic artery, unpaired median sacral artery, and two terminal branches.

Coeliac Trunk (Fig. 12.7)

It is a short, wide vessel (1.25 cm long), which arises from the front of the abdominal aorta immediately below the aortic opening of the diaphragm at the level of the intervertebral disc between T12 and L1 vertebrae. It runs forward and somewhat to the right and immediately divides into following three branches: (a) left gastric artery, (b) common hepatic artery, and (c) splenic artery.

(a) Left Gastric Artery (smallest branch)

It passes upward and to the left to reach the cardiac end of the stomach where it turns forward to run downward along

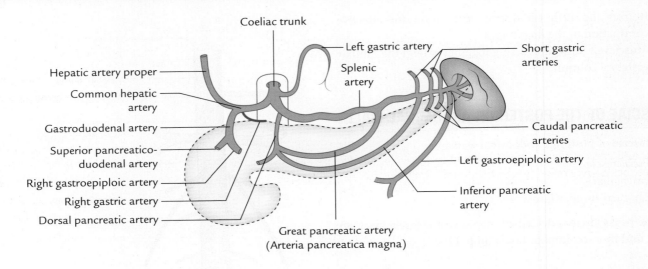

Fig. 12.7 Coeliac trunk.

the lesser curvature of the stomach. It gives rise to esophageal branches at the cardiac end of the stomach and numerous gastric branches along the lesser curvature of the stomach.

(b) Common Hepatic Artery

It is larger than the left gastric artery. It runs downward, forward, and to the right to reach the upper surface of the first part of the duodenum. Here it turns upward and runs in the right free margin of the lesser omentum (as hepatic artery proper) in front of the portal vein and to the left of common bile duct. On reaching the porta hepatis, it terminates by dividing into right and left hepatic arteries.

The common hepatic artery gives rise to the following branches:

1. **Gastroduodenal artery** arises at the upper border of the first of the duodenum. It runs downward behind the duodenum and terminates at its lower border by dividing into **right gastroepiploic** and **superior pancreatic duodenal arteries.**
2. **Right gastric artery** arises at just distal to the origin of gastroduodenal artery. It turns to the left and runs upward along the lesser curvature of the stomach.
3. **Hepatic artery proper** is the continuation of the common hepatic artery. It gives rise to right and left hepatic arteries at the porta hepatis. The *right hepatic artery* gives origin to *cystic artery* to supply the gallbladder. The right and left hepatic arteries supply the right and left physiological lobes of the liver, respectively.

(c) Splenic Artery (largest branch)

It is remarkably tortuous. It runs horizontally to the left, along the upper border of the body and tail of the pancreas, crosses in front of left suprarenal gland and anterior surface of the upper part of kidney to enter the lienorenal ligament through which it reaches the hilum of spleen. Here it divides into five or more segmental branches, which enter the spleen to supply it.

The splenic artery in addition to terminal segmental branches to the spleen gives off the following branches:

1. **Pancreatic branches:** They are numerous and supply whole of the pancreas except the head. The named pancreatic branches are large and constant, *viz.,* (i) **dorsal pancreatic artery** which usually arises from the splenic artery near its origin, (ii) **great pancreatic artery** (arteria pancreatica magna) which enters the body of pancreas and runs along the main pancreatic duct, and (iii) **caudal pancreatic arteries** which supply the tail. The pancreatic branches anastomose freely with each other and one of these is termed **inferior pancreatic artery.**
2. **Short gastric arteries** (3–7 in number): They arise from the terminal part of the splenic artery and supply the fundus of the stomach.
3. **Left gastroepiploic artery:** It arises from the terminal part of the splenic artery near the hilum of spleen and runs along the greater curvature of the stomach, and terminates by anastomosing with the right gastroepiploic artery.

Superior Mesenteric Artery

It arises from the front of the abdominal aorta about 1 cm below the coeliac trunk at the level of lower border of L1 vertebra. At the origin, it is sandwiched between the splenic vein above and the left renal vein below (Fig. 12.7). It is described in detail in Chapter 10 (see page 160).

Inferior Mesenteric Artery
It arises from the front of abdominal aorta about 4 cm above the bifurcation of aorta at the level of L3 vertebra. It is described in detail in Chapter 10 (see page 162).

Median Sacral Artery
It arises from the back of the abdominal aorta just above its bifurcation. It runs downward in the median plane into the pelvis and ends at the coccygeal body in front of the coccyx. Sometimes it gives origin to the fifth lumbar arteries.

Inferior Phrenic Arteries
These are the first branches of the abdominal aorta and arise from it just above the coeliac trunk. They pass superolaterally over the crura of diaphragm near the superior margins of suprarenal glands and ramify on the inferior surface of the diaphragm. They also give off superior *suprarenal arteries* to the corresponding suprarenal glands.

Renal Arteries
These are large wide-bored, straight vessels, which arise at right angles from the sides of the abdominal aorta, just below the origin of the superior mesenteric artery, at the level of the upper part of the L2 vertebra.

The left artery is slightly higher than the right artery whereas the right artery is longer than the left artery. The right artery passes to the right posterior to the inferior vena cava and right renal vein to reach the hilum of right kidney. The left renal artery passes to the left posterior to the left renal vein to reach the hilum of left kidney. It is crossed in front by the inferior mesenteric vein. Each renal artery gives rise to the **inferior suprarenal artery** to the corresponding suprarenal glands. The distribution of the renal arteries within the kidney is described in Chapter 11 (see page 170).

Gonadal Arteries (testicular and ovarian arteries)
The gonadal arteries are long slender vessels. They arise from the front of the aorta a little below the origin of the renal arteries. (Each **testicular artery** runs downward and laterally between the ureter posteriorly and intestines and mesenteric vessels anteriorly to reach the corresponding deep inguinal ring. The **right testicular artery** lies anterior to the inferior vena cava, psoas major, ureter, and external iliac artery, and posterior to the third part of duodenum, right colic, ileocolic and superior mesenteric vessels, and caecum.

The **left testicular artery** lies anterior to the same structures as that of the right testicular artery except the inferior vena cava, but it lies posterior to the third part of duodenum, inferior mesenteric vein, left colic and sigmoidal vessels, and inferior part of the descending colon.

On entering the deep inguinal ring, each artery traverses the inguinal canal as a constituent of the spermatic cord. At the upper pole of testis, it terminates by dividing into branches that supply the testis and epididymis.

The ovarian arteries have origin and course similar to testicular arteries except that they cross the external iliac vessels about 2.5 inferior to their origin, at the pelvic brim to enter the pelvis.

At pelvic brim, each ovarian artery enters the suspensory (infundibulopelvic) ligament of the ovary, runs in it to enter the broad ligament, then runs below the uterine tube medially, and terminates by anastomosing with the uterine artery at the superolateral angle of the uterus. In its course, it supplies the ovary and uterine tube. A branch to the ovary passes through the mesovarium.

Lumbar Arteries
The upper four pairs of these arteries arise from the posterior surface of the abdominal aorta. They pass laterally on the surfaces of the bodies of lumbar vertebrae and then backward deep to the psoas major. The fifth pair of lumbar arteries is usually represented by the lumbar branches of the iliolumbar arteries. But rarely they may arise from the median sacral artery.

Common Iliac Arteries
These are the terminal branches of the abdominal aorta. Each artery begins in front of the body of L4 vertebra about ½ inch (1.25 cm) to the left of the median plane. The left common iliac artery is shorter (4 cm) than the right common iliac artery (5 cm).

Each artery courses downward and laterally and terminates in front of the sacroiliac joint by dividing into external and internal iliac arteries.

1. The **right common iliac artery** passes in front of the commencement of the inferior vena cava. The right common iliac vein is posterior and medial to it.
2. The **left common iliac artery** is lateral to the left common iliac vein. It is crossed in its middle by the inferior mesenteric vessels.

External Iliac Arteries
Each external iliac artery extends downward and laterally as a continuation of the common iliac artery up to the midinguinal point where it enters the thigh behind the inguinal ligament to be continued as the femoral artery.

Each external iliac artery gives rise to two named branches—**inferior epigastric artery** and **deep circumflex iliac artery**.

The **inferior epigastric artery** arises just above the inguinal ligament and runs upward and medially in the extraperitoneal tissue deep to fascia transversalis, passes along the medial margin of the deep inguinal ring, where it is hooked laterally by the ductus deferens/round ligament of the uterus. At the lateral border of rectus abdominis, it pierces fascia transversalis to enter the rectus sheath in front of arcuate line. Within the rectus sheath, it ascends up and ends by anastomosing with the superior epigastric artery at the level of the umbilicus.

The **deep circumflex iliac artery** arises from the lateral side opposite the inferior epigastric and runs laterally along the posterior margin of inguinal ligament. On reaching the anterior superior iliac spine it terminates by anastomosing with the lateral circumflex femoral and superior gluteal arteries.

Internal Iliac Arteries

They are described in Chapter 14, p. 221.

The branches of abdominal aorta are summarized in Flowchart 12.1 and Figure 12.8.

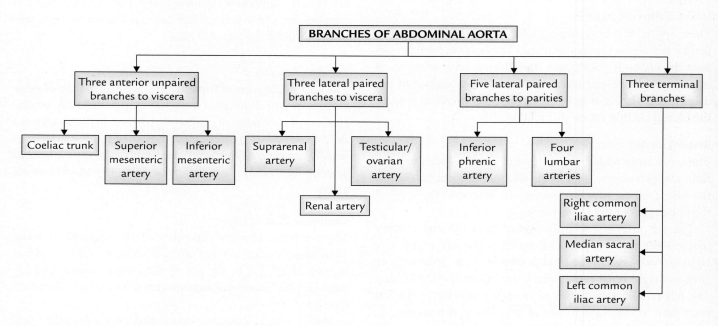

Flowchart 12.1 Branches of the abdominal aorta.

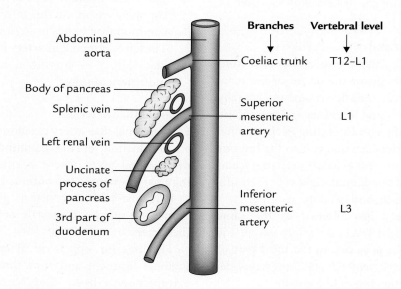

Fig. 12.8 Three ventral branches of the abdominal aorta as seen in left lateral view of a sagittal section through the abdominal aorta. Note: Superior mesenteric artery at its origin is sandwiched between splenic and left renal veins.

Clinical correlation

- **Pulsations of the abdominal aorta:** They can be felt in the median plane on the anterior abdominal wall at the level of L4 vertebra, especially in children and thin-built adults. The abdominal aorta can also be compressed at this site by a backward pressure on the anterior abdominal wall.
- **Aortic aneurysm (Fig. 12.9):** The aortic aneurysm (localized dilatation of the aorta) commonly occurs below the origin of the renal arteries (95%) usually in elderly men. Most common cause of aortic aneurysm is atherosclerosis, which weakens the aortic wall. Clinically, it presents as pulsatile and expansile abdominal mass typically just superior to and to the left of the umbilicus. The origin of renal arteries is an important landmark in the abdominal aortic aneurysm surgery.

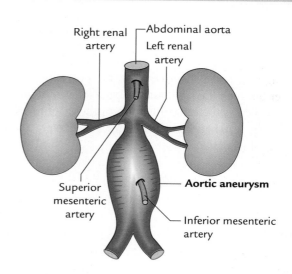

Fig. 12.9 Aortic aneurysm.

INFERIOR VENA CAVA (IVC) (Fig. 12.10)

The IVC is the largest and widest vein of the body. It drains most of the blood from the body below the diaphragm into the right atrium of the heart.

Formation, Course, and Termination

The IVC is formed by the union of right and left common iliac veins in front of the body of L5 vertebra, below the

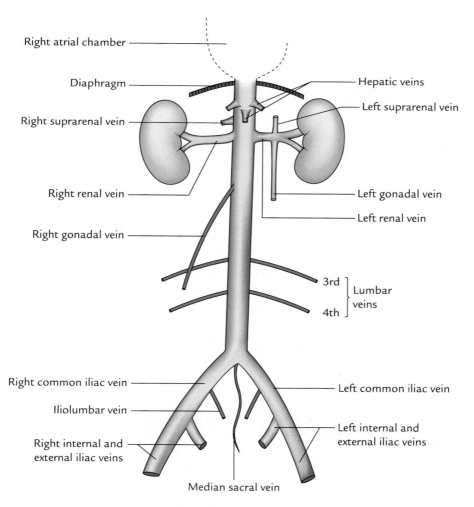

Fig. 12.10 Extent and tributaries of the inferior vena cava.

aortic bifurcation, and behind the right common iliac artery. It ascends in front of the vertebral column on the right side of the aorta. It then arches forward on the right crus of the diaphragm to reach the groove on the posterior surface of the liver between the right and caudate lobes, just above the groove it pierces the central tendon of the diaphragm at the level of T8 vertebra and terminates by entering the right atrium of the heart.

N.B. The IVC extends across the eight vertebrae (L4 to T8) and is about twice the length of the abdominal aorta.

Relations

Anterior: From below upward, the structures anterior to the IVC as it ascends are:

1. Root of the mesentery.
2. Right testicular/ovarian artery.
3. Third part of the duodenum.
4. Head of the pancreas and bile duct.
5. Portal vein (posterior to first of duodenum and in the right free margin of lesser omentum).
6. Posterior surface of the liver between the right and caudate lobes.

Posterior: From below upward, the structures posterior to the IVC as it ascends are:

1. Right sympathetic chain and psoas major.
2. Right renal artery.
3. Right coeliac ganglion.
4. Right suprarenal gland (medial part).
5. Right middle suprarenal vein.
6. Right inferior phrenic artery.

Tributaries

The IVC receives the following tributaries:

1. Three formative veins—two common iliac veins and the median sacral vein. The latter may join the left common iliac vein. Each common iliac vein receives an iliolumbar vein.
2. Three abdominal wall tributaries—inferior phrenic vein and third and fourth lumbar veins. The first and second lumbar veins end in the ascending lumbar vein.
3. Three lateral visceral tributaries—right suprarenal vein, renal veins, and right testicular/ovarian vein. The left suprarenal vein and left gonadal veins drain into the left renal vein.
4. Three anterior visceral tributaries—right, middle, and left hepatic veins.

Compression of the inferior vena cava (IVC): The IVC is commonly compressed by an enlarged uterus during the last trimester of the pregnancy. This causes edema of the ankle and feet, and varicose veins in the lower limb.

The compression and blockage of the IVC by the malignant retroperitoneal tumors result in dilatation of the anastomotic channel between IVC and superior vena cava (**caval–caval shunt**) so that the blood could be returned to the right atrium. Clinically, it presents as the prominent subcutaneous vein called *thoraco-abdominal vein* formed due to dilatation of anastomotic venous channel between the *lateral thoracic vein,* a tributary of the axillary vein, and the *superficial epigastric vein,* a tributary of the femoral vein.

LYMPHATICS AND LYMPH NODES OF THE POSTERIOR ABDOMINAL WALL (Fig. 12.11)

LYMPHATICS

The lymph vessels draining the posterior abdominal wall and most of the abdominopelvic organs except part of the liver terminate in the **cisterna chyli and thoracic duct.** The lymphatic stream is intercepted by a series of lymph node groups before reaching the cisterna chyli and the thoracic duct.

Cisterna Chyli

It is an elongated white lymphatic sac about 5–7 cm long and 4 mm wide. It lies on the front of L1 and L2 vertebrae between the aorta and the azygos vein, hidden by the right crus of the diaphragm. Superiorly it continues as the thoracic duct.

Tributaries
The cisterna chyli receives the following tributaries:

1. Right and left intestinal lymph trunks—from the preaortic lymph nodes, which open in its middle. These trunks drain the lymph from the small intestine, stomach, and liver.
2. Right and left lumbar lymph trunks—from the para-aortic lymph nodes, which open in it inferiorly.
3. A pair of lymph vessels—from the lower intercostal lymph nodes, which open in it superiorly.

LYMPH NODES

These are located along the external iliac arteries, common iliac arteries, and abdominal aorta, and accordingly termed external iliac, common iliac, and aortic lymph nodes.

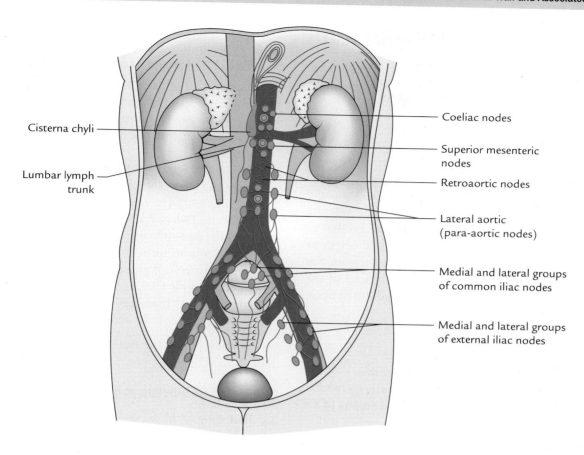

Fig. 12.11 Lymphatics and lymph nodes of the posterior abdominal wall.

External Iliac Nodes

These are 8–10 in number and lie along the external iliac vessels. The *medial nodes* receive the lymph from the pelvic viscera and lower limb, whereas the *lateral nodes* receive the lymph from the territories of inferior epigastric and deep circumflex iliac vessels. Afferents from these node pass into the *common iliac nodes*.

Common Iliac Nodes

These are 4–6 in number and lie along the common iliac vessels (lateral group) and below the bifurcation of the aorta (medial group). The lateral group of nodes receives the lymph from the pelvis and lower limb via external and internal iliac nodes, whereas the medial group of nodes receives the lymph from the pelvic viscera directly and through the *internal iliac and sacral nodes*.

Aortic Lymph Nodes

They are situated along the abdominal aorta and inferior vena cava, and are arranged into two groups—pre-aortic and para-aortic.

1. **Pre-aortic nodes:** The nodes are located around the origin of coeliac, superior mesenteric, and inferior mesenteric arteries and are accordingly named as *coeliac, superior mesenteric, and inferior mesenteric nodes*. They receive the lymph from the organs supplied by these arteries.

   The efferents from pre-aortic nodes form the **intestinal** lymph trunks, which drain into the cisterna chyli.

2. **Para-aortic (lateral aortic) nodes:** They are situated on each side of the abdominal aorta, some nodes of this group lie behind the aorta and called **retroaortic nodes**. The para-aortic nodes are also called **lumbar nodes**. They receive the lymph from suprarenal glands, kidneys and ureters, and testes or ovaries. They also receive the lymph from most of the pelvic organs and the lower extremities through internal iliac, external iliac, common iliac, and other pelvic nodes.

   The efferents from para-aortic nodes form lumbar trunks which drain into the cisterna chyli.

NERVES OF THE POSTERIOR ABDOMINAL WALL

The nerves of the posterior abdominal wall include subcostal nerve, ventral rami of lumbar nerves, and lumbar sympathetic chains.

SUBCOSTAL NERVE

It is the ventral ramus of the 12th thoracic spinal nerve. It enters the abdomen behind the lateral accurate ligament (lateral lumbocostal arch) and runs downward and laterally in front of the quadratus lumborum beneath the anterior layer of thoraco-lumbar fascia. At the lateral border of quadratus lumborum, it pierces the aponeurotic origin of transversus abdominis and enters the plane between the transversus abdominis and internal oblique muscles of the anterior abdominal wall. Its further course and distribution are described in Chapter 3 (see page 41).

LUMBAR PLEXUS (Fig. 12.12)

The lumbar plexus is formed within the substance of the psoas major by the union of ventral rami of L1–L3 lumbar nerves and a larger upper part of the ventral ramus of L4 nerve.

The lower smaller part of the ventral ramus of L4 nerve joins with the ventral ramus of L5 nerve to form the **lumbosacral trunk** which takes part in the formation of sacral plexus.

The ventral ramus of the 4th lumbar nerve is sometimes called *nervi furcalis*, because it forms the connecting link between the lumbar and sacral plexuses.

1. The ventral ramus of the L1 nerve supplemented by a twig from T12 (subcostal) nerve divides into a larger upper branch and smaller lower branch. The larger upper branch gives rise to *iliohypogastric* and *ilioinguinal nerves*.
2. The smaller lower branch joins with a twig from the L2 nerve and forms the *genitofemoral nerve*.
3. The L2, L3, L4 nerves divide into dorsal and ventral divisions. The dorsal divisions of L2, L3, L4 unite to form the *femoral nerve*. The ventral divisions of L2, L3, and L4 join to form the *obturator nerve*. The *accessory obturator* nerve if present is derived from the ventral branches of the L3, L4 nerves.
4. The principal branches of the lumbar plexus are the *femoral nerve* and the *obturator nerve*.

The branches of the lumbar plexus are summarized in Table 12.1.

Course and Distribution of the Branches

1. **Iliohypogastric nerve:** It emerges beneath the lateral border of the psoas major muscle, passes downward and laterally in front of the quadratus lumborum. At the lateral border of quadratus lumborum it pierces aponeurotic origin of the transversus abdominis just

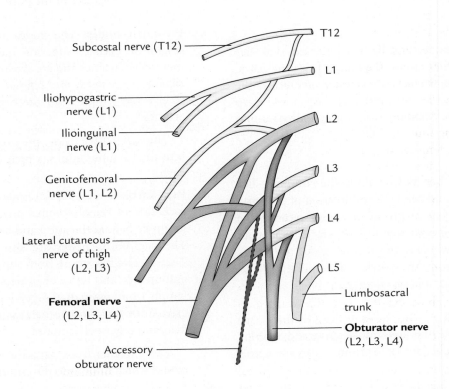

Fig. 12.12 Lumbar plexus of nerves: The dorsal divisions are shown by green colour and ventral divisions by blue colour.

Table 12.1 Branches of the lumbar plexus

Branches	Root value
1. Iliohypogastric nerve	L1
2. Ilioinguinal nerve	L1
3. Genitofemoral nerve	L1, L2 (ventral divisions)
4. Lateral cutaneous nerve of the thigh	L2, L3 (dorsal divisions)
5. Femoral nerve	L2, L3, L4 (dorsal divisions)
6. Obturator nerve	L2, L3, L4 (ventral divisions)
7. Accessory obturator nerve (occasional)	L3, L4 (ventral divisions)

above the iliac crest and runs in the anterior abdominal wall (see page 41). It provides cutaneous innervation to the skin of gluteal region and anterior abdominal wall in the hypogastric region.

2. **Ilioinguinal nerve:** It pursues the same course as the iliohypogastric nerve, but at a slightly lower level. It pierces the transversus abdominis close to the anterior part of the iliac crest (see page 41). It provides motor innervation to internal oblique and transversus abdominis muscles and sensory innervation to the skin on the upper medial aspect of the thigh, root of penis, and scrotum in the male, and mons pubis and labium majus in the female.

3. **Genitofemoral nerve:** It passes forward through the psoas, pierces it and its covering psoas fascia. It runs on the anterior surface of the psoas near its medial border and divides above the inguinal ligament into genital and femoral branches. The *femoral branch* runs along the lateral side of the external iliac artery and enters the femoral sheath, where it lies anterolateral to the femoral artery. It pierces the anterior wall of the sheath to supply the skin over the femoral triangle. The *genital branch* enters the deep inguinal ring and traverses through the inguinal canal along the spermatic cord in the male and the round ligament of uterus in the female. In the male it supplies the cremaster muscle and scrotal skin, and in the female it supplies the skin of mons pubis and labium majus.

4. **Lateral cutaneous nerve of the thigh (Lateral femoral cutaneous nerve):** It emerges beneath the lateral border of the psoas major above the iliac crest, runs downward and laterally across the iliac fossa in front of the iliacus muscle under cover of the iliac fascia. It enters the thigh by passing beneath the lateral end of the inguinal ligament. Sometimes it passes through the inguinal ligament. It provides cutaneous innervation to the upper lateral aspect of the thigh.

5. **Femoral nerve:** It emerges beneath the lateral border of the psoas major below the iliac crest, runs downward and slight laterally in the groove between the psoas major and iliacus under cover of the iliac fascia. It enters the thigh by passing deep to the inguinal ligament where it lies lateral to the psoas sheath. Before entering the thigh it supplies the iliacus muscle. Its course and distribution in the thigh are described in Chapter 22 (see page 340).

6. **Obturator nerve:** It emerges beneath the medial border of the psoas major in the lumbosacral triangle, crosses the anterolateral angle of the ala of sacrum to run downward and forward along the lateral wall of the true pelvis, and finally enters the thigh by passing through the obturator canal. Its course and distribution in the thigh are described in Chapter 23 (see page 347).

7. **Accessory obturator nerve:** It is an inconstant nerve. When present, it accompanies the medial border of the psoas major to enter the thigh. It supplies the pectineus muscles.

ABDOMINAL PART OF THE AUTONOMIC NERVOUS SYSTEM (Fig. 12.13)

The abdominal part of the autonomic nervous system comprises the following two components:

1. Lumbar sympathetic chains.
2. Autonomic plexuses of the posterior abdominal wall.

LUMBAR SYMPATHETIC CHAIN

It is a ganglionated chain situated on either side of the lumbar vertebrae. It commences deep to the medial arcuate ligament of the diaphragm as the continuation of the thoracic sympathetic trunk. It runs vertically downward along the sides of bodies of the lumbar vertebrae and the intervening intervertebral discs overlapped on the right side by the IVC and on the left side by the abdominal aorta. The lumbar arteries lie deep to the chain but the lumbar veins may cross superficial to it. The chain enters the pelvis in front of the ala of sacrum beneath the common iliac vessels, where it continues as the sacral sympathetic chain in front of the sacrum. Inferiorly the right and left sympathetic chain converges and unites in front of the coccyx to form the ganglion impar.

Each lumbar sympathetic chain possesses four ganglia, the first and second often being fused together.

Branches

1. **White rami communicantes:** Anterior primary rami of L1 and L2 lumbar nerves send white rami communicantes to the corresponding lumbar ganglia. A white ramus

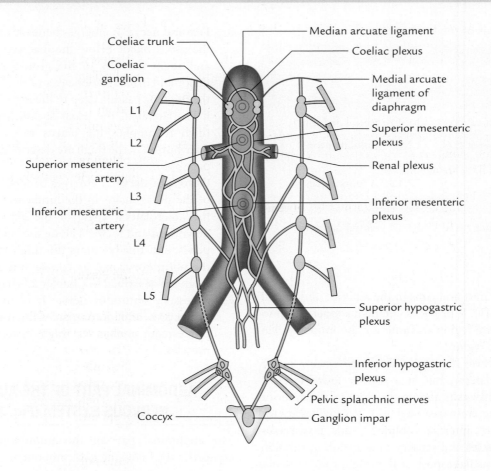

Fig. 12.13 Lumbar sympathetic chain and autonomic plexuses of the posterior abdominal wall.

contains preganglionic nerve fibres and afferent sensory nerve fibres.

2. **Gray rami communicantes:** Gray ramus communicans arise from each lumbar ganglion and get connected to the ventral rami of corresponding lumbar nerves. A gray ramus contains postganglionic fibres.

3. **Lumbar splanchnic nerves:** These are usually four in number and arise as medial branches from corresponding lumbar ganglia. They convey preganglionic motor and viscerosensory (pain) fibres. The upper two lumbar splanchnic nerves join the coeliac and aortic autonomic plexuses, and the lower two joins the superior hypogastric plexus.

AUTONOMIC PLEXUSES OF THE POSTERIOR ABDOMINAL WALL

The preganglionic and postganglionic sympathetic fibres, preganglionic parasympathetic fibres, and visceral afferent fibres form a plexus of nerves around the abdominal aorta. The regional concentrations of this plexus form two major well-demarcated plexuses—the coeliac and superior hypogastric plexuses.

Coeliac Plexus (Solar Plexus)

Location

1. The coeliac plexus is located on the front of the abdominal aorta around the coeliac trunk and origin of the superior mesenteric artery.

2. It is a dense network of fine nerve fibres which connect the two coeliac ganglia.

3. It supplies the sympathetic fibres to all the abdominal organs including gonads.

4. It is the largest of the three great autonomic plexuses.

The **coeliac ganglia** are two irregular masses of nerve cells situated one on each side of the origin of coeliac artery.

Each ganglion is divisible into a large upper part and a lower part. The lower part is more or less detached from the upper part and is called **aorticorenal ganglion.**

Fibre Input

1. *Greater splanchnic nerve* joins the upper part of the coeliac ganglion.

2. *Lesser splanchnic nerve* joins the aorticorenal ganglion.

3. *Preganglionic vagal fibres* derived from the posterior vagal trunk, which contains fibres from both right (chiefly) and left vagus nerves.
4. *Sensory phrenic fibres* reach the plexus along the inferior phrenic artery.

Branches

The coeliac plexus gives rise to a number of secondary plexuses which run along and surround the different branches of aorta. These are as follows:

1. **Phrenic plexus:**
   (a) It accompanies the corresponding interior phrenic artery to the diaphragm. Some filaments pass to the suprarenal gland through superior suprarenal artery.
   (b) It receives one or two branches from the phrenic nerve.
2. **Hepatic plexus:**
   (a) It is the largest secondary plexus derived from the coeliac plexus.
   (b) It receives filaments from left and right vagus nerves and right phrenic nerve.
   (c) It accompanies the hepatic artery and its branches to the liver, gallbladder, and bile duct.
   (d) Its vagal fibres are motor to the musculature gall-bladder and bile duct, and inhibitory to the sphincter of the bile duct.
3. **Left gastric plexus:**
   (a) It accompanies the left gastric artery.
   (b) Its sympathetic nerves are motor to the pyloric sphincter of the stomach.
4. **Splenic plexus:** It accompanies the splenic artery to spleen.
5. **Suprarenal plexus:** It contains mainly preganglionic fibres of greater splanchnic nerve, which synapse with chromaffin cells of the adrenal medulla which are homologous with postganglionic sympathetic neurons. Relative to its size the suprarenal gland has a larger autonomic supply than any other organ in the body.
6. **Renal plexus:** It is formed by the fibres from the aorticorenal ganglion, lowest thoracic splanchnic nerve, first lumbar splanchnic nerve, etc., and supplies the kidney and upper part of the ureter.
7. **Testicular plexus:** It accompanies the testicular artery to the testis. Branches from the plexus also supply the epididymis and vas deferens.
8. **Ovarian plexus:** It accompanies the ovarian artery to supply the ovary and uterine tube.
9. **Superior mesenteric plexus:** It is located around the superior mesenteric artery and contains the superior mesenteric ganglion in its upper part or usually immediately above the origin of superior mesenteric artery. Branches of the plexus supply the superior mesenteric territory.
10. **Abdominal aortic plexus (intermesenteric plexus):**
    (a) It is formed by filaments from the coeliac plexus and ganglia, and first and second lumbar splenic nerves.
    (b) It is situated on the front of the aorta between the origins of superior and inferior mesenteric arteries.
    (c) It consists of 4–12 nerves (intermesenteric) connected by oblique arranged branches.
    (d) It is continuous below with the superior hypogastric plexus.
11. **Inferior mesenteric plexus:** It is formed chiefly from the aortic plexus and distributed to the territory of inferior mesenteric artery.

Superior Hypogastric Plexus (Presacral Nerve)

Location

It lies in front of the bifurcation of the abdominal aorta and body of the fifth lumbar vertebra between the two common iliac arteries. It is often referred to as **presacral nerve** but the plexus is never sufficiently condensed to resemble a single nerve and moreover plexus is prelumbar rather than presacral in position. Therefore, the name presacral nerve appears to be inappropriate.

Formation

It is formed by the union of:

1. Descending fibres of the aortic plexus.
2. Third and fourth lumbar splanchnic nerves.
3. Ascending filaments of inferior hypogastric plexus (carrying fibres of the pelvic splanchnic nerves). These fibres supply the parts of gut derived from the hindgut.

N.B. Below the superior hypogastric plexus divides into right and left hypogastric nerves which descend in front of the sacrum to join the two **inferior hypogastric plexuses** located in the pelvis which also receives twigs from the sacral sympathetic ganglia and pelvic splanchnic nerves (S2, S3, S4).

Functions

1. The parasympathetic fibres have exclusive control on the muscular walls of the bladder, urethra, and rectum. The pelvic splanchnic nerves (**nervi erigentes**) also relax the walls of arteries supplying the erectile tissue, of penis (or clitoris) leading to their erection hence the name *nerve erigentes*.
2. Sympathetic fibres when stimulated cause the epididymis, vas deferens, seminal vesicle, and prostrate to contract and empty their contents into the urethra (ejaculation) and constrict the internal urethral sphincter (involuntary), thus preventing the seminal fluid to enter the urinary bladder during ejaculation.

Clinical correlation

- **Visceral pain:** The viscera are insensitive to cutting, crushing, or burning but visceral pain does occur following excessive distension, spasmodic contraction of smooth muscles, and ischemia of the viscera. The visceral pain is usually referred to the skin supplied by same segmental nerves (referred pain).

- **Lumbar sympathectomy:** It is done for vaso-occlusive disease of lower limb (Buerger's disease). Usually the second, third, and fourth lumbar ganglia are excised along with intermediate chain. This causes adequate vasodilation of the lower limb. Consequently the skin of the lower limb becomes warm, pink, and dry. The first lumbar ganglion is preserved because it plays an important role in ejaculation (keeps the sphincter vesicae closed during ejaculation).

  Removal of first lumbar sympathetic ganglion results in dry coitus.

- **Presacral neurectomy:** In females, it is successful in the cases of *intractable dysmenorrhea* because pain fibres from the body of uterus pass through the presacral nerve (superior hypogastric plexus).

  In males, presacral neurectomy is followed by loss of power of ejaculation although he may have normal erection (intact nervi erigentes).

Golden Facts to Remember

- Key muscle of the posterior abdominal wall — Psoas major
- Commonest site of the aortic aneurysm — Abdominal aorta below the origin of renal arteries
- Largest vein of the body ⎫
- Widest vein of the body ⎭ — Inferior vena cava
- Largest lymphatic sac in the body — Cisterna chyli
- Largest autonomic plexus in abdomen — Coeliac (solar) plexus
- Commonest site of the pheochromocytoma — Adrenal medulla

Clinical Case Study

A 65-year-old man visited his family physician and complained that he feels pain in his both legs when taking long walks. In the past few months, he noticed that cramp-like pain occurs after walking about 100 yards and it disappears on rest and appears again as he walks the same distance. He also told that he experiences difficulty in erection. The arteriography of the abdominal aorta revealed the blockage in the region of its bifurcation. A diagnosis of "**abdominal aorta blockage**" was made.

Questions

1. What is the extent of abdominal aorta? Name its terminal branches.
2. What is the commonest cause of the blockage of aorta?
3. Name the term used for the type of pain felt by the patient in recent times. Give the cause of pain.
4. What is the cause of difficulty in erection in this case?

Answers

1. It extends in front of the vertebral column from T12 to L4 vertebrae. Its terminal branches are right and left common iliac arteries.
2. Advanced arteriosclerosis.
3. Claudication. It occurs as a result of an insufficient amount of blood reaching the legs during walking.
4. Lack of blood entering internal iliac arteries. (Student must remember that blood supply to the penis is derived from the internal iliac arteries.)

Pelvis

The term "pelvis" literally means a basin. It is made up of four bones: two hip (innominate) bones, sacrum, and coccyx, bound to each other by the ligaments (Fig. 13.1).

The functions of the pelvis are:

1. It contains the pelvic viscera (urinary bladder and rectum in both sexes and uterus in female) and protects them.

2. It supports the weight of the body and transmits it to the lower limbs successively through sacrum, sacroiliac joints, innominate bones, and then to femora in the standing position, and ischial tuberosities in the sitting position.

3. During walking the pelvis swings from side to side by rotatory movements at the lumbosacral articulation.

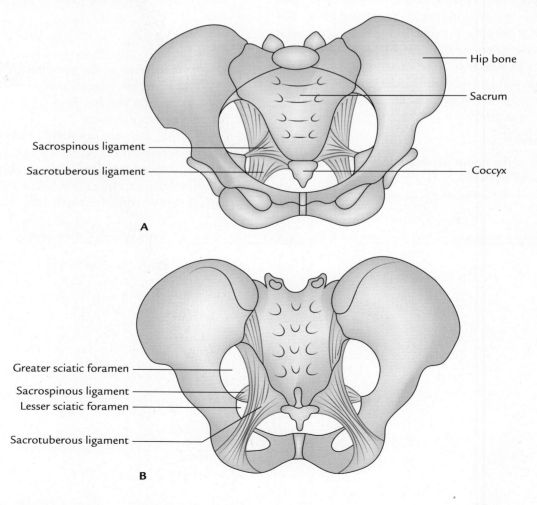

Fig. 13.1 The female pelvis: **A**, front view; **B**, back view.

4. It provides attachments for muscles.
5. In the female, it provides bony support for the birth canal.

BONES OF THE PELVIS

These have been already described in detail in Chapter 2.

JOINTS AND LIGAMENTS OF THE PELVIS

The joints of the pelvis are: (a) symphysis pubis and (b) right and left sacroiliac joints and sacrococcygeal joint (Fig. 13.2).

SYMPHYSIS PUBIS

It is a secondary cartilaginous joint between the bodies of two pubic bones. The articular surfaces are covered by a plate of hyaline cartilage which are then united by a disc of fibrocartilage. The joint is surrounded and strengthened by the fibrous ligaments, especially above and below. The **inferior pubic (arcuate) ligament** is very strong.

SACROILIAC JOINTS

These are generally described as plane synovial joints formed by union of the auricular surfaces of the sacrum and the ilium on each side. The sacroiliac joint is surrounded and strengthened by the following ligaments:

1. Interosseous sacroiliac ligament.
2. Ventral sacroiliac ligament.
3. Dorsal sacroiliac ligament.
4. Iliolumbar ligaments.

N.B. Truly speaking, the two sacroiliac joints are strong, weight-bearing joints, each consisting of two components (Fig. 13.2):

(a) An **anterior plane type of synovial joint** between the auricular surfaces of the ilium and sacrum.
(b) A **posterior syndesmosis** between the tuberosities of the sacrum and ilium.

- The **interosseous sacroiliac ligament** is the **second strongest ligament in the body** and connects the irregular bony tuberosities of the sacrum and ilium behind the auricular surfaces.
- The **ventral sacroiliac ligament** connects the ala and pelvic surface of the sacrum with the adjacent part of the ilium.
- The **dorsal sacroiliac ligament** is made up of strong fibrous bands, which connect the posterosuperior iliac spine of ilium with the intermediate sacral crest.
- The **iliolumbar ligament** connects the transverse process of the L5 vertebra to the ilium.

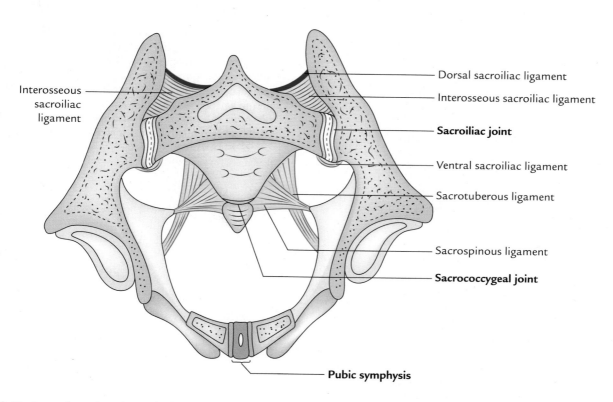

Interosseous sacroiliac ligament

Dorsal sacroiliac ligament
Interosseous sacroiliac ligament
Sacroiliac joint
Ventral sacroiliac ligament
Sacrotuberous ligament
Sacrospinous ligament
Sacrococcygeal joint
Pubic symphysis

Fig. 13.2 Horizontal section through the lesser pelvis to show the sacroiliac joints and pubic symphysis.

- The **sacrotuberous ligament** is a strong broadband of the fibrous tissue. It has broad upper medial end and narrow lower lateral end. The upper end is attached from above downward to the posterior superior iliac spine, posterior inferior iliac spine, lower part of the posterior surface, and lateral border of the sacrum, and adjoining upper part of the coccyx. Its lower end is attached to the medial margin of the ischial tuberosity. Some of the fibres from the lower end are continued on to the ramus of the ischium to form *falciform process*.
- The **sacrospinous ligament** is a triangular sheet of fibrous tissue, with its apex attached laterally to the ischial spine and base attached medially to the side of sacrum and coccyx.

The sacrotuberous and sacrospinous ligaments convert the greater and lesser sciatic notches of the hip bone into greater and lesser sciatic foramina—the two important exits from the pelvis.

Stability of the Sacroiliac Region

The sacrum hangs from sacroiliac joints forming the posterior wall of the pelvis. The body weight tends to cause forward rotation of the upper end of sacrum and concomitant backward rotation of its lower end (Fig. 13.3).

Ligaments resisting forward rotation of the upper end of sacrum are:

1. Interosseous sacroiliac ligament.
2. Posterior sacroiliac ligament.
3. Iliolumbar ligament.

Ligaments resisting the backward relation of the lower end of the sacrum are as follows:

1. Sacrotuberous ligament.
2. Sacrospinous ligament.
3. Sacrococcygeal joint.

These ligaments are already described with the sacroiliac joints.

SACROCOCCYGEAL JOINT

It is a secondary cartilaginous joint between the apex of sacrum and the base of coccyx. The bones are united by thin intervertebral disc. The sacrococcygeal joint is strengthened by *ventral and dorsal sacrococcygeal ligaments*, and *intercornual ligaments* (connecting cornua of sacrum and coccyx). The coccyx moves a little backward during defecation and parturition.

Clinical correlation

- **Prominence of hips in multiparous females:** During pregnancy (particularly in the last trimester), the pelvic joints are relaxed by **relaxin hormone** to provide smooth passage of the baby. After childbirth these ligaments tighten up again but never regain their original efficiency. As a result, the pelvis widens and hips become more prominent in a multiparous female.
- **Gait in late pregnancy:** The body of the fifth lumbar vertebra makes an angle of about 120° with the sacrum. This angle is called **lumbosacral angle**. It opens posteriorly, because the intervertebral disc between L5 and S1 is thicker anteriorly than posteriorly (Fig. 13.4). The forward tilt of the upper end of the sacrum due to weight is prevented by the ligaments. During late pregnancy due to relaxation of ligaments and additional body weight due to gravid uterus, the upper end of the sacrum tilts forward during walking and woman tends to fall forward. This, she prevents by walking with backward tilt of her lumbar vertebral column and shoulders, i.e., she walks like a lord.

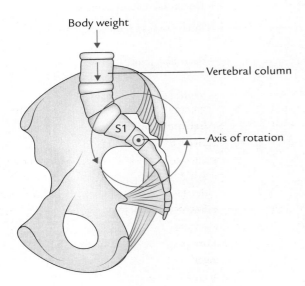

Fig. 13.3 Ligaments resisting rotation of the sacrum. Note weight of the body is transmitted to the sacrum anterior to the axis of rotation of the sacroiliac joint.

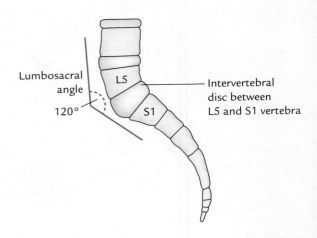

Fig. 13.4 Lumbosacral angle.

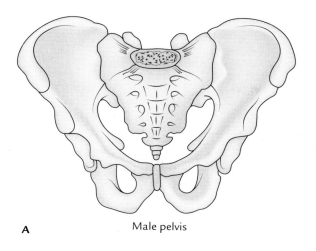
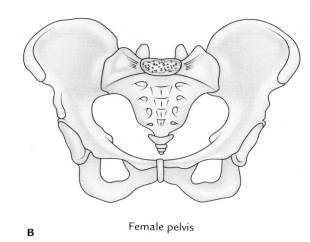

A   Male pelvis   B   Female pelvis

Fig. 13.5 Male and female pelvis.

DIFFERENCES BETWEEN THE MALE AND FEMALE PELVIS (Fig. 13.5)

The differences between the male and female pelvis are principally associated with the following two features:

1. Heavier build and stronger muscles in the male, account for stronger bones and well-defined muscle markings in the male pelvis.
2. To provide passage to the baby during parturition, the pelvic cavity is comparatively wider and shallower in the female.

The sex differences between the male and female pelvis are summarized in Table 13.1 and shown in Figure 13.6.

OBSTETRIC PELVIS (TRUE PELVIS)

The pelvis is divided into the false or greater pelvis above, and true or lesser pelvis below. The plane of division is **pelvic inlet** formed by the sacral promontory behind and linea terminalis at the sides and front. The linea terminalis may be traced as a continuous line from behind forward as the arcuate line of the ilium, the iliopectineal line (pecten), and the pubic crest.

Table 13.1 Differences between the male and female pelvis

	Male	Female
General structure	Heavy and thick	Light and thin
Articular surfaces	Large	Small
Muscle attachments	Well marked	Indistinct
False pelvis	Deep	Shallow
Pelvic inlet	Heart shaped	Oval
Pelvic canal/cavity	"Long segment of a short cone," i.e., long and tapered	"Short segment of a long cone," i.e., short with almost parallel sides
Pelvic outlet	Comparatively small	Comparatively large
First piece of sacrum	Superior surface of the body occupies nearly half the width of base of sacrum	Superior surface of the body occupies about one-third the width of base of sacrum
Sacrum	Long, narrow, with smooth forward concavity	Short, wide, flat, curving forward in the lower part
Sacroiliac articular facet (auricular surface)	Extends down up to the lower border of third piece of sacrum	Extends down only up to the upper border of third piece of sacrum
Subpubic angle (Fig. 13.6; angle between inferior pubic rami	< 90° (angle between the middle and index fingers)	90° or more (angle between the thumb and the index finger)
Inferior pubic ramus	Presents a strong everted surface for attachment of the crus of the penis	This marking is not present
Acetabulum	Large	Small
Ischial tuberosities	Inturned	Everted
Obturator foramen	Larger and oval	Smaller and triangular

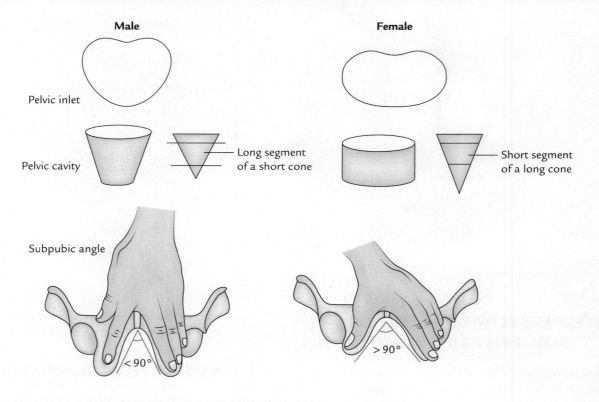

Male

Female

Pelvic inlet

Pelvic cavity — Long segment of a short cone — Short segment of a long cone

Subpubic angle

< 90°   > 90°

Fig. 13.6 Some of the main differences between the male and female pelvis.

The false pelvis is really a part of the abdominal cavity proper. The true pelvis is involved in the process of birth, hence called **obstetric pelvis/true pelvis**. Therefore, the student must know its size, form, and dimensions in detail.

REGIONS OF THE TRUE PELVIS

The true pelvis presents the pelvic inlet, pelvic outlet, and pelvic cavity.

Boundaries of the Pelvic Inlet (Fig. 13.7)

Posteriorly: Sacral promontory and anterior margins of alae of the sacrum.
Laterally: Arcuate and pectineal lines.
In front: Upper margin of pubic symphysis and pubic crests.

Boundaries of the Pelvic Outlet (Fig. 13.8)

Anteriorly: Lower margin of the pubic symphysis.
Anterolaterally: Conjoint ischiopubic ramus on each side.
Laterally: Ischial tuberosity on each side.
Posterolaterally: Sacrotuberous ligament on each side.
Posteriorly: Tip of the coccyx.

Boundaries of the Pelvic Cavity

Anteriorly: Pelvic surfaces of the bodies of pubic bone, pubic rami, and pubic symphysis.
Posteriorly: Pelvic surfaces of the sacrum and coccyx.
Laterally: Pelvic surfaces of the ilium ischium below the arcuate line.

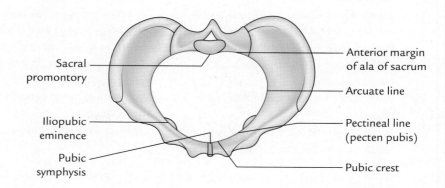

Sacral promontory — — Anterior margin of ala of sacrum

Iliopubic eminence — — Arcuate line

— Pectineal line (pecten pubis)

Pubic symphysis — — Pubic crest

Fig. 13.7 Pelvic inlet.

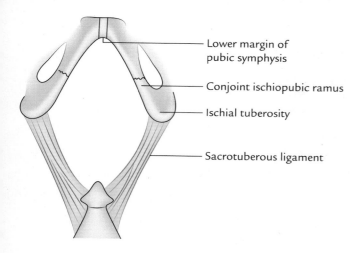

Fig. 13.8 Pelvic outlet.

- Lower margin of pubic symphysis
- Conjoint ischiopubic ramus
- Ischial tuberosity
- Sacrotuberous ligament

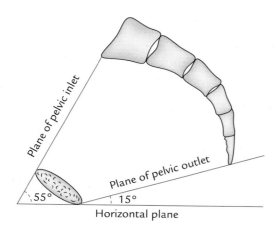

Fig. 13.9 Pelvic inclination.

PELVIC INCLINATION (Fig. 13.9)

The pelvic brim and pelvic outlet do not lie in the horizontal plane when the subject stands erect. The planes of pelvic inlet and pelvic outlet incline downward from behind forward. As a result, the *plane of pelvic inlet* forms an angle of about 55°/60° to the horizontal plane, and the *plane of pelvic outlet* forms an angle of 15° with the horizontal plane (Fig. 13.9).

Pelvic Planes (Fig. 13.10)

Plane of greatest pelvic dimension: It is an imaginary plane passing anteroposteriorly through the middle of pubic symphysis and junction between S2 and S3 vertebrae.

Plane of least pelvic dimension: **Anteroposteriorly** it is an imaginary plane passing through the lower margin of pubic symphysis to the tip of sacrum. **Transversely**, it is an imaginary plane passing through the ischial spines.

OBSTETRICAL PELVIC MEASUREMENTS

PELVIC DIAMETERS

Conjugate Diameters (Fig. 13.11)

1. *External conjugate:* It is the distance between the upper margin of pubic symphysis to the tip of the spine of S1 vertebra.
2. *True conjugate:* It is the distance between the midpoint of sacral promontory to the upper margin of the pubic symphysis. It corresponds to the anteroposterior diameter of the pelvic inlet.
3. *Diagonal conjugate:* It is the distance from midpoint of the sacral promontory to the lower margin of the pubic symphysis. It is the most useful measurement clinically. Normally it measures about 5 inches (12.5 cm). It can be measured roughly by per vaginal (P/V) examination, of course without discomfort to the patient.
4. *Obstetrical conjugate:* It is the shortest distance between the pelvic surface of the pubic symphysis and sacral promontory.

Diameters at the Pelvic Inlet (Fig. 13.12)

1. *Anteroposterior:* It extends from the midpoint of the sacral promontory to the midpoint of the upper margin of pubic symphysis.
2. *Oblique:* It extends from the sacroiliac joint of one side to the iliopectineal eminence of the other side.
3. *Transverse:* It is the maximum transverse diameter of the pelvic inlet (i.e., greatest width of the pelvic inlet).

Diameters at the Mid-pelvic Cavity

1. *Anteroposterior:* It extends from the middle of the pubic symphysis to the middle of 3rd sacral vertebra.
2. *Oblique:* It extends from the lower end of the sacroiliac joint of one side to the middle of the obturator membrane of the other side.
3. *Transverse:* It is the greatest width of the pelvic cavity.

Diameters at the Pelvic Outlet (Fig. 13.13)

1. *Anteroposterior:* It extends from the tip of the sacrum to the lower margin of the pubic symphysis.
2. *Oblique:* It extends from the middle of the sacrotuberous ligament of one side to the junction of ischiopubic ramus of the opposite side.
3. *Transverse:* It extends between the inner aspects of the two ischial tuberosities.

The figures of measurement at pelvic inlet, mid-pelvic cavity, and pelvic outlet of true pelvis can be easily remembered by the students in the form (in cm); they are given in Table 13.2.

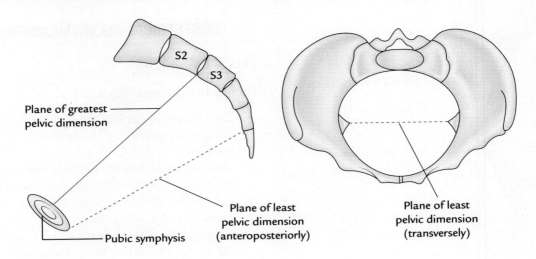

Fig. 13.10 Pelvic planes.

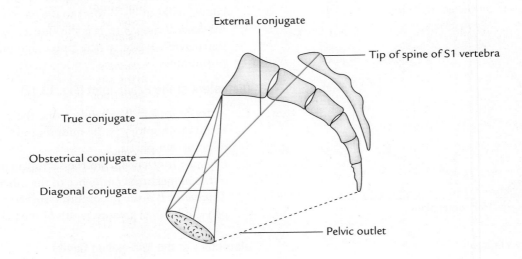

Fig. 13.11 Conjugate diameters.

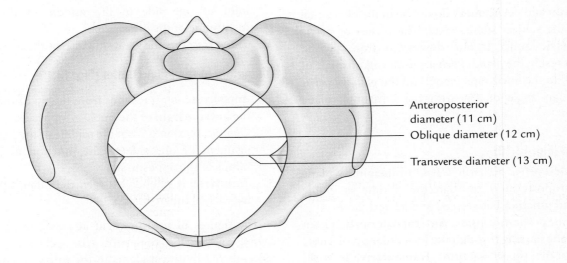

Fig. 13.12 Diameters at the pelvic inlet.

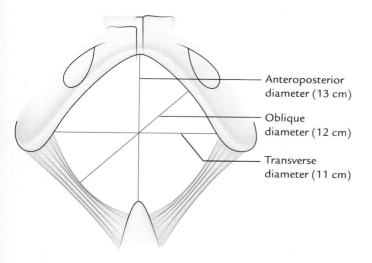

Fig. 13.13 Diameters at the pelvic outlet.

Table 13.2 Obstetrical pelvic measurements (in cm)

Diameter	At inlet	At mid-pelvis	At outlet
Anteroposterior	11	12	13
Oblique	12	12	12
Transverse	13	12	11

Also see the memory box given below.

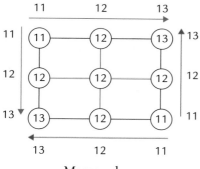

Memory box

N.B. During pelvic measurement the obstetricians ignore the coccyx due to its mobility and they take the tip (apex) of the sacrum as the posterior boundary of the pelvic outlet.

Clinical correlation

- **Adaptation of the fetal head in the pelvis during parturition:** During the process of parturition, the baby's head adapts itself to the dimensions of the pelvic cavity in order to pass through it smoothly. Therefore, during fixation of the head of fetus, the occiput of the head faces toward right/left, i.e., anteroposterior diameter of the head lies transversely at the inlet (13 cm in diameter). Then the head rotates about 90° so that the occiput of the head usually faces anteriorly, i.e., anteroposterior diameter of the head lies anteroposteriorly at the pelvic outlet (13 cm in diameter).

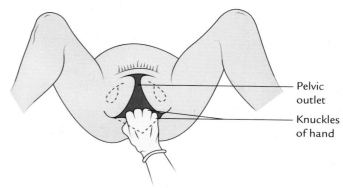

Fig. 13.14 Estimation of the pelvic outlet by knuckles of a clenched fist.

- **Assessment of adequacy of the pelvis during obstetrical examination:** It is done as follows:
- *Transverse diameter of the pelvic outlet* is assessed by measuring the distance between the ischial tuberosities along a plane passing across the anus.
- *Anteroposterior diameter of the pelvic* outlet is measured from the pubis to the sacroiliac joint.
- *Diagonal conjugate* (most important) is assessed by per vaginal examination.
- *Size of the subpubic arch.* In normal gynecoid pelvis, examiner's knuckles (with fist clenched) should be comfortably accommodated between the ischial tuberosities below the pubic symphysis (Fig. 13.14).

TYPES OF THE FEMALE PELVIS

The four types of the female pelvis have been described (after Caldwell and Moloy):

1. Gynecoid.
2. Android.
3. Platypelloid.
4. Anthropoid.

The features of all these types of pelvis are given in Table 13.3.

Morphologically also the pelvis is divided into the following four types:

1. *Mesatipellic (normal):* When transverse diameter of the pelvic inlet is slightly more than the anteroposterior diameter.
2. *Brachypellic (android type):* When anteroposterior diameter of the pelvic inlet is slightly more than the transverse diameter.
3. *Platypellic:* When transverse diameter of the pelvic inlet is much greater than the anteroposterior diameter.
4. *Dolichopellic:* When anteroposterior diameter of the pelvic inlet is much more than the transverse diameter.

Table 13.3 Types of the female pelvis (normal and its variants) and their features

Type	Features
Gynecoid—normal (42%)	• Inlet is transversely oval (transverse diameter is more than anteroposterior diameter) • Spacious roomy pelvic cavity • Suitable for easy passage of the baby during delivery
Android—male type (32%)	• Inlet is heart-shaped (anteroposterior diameter is more than transverse diameter) • Pelvic cavity is funnel-shaped • Outlet reduced in all diameters • May result in obstructed labor
Platypelloid—flat pelvis (2.5%)	• Inlet is anteroposteriorly compressed (transverse diameter is much greater than the anteroposterior diameter) • Poses difficulty in delivery
Anthropoid—ape type (23.5%)	• Inlet is compressed from side-to-side (anteroposterior diameter is much greater than the transverse diameter) • Poses difficulty in smooth delivery

Clinical correlation

Fractures of the pelvis: The pelvis is like a ring. It is very strong and usually requires a direct violence of high velocity to fracture it. The weak sites of the ring are sacroiliac region, pubic rami, and pubic symphysis. Lateral compression of pelvis usually results in fracture through both pubic rami or fracture of pubic ramus on one side associated with dislocation of pubic symphysis. Anteroposterior compression may cause dislocation of pubic symphysis or fracture through pubic rami accompanied by dislocation of the sacroiliac joints. The displacement of part of the pelvic ring indicates that the ring is broken at two places. The soft tissues likely to injure in pelvic fracture are urinary bladder, urethra, and rectum.

Golden Facts to Remember

➤ Strongest ligament of the pelvis	Interosseous sacroiliac ligament
➤ Most important conjugate diameter of the pelvis	Diagonal conjugate
➤ Least diameter of the pelvis	Distance between two ischial spines
➤ Plane of greatest pelvic diameter	Plane passing through the middle of pubic symphysis and junction between S2 and S3 vertebra
➤ Commonest type of the female pelvis	Gynecoid type (42%)
➤ Rare type of the female pelvis	Platypelloid type (2%)
➤ Shallowest wall of the pelvis	Anterior wall

Clinical Case Study

An elder woman was run over by a speeding car as she was crossing the road. She was taken to the emergency department by the police where X-ray examination of the pelvis revealed the disruption of sacroiliac joint and fracture of the body of pubis.

Questions

1. What is the typical fracture of the pelvis?
2. Which viscera are most vulnerable to injury during pelvic fracture?
3. What are stable and unstable fractures of the pelvis?
4. Enumerate the components of the pelvic ring.

Answers

1. The pelvis is like a rigid ring, therefore if it is compressed it tends to break at two places in a *typical fracture of pelvis*. There is fracture of the body of pubic bone on one side and disruption of the sacroiliac joint on the other side.
2. Urinary bladder and urethra.
3. If the pelvic ring breaks at any one point, the fracture will be stable and no displacement will occur. On the other hand, if the pelvic ring breaks at two sites, the fracture will be unstable and displacement will occur.
4. The pelvic ring is made up of (a) pubic rami, (b) ischium, (c) acetabulum, (d) ilium, and (e) sacrum.

CHAPTER 14

Pelvic Walls and Associated Soft Tissue Structures

The walls of pelvis are formed by the bones and ligaments which are partly clothed by the muscles covered with fascia and parietal peritoneum.

The pelvis presents five walls:

- Anterior wall (Fig. 14.1).
- Posterior wall (Fig. 14.2).
- Two lateral walls (right and left, Fig. 14.3).
- Inferior wall (or pelvic floor, Fig. 14.7).

Anterior Wall

The **anterior wall** is the shallowest wall and is formed by the pelvic surfaces of the bodies of the pubic bone, the pubic rami, and the pubic symphysis (Fig. 14.1).

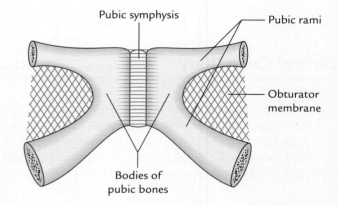

Fig. 14.1 Anterior wall of the pelvis (posterior view).

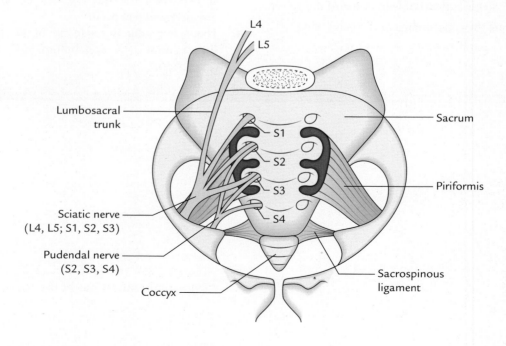

Fig. 14.2 Posterior wall of the pelvis.

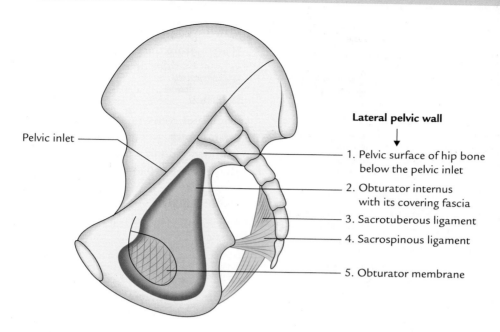

Lateral pelvic wall
↓

1. Pelvic surface of hip bone below the pelvic inlet
2. Obturator internus with its covering fascia
3. Sacrotuberous ligament
4. Sacrospinous ligament
5. Obturator membrane

Pelvic inlet

Fig. 14.3 Lateral wall of the pelvis.

Posterior Wall
The posterior wall is extensive and is formed by the pelvic surfaces of the sacrum and coccyx. It is lined by the piriformis muscles with their covering fascia (Fig. 14.2).

Lateral Wall
The lateral wall is formed by the pelvic surface of the hip bone below the pelvic inlet, the obturator membrane, the sacrotuberous and sacrospinous ligaments, and the obturator internus muscle with its covering fascia (Fig. 14.3).

Inferior Wall (or Pelvic Floor)
The inferior wall is formed by the pelvic diaphragm, which in turn is formed by the levator ani and coccygeus muscles with their covering fasciae. The pelvic diaphragm stretches across the true pelvis and divides it into the main pelvic cavity above and the perineum below. The floor of the pelvic cavity supports the pelvic viscera. The pelvic diaphragm is described on p. 215.

The soft tissue structures on the pelvic walls from deep to superficial, are arranged as follows (Fig. 14.4):

1. Muscles.
2. Nerves.
3. Pelvic fascia.
4. Blood vessels.
5. Peritoneum.

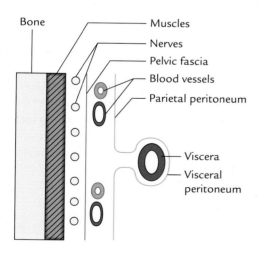

Bone
Muscles
Nerves
Pelvic fascia
Blood vessels
Parietal peritoneum

Viscera
Visceral peritoneum

Fig. 14.4 Arrangement of soft tissue structures on the pelvic walls.

MUSCLES OF THE PELVIS

The muscles of the pelvis are:

1. Obturator internus.
2. Piriformis.
3. Levator ani.
4. Coccygeus.

OBTURATOR INTERNUS (Fig. 14.5)

The obturator internus is a thick, fan-shaped muscle that covers most of the lateral wall of the pelvis.

Origin

It arises from:

(a) Obturator membrane.

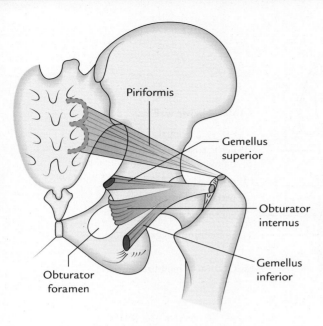

Fig. 14.5 Piriformis and obturator internus muscles.

(b) Margins of the obturator foramen (except at the obturator canal).
(c) Pelvic surface of the ileum between the obturator foramen and the greater sciatic notch.

Insertion

The fibres converge posteroinferiorly to form a strong tendon that hooks around the lesser sciatic notch almost at right angle and crosses the posterior aspect of the hip joint to be inserted into the medial surface of greater trochanter.

Nerve Supply

It is supplied by the **nerve to obturator internus** (L5; S1, S2), a special nerve from the sacral plexus.

Actions

1. It helps to stabilize the hip joint.
2. It is the lateral rotator of femur in erect posture and the abductor of femur when the hip joint is flexed.

N.B. The pelvic surface of the obturator internus is covered by a dense layer of fascia—the **obturator fascia**. Between the body of pubis and the ischial spine, the fascia forms a linear thickening called the **tendinous arch of obturator fascia**.

PIRIFORMIS (Fig. 14.5)

The piriformis is a triangular muscle one on either side on the front of the posterior wall of true pelvis.

Origin

It arises from the pelvic surface of the middle three pieces of sacrum by three digitations.

Insertion

The fibres converge inferolaterally, pass through the greater sciatic notch, to enter the gluteal region where they form a rounded tendon which is inserted into the tip (i.e., top) of the greater trochanter.

Nerve Supply

It is supplied by ventral rami of first and second sacral nerves (S1, S2).

Actions

1. It helps to stabilize the hip joint.
2. It is the lateral rotator of femur when the hip joint is extended and its abductor when the joint is flexed.

LEVATOR ANI (Fig. 14.6)

The two levator ani are the wide curved, thin sheets of muscles. They slope from the side wall of the pelvis toward the median plane where they fuse with each other to form the gutter-like floor of the true pelvis, and separates it from the ischiorectal fossae.

Origin

The levator ani muscle has a linear origin from the pelvic surface of the body of pubis, a tendinous arch of obturator fascia, and the pelvic surface of the ischial spine.

Insertion

The groups of fibres sweep backward, downward and medially to be inserted as follows (Fig. 14.7):

1. The *anterior fibres* form a sling around the prostate (**levator prostatae**) or vagina (**sphincter vaginae**) and are inserted into the perineal body (a mass of fibrous tissue) in front of the anal canal.
2. The *intermediate fibres* (**puborectalis**) form a sling around the anorectal junction to be inserted into the **anococcygeal raphe** (a fibrous raphe which extends from the anorectal junction to the tip of coccyx).
3. The *posterior fibres* (**iliococcygeus**) are inserted into the anococcygeal raphe and the coccyx.

Nerve Supply

(a) It is by the perineal branch of 4th sacral nerve (S4) from its pelvic surface.
(b) It is by the perineal branch of the pudendal nerve (S2, S3) from its perineal surface.

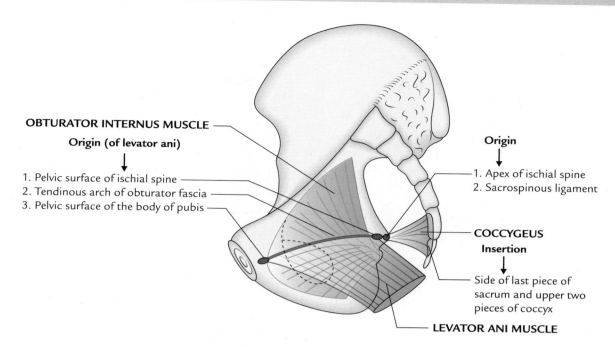

OBTURATOR INTERNUS MUSCLE

Origin (of levator ani)
↓

1. Pelvic surface of ischial spine
2. Tendinous arch of obturator fascia
3. Pelvic surface of the body of pubis

Origin
↓

1. Apex of ischial spine
2. Sacrospinous ligament

COCCYGEUS
Insertion
↓

Side of last piece of sacrum and upper two pieces of coccyx

LEVATOR ANI MUSCLE

Fig. 14.6 Origin of levator ani muscle. (The origin of obturator internus, and origin and insertion of coccygeus muscle are also shown).

Actions

1. The levator ani muscles of two sides together support the pelvic viscera and resist the intra-abdominal pressure during straining and expulsive efforts of the anterior abdominal wall muscles.
2. They also subserve a sphincteric action on the anorectal junction to maintain continence of faeces in both sexes and vagina in female.

COCCYGEUS (ISCHIOCOCCYGEUS)

The coccygeus is a small triangular muscle situated behind the levator ani muscle (Fig. 14.6).

Origin

It arises by its apex from the pelvic surface of ischial spine and sacrospinous ligament.

Insertion

From its base into the sides of upper two pieces of coccyx and the last piece of sacrum.

Nerve Supply

It is by the ventral rami of 4th and 5th sacral nerves (S4, S5).

Actions

1. The coccygeus muscles assist the levator ani muscles to support the pelvic viscera.
2. They can also produce minor movements of the coccyx.

PELVIC DIAPHRAGM (Fig. 14.7)

The pelvic diaphragm is a muscular partition between the true pelvis and the perineum. It forms the gutter-shaped pelvic floor. It is formed by the large levator ani and small coccygeus muscles of two sides and their covering fasciae. It is incomplete anteriorly to allow passage for the urethra in the males, and the urethra and vagina in the females.

Functions

The pelvic diaphragm provides principal support to the pelvic viscera and has a sphincteric action on the rectum and vagina. It also assists in increasing the intra abdominal pressure during defecation, micturition, and parturition. The attachments of the levator ani and coccygeus muscles are already described in this chapter.

Openings

The pelvic diaphragm presents the following openings:

1. **Hiatus urogenitalis:** It is a triangular gap between the anterior fibres of the two levator ani muscles. It transmits the urethra in male, and the urethra and vagina in female. The hiatus urogenitalis is closed from below by the **urogenital diaphragm.**

2. **Hiatus rectalis:** It is a round opening between the perineal body and the anococcygeal raphe. It provides passage to the anorectal junction.

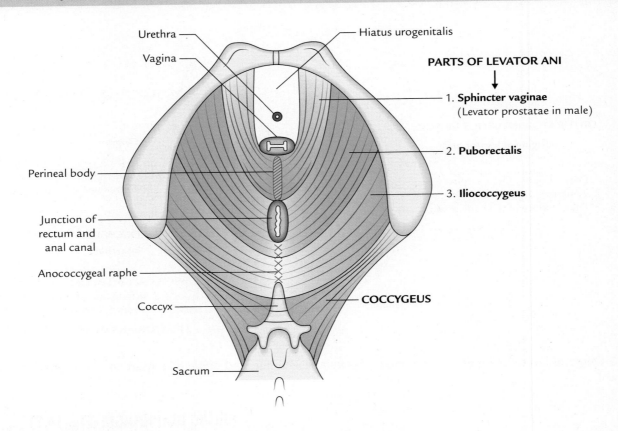

Fig. 14.7 Pelvic diaphragm.

N.B. *Evolution of the pelvic diaphragm:* In quadrupeds, the muscles of pelvic diaphragm are the muscles of tail. The anterior portion of levator ani is called *pubococcygeus* and posterior portion *iliococcygeus*. The pubococcygeus pulls the tail forward, and iliococcygeus and ischiococcygeus move the tail sideways. In human being, with the assumption of upright posture, the pubococcygeus and iliococcygeus together form the levator ani and ischiococcygeus persists as coccygeus muscle.

Clinical correlation

Injury of pelvic diaphragm: The pelvic diaphragm may be injured (tearing of perineal body) during difficult childbirth. As a result it becomes weak and can no longer provide sufficient support to the pelvic viscera. This may lead to uterine prolapse (Fig. 14.8) and rectal prolapse.

PELVIC FASCIA (Fig. 14.9)

The pelvic fascia is present in the form of two layers—parietal layer and visceral layer.

PARIETAL LAYER

It is the continuation of fascia transversalis of the anterior abdominal wall. In the pelvis, it is termed by different names on the basis of structures it lines. These are as follows:

1. **Obturator fascia:** It is a well-defined layer of fascia that covers the obturator internus muscle. It presents a linear

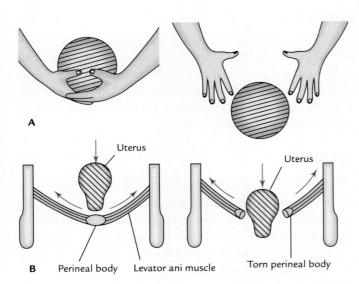

Fig. 14.8 Prolapse of the uterus following tearing of perineal body during difficult birth: **A**, simulative representation, **B**, actual representation.

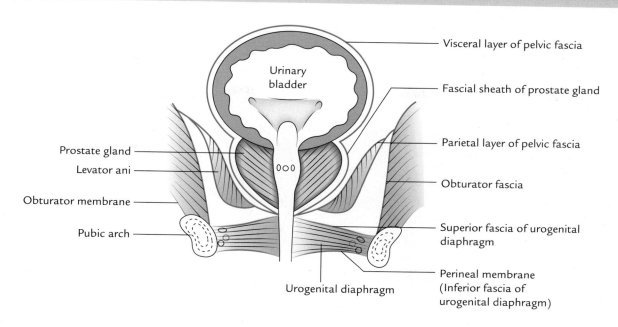

Fig. 14.9 Pelvic fascia as seen in coronal section of the male pelvis.

thickening called *tendinous arch* which provides origin to the levator ani muscle.

2. **Fascia covering piriformis:** It is a thin layer of fascia covering the piriformis. The sacral plexus lies between this fascia and piriformis muscle. The branches of the sacral plexus do not pierce this fascia while passing out of the pelvis.

3. **Superior fascia of pelvic diaphragm:** It covers the superior surface of the pelvic diaphragm.

VISCERAL LAYER

It is condensation of the loose areolar tissue around the extraperitoneal parts of the pelvic viscera and blood vessels. It is loose and thin, around distensible organs (e.g., urinary bladder) but thick around the non-\distensible organs (e.g., prostate gland). Its condensations around the neurovascular structures form the *ligaments of the pelvic organs* which play an important role in supporting the pelvic organs, such as urinary bladder and uterus.

PERITONEUM OF THE PELVIS

The layout of the peritoneum in pelvis can be understood best by tracing it within the pelvis in the sagittal section.

PERITONEUM OF THE MALE PELVIS (Fig. 14.10)

The peritoneum passes down from the anterior abdominal wall on to the superior surface of the urinary bladder. Then, it passes down on the posterior surface of the urinary bladder till it reaches the upper end of seminal vesicle which it covers. Here it turns backward to reach the anterior aspect of the rectum forming a shallow peritoneal pouch called **rectovesical pouch**.

The peritoneum then passes up on the front of the middle third of rectum and front and lateral aspects of the upper third of rectum. It then becomes continuous with the parietal layer of the peritoneum.

PERITONEUM OF THE FEMALE PELVIS (Fig. 14.11)

In the female pelvis, the peritoneum passes down from the anterior abdominal wall on to the superior surface of the urinary bladder; then passes down a little on its posterior surface to be reflected on the anterior surface of the uterus forming the uterovesical pouch. It covers the top of the uterus, passes on its posterior surface and posterior aspect of the posterior fornix of the vagina. Then it is reflected on the anterior aspect of the rectum to form deep *rectouterine pouch*. The relationship of the peritoneum to rectum is same as in male.

NERVES OF THE PELVIS

The nerves of the true pelvis are divided into two groups—somatic nerves and autonomic nerves.

SOMATIC NERVES

The following neural structures are to be studied under this heading:

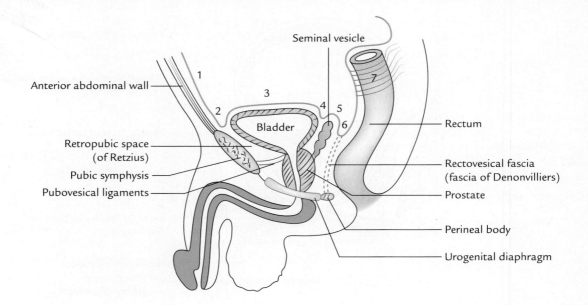

Fig. 14.10 Peritoneum of the male pelvis (sagittal section): 1 = anterior abdominal wall; 2 = back of the pubis; 3 = superior surface of the bladder; 4 = posterior surface of the bladder; 5 = upper ends of the seminal vesicles; 6 = rectovesical pouch; 7 = rectum.

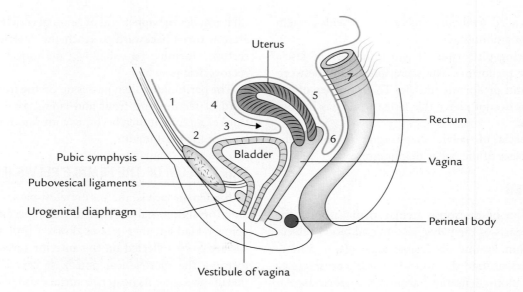

Fig. 14.11 Peritoneum of the female pelvis (sagittal section): 1 = anterior abdominal wall; 2 = back of the pubis; 3 = superior surface of the bladder; 4 = uterovesical pouch; 5 = posterior surface of the uterus and posterior fornix; 6 = rectouterine pouch (of Douglas); 7 = rectum.

1. Lumbosacral trunk.
2. Sacral plexus.
3. Coccygeal plexus.

Lumbosacral Trunk (Fig. 14.12)

It is a thick cord formed by the descending part of the ventral ramus of L4 nerve and entire ventral ramus of L5 nerve. It descends obliquely over the lateral part of the ala of sacrum and enters the pelvis posterior to the pelvic fascia.

Sacral Plexus (Fig. 14.13)

The sacral plexus is formed by the ventral primary rami of L4, L5; S1, S2, S3 nerves.

N.B. The L4 nerve is shared by both the lumbar and sacral plexuses. It bifurcates and its ascending branch takes part in the formation of lumbar plexus, and its descending branch joins the ventral ramus of L5 nerve to form the *lumbosacral trunk* which contributes to the sacral plexus.

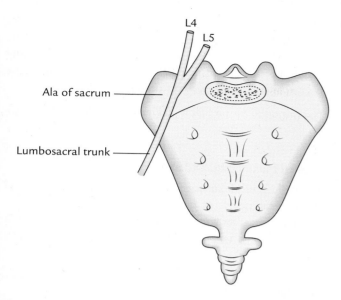

Fig. 14.12 Lumbosacral trunk.

Position and Relations

The sacral plexus lies in front of the piriformis deep to the pelvic fascia in the posterior wall of the true pelvis.

The ventral rami of sacral nerves emerge from ventral sacral foramina and unite in front of the piriformis where they are joined by the lumbosacral trunk.

The lumbosacral trunk and ventral ramus of S1 nerve are separated by the superior gluteal vessels.

The ventral rami of S1, S2 nerves are separated by the inferior gluteal vessels.

Branches

Nerves arising from the roots of plexus

1. Muscular branches: These are short twigs to piriformis (S1, S2) and long branches to levator ani and coccygeus (S3, S4).
2. Pelvic splanchnic nerves (*Nervi erigentes*): They are the slender branches arising from S2, S3, and S4. They

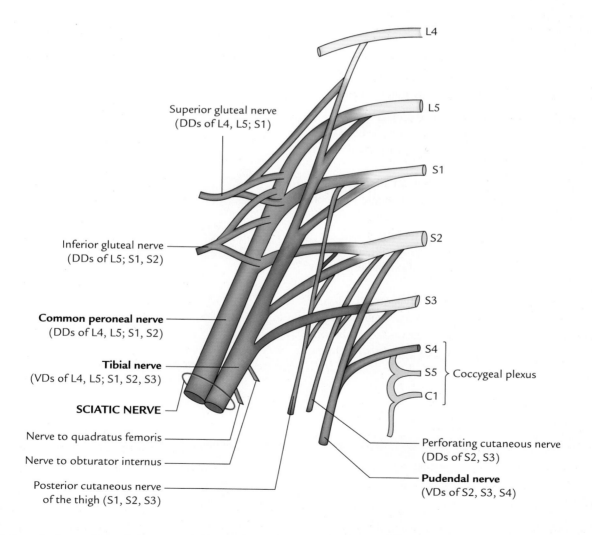

Fig. 14.13 Sacral plexus. Dorsal divisions (DDs) are shown by green colour and ventral divisions (VDs) are shown by blue colour.

provide sacral outflow of the parasympathetic system. They cause constriction of the sphincter vesicae and sphincter ani externus. They also cause dilatation of arteries of the erectile tissue of the penis and clitoris during their erection.

Terminal branches of plexus

1. *Sciatic nerve* (L4, L5; S1, S2, S3): It consists of two nerves (common peroneal and tibial) enclosed in a common sheath:
   (a) The common peroneal nerve is formed by the dorsal divisions of the L4, L5; S1, S2 nerves.
   (b) The tibial nerve is formed by the ventral divisions of the L4, L5; S1, S2, S3 nerves.
2. The sciatic nerve is described in detail on page 361.
3. *Pudendal nerve* (ventral division of S2, S3, S4): It is the lower and smaller terminal branch of the plexus. It is described in detail on page 235.

Branches arising from the pelvic surface of plexus

1. *Nerve to quadratus femoris* (ventral divisions of L4, L5; S1): It passes out of the pelvis through greater sciatic foramen anterior to the sciatic nerve.
2. *Nerve to obturator internus* (ventral divisions of L5; S1, S2): It passes out of the pelvis through greater sciatic foramen between the sciatic and pudendal nerves.

Nerves arising from the dorsal surface of plexus

1. *Superior gluteal nerve* (dorsal divisions of L4, L5; S1): It passes out of the pelvis along the superior gluteal artery above the piriformis.
2. *Inferior gluteal nerve* (dorsal divisions of L5; S1, S2): It passes out of the pelvis through greater sciatic foramen along with the inferior gluteal artery and posterior cutaneous nerve of the thigh below the piriformis.
3. *Posterior cutaneous nerve of the thigh* (S1, S2, and S3): It leaves the pelvis through greater sciatic foramen below the piriformis.
4. *Perforating cutaneous nerve* (dorsal divisions of S2, S3): It descends on the piriformis and coccygeus, passes between coccygeus and levator ani, pierces sacrotuberous ligament and gluteus maximus to supply the gluteal skin.

5. *Perineal branch of fourth sacral nerve:* It descends on the coccygeus, pierces it, and appears in the posterior angle of the ischiorectal fossa at the side of coccyx by passing deep to the sacrotuberous ligament. It supplies the external anal sphincter and skin around it.

The branches of the sacral plexus are summarized in Table 14.1.

Coccygeal Plexus (Fig. 14.13)

It is a small nerve plexus formed by the ventral rami of S4, S5 and coccygeal nerve. It lies on the pelvic surface of the coccygeus. It supplies coccygeus and part of the levator ani. It pierces the coccygeus and supplies the skin from the coccyx to the anus.

AUTONOMIC NERVES

The study of autonomic nerves in the pelvis includes the sympathetic trunks and the inferior hypogastric plexuses.

Sacral Sympathetic Trunks (Fig. 14.14)

The right and left sympathetic trunks descend in the pelvis between the bodies of sacral vertebrae and the pelvic sacral foramina.

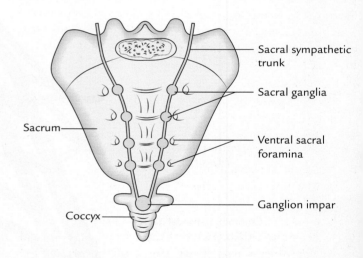

Fig. 14.14 Sacral sympathetic trunks.

Table 14.1 Branches of the sacral plexus

From root	Terminal	From pelvic surface	From dorsal surface
Muscular branches	Sciatic (L4, L5; S1, S2, S3)	Nerve to quadratus femoris (L4, L5; S1)	Superior gluteal nerve (L4, L5; S1)
Pelvic splanchnic nerves	Pudendal (S2, S3, S4)	Nerve to obturator internus (L5, S1; S2)	• Inferior gluteal nerve (L5; S1, S2) • Posterior cutaneous nerve of the thigh (S1, S2, S3) • Perforating cutaneous nerve (S2, S3) • Perineal branch of 4th sacral nerve (S4)

Inferiorly the two trunks converge and unite in the median *ganglion impar* in front of the coccyx.

Ganglia

There are four or five sacral ganglia in each trunk and the common **ganglion impar.**

Branches

1. The gray rami communicate to the ventral rami of all the sacral and coccygeal nerves.
2. The small branches to the median sacral artery.
3. The *sacral splanchnic nerves* to the inferior hypogastric plexus from the upper ganglia and to the rectum from the lower ganglia.
4. The small branches to the coccygeal body from the ganglion impar.

Inferior Hypogastric Plexuses

The two inferior hypogastric plexuses (right and left) are situated by the sides of rectum. Each plexus is composed of both sympathetic and parasympathetic fibres. The nerve cells in it are postganglionic parasympathetic neurons.

It receives postganglionic sympathetic fibres from the superior hypogastric plexus (presacral nerve) and preganglionic parasympathetic fibres from the pelvic splanchnic nerve (S2, S3, and S4). It also receives sensory fibres from the viscera.

Each plexus surrounds the corresponding internal iliac artery and divides into subsidiary plexuses along its visceral branches to supply the pelvic organs. The subsidiary/visceral plexuses are:

1. *Rectal plexus* surrounds the middle rectal artery and supplies the rectum.
2. *Vesical plexus* supplies the urinary bladder, adjoining parts of the ureters and seminal vesicles.
3. *Prostatic plexus* surrounds the prostate and supplies prostate, seminal vesicles and ejaculatory ducts. It also gives rise to *cavernous nerves* of the penis which supply the erectile tissue of bulb and crura of penis.
4. *Uterine and vaginal plexuses* accompany the uterine and vaginal arteries, respectively. The uterine plexus supplies the uterus, uterine tubes, and ovaries. The vaginal plexus supplies the vagina and sends *cavernous nerves* to the erectile tissue of the bulbs of the vestibule and clitoris.

VESSELS OF THE TRUE PELVIS

The vessels of the pelvis are:

1. **Arteries** (superior rectal, internal iliac, median sacral, and ovarian).
2. **Veins** (internal iliac, superior rectal, median sacral and ovarian veins, and pelvic venous plexuses).
3. **Lymph vessels** and associated lymph nodes.

ARTERIES

Superior Rectal Artery

It is the continuation of inferior mesenteric artery. It begins on the middle of left common iliac artery and descends in the medial limb of the sigmoid mesocolon to reach the rectum. It supplies the mucous membrane of rectum and the upper half of the anal canal (For details see page 283).

Internal Iliac Artery (Fig. 14.15)

It is the smaller of the two terminal branches of the common iliac artery. It passes down in the pelvis to the upper margin of the greater sciatic foramen, where it divides into *anterior* and *posterior divisions.*

Branches of the Anterior Division (Fig. 14.15)

1. *Superior vesical artery:* It is the persistent proximal part of the umbilical artery in fetus. It runs forward and medially to supply the upper part of the urinary bladder. It is crossed by the ductus deferens and often gives branch to it. Distally it is continuous with the medial umbilical ligament which represents distal obliterated part of the umbilical artery.
2. *Obturator artery:* It passes forward along the lateral wall of the pelvis along the obturator nerve and leaves the pelvis through the obturator canal. It gives an important pubic branch which anastomoses with the corresponding branch of the inferior epigastric artery on the pelvic surface of the body of pubis. This anastomosis may replace the obturator artery (**accessory obturator artery**).
3. *Inferior vesical artery (vaginal artery in the female):* It runs forward to the base of the urinary bladder. It supplies the base of the bladder, prostate, and seminal vesicles in males. It also gives rise to the artery of the vas deferens.
4. *Middle rectal artery:* It is a small branch which passes medially to the rectum. Commonly it arises with the inferior vesical artery.
5. *Internal pudendal artery:* It is the principal artery of the perineum. It leaves the pelvis through the greater sciatic foramen and passes over the posterior surface of the ischial spine to enter the perineum through the lesser sciatic foramen.
6. *Inferior gluteal artery:* It is the **largest branch** of the anterior division of the internal iliac artery. It passes posteroinferiorly between the ventral rami of S1 and S2 nerves to enter the gluteal region through the greater sciatic foramen.
7. *Uterine artery:* It runs medially on the floor of pelvis along the root of broad ligament, **crosses the ureter superiorly** to reach the lateral fornix of the vagina. Here

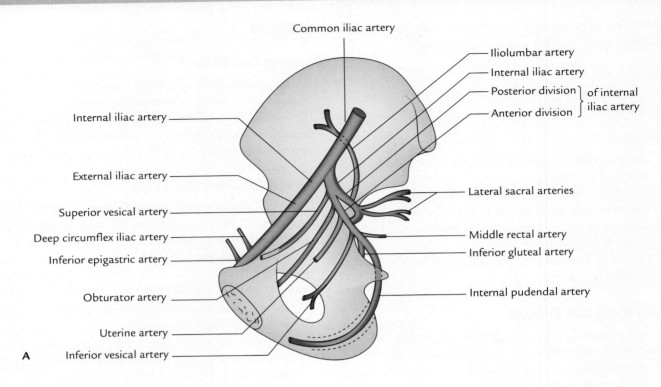

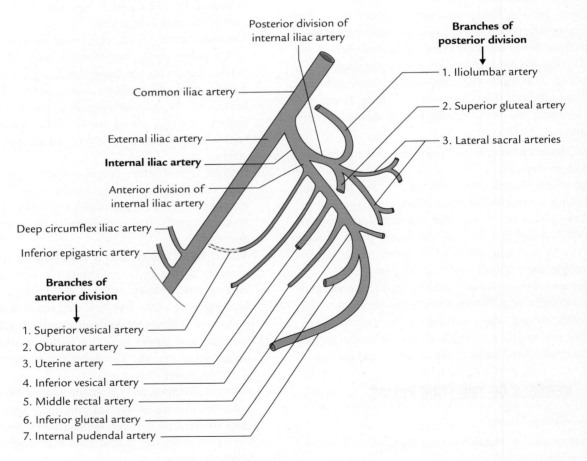

Fig. 14.15 Internal iliac artery: **A**, course and branches in relation to the hip bone; **B**, divisions and branches.

it first ascends upward along the lateral margin of the uterus, then runs along the uterine tube to terminate by anastomosing with the ovarian artery. The uterine artery gives off a vaginal branch.

8. *Vaginal artery:* It corresponds to the inferior vesical artery of the male. It supplies the vagina and the base of the bladder.

N.B. All the branches from anterior division of internal iliac artery are visceral branches *except* inferior gluteal and obturator arteries which are parietal branches.

Branches of the Posterior Division (Fig. 14.15)

1. *Iliolumbar artery:* It ascends upward across the sacroiliac joint behind the external iliac vessels to reach behind the psoas major where it divides into lumbar and iliac branches.
2. *Lateral sacral arteries:* There are usually two (upper and lower) lateral sacral arteries on each side. They run downward and medially over the sacral nerves. Their branches enter the sacral canal through anterior sacral foramina to supply its contents. Their terminations emerge on the dorsal aspect of the sacrum through the dorsal sacral foramina to supply the muscles and skin on the dorsum of sacrum.
3. *Superior gluteal artery:* It first passes backward between the lumbosacral trunk and ventral ramus of S1, then leaves the pelvis through the greater sciatic foramen along with the superior gluteal vessels.

N.B. All the branches of posterior division of internal iliac artery are parietal branches.

The branches of the internal iliac artery are summarized in Table 14.2.

Table 14.2 Branches of the internal iliac artery

Division	Branches
Anterior division	• Superior vesical artery • Obturator artery • Inferior vesical artery (in male) • Middle rectal artery • Internal pudendal artery • Inferior gluteal artery (largest) • Uterine artery (in female) • Vaginal artery (in female)
Posterior division	• Iliolumbar artery • Lateral sacral arteries • Superior gluteal artery

Median Sacral Artery

It arises from the back of aorta just above its bifurcation and descends downward into the pelvis to end in front of the coccyx. It represents the continuation of primitive dorsal aorta.

Ovarian Artery

It arises from the abdominal aorta at the level of L1 vertebra and passes downward and laterally behind the peritoneum. It crosses the external iliac artery at the pelvic brim and enters the pelvis through suspensory ligament of ovary to supply the ovary and lateral one-third of the uterine tube.

N.B. All the arteries of the true pelvis are branches of the internal iliac artery except ovarian and median sacral arteries which arises directly from the abdominal aorta.

VEINS

The *internal iliac vein* runs upward lateral to the internal iliac artery and joins the external iliac vein to form the common iliac vein. Its tributaries correspond to the branches of the internal iliac artery except **umbilical** and **lumbar veins** which drain, respectively, into the portal and common iliac veins.

Note that the superior gluteal vein is the largest tributary of the internal iliac vein except during pregnancy when the uterine veins exceed its size greatly.

The *median sacral veins* accompany the median sacral artery and terminate in the left common iliac vein.

The *superior rectal vein* accompanies the superior rectal artery to become the *inferior mesenteric vein* after crossing the common iliac artery.

The *ovarian vein* forms just below the pelvic inlet by the condensation of the pampiniform plexus around the ovarian artery. On the right side it drains into the inferior vena cava and on the left side into the left renal vein.

LYMPH VESSELS AND LYMPH NODES OF TRUE PELVIS

The **internal iliac lymph nodes** lie along the internal iliac artery. They receive the lymph vessels draining the lymph from all the pelvic contents. They also receive the lymph vessels from deeper structures of the perineum, gluteal region, and back of the thigh. The efferents from those nodes drain into the common iliac nodes.

The **sacral lymph nodes** lie along the median and lateral sacral arteries. They receive the lymph vessels from the posterior wall of the pelvis, rectum, neck of the urinary bladder, prostate, and cervix of the uterus. The efferents from these nodes drain into the common iliac nodes.

In addition to these groups, small nodes are also found in the broad ligament and in the fascial sheaths around the urinary bladder and rectum.

Golden Facts to Remember

➤ Most important function of the pelvic diaphragm	Support of pelvic viscera
➤ Largest and most important muscle of the pelvic floor	Levator ani
➤ Lowest part of the peritoneal cavity in erect posture in male	Rectovesical pouch
➤ Largest branch of the sacral plexus	Sciatic nerve
➤ Largest branch of the anterior division of the internal iliac artery	Inferior gluteal artery
➤ Largest tributary of the internal iliac vein in non-pregnant woman	Superior gluteal vein

Clinical Case Study

A 40-year-old multiparous female attended obstetrics and gynecology OPD and complained that for past one month she feels that something enters in her vagina from above when she strains during defecation. She also complained that she feels pain after coitus. On history taking she told that she has given birth to a baby few months back. On per vaginal examination the obstetrician noticed the **prolapse of the uterus**.

Questions

1. Which structure forms the principal support of the pelvic viscera?
2. Name the muscles which form the pelvic diaphragm.
3. Give the possible cause of uterine prolapse in this case.
4. What are the effects of weak pelvic floor?

Answers

1. Pelvic diaphragm.
2. Levator ani and coccygeus muscles.
3. Injury to the pelvic diaphragm during childbirth.
4. Uterine prolapse, prolapse of vagina, cystocele (herniation of bladder in the vagina), prolapse of rectum, and urinary stress incontinence.

CHAPTER 15
Perineum

The perineum is the lowest region of the trunk below the pelvic diaphragm. It includes all structures that fill the pelvic outlet (Fig. 15.1).

The perineum is traversed by urethra and anal canal in the male, and urethra, vagina, and anal canal in the female. The surface features of the perineum in male are penis, scrotum, and anal orifice, whereas the surface features of the perineum in the female are vulva (female external genitalia) and anal orifice (Fig. 15.1). The median region between vaginal and anal orifices in female, containing perineal body is considered as **gynecological perineum**.

BOUNDARIES

The perineum has superficial and deep boundaries.

Superficial Boundaries
In lithotomy position, the perineum is diamond shaped and is bounded as follows (Fig. 15.2):
Anteriorly: by scrotum in male and mons pubis in female.
Posteriorly: by buttocks.
On each side: by the upper medial aspect of the thigh.

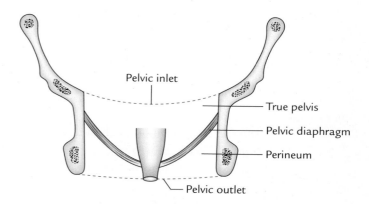

Fig. 15.1 Location of the perineum.

Deep Boundaries
The deep boundaries of the perineum correspond to the boundaries of the pelvic outlet as follows (Fig. 15.3):
Anteriorly: Inferior margin of the pubic symphysis (actually arcuate pubic ligament).
Posteriorly: Tip of the coccyx.

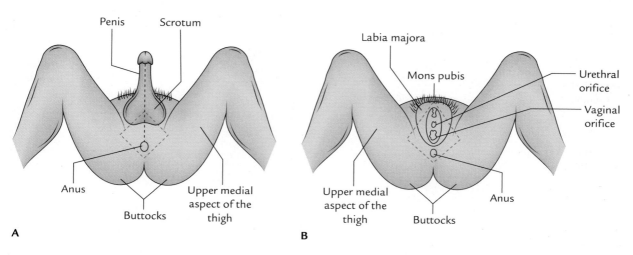

Fig. 15.2 Perineum as seen in lithotomy position (The red broken lines mark the boundaries of pelvic outlet): **A**, male perineum; **B**, female perineum. Interrupted red lines indicate the position of pelvic outlet.

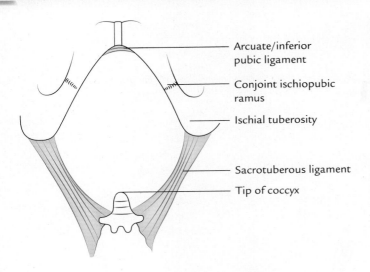

Fig. 15.3 Deep boundaries of the perineum.

On each side:
- *Anterolaterally:* Conjoint ischiopubic ramus.
- *Laterally:* Ischial tuberosity.
- *Posterolaterally:* Sacrotuberous ligament.

DIVISIONS

The perineum is divided into two triangles: (a) anterior urogenital triangle (anterior perineum) and (b) posterior anal triangle (posterior perineum) by a horizontal plane passing through the anterior end of the ischial tuberosities. The urogenital triangle is traversed by the urethra in male and urethra and vagina in female. The anal triangle is traversed by anal canal in both male and female (Fig. 15.4).

UROGENITAL TRIANGLE (ANTERIOR PERINEUM)

It is a triangular area between the ischiopubic rami, in front of a horizontal line joining the anterior ends of two ischial tuberosities. It contains superficial and deep perineal pouches. On the surface, urogenital triangle presents penis and scrotum in male and external genitalia and orifices of urethra and vagina in female.

Cutaneous Innervations (Fig. 15.5)

The cutaneous innervation of the urogenital region is derived from the following nerves:

1. *Dorsal nerve of the penis:* It is a branch of the pudendal nerve and supplies the skin of the penis/clitoris except its root.
2. *Ilioinguinal nerve and genital branch of the genitofemoral nerve:* These nerves supply the skin of the anterior one-third of the scrotum/labium majus and the root of the penis/clitoris.
3. *Perineal branch of the posterior cutaneous nerve of the thigh:* It supplies the skin of the lateral part of the posterior two-third of the scrotum/labium majus.
4. *Posterior scrotal/labial nerves:* These nerves supply the skin of the median part of the urogenital region.

Superficial and Deep Perineal Pouches

A triangular tough fascial sheet called the **perineal membrane** stretches across this triangle and is attached to its sides. The posterior margin of the perineal membrane is fused centrally to the perineal body. The anterior margin of the perineal membrane thickens to form a *transverse perineal ligament.* A small gap between this ligament and the *arcuate pubic ligament* provides passage to the deep dorsal vein of the penis (Fig. 15.6).

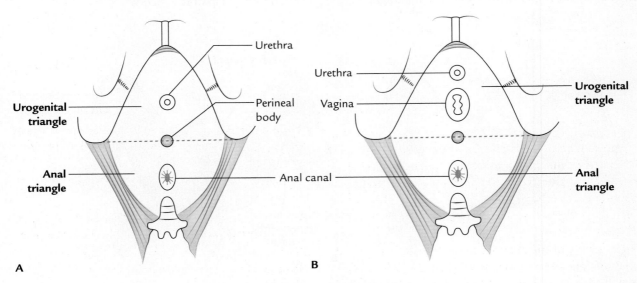

Fig. 15.4 Subdivision of the perineum: **A**, male perineum; **B**, female perineum.

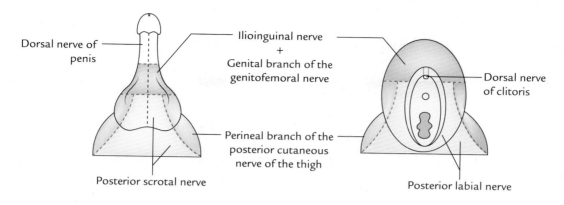

Fig. 15.5 Cutaneous innervation of the urogenital region.

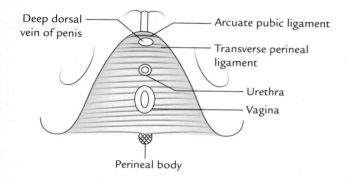

Fig. 15.6 Perineal membrane.

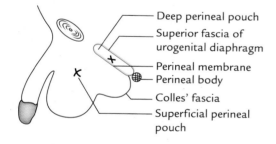

Fig. 15.7 Coronal section of the urogenital region of male perineum showing superficial and deep perineal pouches.

The perineal membrane is pierced by the urethra in male and by the urethra and vagina in female. Above the perineal membrane the urethra is surrounded by a voluntary, sphincter urethrae muscle (**superficial urethral sphincter**). In the female, the superficial urethral sphincter is also pierced by the vagina.

The deep aspect of the external sphincter is covered by a thin fascia which is continuous with the posterior edge of the perineal membrane and is attached at the sides to the ischiopubic rami. Thus, sphincter urethrae is in fact

contained within a fascial capsule which is termed **deep perineal pouch** (Fig. 15.7). This pouch also contains the deep transverse perineal muscles and in male two bulbourethral glands (glands of Cooper) whose ducts pass forward piercing the perineal membrane to open into the bulbous urethra.

The membranous layer of the superficial fascia of abdomen (Scarpa's fascia) surrounds the penis as far as its neck, to form a tube-like **fascia of penis**, the scrotum, and finally in the perineum it fuses with the posterior edge of the perineal membrane.

The perineal part of this fascia is called **Colles' fascia**. Thus, **superficial perineal pouch** is formed between the perineal membrane and Colles' fascia (Fig. 15.7.) It contains the root of penis and some muscles, viz., bulbospongiosus covering the bulb of penis, the ischiocavernosus muscle on each side covering the crus of penis, and the superficial transverse perineal muscle on each side running transversely from the perineal body to the ischial ramus.

The detailed contents of the deep and superficial perineal pouches are given in Tables 15.1 and 15.2, respectively and shown in Figure 15.8.

Table 15.1 Structures within the deep perineal pouch

Male (Fig. 15.8A)	Female (Fig. 15.8B)
Membranous urethra	Urethra and vagina
Deep transversus perinei muscles and sphincter urethrae muscle	Deep transversus perinei muscles and sphincter urethrae muscle
Bulbourethral glands (of Cooper)	No glands
Branches of the internal pudendal artery (arteries to penis)	Branches of the internal pudendal artery (arteries to clitoris)
Branches of the pudendal nerve (dorsal nerve of penis)	Branches of the pudendal nerve (dorsal nerve of clitoris)

Table 15.2 Structures within the superficial perineal pouch

Male (Fig. 15.7)	Female (Fig. 15.6)
Root of penis	Root of clitoris
• Bulb of penis covered by the bulbospongiosus muscles • Crura of penis covered by the ischiocavernosus muscles	• Bulbs of vestibule covered by the bulbospongiosus muscles • Crura of clitoris covered by the ischiocavernosus muscles
Superficial transverse perineal muscles	Superficial transverse perineal muscles
Ducts of bulbourethral glands	Greater vestibular glands (Bartholin glands)
Urethra (within the bulb of penis)	Urethra
Branches of the internal pudendal artery • Perineal artery • Dorsal artery of penis • Deep artery of penis	Branches of the internal pudendal artery • Perineal artery • Dorsal artery of clitoris • Deep artery of clitoris
Branches of the pudendal nerve • Perineal nerve • Dorsal nerve of penis	Branches of the pudendal nerve • Perineal nerve • Dorsal nerve of clitoris

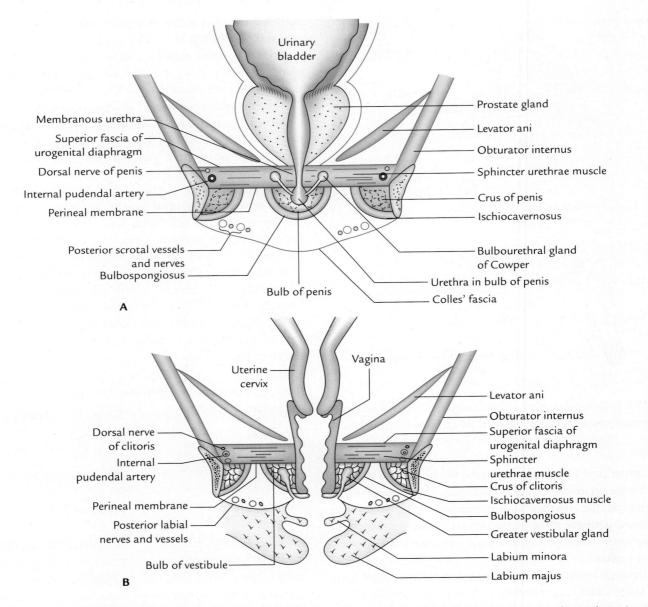

Fig. 15.8 Coronal section of the urogenital region showing contents of the superficial and deep perineal pouches: A, male; B, female.

Relevant Features of the Contents of Deep Perineal Pouch

Membranous urethra

It is 1.5–2 cm long and runs downward and forward through the deep perineal pouch. It pierces the perineal membrane about 2.5 cm behind the pubic symphysis. It is the narrowest and least dilatable part of the urethra.

Sphincter urethrae muscle

It surrounds the membranous part of the urethra in male, and the urethra and vagina in female. Its superficial fibres arise from the transverse perineal ligament and pass backward on either side of the urethra to be inserted into the perineal body. Its deep fibres arise from the inner sides of the ischiopubic rami, pass horizontally to encircle the urethra. The sphincter urethrae muscle forms the voluntary **external urethral sphincter**.

Deep transverse perinei muscle

It is situated posterior to the sphincter urethrae muscle on each side. It arises from the ramus of ischium and inserted into the perineal body.

Bulbourethral glands

They lie one on each side of the membranous urethra. They are about 1 cm in diameter. Their ducts (2.5 cm long) pierce the perineal membrane to open into the bulb of urethra. They contribute a small amount to the seminal fluid.

Branches of the internal pudendal vessels and pudendal nerves

The branches of the internal pudendal vessels and pudendal nerves are described on pp. 235 and 236.

Relevant Features of the Contents of Superficial Perineal Pouch

Root of the penis (Fig. 15.9)

It is described in Chapter 5, p. 60.

Root of the clitoris (Fig. 15.10)

It is made up of three masses of erectile tissue called the **bulb of vestibule** and **right and left crura** of the clitoris. The bulb of vestibule corresponds to the bulb of penis but it is divided into two halves by the vagina (bulbs of vestibule). The bulbs lie one on either side of the vagina and urethra superficial to the perineal membrane. Their tapering anterior ends unite in front of the urethra by a plexus of veins called **bulbar commissure** and continue as a strip of erectile tissue into the glans of the clitoris. Each bulb of vestibule is attached to the inferior surface of the perineal membrane and is covered by the bulbospongiosus muscle.

The crura of the clitoris correspond to the crura of the penis. Each crus is covered by the ischiocavernosus muscle.

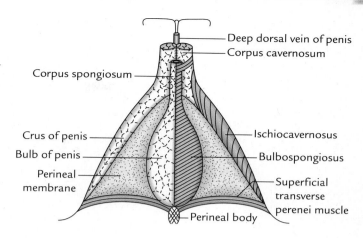

Fig. 15.9 Root of the penis and superficial perineal muscles. The superficial perineal muscles are removed in the left half of the diagram to show crus and bulb of the penis.

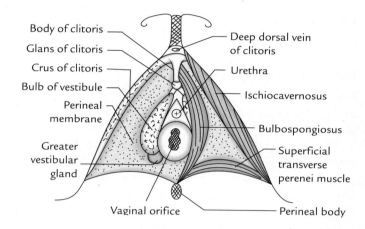

Fig. 15.10 Root of clitoris and superficial perineal muscles. The superficial perineal muscles have been removed in the left half of the diagram to show bulb of the vestibule and greater vestibular gland.

Greater vestibular glands (Bartholin glands; Fig. 15.11)

These are homologous to the bulbourethral glands in male. They are pea shaped and less than 1 cm in diameter. Each gland opens by a single duct 2 cm long into the posterolateral part of the vaginal orifice in the groove between the labium minus and the hymen. The secretions of these glands play a minor role in the lubrication of the lower vagina.

Superficial transverse perineal muscles

They are narrow transverse slips of muscle, one on each side of the perineal body. Each muscle arises from the ischial ramus and runs medially to be inserted into the perineal body.

Branches of the internal pudendal artery and pudendal nerve

The **branches of the internal pudendal artery and pudendal nerve** are described on pp. 235 and 236.

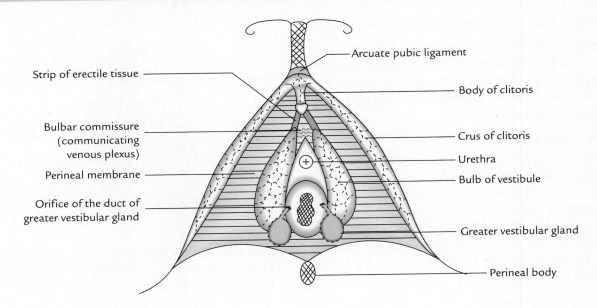

Fig. 15.11 Greater vestibular glands.

Urogenital Diaphragm (Fig. 15.12)

Having described the structures in *the urogenital triangle,* one can easily understand the formation of the urogenital diaphragm.

The urogenital diaphragm is a triangular muscle sheet formed by the sphincter urethrae and deep transversus perinei muscles. On the deeper aspect it is covered by a thin layer of endopelvic fascia called *superior fascia of the urogenital diaphragm,* and on the superficial aspect it is covered by the perineal membrane called *inferior fascia of the urogenital diaphragm* (Fig. 15.12).

This triangular diaphragm occupies the urogenital triangle with its apex behind the pubic symphysis and its sides attached to the ischiopubic rami.

It is pierced by the urethra in male and by the urethra and vagina in female, and contains bulbourethral glands within it in male.

Perineal Membrane (Fig. 15.13)

It is a very strong triangular membrane (fascial sheet) that stretches across the urogenital triangle between the ischiopubic rami at the sides. It intervenes between the superficial perineal pouch below and the deep perineal pouch above.

1. In front, it is thickened to form the **transverse perineal ligament** and is continuous with the superior fascia of the urogenital diaphragm.

2. Behind, it is fixed to the perineal body in the midline and splits into two layers. The upper layer is continuous

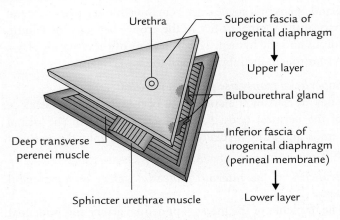

Fig. 15.12 Urogenital diaphragm (in male).

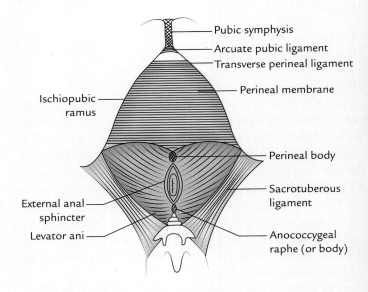

Fig. 15.13 Perineal membrane as seen from below.

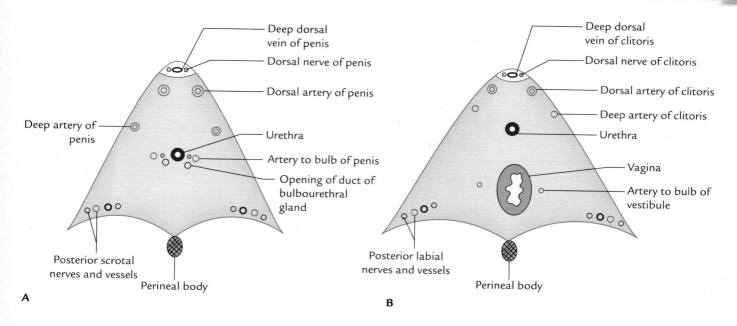

Fig. 15.14 Structures piercing the perineal membrane: **A**, in male; **B**, in female.

with the superior fascia of the urogenital diaphragm; and the lower layer is continuous with Colles' fascia.

Structures Piercing the Perineal Membrane (Fig. 15.14)

1. **Posterior scrotal or labial, nerves and vessels** on each side at the base.
2. **Deep artery of penis or clitoris** near the middle of its attached margin.
3. **Dorsal artery of penis or clitoris** near the anterior part of its attached margin.
4. Urethra in the midline.
5. Ducts of the bulbourethral glands.
6. Artery to the bulb of penis or bulb of vestibule of vagina on each side of the urethra.
7. Vagina (in female) behind the urethra.

Table 15.3 Structures piercing the perineal membrane in male and female

Male (Fig. 15.14A)	Female (Fig. 15.14B)
Urethra	Urethra and vagina
Ducts of the bulbourethral glands	
Artery and nerve to the bulb of penis	Artery and nerve to the bulb of vestibule
Dorsal artery of the penis	Dorsal artery of the clitoris
Deep arteries of the penis	Deep arteries of the clitoris
Posterior scrotal nerves and vessels	Posterior labial nerves and vessels
Branches of the perineal nerve to superficial perinei muscles	Branches of the perineal nerve to superficial perinei muscles

The structures piercing the perineal membrane in male and female are summarized in Table 15.3.

Perineal Body (Fig. 15.15)

The perineal body is a wedge-shaped mass of fibromuscular tissue situated in midline at the junction of urogenital triangle (anterior perineum) and anal triangle (posterior perineum) between the lower ends of vagina and anal canal.

It lies about 1/2 inch (1.25 cm) in front of the anal margin close to the bulb of penis in male and the posterior wall of the vestibule of vagina in female.

The 10 muscles of the perineum converge and interlace in the perineal body. These are as follows:

1. Two superficial transverse perineal muscles.
2. Two deep transverse perineal muscles.
3. Two bulbospongiosus muscles.
4. Two levator ani muscles.
5. One sphincter ani externus.
6. One longitudinal muscle coat of anal canal.

Clinical correlation

- **Damage of perineal body:** The perineal body is extremely important in female in maintaining the integrity of the pelvic diaphragm and providing support to the pelvic organs. It may be damaged during difficult childbirth or cut inadvertently during episiotomy. This may result in prolapse of the uterus, bladder, and rectum.
- **Episiotomy (Fig. 15.16):** It is an incision given in the perineum to enlarge the vaginal orifice to facilitate childbirth.

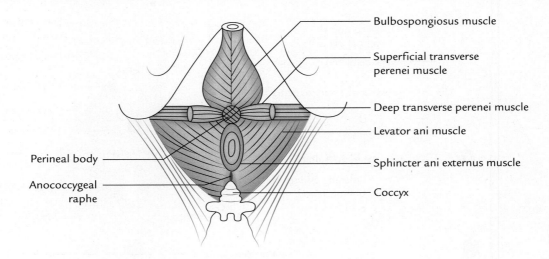

Fig. 15.15 Perineal body. Note various muscles attached to it.

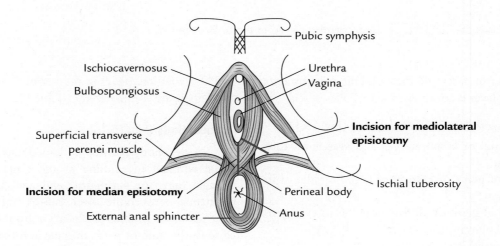

Fig. 15.16 Episiotomy.

(a) *Median episiotomy:* This incision begins at the frenulum of labia minora and proceeds backward in the midline up to the external anal sphincter. It cuts through the skin, vaginal wall, perineal body, and superficial transverse perinei muscle. Inadvertently, it may cut the external anal sphincter.

(b) *Mediolateral episiotomy:* This incision begins at the labia minora and proceeds laterally at an angle of 45°. It cuts through the skin, vaginal wall, and bulbospongiosus muscle.

ANAL TRIANGLE (POSTERIOR PERINEUM)

It is a triangular area bounded in front by a horizontal line joining the anterior ends of ischial tuberosities, laterally by the ischial tuberosities, inferolaterally by the sacrotuberous ligaments, and posteriorly by the coccyx. It contains the anal canal in the middle and ischiorectal fossae one on each side of the anal canal.

Cutaneous Innervation

The cutaneous innervation of the anal region is provided by the following nerves:

- *Inferior rectal nerve (S2, S3, S4):* It supplies the skin around the anus and over the ischiorectal fossae.
- *Perineal branch of S4 nerve:* It supplies the skin posterior to the anus.

Anal Canal

The anal canal is the last 4 cm of the gastrointestinal tract. It lies in the centre of the anal triangle below the pelvic diaphragm and between right and left ischiorectal fossae, which allow its expansion during the passage of faeces.

The anal canal is described in detail in Chapter 19.

Ischiorectal Fossa (Ischioanal Fossa)

The ischiorectal fossa is a wedge-shaped, fat-filled space situated on each side of the anal canal below the pelvic diaphragm (Fig. 15.17). The two fossae communicate with each other behind the anal canal. They help in dilatation of the anal canal, during defecation (i.e., passage of flatus and faeces).

The base of the fossa lies on the skin over the anal region of the perineum and the apex is directed upward and

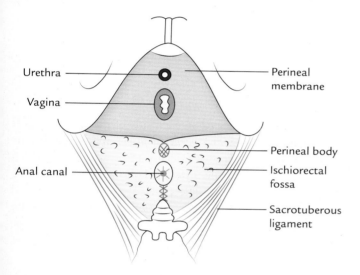

Fig. 15.17 Surface view of the ischiorectal fossa and perineal membrane.

laterally. Each fossa measures about 5 cm in length, 5 cm in width, and 5 cm or slightly more in depth.

Boundaries

These are as follows (Fig. 15.18):

Lateral: Fascia covering the obturator internus muscle and ischial tuberosity.
Medial: Fascia covering the levator ani muscle and external anal sphincter.
Posterior: Sacrotuberous ligament, on the posterior surface of which is gluteus maximus.
Anterior: Posterior border of the perineal membrane.
Floor: Perineal skin.
Roof: Meeting point of the fascia covering obturator internus and inferior fascia of the pelvic diaphragm.

N.B. *Recesses of ischiorectal fossa:* The ischiorectal fossa extends anteriorly above the urogenital diaphragm forming the *anterior recess*, posteriorly deep to sacrotuberous ligament forming the *posterior recess*, and behind the anal canal to be continuous with its opposite fossa forming the *horseshoe-shaped posterior recess*.

Contents (Fig. 15.19)

1. *Ischiorectal pad of fat.*
2. *Inferior rectal nerves and vessels* (running from lateral to medial side).
3. *Perineal branch of fourth sacral nerve* enters the posterior angle of the fossa running over levator ani to reach sphincter ani externus which it innervates.

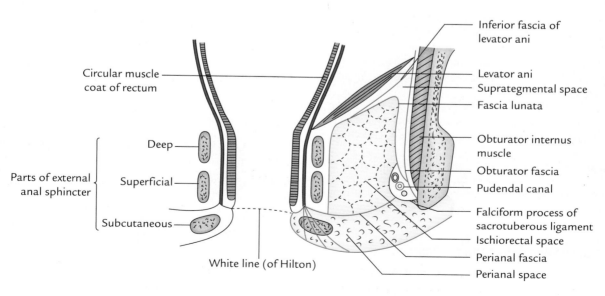

Fig. 15.18 Boundaries of the ischiorectal fossa as seen in coronal section through the anal triangle.

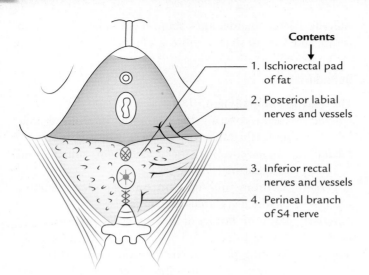

Contents

1. Ischiorectal pad of fat
2. Posterior labial nerves and vessels
3. Inferior rectal nerves and vessels
4. Perineal branch of S4 nerve

Fig. 15.19 Contents of the ischiorectal fossa.

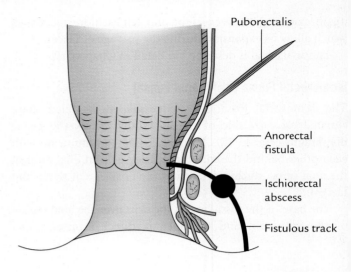

Fig. 15.20 Ischiorectal abscess and anorectal fistula.

4. *Posterior scrotal (or labial) nerves and vessels* cross the anterolateral part of the fossa to enter the urogenital triangle.

Clinical correlation

- **Ischiorectal abscess (Fig. 15.20):** The ischiorectal fossa is prone for infection due to its location. The infection may occur from boils and abrasions of the perianal skin, from lesions within the anal canal, from pelvic infection or rarely via blood. It often forms abscess—the *ischiorectal abscess*.

  The fat in the fossa is loosely arranged; therefore swelling can occur without tension with little pain.

  The infection may readily pass from one fossa to the other through horseshoe-shaped recess behind the anal canal forming *horseshoe-shaped abscess*.

  Since ischiorectal fossa does not contain any important structure, it can be incised fearlessly to drain the abscess.

  In a neglected case, the abscess may burst into the anal canal or on the surface of perineum to form the ischiorectal type of *anorectal fistula* or *fistula in ano*, respectively.
- The fat in ischiorectal fossae provides a cushion-like support to the rectum and anal canal. The loss of this fat in debilitating diseases in children, viz. diarrhea, can cause *rectal prolapse*.
- Occasionally a gap exists between the tendinous origin of the levator ani and obturator fascia. This gap is called **hiatus of Schwalbe**, and through it pelvic organs may herniate into the ischiorectal fossa.

Spaces in the Region of Ischiorectal Fossa

The arrangement of fasciae in this region forms a number of spaces. Only those which have clinical significance are discussed here.

Perianal Space

It is a subcutaneous space on each side of the anal orifice. It is bounded above by the *perianal fascia* and below by the perianal skin. The perianal fascia is a fibrous septum which extends from the white line of Hilton medially to the pudendal canal laterally. The perianal space is subdivided into numerous compartments by fibroelastic septa. The fat in the perianal space is tightly arranged in small loculi. The infection in this space causing **perianal abscess** is therefore very painful.

Pudendal Canal (Alcock's Canal)

It is a fascial canal present in the lateral wall of the ischiorectal fossa about 1 inch (2.5 cm) above the ischial tuberosity (Fig. 15.21). It extends from the lesser sciatic foramen to the posterior limit of the deep perineal pouch (Fig. 15.21). The pudendal canal is formed either by the splitting of the

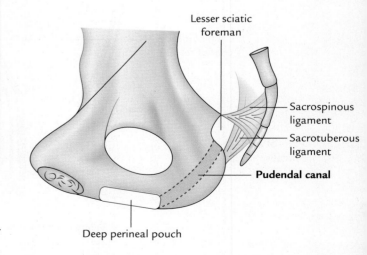

Lesser sciatic foreman

Puborectalis

Anorectal fistula

Ischiorectal abscess

Fistulous track

Sacrospinous ligament

Sacrotuberous ligament

Pudendal canal

Deep perineal pouch

Fig. 15.21 Pudendal canal.

obturator fascia or by separation between the fascia lunata and the obturator fascia.

Contents

1. Pudendal nerve which divides within the canal into the dorsal nerve of penis and the perineal nerve.
2. Internal pudendal vessels.

Pudendal Nerve

The pudendal nerve provides principal innervation to the perineum hence, it is designated as the chief nerve of the perineum.

Origin, course, and distribution (Fig. 15.22)

It arises from ventral rami of S2, S3, S4 nerves in the pelvis. It leaves the pelvis through the greater sciatic foramen below the piriformis muscle, medial to internal pudendal vessels. It crosses the dorsum of ischial spine and immediately disappears through the lesser sciatic foramen to enter the pudendal canal (Alcock's canal) present in the lateral wall of ischiorectal fossa.

In the posterior part of the canal, it gives off the inferior rectal nerve, which crosses the fossa to innervate the external anal sphincter, perianal skin and then divides into the terminal branches, a large perineal nerve and a small dorsal nerve of the penis (or clitoris).

The *perineal nerve* bifurcates almost at once, its deeper branch supplies the sphincter urethrae and other muscles of the urogenital triangle, superficial and deep transverse perineal nerves, ischiocavernosus and bulbospongiosus; its superficial branch/branches innervate the posterior two-third of the scrotum (or labium majus) as the posterior scrotal (or labial nerves).

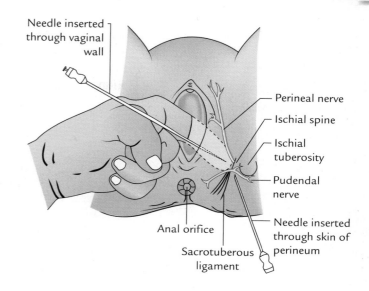

Fig. 15.23 Pudendal nerve block.

The *dorsal nerve of penis (or clitoris)* traverses the deep perineal pouch then passes through a gap between the arcuate pubic and transverse perineal ligaments to reach the dorsum of penis, where it innervates the skin of the body and glands of the penis.

Clinical correlation

Pudendal nerve block (Fig. 15.23): The pudendal nerve is infiltrated with a local anaesthetic where it crosses the ischial spine. The ischial spine is palpated through the vagina. A long needle is inserted through the vaginal wall and guided by a finger to the ischial spine. The needle can also be inserted through the skin of perineum.

When the pudendal block is carried out bilaterally, there is a loss of anal reflex (which is a useful test to know that a successful block is achieved), relaxation of the pelvic floor muscles, and loss of sensation to the vulva and lower one-third of the vagina (for details, see *Clinical and Surgical Anatomy*, 2nd Edition by Vishram Singh).

Internal Pudendal Artery (Fig. 15.24)

It is one of the two terminal branches of the anterior division of the internal iliac artery.

It leaves the pelvis through greater sciatic foramen below the piriformis. It crosses the dorsal surface of the ischial spine (lateral to the pudendal nerve) and enters the perineum through the lesser sciatic foramen, where it passes through the pudendal canal in the lateral wall of the ischiorectal fossa.

Branches

1. **Inferior rectal artery** arises in the pudendal canal, accompanies the inferior rectal nerve and traverses across the ischiorectal fossa to supply the structures in the perianal region.

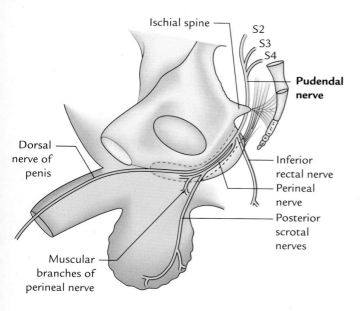

Fig. 15.22 Course and branches of the pudendal nerve.

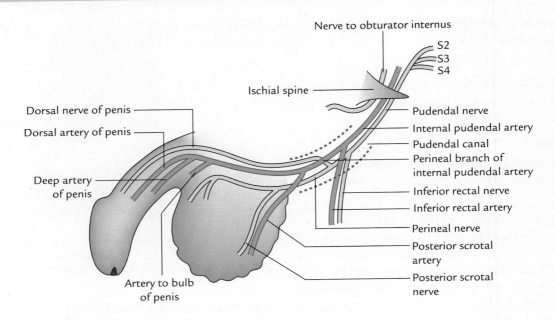

Fig. 15.24 Course and distribution of the pudendal nerve and internal pudendal artery.

2. **Perineal branch** arises in the anterior part of the canal, pierces the perineal membrane to enter the superficial perineal pouch, where it divides into a transverse perineal artery and two posterior scrotal or labial arteries.

3. **Artery to the bulb and urethra** arises in the deep perineal pouch, pierces the perineal membrane and supplies the erectile tissue of the bulb of penis in male or bulbs of vestibule of the vagina in female. It also supplies the urethra in both sexes.

4. **Deep artery of penis or clitoris** pierces the perineal membrane and supplies the erectile tissue, corpora cavernosa.

5. **Dorsal artery of penis or clitoris** pierces the perineal membrane, passes upward between the crura of penis or clitoris and runs on the dorsal surface of the penis or clitoris beneath the fascia of penis (Buck's fascia) lateral to the deep dorsal vein, and medial to the dorsal nerve of penis. It supplies prepuce and glans of penis.

Golden Facts to Remember

- Key structure in the urogenital triangle — Perineal membrane
- Key structure in the perineum ⎫
- Central tendon of the perineum ⎭ — Perineal body
- Chief nerve of the perineum — Pudendal nerve
- Exercises commonly advised to strengthen the perineal muscles — Kegel exercises
- Structures homologous to the bulbourethral gland in females — Greater vestibular glands

Clinical Case Study

A 40-year-old woman visited obstetrics and gynecology OPD and complained of a swelling in the genital region. On examination the doctor found a tense cystic swelling beneath the posterior two-third of her right labium majus and minus. A diagnosis of "**Bartholin's cyst**" was made.

Questions

1. What are Bartholin glands and where are they located?
2. Name the sites of openings of the ducts of these glands.
3. What is Bartholin's cyst? Give its cause.
4. What is the other name of Bartholin glands and what is their function?

Answers

1. There are two (right and left) Bartholin glands. They are located in the superficial perineal pouch, one on either side of the vaginal orifice.
2. Posterolateral part of the vaginal orifice in the groove between the hymen and the labium minus.
3. The Bartholin's cyst is a retention cyst, produced by the retention of its secretion caused by blockage of its duct.
4. Greater vestibular glands. Their secretion helps a bit to lubricate the lower part of the vagina.

Urinary Bladder and Urethra

URINARY BLADDER

The urinary bladder is a muscular reservoir of urine, lying in the anterior part of the pelvis. It is commonly involved in clinical conditions such as retention of urine, cystitis (inflammation of the urinary bladder), calculus, disorder of micturition, and cancer. Hence, its anatomy is of immense importance to clinicians.

LOCATION

The urinary bladder is situated in the anterior part of the lesser pelvis immediately behind the pubic symphysis and in front of rectum in male and uterus in the female (Fig. 16.1). The location of the urinary bladder varies with the amount of urine it contains and with age.

When the bladder is empty it lies entirely within the lesser pelvis but when it becomes distended with urine, it expands upward and forward into the abdominal cavity.

In children, the bladder is an abdominopelvic organ even when it is empty because the pelvic cavity is small and the neck of bladder lies at the level of the upper border of pubic symphysis. It begins to enter the enlarging pelvis at the age of six years but does not become a pelvic organ entirely until after puberty.

Size and Shape

The size and shape of the urinary bladder vary according to the amount of urine that it contains. It is tetrahedral in shape when empty and ovoid in shape when distended.

Capacity

Normally in adult male the capacity varies from 120 to 320 ml. The mean capacity is about 220 ml.

1. An amount of urine beyond 220 ml causes a desire to micturate but the bladder is usually emptied at about 250–300 ml.

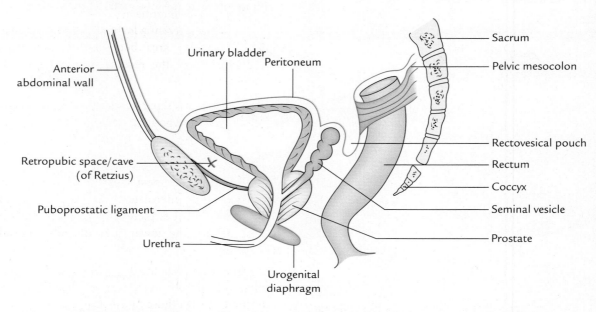

Fig. 16.1 Location of the urinary bladder in male. Also note the reflection of peritoneum in male pelvis.

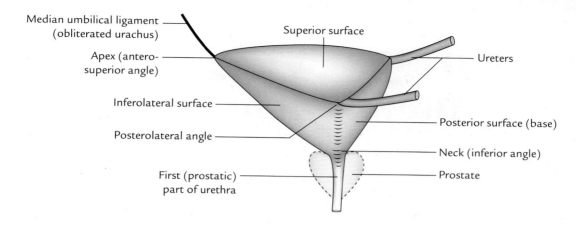

Fig. 16.2 External features of empty bladder (left lateral view).

2. The filling of urine up to 500 ml may be tolerated but beyond this, it causes pain due to tension of its wall. On collection of urine about 800 ml, the micturition is beyond one's voluntary control.

EXTERNAL FEATURES AND RELATIONS
(Figs 16.2 and 16.3)

An empty and contracted bladder as seen in a cadaver is tetrahedral in shape and presents the following external features:

1. Apex.
2. Base.
3. Neck.
4. Three surfaces (superior and two inferolateral surfaces).
5. Four borders (anterior, posterior and two lateral).

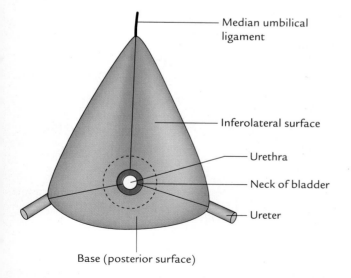

Fig. 16.3 External features of empty urinary bladder (inferior view).

APEX

It provides attachment to the **median umbilical ligament** and lies posterior to the upper margin of the pubic symphysis.

The *median umbilical ligament* is the fibrous remnant of the intra-abdominal part of the allantois (urachus).

BASE (POSTERIOR SURFACE/FUNDUS)

- The urinary bladder is triangular in shape and directed posteroinferiorly toward the rectum.
- Its superolateral angles are joined by the ureters while its inferior angle gives rise to the urethra.

In the *male*, its relations are (Fig. 16.4):

1. **Upper part** is separated from rectum by the rectovesical pouch containing coils of the small intestine.
2. **Lower part** is separated from rectum by the terminal parts of vasa deferentia and seminal vesicles.
   - The vasa deferentia lie medial to the seminal vesicles.
3. The triangular area between the vasa deferentia is separated from the rectum by **rectovesical fascia (of Denonvilliers)**.

In the *female*, it is separated from the cervix of uterus and by the vesicouterine pouch.

NECK

It is the lowest and most fixed part of the bladder. It is situated where the inferolateral and the posterior surfaces of the bladder meet. It is pierced by the urethra. It lies about 3–4 cm behind the lower part of pubic symphysis. Its relations are:

- *In the male*, it rests on the upper surface of the prostate where the smooth muscle fibres of the bladder wall are continuous with those of the prostate.
- *In the female*, it is related to the urogenital diaphragm.

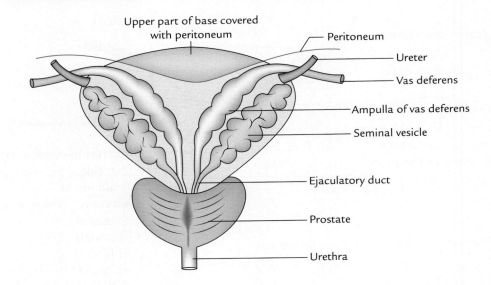

Fig. 16.4 Relation of the base of urinary bladder in the male.

SUPERIOR SURFACE

It is triangular in shape and bounded on each side by the *lateral borders* which extend from ureteric orifices posterolaterally to the apex anteriorly and posteriorly by the *posterior border* which joins the ureteric orifices.

In the male, it is completely covered by the peritoneum which separates it from:

- coils of the ileum, and/or
- sigmoid colon.

Along its lateral borders, the peritoneum is reflected on to the pelvic walls.

In the female, it is covered by the peritoneum except for a small area near the posterior border, which is related to the supravaginal part of the uterine cervix. Here the peritoneum is reflected on to the uterine isthmus forming **vesicouterine pouch.**

INFEROLATERAL SURFACES

Each inferolateral surface slopes downward, forward, and medially to meet its fellow of the opposite anteriorly in the midline.

These surfaces are separated from each other, anteriorly by the *anterior border,* and from the superior surface by the *lateral borders.*

The inferolateral surfaces are devoid of peritoneum and in both male and female are related:

- *In front to* (Fig. 16.5)
  - retropubic space,
  - pubic symphysis, and
  - puboprostatic ligaments.

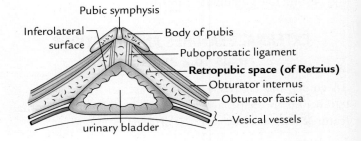

Fig. 16.5 Relations of the inferolateral surfaces of the urinary bladder.

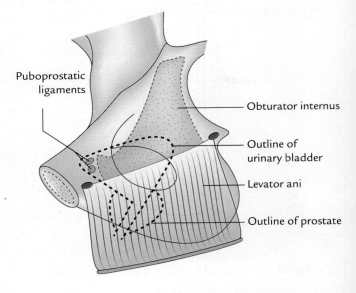

Fig. 16.6 Medial view of lower part of lateral pelvic wall and levator ani muscle. The bladder is superimposed by dotted lines to show relations of its inferolateral surface.

- *Behind to* (Fig. 16.6)
  – obturator internus muscle above, and
  – levator ani muscle below.

N.B. *Retropubic space (cave of Retzius):* It is a perivesical space bounded anteriorly by the posterior aspect of pubic symphysis, and adjoining posterior wall of rectus sheath; posteriorly by inferolateral surfaces of the urinary bladder, superiorly by reflection of peritoneum from the superior surface of urinary bladder to the posterior aspect of the anterior abdominal wall up to the umbilicus, and inferiorly by puboprostatic/pubovesical ligaments (Fig. 16.1).

The relations of the urinary bladder are summarized in Table 16.1.

Clinical correlation

Suprapubic aspiration of the urinary bladder: When the urinary bladder is distended it peels off the peritoneum from the anterior abdominal wall and comes in its direct contact. Now it can be aspirated suprapubically without any damage to the peritoneum. In suprapubic cystostomy, the same condition can be obtained by artificial distension of the urinary bladder.

SUPPORTS OF THE URINARY BLADDER (FIXATION OF THE URINARY BLADDER)

The urinary bladder is anchored firmly at its neck, where it is fixed by its continuity with the prostate and urethra. The fixation of the bladder is also helped by the different ligaments of the urinary bladder.

Table 16.1 Relations of the urinary bladder

Parts	Relations
Base	• Rectovesical pouch in the male • Vesico uterine pouch in the female • Vasa deferentia and seminal vesicles (separated from the rectum by fascia of Denonvilliers)
Superior surface	• Peritoneal cavity containing loops of ileum • Coils of ileum • Sigmoid colon • Uterine cervix (in female)
Anterior surface (inferolateral surfaces)	• Retropubic space • Puboprostatic ligaments • Obturator internus and levator ani muscles
Apex	Median umbilical ligament
Neck	• Prostate gland (in male) • Urogenital diaphragm (in female)

LIGAMENTS (Fig. 16.7)

The ligaments of the bladder are of two types—true and false.

True Ligaments

These are formed by the condensation of pelvic fascia around the neck and the base of the bladder and have a supportive function for the bladder.

1. *Lateral ligaments* (two in number, right and left): They extend from the side (inferolateral surface) of the bladder to the tendinous arch of pelvic fascia.
2. *Puboprostatic ligaments* (four in number, two on each side—lateral and medial): They fix the neck of bladder.
   (a) **Lateral puboprostatic ligament** extends downward and medially from the anterior end of the tendinous arch of pelvic fascia to blend with the upper part of the prostatic sheath.
   (b) **Medial puboprostatic ligament** extends downward and backward from the back of the pubic bone near the pubic symphysis to the prostatic sheath and forms the floor of retropubic space (of Retzius).
   Fascial bands similar to puboprostatic ligaments in the female are termed pubovesical ligaments. They end around the neck of the urinary bladder.
3. *Median umbilical ligament* is the fibrous remnant of the urachus. It extends from the apex of the bladder to the umbilicus. It maintains the bladder in position anteriorly and superiorly.
4. *Posterior ligament* (two in number, right and left): They extend as a sheet of loose areolar tissue from the side of the base of the bladder to the lateral pelvic wall. They enclose the vesical venous plexus.

False Ligaments

These are peritoneal folds and do not have supportive function as performed by true ligaments. They are seven in number.

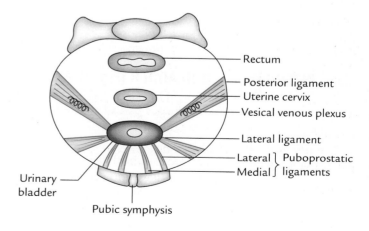

Fig. 16.7 True ligaments of the urinary bladder in the female.

- *Anteriorly* there are three folds:
  Median umbilical fold, the fold of peritoneum over the median umbilical ligament.
  Two medial umbilical folds, the folds of peritoneum over the obliterated umbilical arteries.
- *Laterally* a pair of false lateral ligaments is formed by the reflection of the peritoneum from the bladder to the side wall of the pelvis and forms the floor of paravesical fossae.
- *Posteriorly* a pair of false posterior ligaments is formed. These are the sacrogenital folds which are the folds of peritoneum extending from the side of the bladder, posteriorly, on either side of the rectum, to the anterior aspect of the third sacral vertebra.

MICROSCOPIC STRUCTURE

The bladder wall from within outward is composed of:

- A mucous membrane.
- A muscular coat.
- Adventitia.

Mucous membrane: It is pale pink in colour and covered with a transitional epithelium. It is thrown into folds (rugae) when the bladder is empty. The mucosal area covering the internal surface of the base of the bladder is termed "**trigone.**"

Muscular coat: It constitutes the **detrusor** muscle which consists of three layers of smooth muscle fibres.

- An outer longitudinal layer.
- A middle circular layer.
- An inner longitudinal layer.

There is profuse intermingling of the muscle fibres of these layers and they cannot be separated into three clearly defined layers.

Since the muscle fibres of the bladder wall are mainly concerned with the evacuation of the bladder they are collectively called the "detrusor muscle."

Adventitia: It is made up of fibroelastic tissue.

INTERIOR OF THE BLADDER (Fig. 16.8)

1. In an empty bladder, the greater part of mucosa shows irregular folds (rugae) because it is loosely attached to the subjacent muscular layer.
2. Over a small triangular area, immediately above and behind the internal orifice of the urethra (**trigone of the bladder**), the mucous membrane is firmly bound to the muscular coat and therefore is smooth. The limits of trigone are defined superiorly by the openings of the ureters and inferiorly by the urethra.

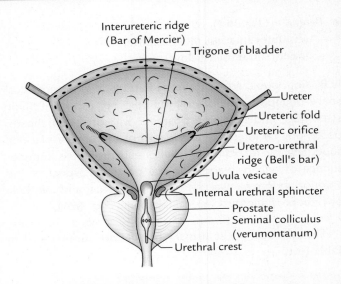

Fig. 16.8 Interior of the urinary bladder as seen in the coronal section.

The trigone of urinary bladder presents the following features:

1. *Anteroinferior angle*, formed by the internal orifice of the urethra.
2. *Two posterosuperior angles*, formed by openings of the ureters.
3. *Uvula vesicae*, a slight elevation in the mucous membrane immediately above and behind the internal urethral orifice. It is produced by the median lobe of prostate.
4. *Interureteric ridge/crest* (**bar of Mercier**) forms the superior boundary of trigone and connects the two ureteric orifices. It is produced by the continuation into the bladder wall of the inner longitudinal coats of the ureters.

    The lateral ends of this ridge extend beyond the openings of the ureter as **ureteric folds** (produced by the ureters as they run obliquely through the bladder wall).

N.B. The **interureteric ridge (bar of Mercier)** serves as a guide to locate the orifices of the ureter during cystoscopy.

5. *Two uretero-urethral ridges (Bell's bars)* extend from the ureteric orifice to the urethral orifice. They are produced by longitudinal fibres of the ureter which extends behind the ureteric orifice down on each side of trigone toward the middle lobe of the prostate.

ARTERIAL SUPPLY

It is by the following arteries:

1. The principal arteries supplying blood to the bladder are superior and inferior vesical arteries which are the branches of anterior division of internal iliac arteries.
2. The other arteries which make small contribution in supplying the lower part of the bladder are:
   (a) Obturator and inferior gluteal arteries.
   (b) Uterine and vaginal arteries in the female.

VENOUS DRAINAGE

The veins of the bladder do not follow the arteries. They form a complicated plexus on the inferolateral surfaces near the prostate called **vesical venous plexus**.

1. This plexus passes backward in the posterior ligaments of the urinary bladder to drain into the internal iliac veins.
2. It communicates:
   (a) In the male with the prostatic venous plexus.
   (b) In the female with the veins at the base of broad ligament.

LYMPHATIC DRAINAGE

The lymphatics of the bladder drain chiefly into the **external iliac lymph nodes**. Some lymph vessels also drain into the *internal iliac lymph nodes* including nodes in the obturator fossa.

NERVE SUPPLY (Fig. 16.9)

Motor Innervation

It is provided by the parasympathetic, sympathetic, and somatic fibres.

1. *Parasympathetic fibres (nervi erigentes)* are derived from S2, S3, S4 (spinal micturition centre) segments of the spinal cord. They are motor to the detrusor muscle and inhibitory to the sphincter vesicae (internal urethral sphincter).
2. *Sympathetic fibres* are derived from T11, T12 thoracic and L1, L2 lumbar segments of the spinal cord.
   They are inhibitory to the detrusor and motor to the sphincter vesicae.
3. *Somatic fibres (pudendal nerve)* are derived from S2, S3, S4 spinal segments. They are motor to the external urethral sphincter.

N.B. The *sympathetic innervation* is responsible for the filling of the bladder and *parasympathetic innervation* for the emptying of the bladder. The *somatic innervation* is responsible for voluntary control of micturition.

Sensory Innervation

The majority of sensory fibres run along the parasympathetic fibres (pelvic splanchnic nerves/nervi erigentes; S2, S3, S4). Some fibres also run with the sympathetic fibres. The

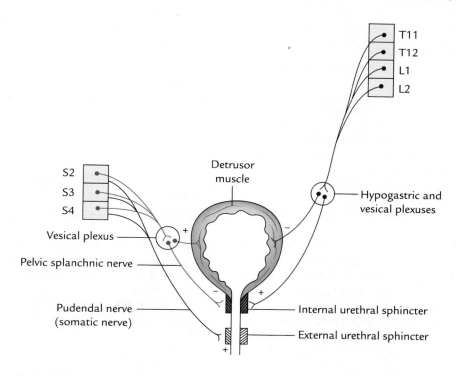

Fig. 16.9 Innervation of the urinary bladder (sympathetic innervation: blue lines; parasympathetic innervation: red lines; somatic innervation: black lines).

division of sympathetic fibres (presacral neurectomy does not alleviate bladder pain because pain fibres are carried by both sympathetic and parasympathetic fibres.

N.B. Two kinds of fibres are recognized:

1. Fibres concerned with pain.
2. Fibres concerned with conscious awareness of filling of the bladder.
   • The pain fibres run in the anterolateral white columns of the spinal cord.
   • The fibres concerned with the awareness of filling of the bladder lie in the posterior columns of the spinal cord.

Clinically, this accounts for the fact that awareness of the bladder being filled and desire to micturate remain normal after bilateral anterolateral cordotomy for the relief of pain.

Clinical correlation

- **Trabeculated bladder:** It results due to chronic obstruction to the outflow of the urine by enlarged prostate or stricture of the urethra. The bladder becomes distended and its musculature hypertrophies. Its muscular fasciculi increase in size and interface in all the directions giving rise to an open weave appearance of the bladder wall, known as the "**trabeculated bladder.**"
- **Suprapubic cystostomy:** It is an extraperitoneal approach to open the cavity of the urinary bladder. It is done for: Drainage purposes, treatment of intravesical conditions, viz., vesical stones, etc., and removal of the prostate.

  The bladder is distended (if not the case of retention of urine) with about 300 ml of fluid. As a result, the anterior aspect of bladder comes in direct contact with the anterior abdominal wall. The bladder can be now approached through anterior abdominal wall without entering into the peritoneal cavity.
- **Neurogenic bladder:** Micturition is essentially a reflex action involving the sensory and motor (sympathetic and parasympathetic) pathways being mediated by the lower micturition centre (S2, S3, S4). The voluntary control over this reflex is exerted by the higher centre (cerebral cortex) through upper motor neurons of pyramidal tract.

  Any defect in this neural mechanism of micturition leads to *neurogenic bladder.*

  The neurogenic bladder lacks the normal neural control of micturition.

  The types of neurogenic bladder are:

  (a) Automatic reflex bladder: It results from complete transection of the cord above the lower micturition centre (S2, S3, S4) involving pyramidal tracts (upper motor neurons) clinically it presents as:
  - The voluntary inhibition and initiation of micturition are lost.
  - The bladder empties reflexly every 1 to 4 hours. When the filling reaches a certain level, the detrusor muscle contracts reflexly as in early infancy. This is called *automatic* or *reflex bladder*.

  (b) Autonomous bladder: It Results from the destruction of S2, S3, S4 segments of the spinal cord (lower centre of micturition). Clinically it presents as:
  - The reflex and nervous control of micturition is lost. The bladder wall becomes flaccid and capacity of bladder is greatly increased. The result is continuous dribbling and this type of bladder is called an autonomous bladder.
  - The bladder may be emptied by the manual compression or by the abdominal muscular contraction.

  N.B.
  - Interruption of sensory side of reflex (e.g., tabes dorsalis) leads to **atonic neurogenic bladder** with residual urine.

    A large amount of urine collects without any reflex contraction.
  - In lesions above S2 and below T4–T6, the sympathetic innervation is intact and the patient therefore becomes aware when the bladder is full.

DEVELOPMENT

The urinary bladder develops from the following sources:

1. Whole of bladder except its apex develops from vesicourethral canal (upper part of urogenital sinus).
2. *Apex of the bladder* is derived from the proximal part of the allantoic diverticulum.
3. *Mucous membrane of trigonum vesicae* is derived from the mesoderm of the incorporated lower ends of the mesonephric ducts.
4. *Mucous membrane in the rest of the bladder* is derived from the endoderm of the vesicourethral part of the cloaca.
5. Muscle and serous coat of the bladder are derived from the splanchnic layer of the lateral plate mesoderm.

Clinical correlation

- **Congenital anomalies** are defective obliteration of urachus (Fig. 16.10).
- **Urachal fistula:** The urachus is the abdominal part of allantois extending from the apex of the bladder to the umbilicus. It normally obliterates and forms the *median umbilical ligament* but rarely remains patent resulting in the *urachal fistula,* which may lead to discharge of the urine through umbilicus. Clinically it presents as discharge of urine from the umbilicus.
- Sometimes the intermediate part of the urachus fails to obliterate and forms the **urachal cyst.**
- If distal part of urachus fails to fibrose, it leads to formation of **urachal sinus.**

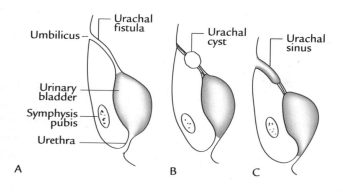

Fig. 16.10 Congenital anomalies due to defective obliteration of allantois. (*Source:* Fig. 9.34, Page 485, *Clinical and Surgical Anatomy*, 2e, Vishram Singh. Copyright Elsevier 2007, All rights reserved.)

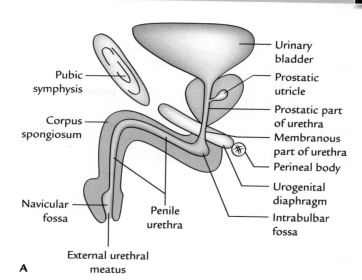

URETHRA

The urethra is a tubular passage, which transmits urine and seminal fluid in males and only urine in females. The study of urethra is important clinically to perform procedures of catheterization and cystoscopy. The urethral rupture is also common.

MALE URETHRA (Fig. 16.11)

The male urethra is about 18–20 cm long.

It extends from the internal urethral orifice at the neck of the urinary bladder to the external urethral orifice (EUO) at the tip of the glans penis.

In flaccid state of the penis, the long axis of the urethra presents two curvatures and is therefore S-shaped. In erect state of the penis, the distal curvature disappears and as a result it becomes 'J-shaped'.

PARTS

According to its location, the urethra is divided into the following three parts:

1. Prostatic part (passes through the prostate).
2. Membranous part (passes through the urogenital diaphragm).
3. Spongy or penile part (passes through the corpus spongiosum of penis).

Prostatic Part of the Urethra (3 cm Long)

As its name implies it traverses through the anterior part of the prostate. It is the **widest and most dilatable part** of the male urethra. It is fusiform in the coronal section. The inner aspect of its posterior wall presents the following features (Fig. 16.12):

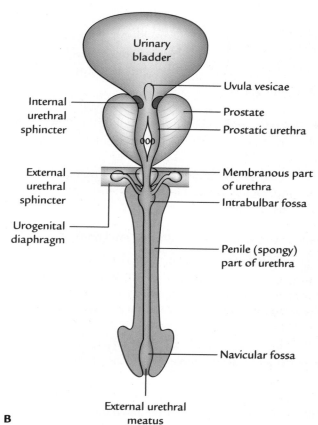

Fig. 16.11 Male urethra: **A**, left view in the sagittal section; **B**, anterior view (urethra straightened and cut open).

1. *Urethral crest*, a median longitudinal ridge of the mucous membrane.
2. *Colliculus seminalis (verumontanum)*, an elevation on the middle of the urethral crest. The prostatic utricle opens on its summit by a slit-like orifice. On either side of the orifice of the prostatic utricle opens the ejaculatory ducts.

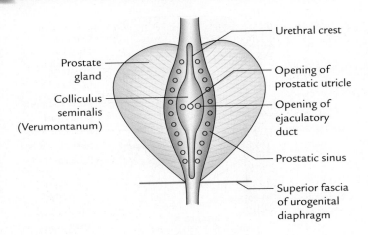

Fig. 16.12 Features of the posterior wall of the prostatic urethra.

3. *Prostatic sinuses*, vertical grooves one on each side of the urethral crest. Each sinus presents 15–20 openings of the prostatic glands.

N.B. *Prostatic utricle:* It is a mucous cul-de-sac (5.5 cm long) in the substance of the median lobe of the prostate. It develops from united caudal ends of the two Müllerian ducts; hence it corresponds to (i.e., homologous to) the uterus and vagina of the female. It is also termed *vaginus masculinus.*

Membranous Part of the Urethra (2 cm Long)

It traverses through the urogenital diaphragm and pierces the perineal membrane about 2.5 cm below and behind the pubic symphysis. It is surrounded by the sphincter urethrae muscle, which serves as the voluntary external sphincter of the bladder.

With the exception of external urethral orifice, it is the **narrowest and least dilatable part** of the urethra. Numerous mucous glands are often found in it. In cross section, its lumen is star-shaped.

Spongy Part of the Urethra (15 cm Long)

It traverses through the corpus spongiosum of the penis. It first passes upward and forward in the bulb of penis to lie below the pubic symphysis. Then it bends downward and forward, and traverses the corpus spongiosum in the free part of the penis and terminates as the external urethral orifice just below the tip of glans penis.

It presents two dilatations: (a) in the bulb of penis to form **intrabulbar fossa** (3 cm long) and (b) in the glans penis to form **navicular fossa/terminal fossa** (1.25 cm long).

In cross section, the shape of the spongy urethra differs in different parts, *viz.*, trapezoid-shaped in the bulb, like a transverse slit in the body and like a vertical slit at the external urethral orifice.

- The small simple tubular mucous glands called **urethral glands** (**Littre's glands**) open in the entire spongy part of the urethra except in the terminal fossa.
- The pit-like small mucous recesses, the urethral lacunae (of Morgagni) project from the entire spongy part of the urethra except in the terminal fossa. The lacunae receive the openings of urethral glands. One lacuna present in the roof of terminal fossa is called **lacuna magna** or **sinus of Guerin**.

The external urethral orifice is the narrowest part of the male urethra. It is in the form of a sagittal slit about 6 mm long.

The features of different parts of the male urethra are summarized in Table 16.2 and shown in Figure 16.13.

N.B. The lumen of the male urethra is irregular, i.e., it has different shapes in different parts. This makes the urine projectile in nature and provides a spiral twist to the urinary flow. As a result, the early separation of droplets of urine does not occur which prevents the wetting of the clothes.

Table 16.2 Different parts of the male urethra

Features	Prostatic part	Membranous part	Spongy part
Location	Within prostate	Within urogenital diaphragm	Within penis (corpus spongiosum)
Length	3 cm	1.5–2 cm	15 cm
Shape in cross section	Horseshoe shaped	Star-shaped	In the bulb—trapezoid In the body—transverse slit At external urethral orifice—vertical slit
Diameter and dilatability	Widest and most dilatable	Narrowest and least dilatable	Mostly uniform diameter with medium dilatation
Openings	• Prostatic utricle • Ejaculatory ducts • Prostatic glands	Minute mucous glands	Urethral glands (Littre's glands)

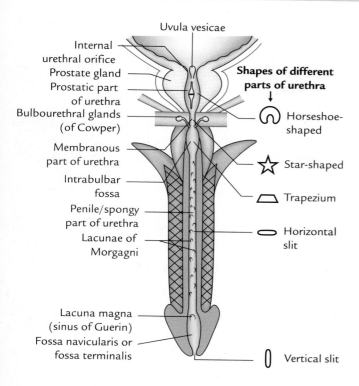

Fig. 16.13 Different parts of the male urethra and their shapes.

URETHRAL MUCOSA

The urethral mucosa presents regional variations as follows:

1. *Prostatic urethra* above the seminal colliculus is lined by transitional epithelium and below it by stratified columnar epithelium.

2. *Membranous urethra* is lined by stratified columnar epithelium.
3. Spongy urethra up to navicular fossa is lined by stratified columnar epithelium. The navicular fossa and external urethral orifice are lined by stratified squamous epithelium.

Clinical correlation

- **Rupture of the urethra:** The rupture of the urethra leads to extravasation of urine. The commonest site of rupture is bulb of the penis, just below the urogenital diaphragm following a fall astride a sharp object. The urethra is crushed against the edge of the pubic bones. The urine extravasates into the superficial perineal pouch and passes forward over the scrotum, penis, and anterior part of the anterior abdominal wall deep to membranous layer of the superficial fascia (**superficial extravasation**; Fig. 16.14A). If the urethra ruptures above urogenital diaphragm urine escapes above the deep perineal pouch and may pass upward around the prostate and bladder in the extraperitoneal space (**deep extravasation**; Fig. 16.14B).
- **Catheterization of the male urethra:** It is done in the patients who are unable to pass urine and their bladders are distended due to retention of urine leading to severe discomfort and pain in the hypogastric region. While passing the catheter one should remember the normal curvatures of the urethra. Further one should know that immediately above the external urethral meatus the urethra presents a large mucosal recess guarded by a mucosal fold, which may catch the tip of catheter. The catheter/iron bougie should therefore always be introduced into the urethra with its beak turned downward. Otherwise the forceful insertion of catheter may create a false passage in urethra or rupture it.

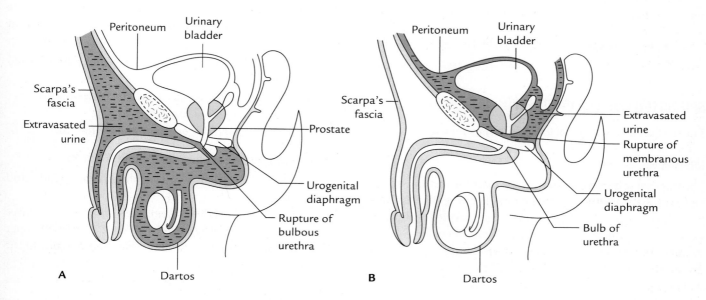

Fig. 16.14 Rupture of urethra: A, rupture of the bulbous urethra leading to superficial extravasation; B, rupture of the urethra above the urogenital diaphragm leading to deep extravasation. The orange coloured areas represent the extravasated of urine.

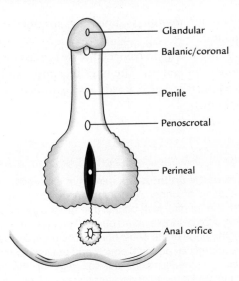

Fig. 16.15 Types of Hypospadias. (*Source*: Fig. 9.27, Page 478, *Clinical and Surgical Anatomy*, 2e, Vishram Singh. Copyright Elsevier 2007, All rights reserved.)

- **Hypospadias:** It is a congenital anomaly in which external urethral orifice is located on the inferior/ventral aspect of penis instead at the tip of the glans penis. It occurs due to failure of the fusion of urethral folds. Depending upon the location of external urethral orifice (EUO), the hypospadias are classified into 5 types (Fig. 16.15):
1. *Glandular:* If external urethral orifice opens on the under surface of the glans.
2. *Balanic:* If urethral orifice opens at the base of glans penis.
3. *Penile:* If urethral orifice opens on ventral aspect of the body of penis.
4. *Penioscrotal:* If urethral orifice opens at the junction of penis and scrotum.
5. *Perineal:* If urethral orifice opens as sagittal slit on ventral aspect of scrotum.

SPHINCTERS OF THE URETHRA

The urethra has two sphincters—internal and external.

Internal Sphincter

The internal sphincter surrounds the internal urethral orifice and is probably formed from the muscle of the bladder wall. It is involuntary in nature and often termed **sphincter vesicae**. It is supplied by the sympathetic fibres from lower thoracic and upper lumbar segments of the spinal cord (T11 to L2). It relaxes during urination but closes (i.e., contracts) during ejaculation (to prevent the retrograde entry of semen into the bladder).

Table 16.3 Differences between the internal and external sphincters of the urethra

Internal urethral sphincter	External urethral sphincter
• Surrounds the internal urethral orifice	• Surrounds the membranous part of urethra
• Derived from the bladder musculature of trigonal region	• Derived from the sphincter urethrae muscle
• Innervated by the sympathetic fibres (T11–L2 segments)	• Innervated by the somatic fibres (S2, S3, S4 segments)
• Involuntary	• Voluntary

External Sphincter (or Sphincter Urethrae)

The external sphincter surrounds the membranous part of the urethra and is derived from the sphincter urethrae muscle. It is voluntary in nature and is supplied by the pudendal nerve (S2, S3, S4).

The differences between the internal and external sphincters of the urethra are given in Table 16.3.

FEMALE URETHRA

The female urethra is about 4 cm long. It begins at the internal urethral orifice at the neck of bladder and passes downward and forward embedded in the anterior wall of the vagina through urogenital diaphragm. It pierces the perineal membrane, and opens in the vestibule of vagina in front of the vaginal orifice. In the vestibule of vagina, the urethral orifice is situated in front of the vaginal orifice and about 2.5 cm behind the glans of clitoris.

Shape of the Female Urethra

In cross section, the shape of female urethra differs in different parts:

1. *In the upper part*, it is *crescentic* with convexity directed forward.
2. *In the middle part*, it is *star-shaped* (stellate-shaped).
3. *In the lower part*, it is a *transverse slit*.
4. *At the external urethral orifice*, it is a *sagittal slit*.

Glands and Lacunae around the Female Urethra

1. *Urethral glands:* These are small tubular glands and surround the entire urethra.
2. *Paraurethral glands (of Skene):* These are relatively large mucous glands and aggregated on each side of the upper part of the urethra. These glands are homologous to the male prostate.
3. *Urethral lacunae:* These are pit-like mucous recesses along the entire urethra.

Clinical correlation

- The female urethra is easily dilatable, hence catheter/cystoscope can be easily negotiated.
- *Urinary tract infections* are much more common in females due to shortness of the urethra and presence of its orifice on the surface close to the vaginal and anal orifices. Therefore, females must take bath at least once a day.
- *Urinary incontinence* is common in females because in them external urethral sphincter is a tenuous structure and is further weakened during childbirth.

Golden Facts to Remember

➤ Most fixed part of the urinary bladder	Neck of the urinary bladder
➤ Most common tumor of the urinary bladder	Transitional cell carcinoma (>90%)
➤ Widest and most dilatable part of the male urethra	Prostatic part
➤ Narrowest and least dilatable part of the male urethra	Membranous part
➤ Narrowest part of the male urethra	External urethral orifice (EUO)
➤ Uterus and vagina in the male is represented by	Prostatic utricle
➤ Prostate gland in the females is represented by	Paraurethral glands (of Skene)

Clinical Case Study

An inebriated 37-year-old man was involved in a verbal fight with a woman, using unparliamentary language. Seeing this, the woman's husband came and gave the man a severe blow in the lower part of his anterior abdominal wall. Following the blow, the man doubled up with pain and collapsed on the road. Police was called and they took him to the emergency department of a nearby hospital. The man was in a state of shock and complained of pain in the lower abdomen. He did not pass urine since he received the blow. A diagnosis of **ruptured urinary bladder** was made.

Questions

1. Give the types of rupture of urinary bladder.
2. Which wall of the urinary bladder is commonly involved in intraperitoneal rupture?
3. Which wall of the urinary bladder is involved in extraperitoneal rupture?

Answers

1. Intraperitoneal and extraperitoneal.
2. Superior wall. It occurs most commonly when the bladder is full and has extended up into the abdomen.
3. Anterior wall below the level of peritoneal reflection. It mostly occurs in fracture of the pelvis when bony fragments pierce the bladder wall.

CHAPTER 17

Male Genital Organs

The male genital organs are divided into two groups: internal and external. The external genital organs are already described in Chapter 5.

The internal genital organs (Fig. 17.1) include:

1. Testes and epididymis.
2. Prostate.
3. Bulbourethral glands.
4. Seminal vesicles.
5. Ejaculatory ducts and penis.
6. Vasa deferentia (deferent ducts).

The testis and epididymis are described along with external genital organs in Chapter 5.

PROSTATE

The prostate is a pyramidal-shaped, fibromuscular glandular organ which surrounds the prostatic urethra. The prostate gland secretes acid phosphatase, fibrinolysin, citric acid, amylase, prostate-specific antigen (PSA), and prostaglandins. Its secretions form the bulk of the seminal fluid. Its female homologue is paraurethral glands (of Skene).

LOCATION (Fig. 17.2)

The prostate is located in the lesser pelvis below the neck of the urinary bladder and above the urogenital diaphragm. It

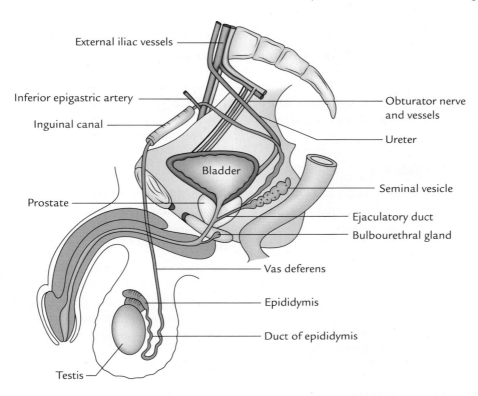

External iliac vessels

Inferior epigastric artery

Inguinal canal

Obturator nerve and vessels

Ureter

Bladder

Seminal vesicle

Prostate

Ejaculatory duct

Bulbourethral gland

Vas deferens

Epididymis

Duct of epididymis

Testis

Fig. 17.1 Male reproductive organs. Note the course and relations of vas deferens, in the four regions (*viz.*, scrotum, spermatic cord, inguinal canal, and pelvis) traversed by it.

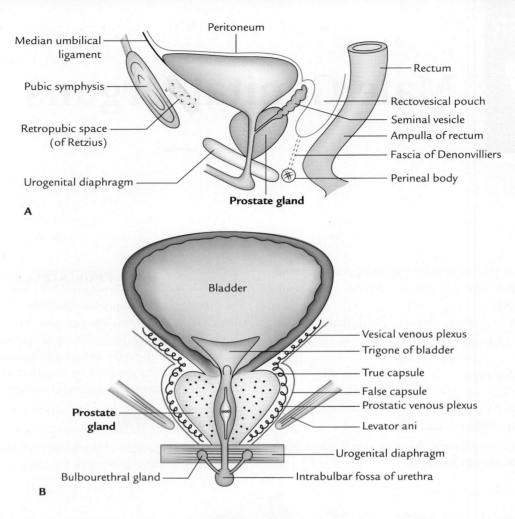

Fig. 17.2 Location of the prostate gland: **A**, as seen in the sagittal section; **B**, as seen in the coronal section.

lies behind the lower part of the pubic symphysis and in front of the rectal ampulla. It is embraced on each side by the levator ani muscle.

SHAPE, SIZE, AND MEASUREMENTS

The prostate is like an inverted cone in shape and resembles a chestnut in appearance. It presents the following measurements:

Weight: 3 g.
Width (at base): 4 cm.
Length: 3 cm.
Thickness: 2 cm.

N.B. The prostate belongs to the category of organs which have more width than length, such as caecum, coeliac trunk, etc.

EXTERNAL FEATURES AND RELATIONS

The prostate presents the following external features:

1. Apex.
2. Base.
3. Four surfaces (anterior, posterior and two inferolateral).

Apex

It is directed downward and rests on the superior surface of the urogenital diaphragm.

Base

It is directed upward and surrounds the neck of the urinary bladder with which it is continuous structurally. The junction is marked by a circular groove. The base is pierced by the urethra in the median plane at the junction of its anterior one-third and posterior two-third.

Surfaces

Anterior surface: It is narrow and convex from side to side. It is situated 2 cm behind the pubis symphysis. It is separated from the symphysis by the retropubic space (of Retzius)

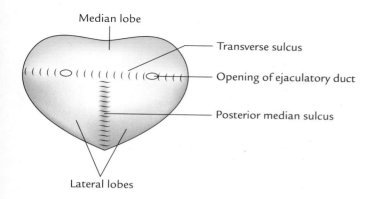

Fig. 17.3 Features of the posterior surface of the prostate.

filled with extraperitoneal fat. A little above the apex, this surface is pierced by the urethra.

Posterior surface: It is broad and flat and lies in front of the ampulla of the rectum, from which it is separated by the fascia of Denonvilliers. The posterior surface is divided into small upper and larger lower areas by a transverse sulcus, which is pierced on each side of the median plane by the ejaculatory duct. The upper areas represent the median lobe and the lower area is divided by a median sulcus into two lateral lobes (Fig. 17.3).

Inferolateral surfaces: These are related to the anterior fibres of levator ani (levator prostate).

LOBES OF THE PROSTATE (Fig. 17.4)

The prostate is divided into five lobes:

1. Anterior lobe (isthmus).
2. Posterior lobe.
3. Median lobe.
4. Two lateral lobes.

Anterior Lobe

The anterior lobe lies in front of the urethra and connects the two lateral lobes. It is devoid of the glandular tissue and often called isthmus.[1]

Posterior Lobe

The posterior lobe lies behind the ejaculatory ducts and median lobe and connects the two lateral lobes. The primary carcinoma of the prostate begins in this lobe.

Median Lobe (Middle Lobe)

The median lobe is wedge-shaped and lies behind the upper part of the urethra and in front of ejaculatory ducts. Its

base produces an elevation at the apex of trigonum vesicae called uvula vesicae. The median lobe normally projects into the prostatic urethra raising a ridge called urethral crest.

It contains much of the glandular tissue and is a common site of adenoma.

Lateral Lobes

The lateral lobes lie one on each side of the urethra. On the posterior surface of the prostate, two lateral lobes are separated from each other by posterior median sulcus. The lateral lobes contain some glandular tissue and therefore adenoma may arise here in the old age.

STRUCTURES WITHIN THE PROSTATE

These are as follows:

1. *Prostatic urethra* traverses vertically downward through the gland at the junction of its anterior one-third and posterior two-third and opens on the anterior surface just above the apex.
2. *Ejaculatory ducts* traverse the gland posterolateral to the median lobe and open in the urethra.
3. *Prostatic utricle* is a mucous cul-de-sac about 6 mm long which extends upward and backward from the prostatic urethra, behind the median lobe.

CAPSULES OF THE PROSTATE (Fig. 17.5)

The prostatic capsules are two in number in normal gland and three in number if gland is affected by benign hypertrophy of the prostate.

1. *True capsule:* It is formed by the condensation of peripheral fibrous stroma of the gland, hence intimately related to the gland.
2. *False capsule (prostatic sheath):* It is derived from the pelvic fascia. It is outside the true capsule and envelops the prostate gland and urinary bladder in the same compartment.
3. *Surgical/pathological capsule:* When the adenoma of the gland enlarges, the peripheral part of the organ becomes compressed. This compressed part of the gland is called surgical or pathological capsule.

N.B. The **prostatic venous plexus** lies between the true and false capsules except on the posterior surface of the gland. (cf. the venous plexus of the thyroid gland lies deep to both true and false capsules).

---

[1]Truly speaking, it is not a lobe but a band of fibrous tissue connecting two lateral lobes.

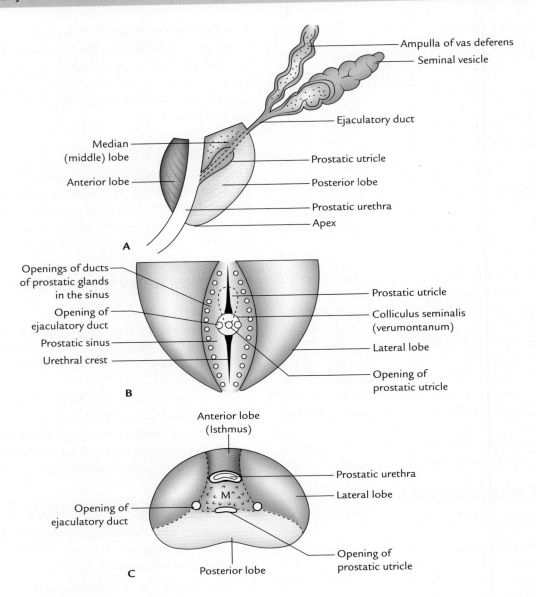

Fig. 17.4 Lobes of the prostate gland as seen in sections through different planes: **A**, left view of a sagittal section; **B**, coronal section through the posterior half of the gland; **C**, horizontal section (M = median lobe).

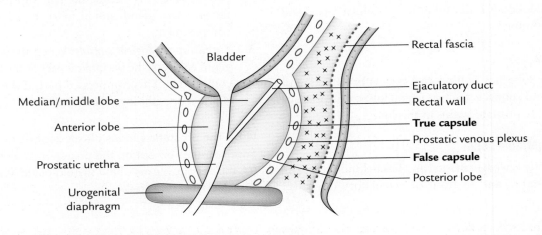

Fig. 17.5 Capsules of the prostate gland as seen in the sagittal section.

SUPPORTS OF THE PROSTATE

These are:

1. *Urogenital diaphragm:* The apex of the gland rests on it and the prostatic sheath (false capsule) is continuous with its superior fascia.
2. *Two pairs of puboprostatic ligaments:* They extend from the prostatic sheath (false capsule) to the back of the pubic bones. The medial pair lies near the apex of the gland and the lateral pair close to the base.
3. *Rectovesical fascia of Denonvilliers:* The posterior aspect of prostatic sheath adheres to this fascia posteriorly.

N.B. *Fascia of Denonvilliers (rectovesical fascia):* It is a fascial septum between prostate and ampulla of the rectum and extends from the floor of rectovesical pouch to the perineal body. Origin of the fascia has a developmental basis. In foetus, the rectovesical pouch is deep and separates the prostate from the rectum. In later life, two layers of the peritoneum between prostate and rectum fuse to form this fascia. The carcinoma prostate only rarely penetrates this fascial barrier so that involvement of the rectum is unusual.

STRUCTURE OF THE PROSTATE

The prostate gland is made up of fibrous tissue (1/4), muscular tissue (1/4), and glandular tissue (1/2). The glandular tissue consists of tubuloalveolar glands arranged in three concentric groups (mucosal, submucosal, and main); all of them open into the urethra. The fibromuscular tissue forms the stroma and the glandular tissue forms the parenchyma of the prostate gland. The lumen of tubuloalveolar gland contains small colloid masses called corpora amylacea.

Structural Zones of the Prostate Gland

Histologically, the prostate gland does not show the lobular pattern as generally described in *Gross Anatomy;* instead there are two well-defined concentric zones separated by an ill-defined irregular fibrous layer. The zones are absent anteriorly (Fig. 17.6).

1. *Outer zone:* The larger outer zone is composed of long-branching glands (prostatic gland proper). The ducts of these glands curve backward and open in the prostatic sinus below the colliculus seminalis. This zone is the common site of carcinoma prostate.
2. *Inner zone:* The smaller inner zone is composed of outer submucosal glands, which open in the prostatic sinus at the level of colliculus seminalis. Deep to these glands are simple mucosal glands (suburethral glands), which are short and open all around the urethra above the level of colliculus seminalis.

All hypertrophies of the prostate arise from these mucosal (suburethral/subcervical) glands. Therefore, the inner zone of prostate is the common site of benign prostatic hypertrophy (BPH).

ARTERIAL SUPPLY

The prostate gland is supplied by the branches of inferior vesical, middle rectal, and internal pudendal arteries.

VENOUS DRAINAGE

The veins from the prostate form a rich venous plexus around the sides and base of the gland and occupy the space between the true and false capsules. It receives the deep

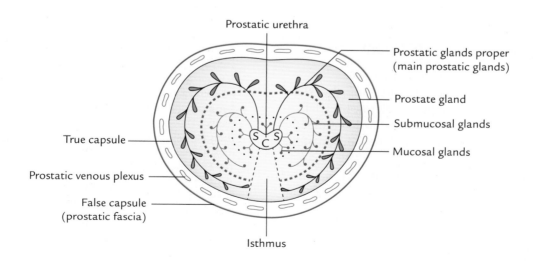

Fig. 17.6 Horizontal section of the prostate gland showing its structural zones. Note mucosal, submucosal, and main prostatic glands arranged into three concentric layers (S = prostatic sinus, C = colliculus seminalis (urethral crest)).

dorsal vein of the penis in front and is continuous above with the vesical venous plexus.

The mode of venous drainage from the prostatic venous plexus follows two pathways:

1. Into internal iliac veins through the posterior ligaments of the urinary bladder.
2. Into internal and external vertebral venous plexus (of Batson) through veins passing through anterior sacral foramina. The communication between the vesical and vertebral venous plexuses is valveless.

N.B. The venous drainage of the prostate follows two pathways:
(a) Prostatic venous plexus → internal iliac veins → IVC. This pathway explains the metastasis of cancer prostate into the heart and lungs.
(b) Prostatic venous plexus → vertebral venous plexus (of Batson) → intracranial dural venous sinuses. This pathway explains the metastasis of cancer prostate into the vertebral column and brain.

LYMPHATIC DRAINAGE

The lymphatics from the prostate drain into the internal iliac, external iliac, and sacral groups of the lymph nodes.

NERVE SUPPLY

The prostate is supplied by the following nerves:

1. The *sympathetic supply* is provided by the *superior hypogastric plexus*. The preganglionic sympathetic fibres arise from L1 and L2 spinal segments.
2. The *parasympathetic supply* is provided by the *pelvic splanchnic nerves* which convey preganglionic fibres from S2, S3, S4 spinal segments.

DEVELOPMENT OF THE PROSTATE GLAND

The prostate develops from the following sources:

1. The parenchyma (glandular portion) of the gland develops in the third month of intrauterine life (IUL) as a series of endodermal buds (outgrowths) from the lining of primitive urethra and adjoining portion of the urogenital sinus.
2. The *stroma of the gland* develops in the 4th month of IUL from the surrounding mesenchyme derived from the splanchnic layer of mesoderm.

CHANGES IN THE PROSTATE WITH AGE

The age-related changes in prostate are as follows:

1. *In childhood,* the prostate gland is small and is composed mainly of fibromuscular stroma and rudiments of ducts.

2. *At puberty,* there is a sudden increase in the size of gland under the influence of male hormone (testosterone). It becomes double of its prepubertal size. There is rapid proliferation of prostatic follicles which start secretion.
3. *During the third decade,* there are irregular epithelial infoldings in the lumen of the follicles, making them irregular.
4. *During the fourth decade,* the size of prostate remains constant. The epithelial infoldings in the lumen gradually disappear and amyloid concretions (amyloid bodies) appear in the follicles.
5. *During the fifth decade* (i.e., after 50 years of age), some degree of prostatic hypertrophy is invariably present. It is as much a sign of aging as the graying of hair. In some cases, the gland, however, is reduced in size called *senile atrophy.*

Clinical correlation

- **Benign prostatic hypertrophy (BPH):** After 50 years of age, the prostate gland is enlarged due to hypertrophy of median lobe (hypertrophy of subcervical glands of Albarran) forming an adenoma. The BPH commonly involves the median lobe, which compresses the prostatic urethra and obstructs the urine flow. The enlargement of uvula vesicae due to enlarged median lobe results in the formation of **postprostatic pouch of stagnant urine** in the urinary bladder behind the internal urethral orifice (Fig. 17.7). Clinically BPH presents as: (a) increased frequency of urination, (b) urgency of urination, (c) difficulty in starting and stopping urination, and (d) a sense of incomplete emptying of the urinary bladder.

  The surgical removal of adenoma is called **prostatectomy**. The adenoma is enucleated, leaving behind both the capsules and the prostatic venous plexus between them.

  After prostatectomy, the patient becomes sterile because the mechanism of internal urethral sphincter is disturbed and semen enters into the urinary bladder during ejaculation.

  There are several surgical approaches of prostatectomy, viz., suprapubic, retropubic, perineal, and transurethral.

  Most adenomatous enlargements of the prostate are nowadays resected transurethrally.

- **Prostatic carcinoma:** It usually occurs after the age of 50 years. The carcinoma is commonly found in the outer (peripheral) zone which usually involves the posterior lobe. Clinically, it presents as:
  (a) Pain in perineum.
  (b) Urinary obstruction.
  (c) Difficulty in urination.

  For diagnosis, per rectal examination reveals irregular, hard, fixed prostate, and absence of median groove in its posterior surface. The serum levels of acid phosphatase and prostate specific antigen (PSA) are used in diagnosis and management of prostate cancer.

  The metastasis of prostatic carcinoma commonly occurs in the lumbar vertebrae and pelvis.

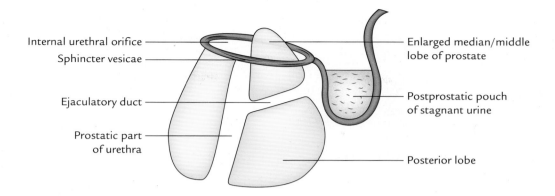

Fig. 17.7 Sagittal section of enlarged prostate gland involved in benign hypertrophy. Note the position of median lobe and presence of postprostatic bladder pouch filled with stagnant urine.

SEMINAL VESICLES

The seminal vesicles are two coiled sacculated tubes about 2 inches (5 cm) long which can be unraveled to three times of this length (Fig. 17.8). They lie extraperitoneally on each side, at the base of the urinary bladder, lateral to the termination of the vas deferens and in front of the rectum. The lower narrow end of seminal vesicle (duct of seminal vesicle) joins the ductus deferens to form the *ejaculatory duct.*

The seminal vesicles, as their name implies, do not form a reservoir for sperms. Their secretions form a large amount of the seminal fluid. The secretion of seminal vesicles is slightly alkaline, containing fructose, choline, and a coagulating enzyme called vesiculose.

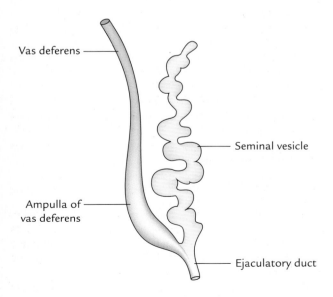

Fig. 17.8 The unraveled seminal vesicle.

EJACULATORY DUCTS

There are two ejaculatory ducts one on each side of the median plane at the lower part of the bladder base. Each duct traverses anteroinferiorly through the upper posterior half of the prostate and along the side of prostatic utricle to open in the posterior wall of prostatic urethra on the seminal colliculus (verumontanum) on either side of the opening of *prostatic utricle.*

VASA DEFERENTIA (DEFERENT DUCTS)

These are two in number (right and left). *Each vas deferens is a thick-walled muscular tube which transports spermatozoa from the epididymis to the ejaculatory duct.* The vas deferens is about 18 inches (45 cm) long and has a narrow lumen except in the terminal part which is sacculated—the *ampulla of vas deferens.*

COURSE AND RELATIONS

External Course of Vas Deferens

It begins at the inferior pole of the testis as direct continuation of the duct of epididymis and ascends upward behind the testis and medial to the epididymis. It enters the spermatic cord, where it lies in its posterior part, which is the usual site of vasectomy. It passes through inguinal canal

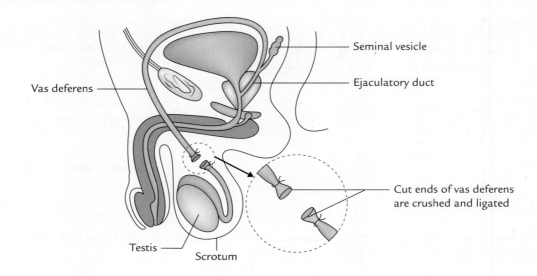

Fig. 17.9 Vasectomy (medial view from left).

and enters the abdominal cavity by passing through the deep inguinal ring located lateral to the inferior epigastric artery.

Internal Course of Vas Deferens

It hooks around the lateral side of the inferior epigastric artery and passes backward and medially across the external iliac vessels and enters the lesser pelvis. In the lesser pelvis, it runs downward and backward on the lateral pelvic wall crossing successively obliterated umbilical artery, obturator nerve, and vessels. Then it crosses above and medial to the terminal part of the ureter and makes an angular bend downward and medially. Thereafter, it passes behind the base of the bladder in front of the rectal ampulla and on the medial side of the seminal vesicle. This part of the vas deferens is enlarged and sacculated to form an ampulla which probably stores the semen. Finally it converges to reach the base of prostate where it joins the duct of the seminal vesicle to form the ejaculatory duct, immediately posterior to the neck of the bladder.

ARTERIAL SUPPLY

The vas deferens is supplied by the following arteries:

1. *Artery to vas deferens*, a branch of superior vesical artery.
2. *Artery to vas deferens*, a branch of inferior vesical artery.
3. *Artery to vas deferens*, a branch of middle rectal artery.

VENOUS DRAINAGE

The veins from vas deferens join the vesical venous plexus which in turn drains into the internal iliac veins.

NERVE SUPPLY

It is primarily by the parasympathetic fibres from the pelvic splanchnic nerves.

Clinical correlation

Vasectomy: This is a common method of male sterilization. It is a minor operation done under local anesthesia. In this procedure, a short segment of each vas is excised. The cut ends are crushed and ligated (Fig. 17.9). The vas deferentia are approached through a median incision in the upper part of the scrotum below the penis. As a result, seminal fluid ejaculated a week after vasectomy, will not contain sperms and hence pregnancy cannot occur. The sperms which continue to be produced undergo degeneration and are absorbed in the epididymis.

The growth of interstitial cells is not affected, therefore testes continue to produce testosterone and the individual's potency is not affected.

Reversal of vasectomy is possible. The cut ends are united and recanalization is done if required. However, it is successful in only favorable cases, i.e., individuals with less than 30 years of age and if this procedure is performed within seven years of vasectomy.

Golden Facts to Remember

▶ Common site of benign prostatic hypertrophy of the prostate (BPH)	Median lobe of the prostate
▶ Common site of prostatic cancer	Posterior lobe
▶ Most of the seminal fluid is formed by the secretions of	Prostate gland
▶ Prostatism	Symptom complex consisting of frequency, urgency, and difficulty of micturition
▶ Most common approach to remove adenoma of prostate	Transurethral

Clinical Case Study

A 67-year-old man was admitted in hospital with history of pain in the perineum, with difficulty, urgency, and frequency in micturition. Per-rectal examination revealed an enlargement of the prostate. It was smooth and non-nodular. The investigations ruled out carcinoma prostate. The diagnosis of "benign prostatic hypertrophy of prostate (BPH)" was made.

Questions

1. What is benign prostatic hypertrophy?
2. What are the common sites of occurrence of the benign prostatic hypertrophy and carcinoma of prostate?
3. What are the posterior relations of the prostate?
4. What are the two anatomical capsules of prostate? Name the structure present between them.
5. What is surgical/pathological capsule?

Answers

1. It is the enlargement of prostate due to the hypertrophy of the periurethral glands of median lobe, forming an adenoma.
2. Median lobe of prostate is the common site of BPH and posterior lobe is the most common site of carcinoma of prostate.
3. Posteriorly, the prostate gland is related to *fascia of Denonvilliers* which separates it from the ampulla of rectum. The ejaculatory ducts also pierce the posterior surface.
4. The prostate gland is enclosed in two capsules: an inner true capsule and an outer false capsule. The *prostatic venous plexus* lies between the two capsules.
5. When benign adenomatous hypertrophy of prostate occurs, the normal peripheral part of the gland becomes compressed. This compressed part of the gland around the adenoma is called *surgical or pathological capsule.*

Female Genital Organs

The female genital organs are divided into two groups: internal and external (Fig. 18.1). The **internal genital organs** are situated within the pelvis and include (a) a pair of **ovaries**, (b) a pair of **uterine tubes**, (c) a single **uterus**, and (d) a single **vagina**. The **external genital organs** in the female are collectively called the vulva and consist of (a) **mons pubis**, (b) a pair of **labia majora** and **minora**, (c) a single **clitoris**, (d) vestibule of vagina, and (e) a pair of greater vestibular glands. They form the superficial features of the female perineum.

INTERNAL GENITAL ORGANS

OVARIES

The ovaries are female gonads (homologous of testes in the male) which produce female gametes called oocytes (ripe ova). The ovaries are almond-shaped and grayish pink in colour. Each ovary is about 4 cm long, 2 cm wide and 1 cm thick.

LOCATION

In nulliparous adult women, each ovary lies in the *ovarian fossa* on the lateral pelvic wall below the pelvic brim (Fig. 18.2). The **ovarian fossa** is a slight peritoneal depression bounded:

- *Posteriorly* by the ureter and internal iliac vessels.
- *Anteriorly* by the external iliac vessels.
- *Inferiorly* by the uterine tubes (in the free margin of broad ligament).

The obturator nerve and vessels cross the floor of the fossa.

Peritoneal Relations (Fig. 18.3)

Each ovary is attached to the posterior surface of the broad ligament by a short peritoneal fold called *mesovarium.* Through mesovarium, ovarian vessels enter the hilus of ovary.

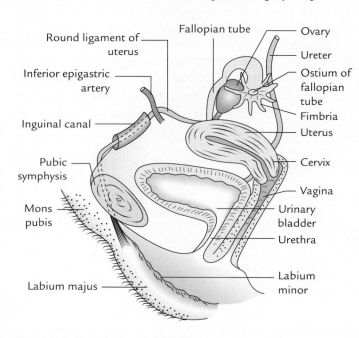

Fig. 18.1 Female genital organs.

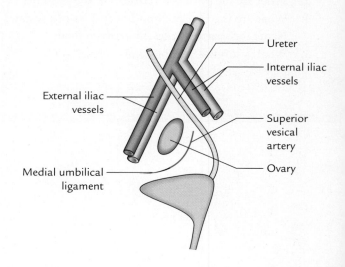

Fig. 18.2 Location of ovary in the ovarian fossa. Note the boundaries of ovarian fossa.

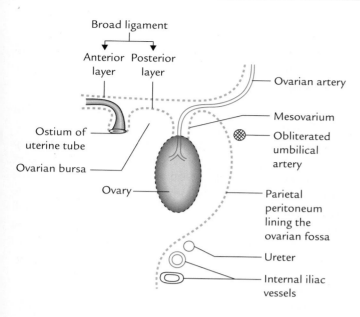

Fig. 18.3 Peritoneal relations of the ovary.

Each ovary is almost entirely covered by the peritoneum except along the mesovarian border where two layers of the covering peritoneum are reflected on the posterior layer of the broad ligament.

The mesovarium acts as a hilum of the ovary and conveys blood vessels and nerves to the ovary. The peritoneal layers of the mesovarium become continuous with the germinal

epithelium of the ovary. The junction between the flattened mesothelium of peritoneum and the cuboidal germinal epithelium of ovary is marked by **white line of ovary** (**line of Furre**).

EXTERNAL FEATURES AND RELATIONS (Fig. 18.4)

Before the onset of ovulation the surfaces of the ovary are smooth, but after puberty they become nodular. *The external features of the ovary are always described as seen in a nulliparous woman.* In anatomical position, the long axis of the ovary is almost vertical so that it has an upper pole and a lower pole. The ovary presents the following external features (Fig. 18.4A):

1. Two extremities or poles.
2. Two surfaces.
3. Two borders.

N.B. In multiparous women (after one or more deliveries), the long axis of ovary becomes horizontal and its surfaces become irregular (Fig. 18.4B).

Extremities (or Poles)

1. *Superior extremity:* It is broader than the lower extremity and is related to the uterine tube and the external iliac vein. It provides attachment to a fold of peritoneum called **suspensory ligament of ovary** which contains ovarian vessels and nerves.

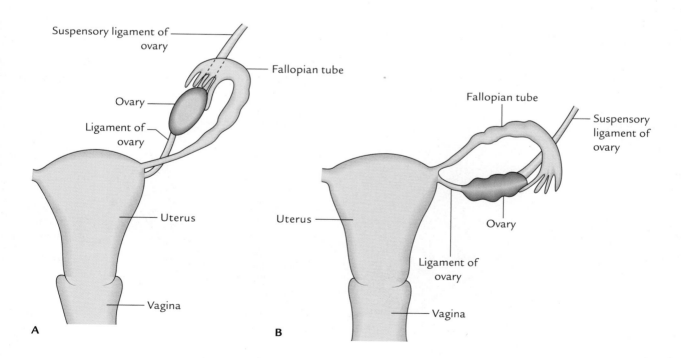

Fig. 18.4 Position of ovary: A, in a nulliparous woman it is vertical and its surfaces are smooth; B, in a multiparous woman it is horizontal and its surfaces are irregular.

2. *Inferior extremity (or pole):* It is narrower than the upper extremity and is related to the pelvic diaphragm. It is connected to the lateral angle of the uterus posteroinferior to the attachment of fallopian tube by the ligament of ovary.

Surfaces

1. *Lateral surface:* It is convex and is in contact with the parietal peritoneum lining the *ovarian fossa.* This surface separates the ovary from extraperitoneal tissue, and obturator nerve and vessels.
2. *Medial surface:* To a large extent, this surface is covered by the uterine tube, from which it is separated by a peritoneal recess called *ovarian bursa.*

Borders

1. *Anterior (mesovarian) border:* It is straight and attached to the posterior layer of broad ligament by a short fold of peritoneum called **mesovarium**.
2. *Posterior (free) border:* It is convex and is directed toward the uterine tube and is related to the ureter.

N.B. *Relationship of the ovary with the fallopian tube:* The uterine tube arches over the ovary running along its mesovarian border. It curves over its superior extremity then passes downward on its free border and medial surface and makes direct contact with the ovary by one of its fimbriae called *ovarian fimbria.*

STRUCTURE

Histologically, it is divided into two parts—cortex and medulla (Fig. 18.5).

Cortex

The cortex is the thick peripheral part and contains ovarian follicles in different stages of maturity.

It is covered by the germinal epithelium which is made up of a single layer of cuboidal cells in younger age. In the later life, the epithelial cells become flattened. The germinal epithelium becomes continuous with the peritoneum at the mesovarian border. Immediately beneath the germinal epithelium, the connective tissue of the cortex is condensed to form a whitish tough fibrous tissue layer called *tunica albuginea.*

Medulla

The medulla lies deep to the cortex. It consists of loose connective tissue containing relatively large blood vessels, particularly veins.

ARTERIAL SUPPLY (Fig. 18.6)

The ovary is mainly supplied by an *ovarian artery* which arises from the aorta at the level of L1 vertebra. It reaches the ovary after passing successively through the suspensory ligament of ovary, mesosalpinx, and mesovarium. It terminates by anastomosing with the uterine artery. The ovary is also supplied by an ovarian branch of the uterine artery through the mesovarium.

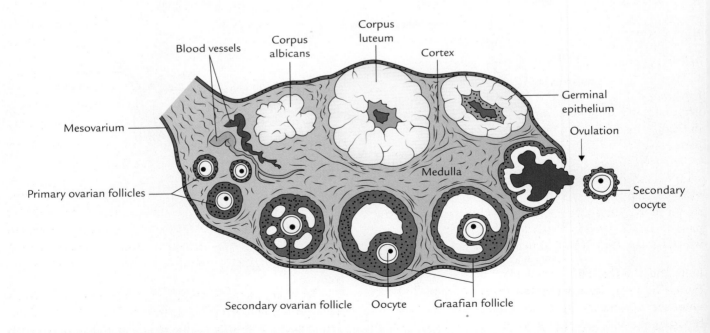

Fig. 18.5 Structure of the ovary.

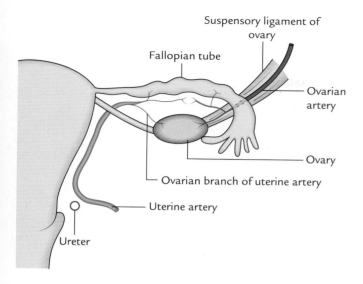

Suspensory ligament of ovary

Fallopian tube

Ovarian artery

Ovary

Ovarian branch of uterine artery

Uterine artery

Ureter

Fig. 18.6 Arterial supply of the ovary.

VENOUS DRAINAGE

The veins of the ovary emerge from the hilum and form the *pampiniform plexus* around the ovarian artery, from which a single ovarian vein is formed near the superior aperture of the pelvis/pelvic inlet. The right ovarian vein drains into the inferior vena cava while the left ovarian vein drains into the left renal vein.

LYMPHATIC DRAINAGE

The lymphatics from the ovary follow the ovarian vein and drain into the **pre-aortic and para-aortic lymph nodes** (from the bifurcation of aorta to the level of renal vessels).

NERVE SUPPLY

The ovary is innervated by the postganglionic sympathetic (T10, T11) and parasympathetic (S2, S3, S4) fibres, derived from abdominal autonomic plexuses. The role of autonomic nerves to the ovary is unclear. Although generally it is thought that sympathetic fibres are vasomotor and parasympathetic fibres are vasodilators.

The visceral afferent fibres from the ovary run along the sympathetic pathways to the spinal segments T10, T11. The ovarian pain is referred in the umbilical region being supplied by T10 spinal segment. The intractable ovarian pain can be alleviated by transecting the suspensory ligament, which contain the afferent (general visceral afferent) fibres.

N.B. The blood vessels, lymphatics, and nerves pass over the pelvic inlet, cross the external iliac vessels, and then enter the suspensory ligament of the ovary (lateral end of broad ligament) and finally enter the hilum of ovary via the mesovarium.

FUNCTIONS

The functions of the ovaries are as follows:

1. *Production of oocytes (female gametes):* During the reproductive life of females (30–45 years), ovaries produce alternatively one ripe ovum per menstrual cycle (of 28 days). The ovum develops into a small cystic follicle called Graafian (ovarian) follicle, which ruptures approximately in the middle of menstrual cycle, i.e., 14th day, and releases the ovum into the peritoneal cavity. After ovulation, the empty Graafian follicle is converted into a mass of specialized tissue called *corpus luteum.*

2. *Production of hormones:* The ovaries produce two hormones—progesterone and estrogen. The progesterone is secreted by the luteal cells and estrogen by the follicular cells.

DEVELOPMENT

The ovary, one on each side, develops within the abdominal cavity from a **genital ridge** on the posterior abdominal wall. The genital ridge is formed by the thickening of coelomic epithelium that covers the medial side of mesonephros. It receives primordial germ cells derived from the wall of the yolk sac.

The ovary then descends into the pelvis. The descent involves the gubernaculum (a band of fibromuscular tissue) and processus vaginalis (a process of the peritoneum formed due to its evagination).

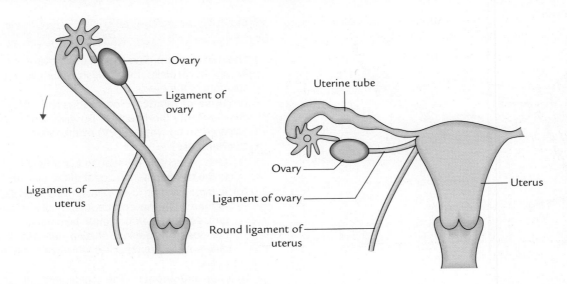

Fig. 18.7 Descent of an ovary and its relationship to the developing uterine tube and uterus. Note the formation of ligament of the ovary and round ligament of the uterus.

The gubernaculum extends from the ovary to the junction of the uterus and uterine tube (forming the *ovarian ligament* in adult) and then continues in the labium majus (forming the round ligament of the uterus in the adult). The processus vaginalis is obliterated in the adult (Fig. 18.7).

Clinical correlation

- **Ovarian dysgenesis:** Congenital absence of one or both ovaries is found in Turner's syndrome.
- **Ectopic ovaries:** The ovary may fail to descend into the pelvis or very rarely may be drawn downward with the round ligament of the uterus into the inguinal canal or even into the labium majus.

UTERINE TUBES (FALLOPIAN TUBES)

The uterine tubes are a pair of ducts which transmit ova from the ovaries to the uterine cavity. Each tube is about 10 cm long and lies in the upper free margin of the broad ligaments of the uterus.

EXTERNAL FEATURES

Each tube presents two ends and four parts (Fig. 18.8).

Ends

Medial End

It opens into the lateral angle of the uterine cavity. The uterine opening (ostium) is 1 mm in diameter.

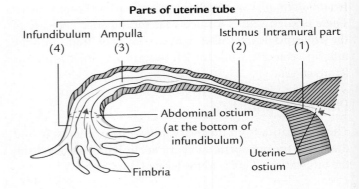

Fig. 18.8 Parts of the uterine tube.

Lateral (fimbriated) End

It communicates with the peritoneal cavity close to the ovary by piercing the posterior layer of the broad ligament.

1. It curves downward and inward partly to encircle the ovary.
2. The abdominal ostium is 3 mm in diameter and its margin possesses irregular small fingerlike processes called fimbriae, hence it is also known as fimbriated end.

Parts

From lateral to medial end, the fallopian tube is divided into four parts: infundibulum, ampulla, isthmus, and intramural.

Infundibulum (1 cm long)

1. It is the funnel-shaped lateral-most part which projects beyond the broad ligament of uterus.

2. It overlies the ovary and presents an abdominal ostium.
3. The circumference of the funnel is prolonged by varying number of irregular processes called fimbriae. One fimbria longer and more deeply grooved than the others is closely applied to the tubal extremity of the ovary and is called an **ovarian fimbria**. The ovarian fimbria acts as a sensor to time the release of ovum. Just before the release of ovum fimbriae start sweeping the surface of ovary and facilitate the entrance of ovum into the fallopian tube.

Ampulla (5 cm long)

1. It is the widest and longest part of the tube and forms rather more than one-half of the entire tube.
2. It is thin walled and tortuous.
3. It is the site of fertilization of ovum.

Isthmus (2.5–3 cm)

1. It is the narrowest part and lies just lateral to the uterus.
2. It is round and cord-like due to thick muscular wall.

Intramural (Interstitial) Part (1 cm long)

It is the segment of uterine tube that traverses the uterine wall at the junction of fundus and body. It lies within the wall of the uterus, hence the name intramural.

STRUCTURE OF THE UTERINE TUBE

From outside inward, the uterine tube consists of three coats: serous, muscular, and mucous.

1. The **serous coat** is derived from the peritoneum.
2. The **muscular coat** is made up of smooth muscle which is arranged into inner circular and outer longitudinal layers.
3. The **mucous coat** consists of lining epithelium and underlying lamina propria.

The mucous membrane lining the tube presents about six primary longitudinal folds which in turn give rise to a number of secondary and tertiary folds. As a result the lumen of the tube becomes highly irregular. This arrangement helps to provide nutrition to the zygote from all sides.

The lining epithelium is simple, ciliated columnar. It consists of two types of cells: ciliated columnar cells and non-ciliated secretory cells. The secretion of secretory cells provides nutrition to the fertilized ovum. The cilia of ciliated cells beat toward the uterine cavity and help in the transport of the fertilized ovum.

ARTERIAL SUPPLY

The fallopian tube is supplied by two arteries: ovarian and uterine arteries. Usually the medial two-third of the tube is supplied by the uterine artery and lateral one-third by the ovarian artery.

VENOUS DRAINAGE

The veins correspond to arteries, thus venous blood is drained by the ovarian and uterine veins.

LYMPHATIC DRAINAGE

The lymph vessels follow the veins and drain into internal iliac lymph nodes, pre-aortic and para-aortic lymph nodes.

NERVE SUPPLY

The tubes are supplied by both sympathetic and parasympathetic fibres. The sympathetic fibres are derived from ovarian and superior hypogastric plexuses. The preganglionic sympathetic fibres are derived from the T11–L2 spinal segments. The preganglionic parasympathetic fibres to the lateral part of the tube are derived from the vagus nerve and to the medial part from the pelvic splanchnic nerves (S2, S3, S4 spinal segments).

Clinical correlation

- **Salpingitis:** The inflammation of the uterine tube (or salpinx) is called salpingitis (salpinx: trumpet-like). It is the commonest cause of tubal block leading to secondary sterility in female. In recent times, the incidence of tubal block has increased in modern females probably because they miss morning bath in order to report on duty in time and waste time in make-up. Tubal infection usually occurs due to upward spread of infection from vagina and uterus. The patency of tubal block is tested by the following tests:
  (a) *Insufflation test* (or Rubin's test): Air is pushed into the uterus, and if tube is patent, the air leaks into the peritoneal cavity. The leakage of air produces hissing or bubbling sound which can be heard by a stethoscope over the iliac fossa.
  (b) *Hysterosalpingography:* It is a radiological technique in which a radiopaque substance (e.g., Lipiodol) is injected into the uterus by a suitable canula. It outlines the uterine cavity and uterine tubes, and if tubes are patent, the contrast medium spills into the peritoneal cavity.
- **Ectopic pregnancy:** It is commonest in the uterine tube (tubal gestation) and is usually associated with *intraperitoneal hemorrhage*, one of the causes of acute abdominal emergency in women of childbearing age. The hemorrhage occurs due to rupture of the tube caused by enlarging conceptus.
- **Tubectomy:** It is an operation for the female sterilization. In this procedure, each fallopian tube is ligated at two points and the segment of tube between the ligatures is resected. This prevents the meeting of male and female gametes, hence no fertilization. This is the ideal method of family planning in female.

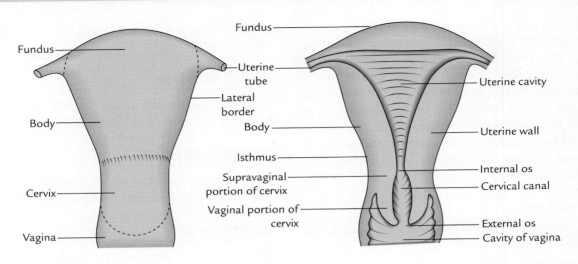

Fig. 18.9 Subdivisions of the uterus.

UTERUS

Synonym: Latin *uterus*; Greek *hystera*: womb; (viz., use of terms such as hysterectomy).

The uterus is a childbearing organ in females. It provides a suitable site and environment for implantation of a fertilized ovum and development of the embryo.

1. It is a hollow thick-walled, muscular organ with a narrow lumen.
2. It is situated obliquely in the lesser pelvis between urinary bladder and rectum.
3. Its long axis is horizontal if the bladder is empty in the *erect* posture.
4. Superiorly, on each side, it communicates with the uterine tube and inferiorly with the vagina (Fig. 18.9).

Shape and Size

It is *pear-shaped*, being flattened anteroposteriorly.

Measurements
Length: 3 inches (7.5 cm).
Breadth (at fundus): 2 inches (5 cm).
Thickness: 1 inch (2.5 cm).
Weight: 30–40 g.

SUBDIVISIONS/PARTS OF THE UTERUS (Fig. 18.9)

The uterus is divided into two main parts: (a) the large upper pear-shaped part—the **body** and (b) a small lower cylindrical part—the cervix. The body forms upper 2/3rd of uterus and **cervix** forms the lower 1/3rd of the uterus. The junction between the body and cervix is marked by a circular constriction called **isthmus**. It is well marked anteriorly. The uterine tubes are attached to the upper part of the body. The

point of fusion between the uterine tube and body is called cornu of the uterus.

Body

The upper expanded dome-like end of the body is called fundus. It is situated above the imaginary horizontal plane passing through the openings of the uterine tubes. The fundus is convex on all sides and covered by the peritoneum.

The body extends from the fundus to the isthmus and contains the **uterine** cavity. It is flattened anteroposteriorly and presents anterior and posterior surfaces, and right and left lateral borders.

Anterior surface: It is flat and directed downward and forward. It is covered by the peritoneum up to the isthmus, where it is reflected on to the upper surface of the urinary bladder forming the **uterovesical pouch** (Fig. 14.11).

Posterior surface: It is convex and directed upward and backward. It is covered by the peritoneum which extends downward up to the posterior fornix of the vagina, where it is reflected on the anterior aspect of rectum forming **rectouterine pouch** (or **pouch of Douglas**) (Fig. 14.11).

Right and left lateral border: Each lateral border is rounded and related to the uterine artery. It is non-peritoneal for it provides attachment to the broad ligament of uterus. The uterine tube enters the uterus at the upper end of this border. Here the round ligament of the uterus is attached anteroinferior to the tube and the ligament of the ovary is attached posteroinferior to the tube (Fig. 18.10).

Cervix

It is the lower cylindrical part. Its lower part projects into the upper part of the vagina through its anterior wall. Thus, the

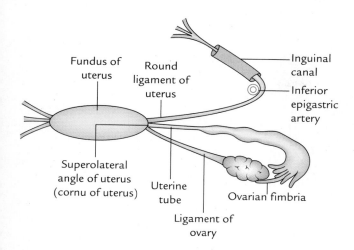

Fig. 18.10 Attachments of the uterine tube, round ligament of uterus, and ligament of ovary to the superolateral angle of uterus, i.e., upper end of the rounded lateral border of the uterine body.

cervix is divided into two parts: (a) upper supravaginal part and (b) lower vaginal part.

Clinically, the **isthmus** is formed by the upper one-third (nearly 0.8 mm) of the supravaginal cervix which is structurally similar to the uterus and forms what is called **"lower uterine segment"** by the obstetricians.

NORMAL POSITION AND AXES OF THE UTERUS (Fig. 18.11)

Normally the uterus lies in position of anteversion and anteflexion.

- *Anteversion:* The long axis of the cervix is normally bent forward on the long axis of vagina forming an angle of about 90°. This position is called the position of *anteversion.*
- *Anteflexion:* The long axis of the body of uterus is bent forward at the level of isthmus (internal os) on the long axis of cervix forming an angle of 170°. This position of the uterus is known as *anteflexion.*

N.B. The *angle of anteversion* is a forward angle between the long axis of cervix and the long axis of vagina. It measures about 90°.

The *angle of anteflexion* is a forward angle between the long axis of the body of uterus and the long axis of the cervix at the isthmus. It measures about 170°. However, most of the Indian books of anatomy describe it as 120°.

RELATIONS OF THE UTERUS (Fig. 18.12)

Anteriorly

1. The *body of uterus* is related to the uterovesical pouch and the superior surface of urinary bladder.

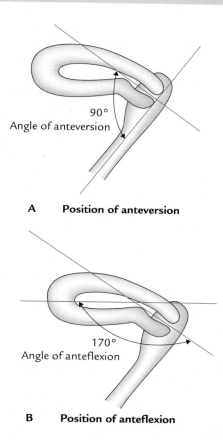

Fig. 18.11 Position of the uterus: A, angle of anteversion (angle between long axis of the vagina and long axis of the cervix); B, angle of anteflexion (angle between long axis of the cervix and long axis of the body of uterus).

2. The *supravaginal portion of cervix* is related to the posterior surface of urinary bladder.
3. The *vaginal portion of cervix* is related to the anterior fornix of the vagina.

Posteriorly

1. The *body of uterus* is related to the rectouterine pouch with coils of ileum and sigmoid colon in it.
2. The *supravaginal portion of cervix* is related to the rectouterine pouch with coils of ileum and sigmoid colon in it.
3. The *vaginal portion of cervix* is related to posterior fornix.

Laterally

1. The *body of uterus* is related to the broad ligament and uterine artery and vein.
2. The *supravaginal portion of cervix* is related to the ureter and uterine artery.
3. The *vaginal portion of cervix* is related to the lateral fornices of the vagina.

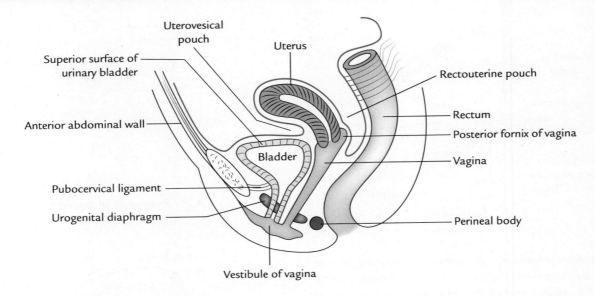

Fig. 18.12 Relations of the uterus.

CAVITY OF THE UTERUS (Fig. 18.13)

The cavity of uterus is small in comparison to its size due to its thick muscular wall. It is divided into two parts: cavity of the body and cavity of the cervix.

Cavity of the Body (Uterine Cavity Proper)

1. It is a **triangular** in coronal section (Fig. 18.13A). The apex of this cavity is continuous below with the *cervical canal* through *internal os*. The implantation commonly occurs in the upper part of its posterior wall.
2. It is a mere **slit** in sagittal section, because the uterus is compressed anteroposteriorly and its anterior and posterior walls are almost in contact.

Cavity of the Cervix (Cervical Canal)

It is a *spindle-shaped canal*, being broader in the middle and narrow at the ends. It communicates anterosuperiorly with the cavity of body of uterus through *internal os* and inferiorly with the cavity of vagina through *external os* (*ostium uteri*).

In nulliparous women (women who have not given birth to a baby) the external os is small and circular, whereas in multiparous women (women who have given birth to two or more babies) the external os is large and transverse, and presents anterior and posterior lips (Fig. 18.13B).

N.B. *Arbor vitae uteri:*
- Both anterior and posterior walls of the cervical canal present a longitudinal fold of mucous membrane. From each of these ridges a number of oblique folds like the fronds of a palm leaf (plicae palmatae) ascend laterally, giving the appearance of branches from the stem of a tree, hence the name *arbor vitae uteri*.

- The folds on the two walls are not opposed but fit between one another (interlocking) so as to close the cervical canal.

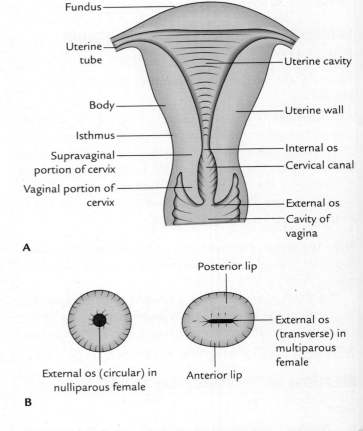

Fig. 18.13 A, Different parts of the uterus; B, shapes of external os in nulliparous and multiparous females.

LIGAMENTS

The ligaments of the uterus are classified into two types: false and true.

The false ligaments are peritoneal folds whereas the true ligaments are fibromuscular bands (Table 18.1). The false ligaments do not provide support to the uterus while true ligaments provide support to the uterus.

False Ligaments (Peritoneal Folds)

Broad Ligaments

These are the broad folds of peritoneum passing from the side of the uterus to the lateral wall of the pelvis on each side.

Together with the uterus they form a septum across the pelvic cavity, dividing it into a small anterior part containing bladder and a large posterior part containing rectum, coils of ileum, and sigmoid colon.

External features

Each broad ligament presents two surfaces and two borders. The details are given in Table 18.2.

Parts of the broad ligament

The broad ligament is subdivided into following four parts:

1. *Mesosalpinx:* It is the part of broad ligament between the fallopian tube and the ligament of the ovary.
2. *Mesometrium:* It is the part of broad ligament extending from the pelvic floor to the ovary, the ligament of ovary, and the body of uterus.
3. *Mesovarium:* It is the fold of posterior (or upper) layer of broad ligament extending to the ovary to be attached with it. It lies just below and behind the ampullary part of the uterine tube.
4. *Infundibulopelvic ligament* (also called *suspensory ligament of ovary*): It is that part of the broad ligament which:
   - Extends from the infundibulum of the tube and the upper pole of the ovary to the lateral wall of the lesser pelvis.
   - Contains the ovarian blood vessels, nerves, and lymph vessels.
   - Is continued laterally over the external iliac vessels as a distinct fold.

Contents of the broad ligament (Fig. 18.14)

The broad ligament contains the following structures:

1. *One tube*
   - Uterine tube.
2. *Two ligaments*
   - Round ligament of uterus.
   - Ligament of ovary.
3. *Two arteries*
   - Uterine artery.
   - Ovarian artery.
4. *Two plexuses of nerves*
   - Uterovaginal plexus.
   - Ovarian plexus.
5. *Three embryological remnants*
   - Epoophoron and its duct (Gartner's duct).
   - Paröophoron.
   - Vesicular appendices.
6. *Other structures*
   - Lymph vessels and lymph nodes.
   - Fibroareolar tissue.
   - Uterovaginal and ovarian nerve plexuses.

Uterovesical Fold (Anterior Ligament)

It is the fold of peritoneum, which is reflected from the front of the uterus on to the upper surface of the bladder at the level of isthmus.

Rectovaginal Fold (Posterior Ligament)

It is the fold of peritoneum which is reflected from the back of the posterior fornix of vagina on to the front of rectum.

Table 18.1 Ligaments of the uterus

False ligaments	True ligaments
Broad ligaments } Rectouterine folds } Paired	Round ligaments } Transverse cervical ligaments } Uterosacral ligaments } Pubocervical ligaments } Paired
Uterovesical fold (anterior ligament) } Rectovaginal fold (posterior ligament) } Unpaired	

Table 18.2 External features of the broad ligament of the uterus

Features	When the bladder is empty	When the bladder is distended
Two surfaces	• Superior • Inferior	• Posterior surface • Anterior surface
Two borders	• Anterior free border • Posterior attached border	• Upper free border • Inferior attached border (base of broad ligament)

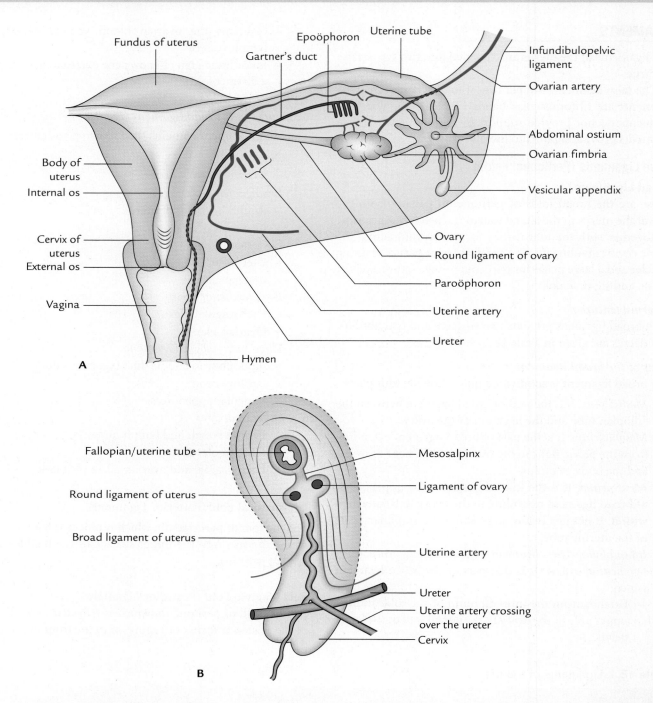

Fig. 18.14 Contents of the broad ligament: **A**, posterior aspect of the right broad ligament of the uterus. The posterior layer of the ligament has been removed to show the contents; **B**, sagittal section through the broad ligament of the uterus showing structures that lie within the broad ligament.

Rectouterine Fold

On each side, it is a semilunar fold of peritoneum extending between the cervix and the rectum. It forms the lateral boundary of rectouterine pouch (of Douglas).

N.B. *Rectouterine pouch (of Douglas):* It is the most dependent part of the pelvic peritoneal cavity. It is bounded in front by the supravaginal part of cervix and posterior fornix of vagina, behind by the middle third of the rectum, and on each side by the rectouterine fold. Its floor lies about 5.5 cm above the anal orifice and 7.5 cm above the vaginal orifice.

The collection of pus or blood in this pouch can be removed by giving an incision in the posterior fornix of vagina (**posterior colpotomy**).

True Ligaments (Fibromuscular Bands)

These ligaments provide support to the uterus, hence described under the heading, supports of the uterus (see page 273).

ARTERIAL SUPPLY (Fig. 18.15)

The uterus is supplied mainly by *two uterine arteries* and partly by *two ovarian arteries.*

The **uterine artery** is a branch of anterior division of internal iliac artery. It runs medially across the pelvic floor in the base of the broad ligament, towards the uterine cervix. It crosses the ureter from above lateral to the cervix above the lateral to the fornix of the vagina. Then it ascends along the side of the uterus. At the superolateral angle of uterus it turns laterally, runs along the uterine tube, and terminates by anastomosing with the ovarian artery.

Branches and Distribution

1. **Close to the cervix** after crossing the ureter, it gives rise to ureteric, vaginal, and cervical branches. The cervical branches form circular anastomosis around the isthmus.
2. **Along the side of body of the uterus** it gives off arcuate (coronary) branches which run transversely on the anterior and posterior surfaces of the body of uterus and anastomoses with their counter parts along the midline.
3. **Along the fallopian tube** it gives off tubal branches and few ovarian twigs.

The uterine artery thus supplies uterus, vagina, medial two-third of uterine tube, ovary, ureter, and structures within the broad ligament.

N.B. *Intrinsic uterine circulation* (Fig. 18.16):
- The arcuate (coronary) arteries (branches of the uterine arteries) of two sides anastomose on the anterior and posterior surfaces of the body of the uterus in the midline.

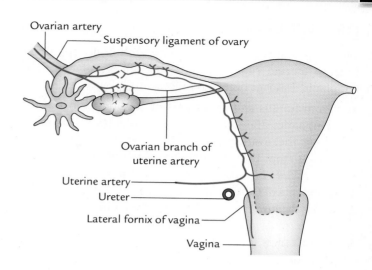

Fig. 18.15 Arterial supply of the uterus.

- The **radial arteries** arise from the arcuate arteries and pierce the myometrium centripetally and anastomose with each other to form stratum vasculare in the middle layer of muscular coat.
- From stratum vasculare, two sets of branches, basal and spiral, arise to supply the endometrium. The functional zone of the endometrium which is cast off during menstruation is supplied by the **spiral arteries**, whereas the basal zone of the endometrium which helps in the regeneration of the denuded endometrium is supplied by the **basal arteries**.

VENOUS DRAINAGE

The veins of the uterus correspond to arteries. They form venous plexus along the lateral borders of the uterus, which drains into internal iliac veins through uterine and vaginal veins.

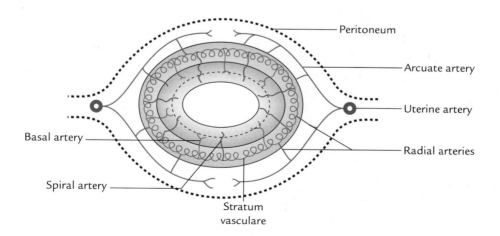

Fig. 18.16 Intrinsic circulation of the uterus.

LYMPHATIC DRAINAGE (Fig. 18.17)

The lymphatic drainage of the uterus is clinically important because uterine cancer spreads through lymphatics. The lymphatic drainage occurs as follows:

1. **From fundus and upper part of the body**, most of the lymphatics drain into *pre- and para-aortic lymph nodes* along the ovarian vessels. However, a few lymphatic vessels from the lateral angles of the uterus drain into *superficial inguinal lymph nodes* along the round ligaments of the uterus.
2. **From the lower part of the body**, the lymph vessels drain into *external iliac nodes* via broad ligament.
3. **From cervix**, on each side the lymph vessels drain in three directions:
   (a) **Laterally**, the lymph vessels drain into *external iliac and obturator nodes* by passing parametric tissue, few of these vessels are intercepted by *paracervical nodes*.
   (b) **Posterolaterally**, the lymph vessels drain into *internal iliac nodes* by passing along the uterine vessels.
   (c) **Posteriorly**, the lymph vessels drain into *sacral nodes* by passing along the uterosacral ligaments.

NERVE SUPPLY

The uterus is richly innervated by both sympathetic and parasympathetic fibres.

1. The **sympathetic fibres** are derived from T12–L2 spinal segments. The sympathetic fibres cause uterine contraction and vasoconstriction.
2. The **parasympathetic fibres** are derived from S2–S4 spinal segments. The parasympathetic fibres inhibit the uterine muscles and cause vasodilatation.
   Strictly speaking, the autonomic control of uterine activities is meager. In fact the uterine activities are mostly under hormonal control.
3. Visceral afferents carrying pain from the uterus take two pathways:
   (a) From the body of uterus, they follow sympathetic pathways. Hence, pain associated with uterine spasm is referred to the T12–L2 dermatomes (e.g., midback, pubic and inguinal regions, and anteromedial aspect of the thigh).
   (b) From the cervix, they cause along the *pelvic splanchnic nerves*, hence pain associated with cervical dilatation is referred to the sacral dermatomes (e.g., perineum, gluteal region, and posterior aspect of the thigh).

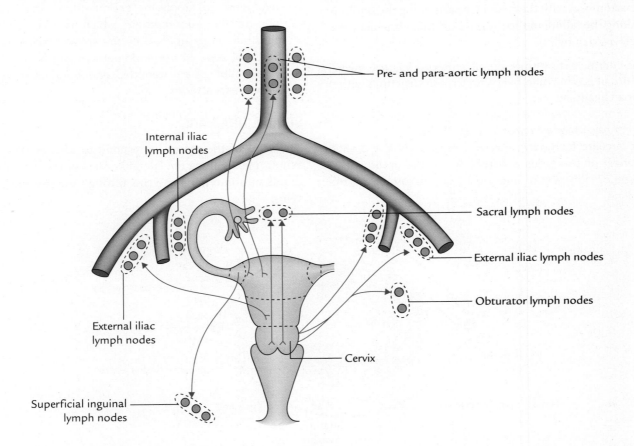

Pre- and para-aortic lymph nodes

Internal iliac lymph nodes

Sacral lymph nodes

External iliac lymph nodes

Obturator lymph nodes

External iliac lymph nodes

Cervix

Superficial inguinal lymph nodes

Fig. 18.17 Lymphatic drainage of the uterus.

STRUCTURE

The wall of the body of uterus consists of three layers. From superficial to deep these are:

1. **Perimetrium:** It is peritoneal covering of the uterus derived from broad ligament.
2. **Myometrium:** It is the thickest layer and consists of compactly arranged smooth muscle bundles.
3. **Endometrium:** It is the mucosal lining of the body of the uterus. It shows cyclic changes.

The structure of cervix is different from body for it is not lined by the endometrium and it does not show cyclic changes.

SUPPORTS OF THE UTERUS

The uterus is kept in position and prevented from sagging down by a number of structures providing support to it. The supports of the uterus are subdivided into two types: chief or primary supports and accessory or secondary supports.

Primary Supports

1. Muscular
   (a) Pelvic diaphragm (page 215).
   (b) Perineal body (page 231).
   (c) Urogenital diaphragm (page 230).
2. Visceral
   (a) Urinary bladder (page 238).
   (b) Vagina (page 274).
   (c) Uterine axis (page 267).
3. Fibromuscular (Fig. 18.18)

(a) Transverse cervical ligaments (of Mackenrodt).
(b) Pubocervical ligaments.
(c) Uterosacral ligaments.
(d) Round ligaments of the uterus.

Secondary Supports

1. Broad ligaments (page 269).
2. Uterovesical fold of peritoneum.
3. Rectovaginal fold of peritoneum.

The following text deals with only fibromuscular supports because others are described elsewhere on pages given in the brackets.

Transverse Cervical Ligaments (Mackenrodt's Ligaments)

They are the most important ligaments of the uterus, hence often called *cardinal ligaments*. They are formed by the condensation of pelvic fascia around the uterine vessels.

Each ligament forms a fan-shaped fibromuscular band which extends from the lateral aspect of cervix and upper vaginal wall to the lateral pelvic wall. They form a hammock which supports the uterus and prevent its downward displacement.

N.B. The tightening of Mackenrodt's ligament is commonly done in surgical repair of the prolapsed uterus.

Pubocervical Ligaments

These are a pair of fibrous bands which extend from the cervix to the posterior aspects of the pubic bones, along the inferolateral surfaces of the urinary bladder. They correspond to puboprostatic ligaments in male.

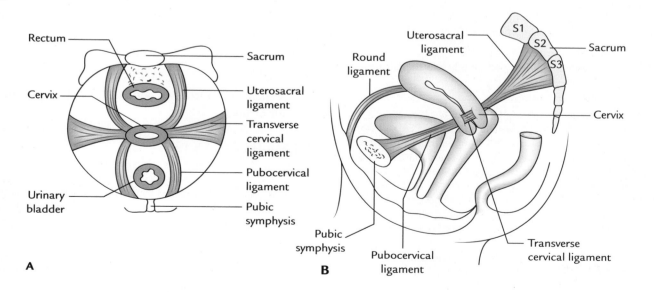

Fig. 18.18 Ligamentous (fibromuscular) supports of the uterus: **A**, as seen from above; **B**, lateral view. Note all these ligaments except the round ligaments are formed by the condensation of visceral layer of pelvic fascia.

Uterosacral Ligaments

These are a pair of fibrous bands which extend from the cervix to the second and third sacral vertebrae, and pass on each side of the rectum.

They lie underneath the rectouterine folds of peritoneum which form the lateral boundaries of the rectouterine pouch.

These ligaments pull the cervix backward against the forward pull of the round ligaments and help in the maintenance of anteflexed and anteverted positions of the uterus.

Round Ligaments of the Uterus (Ligament Teres Uteri)

These are a pair of long (10–12 cm) fibromuscular bands which lie between the two layers of broad ligament.

Each ligament begins at the lateral angle of the uterus, passes forward and laterally between the two layers of broad ligament, enters the deep inguinal ring after winding around the lateral side of the inferior epigastric artery. It traverses the inguinal canal, emerges through the superficial inguinal ring, and splits into numerous thread-like fibrous bands which merge with the fibroareolar tissue of the labium majus.

These ligaments pull the fundus forward and help to maintain the anteversion and anteflexion of the uterus.

Clinical correlation

- **Cervical carcinoma:** It is the most common cancer in females (11%). The second commonest cancer in females is breast cancer (about 8%). It is rare before 20 years of age and reaches its peak between the ages 45 and 55 years. 80% cervical cancers are squamous cell carcinoma and are related to sexual activity. Early sexual exposure and promiscuity are prominent factors.
- It spreads directly to adjacent structures and metastasizes via lymphatics to pelvic lymph nodes and then to the pre-aortic and para-aortic lymph nodes.

Clinical features

1. Abnormal vaginal bleeding particularly intermenstrual.
2. Postcoital bleeding.
3. Pain, anorexia, and weight loss.
4. *Fibroids/fibromyomas of uterus:* These are benign tumors arising from myometrial cells. They are found in about one-fifth of women above 35 years of age. They are usually multiple and may undergo degenerative charges. They undergo atrophy after menopause. Clinically they present as abnormal bleeding (hypermenorrhea) and irregular contour of the uterus on bimanual palpation. They are often asymptomatic. Small asymptomatic fibroids require no treatment. If large, *hysterectomy* (removal of uterus) is the treatment of choice.
5. *Caesarean section:* It is the surgical procedure for delivering the baby by cutting open the abdomen and uterus in cases where vaginal delivery is not possible. The term caesarean section is so named because the Roman Emperor Julius Caesar was supposedly born by this surgical procedure.

VAGINA

Synonym: Greek *Kolpos*: vagina; use of terms such as colpotomy and colporrhaphy.

The vagina is a female organ of copulation and forms the lower part of the birth canal. The term vagina means sheath (cf. vagina forms sheath around the penis during copulation).

It extends upward and backward from the vestibule of vagina (a cleft between the labia minora) to the uterus. It lies between the bladder and urethra in front and rectum and anal canal behind.

The axis of the vagina corresponds with the axis of the pelvic outlet.

SIZE AND SHAPE

Length: The anterior wall of the vagina is 7.5 cm long whereas posterior wall is 9 cm long.
Width: It gradually increases from below upward. The diameter at the upper end is roughly double in size to that at the lower end.
- Diameter at the upper end: 5 cm.
- Diameter at the lower end: 2.5 cm.
Lumen of vagina in cross section:
- In the lower one-third: H-shaped.
- In the middle one-third: Transverse slit.
- In the upper one-third: Round/circular.

FORNICES OF VAGINA

The upper part of the vagina surrounds the cervix of the uterus. The circular area of vaginal lumen around the cervix is called fornix of vagina. It is a short distance above the external os, and deep behind than in front. For the sake of description, the fornix of vagina is divided into four parts:

- Anterior part/anterior fornix.
- Posterior part/posterior fornix.
- Two lateral parts/lateral fornices.

The posterior fornix is about 2 cm deeper than the anterior fornix.

RELATIONS (Fig. 18.19)

Anteriorly

1. The *upper half* is related to the base of urinary bladder.
2. The *lower half* is related to the urethra which is actually embedded in it.

Posteriorly

1. The *upper one-fourth* is related to the rectouterine pouch (or pouch of Douglas).
2. The *middle two-fourth* is related to the ampulla of rectum from which it is separated by loose connective tissue.

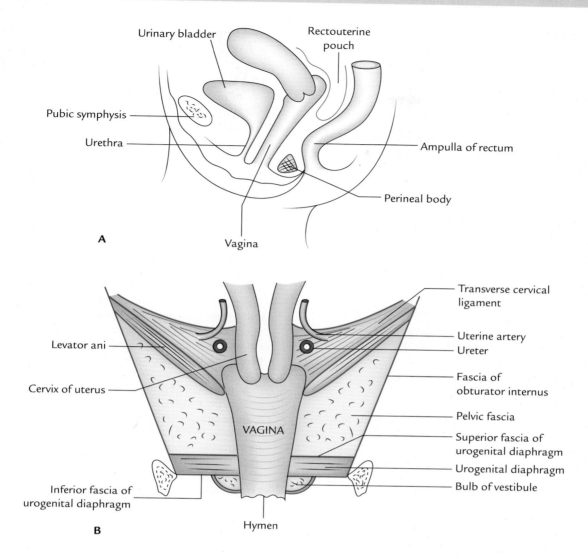

Fig. 18.19 Relations of the vagina: **A**, as seen in the sagittal section; **B**, as seen in the coronal section.

3. The *lower one-fourth* is related to the perineal body separating it from the anal canal.

Laterally

1. The *upper part* is related to the ureters which are close to the lateral fornices and are crossed by the uterine artery.
2. The *middle part* is related to the anterior fibres of levator ani (pubococcygeus part) and pelvic fascia.
3. The *lower part* is related to urogenital diaphragm, bulb of vestibule, bulbospongiosus, and greater vestibular gland (of Bartholin).

STRUCTURE

The wall of vagina consists of the following three layers:

1. An *outer adventitial layer* is made up of loose connective tissue. It contains blood vessels, lymphatics, and nerves.

2. A *muscular layer* is made up of smooth muscle which consists of an outer longitudinal layer and inner circular layer.

3. *Mucous lining:*
   (a) Epithelium is stratified, squamous, non-keratinized containing glycogen in adult women.

   The fluid in the vagina is kept acidic by fermentive action of certain bacteria (*Döderlein's bacilli*) on glycogen, forming lactic acid.

   (b) Lamina propria is dense and contains many elastic fibres.

   There are no glands in the vaginal mucous membrane, but it is kept moist or lubricated by mucous derived from the glands of cervix.

The combination of muscular layer and a highly elastic lamina propria permits the gross distension of the vagina during parturition (childbirth).

Hymen of Vagina

It is an incomplete mucous fold closing the vaginal cavity close to the external orifice of the vagina. The hymen presents various shapes—annular, crescentic, or cribriform. During coitus the hymen ruptures and becomes fissured producing tags of mucous membrane called caruncles.

Rarely the hymen is a complete membrane and obstructs discharge of the blood during menstruation leading to hematocolpos.

N.B. The features of hymen are examined for the medicolegal purpose to confirm virginity.

ARTERIAL SUPPLY

The vagina is a highly vascular organ and is supplied by the following arteries:

1. Vaginal artery, a branch of the internal iliac artery (main artery).
2. Vaginal branch of uterine artery.
3. Internal pudendal artery.
4. Middle rectal artery.
5. Inferior vesical artery.

The vaginal branches of uterine internal iliac arteries anastomose to form midline longitudinal vessels (**azygos vaginal arteries**) along the anterior and posterior vaginal walls.

VENOUS DRAINAGE

The veins of the vagina form a rich venous plexus known as *pampiniform plexus* at the sides of vagina which drains through *vaginal veins* into the internal iliac veins.

LYMPHATIC DRAINAGE

The lymphatics of vagina are divided into three groups:

1. *From upper one-third of vagina*, lymphatics accompany the uterine artery to drain into internal and external iliac nodes.
2. *From middle one-third of vagina*, lymphatics accompany the vaginal artery to drain into internal iliac nodes.
3. *From lower one-third* (strictly speaking vagina below the hymen) of lymphatics accompany those from the vulva to drain into the medial group of superficial inguinal nodes.

NERVE SUPPLY

1. The *upper two-third of vagina* is insensitive to pain, touch, and temperature but it is sensitive to stretch. It is supplied by the sympathetic (L1, L2 spinal segments) and parasympathetic (S2, S3 spinal segments) fibres.

2. The *lower one-third of vagina*, including *region of vaginal orifice*, is extremely sensitive to touch. It is supplied by the pudendal nerve via inferior rectal and posterior labial branches of perineal nerve.

Clinical correlation

*   **Per vaginal (PV) examination** is done to estimate the different pathological conditions by palpating the pelvic organs.
*   **Vaginitis (infection of vagina)** is uncommon in healthy adult females because the vagina is self-sterilizing in adult due to its acidic medium (pH = 4.5) in which organisms are unable to grow. In the child, the normal defence mechanism of the vagina is absent.

    The acidic medium is due to the presence of *Döderlein's bacilli* producing lactic acid from glycogen in the vaginal epithelial cells which is dependent upon the activity of estrogen on the cells causing growth and maturation. After menopause the vaginal epithelium atrophies. Therefore, vaginitis is common in children and old women (after menopause).
*   **Prolapse:** The prolapse of anterior vaginal wall may drag the urinary bladder (*cystocele*) or urethra (*urethrocele*). The prolapse of the posterior vaginal wall drags the rectum (rectocele).
*   **Culdocentesis:** It is a clinical procedure in which a needle is passed through the posterior fornix of vagina into the rectouterine pouch (of Douglas) to drain the pus accumulated in this pouch in pelvic inflammatory disease or blood following rupture of the fallopian tube due to ectopic tubal pregnancy. Nowadays this procedure is used to obtain a fluid sample for collecting oocytes for in vitro fertilization.

EXTERNAL GENITAL ORGANS

The female external genitalia (or vulva/pudendum) consists of a vestibule of vagina and its surrounding structures such as mons pubis, labia majora, labia minora, clitoris, and pair of greater vestibular glands.

Vestibule of Vagina

It is an elliptical space between the labia minora. It contains *urethral orifice* anteriorly and *vaginal orifice* (*vaginal introitus*) posteriorly. The latter is incompletely covered by hymen. In addition to the above openings, it also contains the openings of *greater vestibular glands* (*of Bartholin*), *lesser vestibular glands,* and *paraurethral glands* (*of Skene*).

Mons Pubis

It is an elevation of skin over the pubic symphysis with underlying thick fat pad. The anterior ends of two labia major unite on its sides. It acts as cushion during coitus.

Labia Majora

These are folds of hairy skin with underlying fat pads which unite anteriorly to form the mons pubis.

Labia Minora

These are two thin folds of hairless skin located medial to the labia majora. They enclose the vestibule of vagina. Two labia minora are continuous anteriorly with the prepuce and frenulum of the clitoris; and posteriorly with the *fourchette* which connect the labia minora with the vaginal orifice.

Clitoris

It is a small erectile structure (less than 2 cm in length) located into the anterior margin of the vestibule of vagina. *It is homologous of the penis in male but does not transmit urethra.* The body of clitoris is formed by two corpora cavernosa which are continuous with the crura. The glans of clitoris is formed by the fusion of anterior ends of the bulbs of the vestibule. There is no corpus spongiosum in the body of clitoris. The corpus spongiosum in female is represented by bulbs of the vestibule and glans of clitoris.

The clitoris is richly innervated by sensory receptors which function to initiate and intensify sexual pleasure.

Golden Facts to Remember

► Least movable part of the uterus	Cervix
► Commonest site of fertilization	Ampulla of the uterine tube
► Most important ligaments of the uterus	Transverse cervical ligaments (of Mackenrodt)
► Most common cancer in the female	Cervical cancer
► Largest birth canal	Vagina
► Commonest site of implantation	Posterior wall of the body of uterus
► Most important surgical relation of the uterine artery	Where it crosses the ureter anterosuperiorly (from lateral to medial side)

Clinical Case Study

A 55-year-old woman complained that for the past 2 months she has been feeling the sensation of something coming down into the vagina. She also complained of dribbling of urine on forceful coughing and frequency of micturition. On PV examination, the gynecologist found the descent of cervix into the vagina and cystocele. A diagnosis of "**uterovaginal prolapse**" was made.

Questions

1. What is the normal position of the uterus?
2. What is the commonest cause of prolapse uterus?
3. Name the three chief supports of the uterus.
4. What is the angle of anteversion and what is the angle of anteflexion? Give their measurements.

Answers

1. Anteverted and anteflexed.
2. Relaxation of the pelvic diaphragm due to tear of perineal body in adult and loss of muscle tone in old age.
3. Pelvic diaphragm, perineal body, and transverse cervical ligaments (of Mackenrodt).
4. Angle of anteversion is the forward angle between the long axis of the vagina and the long axis of the cervix.

   Angle of anteflexion is the forward angle between the long axis of the cervix and the long axis of the body of uterus.

   The angle of anteversion measures about 90° and the angle of anteflexion measures about 120°–170°.

Rectum and Anal Canal

RECTUM

The rectum is the distal part of the large intestine between the sigmoid colon and the anal canal. In Latin, the word "rectum" means straight; but the rectum is straight in quadrupeds and not in men. Although the rectum is a part of the large intestine, it is devoid of taenia coli, sacculations and appendices epiploicae—the cardinal features of the large intestine.

The distension of the rectum initiates the desire to defecate.

LOCATION

It is situated in the posterior part of the lesser pelvis in front of the lower three pieces of the sacrum and the coccyx (Fig. 19.1) and behind the urinary bladder in the male and uterus in the female.

Measurements

The rectum is 5 inches (12 cm) long. The diameter of the rectum is not uniform throughout. In the upper part it is 4 cm as that of the sigmoid colon. In the lower part, it forms a dilatation called **rectal ampulla**. When empty the anterior and posterior walls of the rectum are in contact and cross section of the rectum presents lumen in the form of a transverse slit.

EXTENT AND COURSE

The rectum begins as a continuation of the sigmoid colon in front of the third sacral vertebra and becomes continuous with the anal canal about 2–3 cm in front and a little below the tip of the coccyx. The *rectosigmoid junction* is indicated by the lower end of the sigmoid mesocolon.

From its beginning in front of S3 vertebra, first it runs downward and backward, then vertically downward, and finally downward and forward. About 2.5 cm in front and a little below the tip of coccyx, it abruptly turns downward and backward to become continuous with the anal canal. The *anorectal junction* corresponds with the apex of prostate in male.

To summarize the direction of the course is as under:

- *In the upper third*—rectum is directed downward and backward.
- *In the middle third*—rectum is directed vertically downward.
- *In the lower third*—rectum is directed downward and forward.

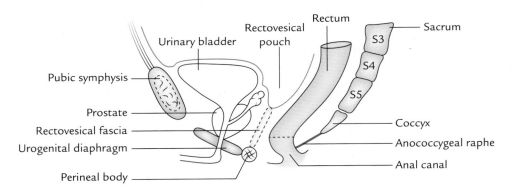

Fig. 19.1 Location of the rectum (as seen in the sagittal section through the male pelvis).

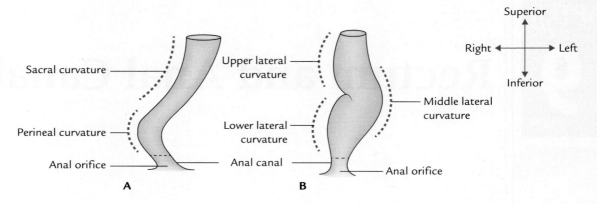

Fig. 19.2 Curvatures (flexures) of the rectum: **A**, anteroposterior curvatures; **B**, lateral curvatures.

CURVATURES (FLEXURES OF THE RECTUM)

The rectum presents curvatures in both anteroposterior and lateral planes (Fig. 19.2).

ANTEROPOSTERIOR CURVATURES

These are two in number, an upper **sacral curvature** and a lower **perineal curvature**.

1. *Sacral curvature* corresponds to the concavity of the sacrum and coccyx.
2. *Perineal curvature* corresponds to the forward bend of the anorectal junction. It is maintained by the puborectal sling derived from the levator ani (Fig. 19.3).

LATERAL CURVATURES

These are three in number and present in the form of two convexities to the right side and one convexity to the left side.

1. *Upper lateral curve* is convex to the right at the junction of S3, S4 vertebrae.
2. *Middle lateral curvature* is convex to the left at the sacrococcygeal junction. It is the most prominent curvature.

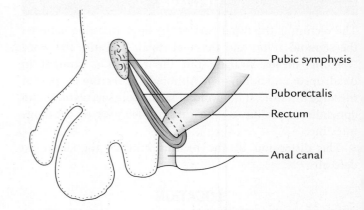

Fig. 19.3 Puborectal sling of the levator ani.

3. *Lower lateral curvature* is convex to the right at the level of tip of the coccyx.

PERITONEAL RELATIONS OF THE RECTUM (Fig. 19.4)

The peritoneal relations of the rectum are as under:
*   *Upper one-third of the rectum* is covered with the peritoneum on the front and sides.

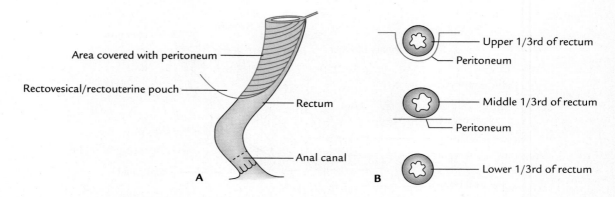

Fig. 19.4 Peritoneal relations of the rectum: **A**, in sagittal section; **B**, in cross sections of the levels of upper 1/3rd, middle 1/3rd, and lower 1/3rd.

- *Middle one-third of the rectum* is covered with the peritoneum only on the front.
- *Lower one-third of the rectum (ampulla)* is not covered by the peritoneum at all.

N.B. The ampulla of rectum lies below the level of rectovesical pouch in the male and rectouterine pouch in the female.

RELATIONS

Anterior Relations

The anterior relations of the rectum differ in male and female. They are given in Table 19.1.

Posterior Relations (Figs 19.5 and 19.6)

The posterior relations are same in both male and female. They are given in Table 19.2.

Lateral Relations

1. *Upper part of rectum* is related to pararectal fossae containing coils of small intestine and sigmoid colon.
2. *Lower part of rectum* is related to levator ani muscles which intimately surround it and provide support.

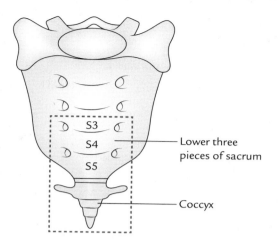

Fig. 19.5 Parts of the sacrum and coccyx covered by the rectum.

INTERIOR OF THE RECTUM

The interior of the rectum presents two types of mucosal folds—temporary and permanent.

- *Temporary folds* are mostly longitudinal and found in the lower part of the rectum. They disappear when rectum distends.

Table 19.1 Anterior relations of the rectum in male and female

Portion of rectum	Relations	
	In male	In female
Upper two-third of rectum (peritoneal)	Rectovesical pouch and coils of the small intestine and sigmoid colon within it	Rectouterine pouch and coils of the small intestine and sigmoid colon within it
Lower one-third of rectum/ ampulla (non-peritoneal)	• Base of the urinary bladder • Ureters (terminal parts) • Seminal vesicles • Ampullae of vas deferens • Prostate (All these structures are separated from the rectum by the well-defined rectovesical fascia of Denonvilliers)	Vagina (lower part) (It is separated from rectum by an ill-defined rectovaginal fascia)

Table 19.2 Posterior relations of the rectum in male and female

Posterior relations	
In the midline	On each side of midline
• Lower three pieces of sacrum • Coccyx • Anococcygeal raphe • Ganglion impar • Median sacral vessels • Superior rectal artery (opposite S3 vertebra only) • Fascia of Waldeyer*	• Piriformis ⎫ • Coccygeus ⎬ Mostly of the left side • Levator ani • Sympathetic chains • Anterior primary rami of S3, S4, S5, and coccygeal nerve (Co1) • Pelvic splanchnic nerves • Lateral sacral vessels

*The *fascia of Waldeyer* is a connective tissue by which rectum (ampulla) is attached to the sacrum and coccyx.

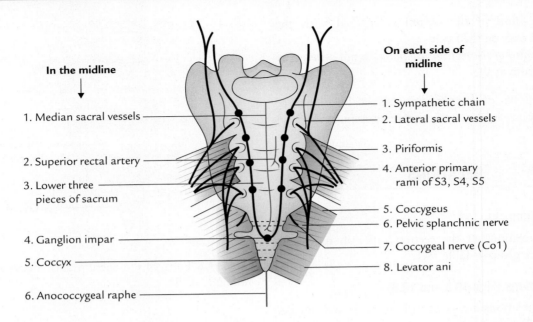

In the midline
↓
1. Median sacral vessels
2. Superior rectal artery
3. Lower three pieces of sacrum
4. Ganglion impar
5. Coccyx
6. Anococcygeal raphe

On each side of midline
↓
1. Sympathetic chain
2. Lateral sacral vessels
3. Piriformis
4. Anterior primary rami of S3, S4, S5
5. Coccygeus
6. Pelvic splanchnic nerve
7. Coccygeal nerve (Co1)
8. Levator ani

Fig. 19.6 Posterior relations of the rectum.

- *Permanent folds (or Houston's valves; Fig. 19.7)* are semilunar (crescentic) transverse folds situated against the concavities of the lateral curvatures of the rectum. They are formed by the reduplication of the mucous membrane containing submucous tissue and thickening of circular smooth muscle of the rectal wall. They are permanent and become more prominent when the rectum is distended. According to Houston, they are four in number and are numbered from above downward as follows:

  1. *First fold (or upper fold)* lies near the upper end close to the rectosigmoid junction. It projects from the right or left wall.

  2. *Second fold* lies about 1 inch (2.5 cm) above the third fold and projects from the left rectal wall along the concavity of upper lateral curvature.

  3. *Third valve* is the largest, most constant, and most important. It projects from the anterior and right wall of the rectum along the concavity of middle lateral curvature. It lies at the level of upper end of ampulla.

  4. *Fourth valve* projects from the left wall of the rectum along the concavity of lower lateral curvature. It lies about 2.5 cm below the third valve.

N.B. The transverse folds of the rectum (rectal valves) provide support to hold the faeces and prevent the excessive

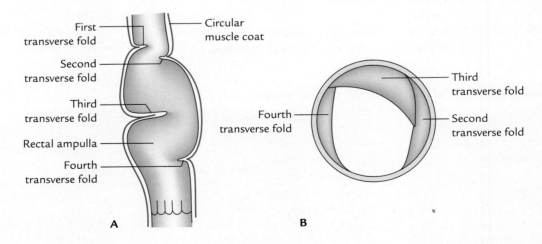

First transverse fold
Second transverse fold
Third transverse fold
Rectal ampulla
Fourth transverse fold
Circular muscle coat
Fourth transverse fold
Third transverse fold
Second transverse fold

A

B

Fig. 19.7 Transverse folds within the lumen of the rectum: A, as seen from above; B, as seen in the coronal section of the rectum.

distension of the rectal ampulla. They can be seen *per anum* with the aid of a speculum.

ARTERIAL SUPPLY (Fig. 19.8)

The rectum is supplied by the following arteries:

1. *Superior rectal artery* (chief artery of the rectum), a continuation of the inferior mesentery artery.
2. *Middle rectal arteries* (2 in number). Each is a branch from the anterior division of the internal iliac artery.
3. *Inferior rectal arteries* (2 in number). Each is a branch of internal pudendal artery.
4. *Median sacral artery,* a branch of the abdominal aorta.

Superior Rectal Artery

It is the chief/principal artery of the rectum and supplies entire mucous membrane up to the anal valves, and the musculature of the upper part of the rectum. It is the continuation of the inferior mesenteric artery (at the pelvic brim) and reaches the back of the rectosigmoid junction opposite the S3 vertebra, where it divides into right and left branches. The right branch further divides into anterior and posterior branches. The branches of both sides subdivide into smaller branches, which pierce the rectal wall and form looped anastomoses in the submucous coat of the lower part of the rectum. From this plexus, straight vessels descend in the anal columns and anastomoses with the branches of the inferior rectal artery at the pectinate line.

Middle Rectal Arteries

The middle rectal artery is a branch of anterior division of the internal iliac artery and passes downward and medially through the lateral ligament of the rectum and supplies the lower part of the rectum. The middle rectal arteries are unimportant because they supply only the superficial coats of the rectum.

Inferior Rectal Arteries

The inferior rectal artery is a branch of the internal pudendal artery. It passes across the ischiorectal fossa to supply the perianal skin, anal sphincters, and anastomoses with the branches of the superior rectal artery at the pectinate line.

Median Sacral Artery

It is a small branch, which arises from the posterior aspect of the aorta near its lower end. It descends in the median plane to supply the posterior wall of the anorectal junction.

VENOUS DRAINAGE

The venous blood from the rectum is drained by the following veins (Fig. 19.9):

1. Superior rectal vein.
2. Middle rectal veins (two in number).
3. Inferior rectal veins (two in number).

The rectal veins arise from **internal and external venous plexuses of the rectum and anal canal.**

The **internal venous plexus** is present in the submucous coat and surrounds the anal canal above Hilton's line. The **external venous plexus** is present between the perianal skin and the subcutaneous part of the external anal sphincter. It surrounds the anus. The internal and external venous plexuses communicate with each other.

Thus, the lower part of the rectum and the anal canal are surrounded by a venous plexus called *annulus hemorrhoidalis.*

Superior Rectal Veins

The tributaries of this vein begin in the anal canal from the *internal rectal venous plexus* in the form of six veins. They pass upward through the anal columns and submucous coat of the rectum, and unite to form the superior rectal vein which pierces the muscular coat of posterior rectal wall about 3 inches (7.5 cm) above the anus. The superior rectal vein continues upward as the inferior mesenteric vein which drains into the splenic vein (portal system).

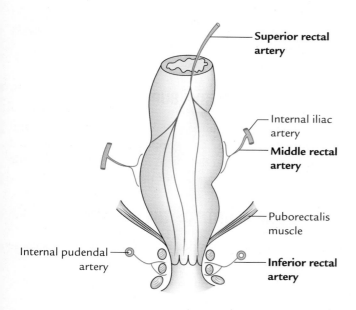

Fig. 19.8 Arterial supply of the rectum and anal canal.

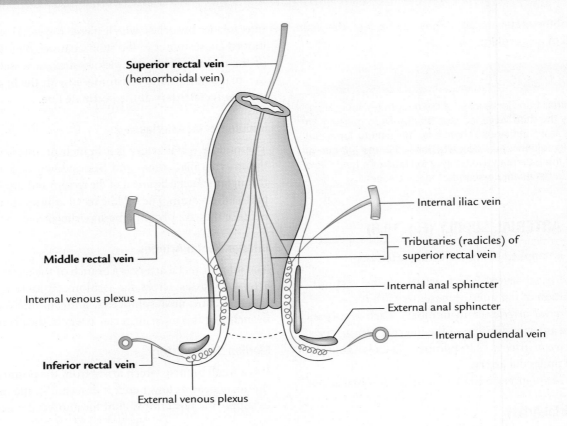

Fig. 19.9 Venous drainage of the rectum and anal canal.

Middle Rectal Veins

These veins arise one on each side from the middle of venous plexus, pass along the lateral pelvic wall, and drain into the internal iliac vein (systemic vein).

Inferior Rectal Veins

These veins arise from the lower part of the plexus. Each vein extends across the ischiorectal fossa and drains into the internal pudendal vein on the corresponding side.

N.B. The superior rectal vein, a tributary of portal vein forms anastomosis with middle and inferior rectal veins the tributary of inferior vena cava at the level of mid-anal canal (one of the important sites of portocaval anastomosis).

LYMPHATIC DRAINAGE (Fig. 19.10)

- *Lymphatics from the upper half* accompany the superior rectal vessels and drain into the **inferior mesenteric nodes**. A few of these vessels are intercepted by the *pararectal lymph nodes* situated on each side of the rectosigmoid junction.
- *Lymphatics from the lower half* accompany the middle rectal vessels and drain into the **internal iliac nodes**.

Clinical correlation

The lymphatics of the rectum are mostly arranged longitudinally in contrast to the lymphatics of most of the small and large intestines, where they are arranged transversely around the gut.

Therefore, when the carcinoma of the rectum spreads along lymphatics it does not cause rectal obstruction unlike the rest of the gut.

NERVE SUPPLY

The rectum is supplied by both sympathetic and parasympathetic fibres. The sympathetic fibres are derived from L1, L2 segments of the spinal cord and parasympathetic fibres from S2, S3, S4 segments of the spinal cord.

SUPPORTS OF THE RECTUM

The rectum is kept in position and prevented from prolapse by the following structures:

1. *Pelvic diaphragm:* It is formed by the levator ani muscles. The puborectalis sling of this diaphragm surrounds the anorectal junction and maintains the anorectal flexure.

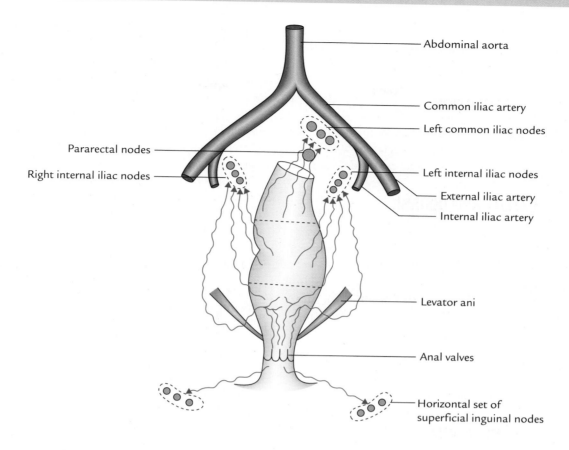

Fig. 19.10 Lymphatic drainage of the rectum and anal canal.

2. *Fascia of Waldeyer:* It is a connective tissue behind the rectum. It extends from the lower part of rectal ampulla to the sacrum and coccyx. It contains perirectal fat, lymph nodes, lymphatics, and superior rectal vessels.

3. *Lateral ligaments of the rectum:* These are fibrous bands formed by the condensation of pelvic fascia one on each side of the rectum. They attach the rectum to the posterolateral walls of the lesser pelvis and contain the middle rectal vessels.

4. *Rectovesical fascia of Denonvilliers.*

5. *Reflection of pelvic fascia* from parietal to visceral layers around the rectum.

6. *Pelvirectal and ischiorectal fat* act as a loose packing material around the rectum and anal canal.

7. Pelvic peritoneum and related vascular pedicles.

8. Perineal body.

Clinical correlation

Prolapse of rectum: It is the protrusion of the rectum through the anus. The prolapse may be incomplete or complete.

(a) *Incomplete prolapse (mucous prolapse):* It is the protrusion of rectal mucosa through the anus and occurs due to excessive straining during defecation. This is due to imperfect support of the rectal mucosa by the submucosa.

(b) *Complete prolapse (procidentia):* In this condition, whole thickness of the rectal wall protrudes through the anus. The causative factors are laxity of the pelvic diaphragm, excessively deep rectovesical or rectouterine pouch and inadequate fixation of the rectum in its presacral bed.

Clinically, it presents as (a) protrusion of the bowel through the anus, (b) mucous discharge and bleeding, (c) pain, and (d) anal incontinence (due to stretching of internal and external anal sphincters).

ANAL CANAL

The anal canal is the terminal part (3.8 cm long) of the large intestine, situated in the perineum below the pelvic diaphragm. Like rectum it is devoid of sacculations, taenia coli, and appendices epiploicae. It is surrounded by an inner involuntary sphincter and an outer voluntary sphincter, whose tone keeps the anal canal closed except during the defecation.

LOCATION

The anal canal is located in the anal triangle of the perineum between the right and left fat-filled ischiorectal fossae. These fossae allow the expansion of the anal canal during defecation.

EXTENT AND COURSE

The anal canal begins at the *anorectal junction*, passes downward and backward, and opens at the **anal orifice,** which is situated in the *natal cleft* (cleft between the buttocks) about 4 cm below and in front of the tip of coccyx. The skin surrounding the anal orifice is pigmented and thrown into radiating folds due to a pull exerted by underlying subcutaneous muscle—the **corrugator cutis ani.**

N.B. The anorectal junction is surrounded by puborectalis which pulls it forward producing, forward convexity and backward bend of 90° (perineal flexure).

RELATIONS

These are as follows:

Anteriorly:
● Perineal body.
● Bulb of penis and spongy urethra in male and lower part of the vagina in female.

Posteriorly:
● Anococcygeal raphe.
● Tip of coccyx.
● Fibrofatty tissue between the perineal skin and the anococcygeal raphe.

Laterally (on each side): Ischiorectal fossa.

INTERIOR OF THE ANAL CANAL (Fig. 19.11)

The anal canal is divided into upper and lower parts by the **pectinate line**. The pectinate line represents the embryological site of attachment of the anal membrane.

The upper part of the anal canal extends from the anorectal junction to the pectinate line; and the lower part of the anal canal extends from the pectinate line to the anal verge.

The upper and lower parts of the anal canal are different in development, blood supply, lymphatic drainage, and nerve supply. The differences between the upper and lower anal canals are given in Table 19.3.

FEATURES IN THE UPPER PART OF ANAL CANAL

The upper part of the anal canal (15 mm long) presents the following features:

1. *Anal columns (columns of Morgagni):* These are permanent longitudinal mucous folds numbering 6 to 10. They contain radicles of the superior rectal vein.
2. *Anal valves (valves of Morgagni):* These are crescentic folds of the mucous membrane which connect the lower

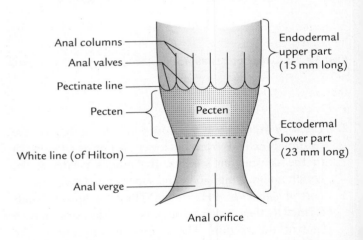

Fig. 19.11 Interior of the anal canal.

Table 19.3 Differences between the upper and lower anal canals

Features	Upper anal canal	Lower anal canal
Development	From endoderm of the hind gut	From ectoderm of proctodeum
Innervation	Autonomic nerves, hence insensitive to pain and temperature	Somatic nerves, hence sensitive to pain and temperature
Epithelial lining	Simple columnar	Stratified squamous
Arterial supply	Superior rectal artery	Inferior rectal artery
Venous drainage	Superior rectal vein draining into portal system	Inferior rectal vein draining into caval system
Lymphatic drainage	Internal iliac lymph nodes	Superficial inguinal lymph nodes (horizontal set)
Hemorrhoids	Internal hemorrhoids	External hemorrhoids

ends of adjacent anal columns. The free margins of these valves are directed upward. The position of these valves is indicated by the wavy pectinate line (also called dentate line).

3. *Anal sinuses:* These are vertical recesses between the anal columns and above the anal valves. The ducts of **tubular anal glands** present in the submucosa open in the floor of anal sinuses.

FEATURES IN THE LOWER PART OF ANAL CANAL

The lower anal canal is further divided into two regions: upper and lower.

(a) *Upper region (often called pecten):* It is 15 mm long and extends from the pectinate line to Hilton's line. It is lined by the non-keratinized stratified squamous epithelium. The mucous lining in this region appears bluish in colour due to underlying dense venous plexus and is adherent to the underlying structures.

(b) *Lower region of lower anal canal:* It is about 8 mm in extent and lined by the true skin containing sweat and sebaceous gland. It shows pigmentation. In adult males, coarse hairs are often found around the anal orifice.

N.B. *Hilton's line:* The white line of Hilton is situated at the junction of the subcutaneous external anal sphincter and the lower end of internal anal sphincter, and represented by the anal intersphincteric groove. It presents the following features:

• It demarcates mucocutaneous junction.
• It appears white because it lies between the bluishpinkish area above and blackish skin below, hence the name **white line of Hilton**.

ANAL SPHINCTERS (Fig. 19.12)

There are two sphincters, (internal and external), around the anal canal, which provide powerful sphincteric mechanism at the distal end of the gastrointestinal tract.

INTERNAL SPHINCTER

1. It is formed by thickened circular muscle coat of the anal canal and surrounds the upper two-third of the canal.
2. Above, it is continuous with the circular muscle coat of the rectum and below reaches up to the level of the white line of Hilton.
3. It is surrounded by the deep and superficial parts of the external anal sphincter.

EXTERNAL SPHINCTER (Figs 19.12 and 19.13)

The external anal sphincter as the name implies is outside the internal anal sphincter. It surrounds the whole length of the anal canal and consists of three parts: deep, superficial, and subcutaneous.

Deep Part

The deep part surrounds the upper part of the internal sphincter. It has no bony attachments. The puborectalis blends with the deep part of external sphincter behind and forms a sling around the anorectal junction, which is attached anteriorly to the back of the pubis. In the resting state, the anorectal tube is angled forward at this level and contraction of puborectalis sling will increase this angle, an important factor in the continence mechanism.

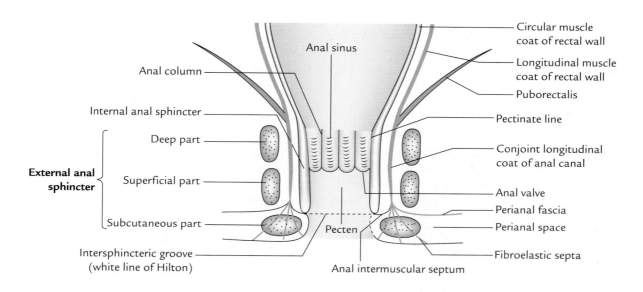

Fig. 19.12 A coronal section of anal canal showing internal and external anal sphincters.

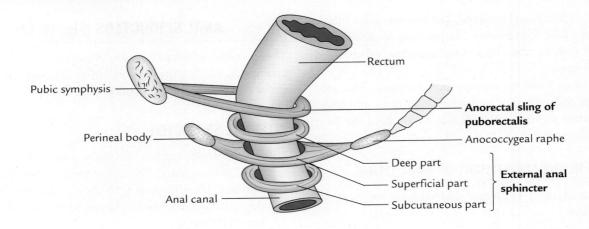

Fig. 19.13 Anorectal sling and different parts of the external anal sphincters.

Superficial Part

The superficial part is elliptical in shape. It arises from the tip of coccyx and anococcygeal raphe behind, surrounds the lower part of internal sphincter and then gets inserted into the perineal body in front.

Subcutaneous Part

The subcutaneous part lies below the internal sphincter in the perianal space and surrounds the lower part of the anal canal. It has the form of flat band, about 15 mm broad. It has no bony attachment. It is traversed by fibroblastic septa derived from the conjoint longitudinal coat.

Nerve Supply of the Sphincter

1. The *internal sphincter* is made up of smooth muscle and supplied by the autonomic nerve fibres (sympathetic and parasympathetic), hence it is involuntary.
2. The *external anal sphincter* is made up of striated muscle and hence, supplied by the somatic nerve—inferior rectal nerve and perineal branch of 4th sacral nerve. It is therefore under voluntary control.

N.B.

- *Anorectal ring:* While doing per rectal examination, the muscular ring on which the flexed finger rests just over an inch above the anal margin is the "anorectal ring". It is formed by the fusion of the deep part of the external sphincter, the internal sphincter, and puborectalis, and demarcates the junction between the anal canal and the rectum. Surgical excision of this ring results in incontinence.
- *Conjoint longitudinal coat of the anal canal:* It is formed at the anorectal junction by the fusion of *puborectalis* and longitudinal muscle coat of the rectal wall. It runs

vertically downward between the internal and external anal sphincters, and at the level of white line it breaks up into a number of fibroelastic septa which fan out, traverse through the subcutaneous part of the anal canal to be attached to the skin around the anal orifice. The most lateral of these septa forms **perianal fascia** which passes laterally to be attached to obturator fascia enclosing the pudendal canal. The space between the perianal fascia and the skin is called **perineal space**. The most medial septum of the conjoint longitudinal coat forms the *anal intermuscular septum*, which passes medially and gets attached to Hilton's line.

SURGICAL SPACES RELATED TO THE ANAL CANAL

These are two ischiorectal fossae, perianal space, and submucous space of the anal canal.

- *Ischiorectal spaces or fossae:* They lie one on each side of the anal canal and are filled with fat.
- *Perianal space:* It surrounds the anal canal below Hilton's line. It lies between the perianal fascia and skin. It contains the subcutaneous part of anal sphincter, lobulated fat, external rectal venous plexus, and terminal branches of the inferior rectal nerve and vessels. The **perianal abscess** is very painful.
- *Submucous space of anal canal:* It lies above the white line of Hilton between the mucous membrane and the internal anal sphincter, and contains *internal rectal venous plexus*.

ARTERIAL SUPPLY

The upper part of anal canal is supplied by the *superior rectal artery* and the lower part of anal canal is supplied by the *inferior rectal artery*.

VENOUS DRAINAGE

The upper part of the anal canal is drained into the portal venous system by the superior rectal vein and the lower part of the anal canal is drained into the caval (systemic) system by inferior rectal veins.

LYMPHATIC DRAINAGE

The upper part of the anal canal drains into the internal iliac nodes whereas the lower part drains into the horizontal group of superficial inguinal nodes. Therefore, the pectinate line forms the *"water shed line"* of the anal canal.

DEVELOPMENT

The upper part of the anal canal is endodermal in origin and develops from *anorectal canal* (dorsal part of cloaca) and lower part of the anal canal is ectodermal in origin and develops from *proctodeum*. The *anal membrane* separating the two parts breaks down at birth. Its remains are represented by the pectinate line in the anal canal. The *anal valves* are said to be the remains of the anal membrane.

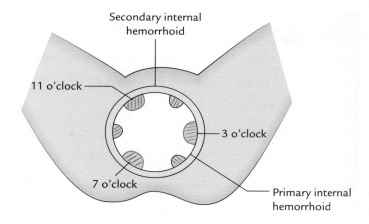

Fig. 19.14 Location of the internal hemorrhoids.

Clinical correlation

- **Hemorrhoids (or piles):** These are variceal dilatations of the *submucosal anal and perianal venous plexuses*. They are classified into two types:

  (a) *Internal hemorrhoids (or true piles):* These are the saccular dilatations of the tributaries of the superior rectal (hemorrhoidal) vein above the pectinate line in portal obstruction. The internal hemorrhoids may be primary or secondary. The primary piles are formed due to dilatations of main tributaries/radicles of the superior rectal vein which lie in the anal columns which occupy the left lateral, right posterior, and right anterior positions. The dilatations of radicles of superior rectal vein in other positions are termed secondary piles. The location of primary piles corresponds to the 3 o'clock, 7 o'clock, and 11 o'clock positions of the anal wall, when viewing the interior of anal canal in lithotomy position (Fig. 19.14).

    Anatomically each hemorrhoids/pile consists of a fold of mucosa and submucosa containing a varicose radicle of the superior rectal vein and a terminal branch of the superior rectal artery.

    They are painless but bleed profusely on straining during defecation (passing stool).

    Types: Initially they are confined within the anal canal (1st degree), gradually they enlarge and prolapse during defecation (2nd degree), and finally remain prolapsed (3rd degree).

  (b) *External hemorrhoids (or false piles):* These are dilatations of the tributaries of inferior rectal vein below the pectinate line. They are covered by the mucous membrane of the lower half of the canal. They are very painful and do not bleed on straining during defecation.

    The so-called thrombosed external pile is a small tense hematoma at the anal margin caused due to rupture of the subcutaneous vein. Therefore, it should be truly termed perianal hematoma.

- **Fissure in anorectal canal:** It is caused by rupture of one of the anal valves (valves of Morgagni) by the passage of hard fecal mass. They occur posteriorly in the midline and are very painful because the inferior aspect of the valve is lined by the mucous membrane/skin of the lower half of anal canal supplied by the somatic nerves.

- **Fistula in anorectal canal:** It is caused by the rupture of an abscess around the canal. The abscess opens spontaneously internally into the anal canal and externally on the surface and the track becomes epithelialized. Low-level anal fistula passing through the lower part of the superficial anal sphincter is the most common.

Golden Facts to Remember

► Most prominent lateral curvature of the rectum	Middle lateral curvature (being convex to the left)
► Most important Houston's valve	Third transverse rectal fold of the mucous membrane
► Chief artery of the rectum	Superior rectal artery
► Chief vein of the rectum	Superior rectal vein
► Location of primary internal piles in lithotomy position	3, 7, and 11 o'clock positions

Clinical Case Study

A 55-year-old woman complained that for the past 1 year she had frequently passed blood-stained stools and recently she noticed that one rounded mass protrudes out from her anus during straining at stool.

After defecation, she is able to push it back inside the anus. The proctoscopic examination revealed three pink coloured swellings located at 3, 7, and 11 o'clock positions with the patient in lithotomy position. The swellings bulged downward when the patient was asked to strain. A diagnosis of **internal hemorrhoids** was made.

Questions

1. What are the internal hemorrhoids?
2. What is the site of occurrence of internal piles?
3. What are the external hemorrhoids?
4. Why the internal hemorrhoids are painless, and the external hemorrhoids are painful?

Answers

1. These are the saccular dilatations of the radicles of superior rectal vein due to portal hypertension.
2. Above the pectinate line.
3. These are saccular dilatations of the radicles of inferior rectal vein.
4. This is because mucous membrane overlying internal hemorrhoids is supplied by the autonomic nerves and mucous membrane/skin covering the external piles is supplied by the somatic nerves.

Introduction to the Lower Limb

The lower limbs/extremities of the body are specialized for transmission of body weight and locomotion. A brief description of comparative anatomy of limbs immensely facilitates the understanding of their structure and function (see page 2, Textbook of Anatomy: *Upper Limb and Thorax* by Vishram Singh).

PARTS/REGIONS

For descriptive purposes, the lower limb is divided into six parts or regions (Fig. 20.1):
- Gluteal region.
- Thigh or femoral region.
- Knee or knee region.
- Leg or leg region.
- Ankle or talocrural region.
- Foot or foot region.

Gluteal Region

The gluteal region lies on the back and side of the pelvis. It consists of two parts: the rounded prominent posterior region called **buttock** and lateral less prominent region called **hip** or **hip region**.

The **buttock** is bounded superiorly by the *iliac crest*, medially by the *intergluteal cleft*, and inferiorly by the *gluteal fold*. The bulk of it forms the gluteal muscles. The **hip region** overlies the hip joint and greater trochanter of the femur.

Thigh or Femoral Region

The femoral region lies between the gluteal, abdominal, and perineal regions proximally and the knee region distally. The bone of the thigh is **femur**, which articulates with the hip bone at the hip joint and upper end of the tibia and patella at the knee joint.

The abdomen is demarcated from the thigh anteriorly by the inguinal ligament and medially by the ischiopubic ramus. This junction between the abdomen and thigh is termed **inguinal region** or **groin**. The gluteal fold is the upper limit of the thigh posteriorly. The lower part of the back of thigh and back of the knee is termed **ham** (*L. poples*).

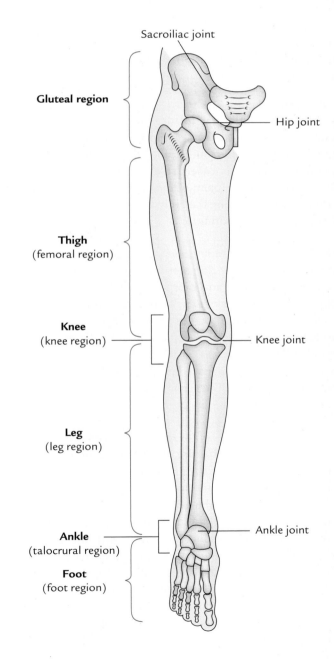

Fig. 20.1 Parts/regions of the lower limb.

Knee or Knee Region

The knee region includes prominences (condyles) of the femur and tibia, head of fibula, and patella (knee cap). The **patella** lies in front of the distal end of femur and medial and lateral femorotibial joints. The posterior aspect of the knee presents a well defined hollow called **popliteal fossa**.

Leg or Leg Region

The leg region lies between the knee and ankle regions. The leg contains two bones: a long and thick medial bone—the **tibia**, and long and narrow lateral bone—the **fibula**. The prominence on the posterior aspect of the leg formed by a large triceps surae muscle is called **calf** (*L. sura*).

Ankle or Talocrural Region

The ankle region includes distal part of the leg, and prominences (malleoli) of tibia and fibula. The ankle joint is located between the malleoli and the talus.

Foot or Foot Region

The foot is the distal part of the lower limb. It contains 7 tarsals, 5 metatarsals, and 14 toe bones (phalanges). The superior surface of the foot is called **dorsum of the foot** and its inferior surface is called **sole of the foot**. The sole is homologous with the palm of the hand. The foot provides a platform for supporting the body weight when standing and plays a key role in locomotion.

N.B. The foot has undergone maximum changes during evolution. In the lower primates (e.g., apes and monkeys), it is a prehensile organ and grasp the boughs with their feet. They can oppose their great toes over the lesser toes. In humans, the great toe comes to lie in line with other toes and loses its power of opposition. It is greatly enlarged to provide principal support to the body. Its four lesser toes because of loss of prehensile function have become vestigial and reduced in size. The tarsal bones have become large, strong, and wedge-shaped to provide stable support.

The four major parts of the lower limb are summarized in Table 20.1. The basic structure of the lower limb is similar to that of upper limb, but it is modified to support the weight of the body and for locomotion.

The lower limb joins the **pelvic girdle** at the hip joint. This girdle is formed by the two hip bones which join anteriorly at the pubic symphysis and posteriorly with the sacrum at the sacroiliac joints. The lower limb is supported by the heavy bones. The **femur** (largest and strongest bone of the body) articulates superiorly with the pelvis at the hip joint and inferiorly with the upper end of tibia at the knee joint. The tibia and fibula articulate with each other at proximal, intermediate, and inferior tibiofibular joints. The distal ends of these bones articulate with the talus to form the ankle joint.

Table 20.1 Parts of the lower limb

Parts	Bones	Joints
Gluteal region (on side and back of pelvis)	Hip bone	Sacroiliac joint
Thigh (from hip to knee)	Femur	• Hip joint • Knee joint
Leg (from knee to ankle)	• Tibia • Fibula	• Tibiofibular joints • Ankle joint
Foot (from heel to toes)	• Tarsals (7) • Metatarsals (5) • Phalanges (14)	• Intertarsal joints (e.g., subtalar talocalcaneonavicular, transverse tarsal, etc.) • Intermetatarsal joints • Metatarsophalangeal joints • Interphalangeal joints

BONES

The bones of the lower limb are described in detail in Chapter 21.

Transmission of the Body Weight through Lower Limb

The body weight is transferred from the vertebral column through sacroiliac joints to the pelvic girdle and from pelvic girdle through the hip joints to the femurs (Fig. 20.2).

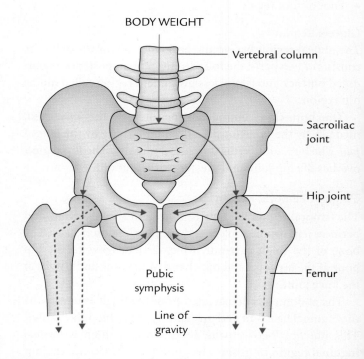

Fig. 20.2 Transmission of body weight from vertebral column to the femurs.

To support the erect posture efficiently, the femurs are oblique being directed inferomedially within the thighs so that during standing the knees are close to each other and placed directly below the trunk. As a result, the centre of gravity falls to the vertical lines of the supporting legs and feet.

A little description of comparative anatomy will make it easy to understand. In quadrupeds, the femurs are vertical and knees are apart with trunk suspended between the limbs (Fig. 20.3).

The body weight is transferred from the knee joint to the ankle joint by the tibia. The fibula does not articulate with the femur, hence does not transfer any weight. At the ankle, the weight born by the tibia is transformed to the talus—the keystone of the longitudinal arch of the foot. The longitudinal arch formed by the tarsals and metatarsals, evenly distribute the weight between the heel and foot when standing. In this way the foot provides a flexible but stable platform to support the body. The weight-bearing points of the foot are medial process of the calcaneus posteriorly and six equal pillars anteriorly formed by the heads of four lateral metatarsals and two sesamoid bones (one on each side of V-shaped ridge) below the head of first metatarsal (Fig. 20.4).

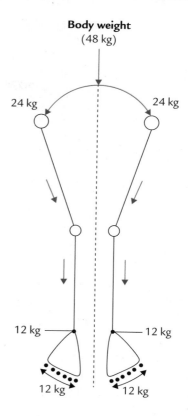

Fig. 20.5 Distribution of weight to the feet.

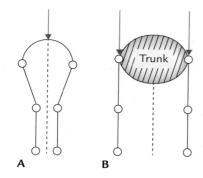

Fig. 20.3 Comparison of arrangement of the lower limb bones in humans (A) and quadrupeds (B).

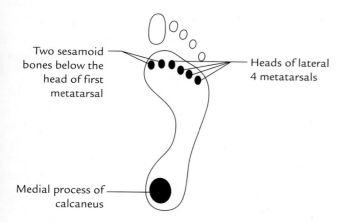

Fig. 20.4 Weight-bearing points of the foot.

Mode of Weight Distribution to the Feet (Fig. 20.5)

The body weight of a person weighing say 48 kg when standing (in fundamental position) is distributed as follows:
- 24 kg goes to each lower limb.
- In each limb, 12 kg goes to the medial process of calcaneus and 12 kg to the metatarsals.
- The metatarsals present six points of equal contact with the ground, viz., heads of lateral four metatarsals and two sesamoid bones below the head of first metatarsal each supporting 2 kg. Thus, the great toe supports the double load of body weight as compared to the other toes of the foot.

N.B. The line of gravity of the body passes through the cervical vertebrae, anterior to the thoracic vertebrae, through the lumbar vertebrae, anterior to the sacrum, posterior to the hip joints, and anterior to the knee and ankle joints (Fig. 20.6).

MUSCLES

The muscles of the lower limb are strong and movements produced by them are coarse than those produced by the muscles of the upper limb.

The major muscles in the gluteal region are gluteus maximus, gluteus medius, and gluteus minimus. The gluteal muscles mainly rotate the thigh laterally.

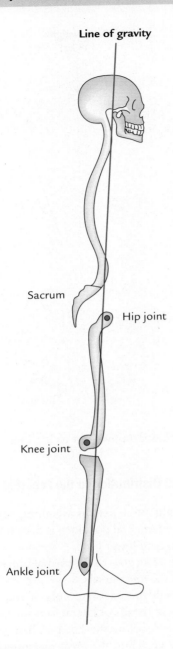

Line of gravity

Sacrum

Hip joint

Knee joint

Ankle joint

Fig. 20.6 Line of gravity.

In the thigh and leg, the deep fascia forms intermuscular septa and divide these regions into underlying compartments. The thigh is divided into **anterior, medial, and posterior compartments**. The muscles in the anterior compartment are primarily extensor of the knee joint. The main muscle in this compartment is **quadriceps femoris**, which consists of four parts: vastus lateralis, vastus medialis, vastus intermedius, and rectus femoris. The muscles of medial compartment of the thigh are adductors of the hip joint. The muscles of posterior compartment of the thigh are called **hamstring muscles**. They are extensors of the hip joint and flexors of the knee joint.

The leg is divided into **anterior, lateral,** and **posterior compartments**. The muscles of the anterior compartment are primarily dorsiflexors of the ankle and extensors of the toes. The muscles of lateral compartment plantarflex and evert the foot. The muscles of posterior compartment are divided into superficial and deep groups by **transverse fascia of the leg.** The superficial muscles, e.g., gastrocnemius, and soleus, which together form the **triceps surae** which is inserted by a long thick tendon (**tendoachillis**) into calcaneus. They act on calcaneus to plantarflex the foot. The muscles of deep group flex the toes and plantarflex the ankle.

The foot has 20 individual muscles, out of which 18 are located in the sole and only two are located on the dorsum of the foot. The muscles of the sole are arranged into four intricate layers. Despite their layered arrangement, the muscles of sole function primarily as a group during the support phase of the stance, maintaining the arches of the foot.

N.B. The **antigravity muscles** of the lower limb are far better developed than those of the upper limb because they lift up the whole body to attain the erect posture and in walking up the staircase. These muscles are: gluteus maximus (extensor of the hip), quadriceps femoris (extensor of the knee), and gastrocnemius, and soleus (plantarflexors of the ankle). They have extensive origin and bulky muscle belly.

Clinical correlation

Intramuscular injection: The muscles commonly used for intramuscular injection in the lower limb are: (a) **gluteus medius** of gluteal region in adults (most common site) and (b) **vastus lateralis** muscle of the thigh region in children.

NERVES

The nerves of the lower limb are derived from **lumbar plexus of nerves (L1 – L4)** within the posterior abdominal wall and **sacral plexus** of nerves (L4 – S4) in the posterior pelvic wall. The nerves of the lower limb are: femoral, obturator, sciatic, tibial, and common peroneal nerves (Fig. 20.7).

1. **Femoral nerve:** It is present on the front of the thigh and innervates the anterior thigh muscles.
2. **Obturator nerve:** It is present on the medial side of the thigh and innervates the adductors of the thigh.
3. **Sciatic nerve** (largest and thickest nerve in the body): It is present in the gluteal region and the back of the thigh. It supplies muscles on the back of the thigh. In the lower part of the back of thigh, it divides into tibial and common peroneal nerves.
4. **Tibial nerve:** It is present on the back of the leg and supplies all the muscles on the back of the leg. At the ankle,

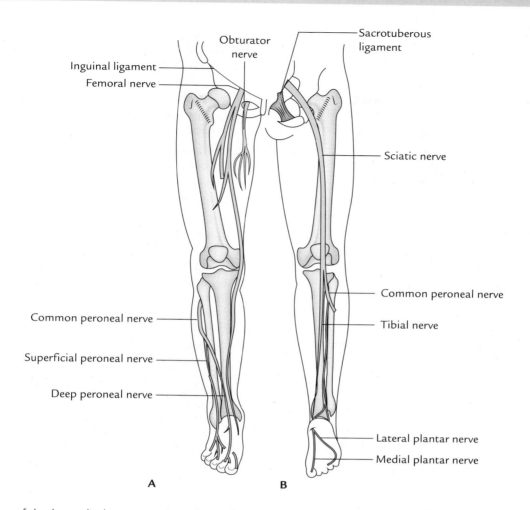

Obturator nerve

Sacrotuberous ligament

Inguinal ligament

Femoral nerve

Sciatic nerve

Common peroneal nerve

Common peroneal nerve

Tibial nerve

Superficial peroneal nerve

Deep peroneal nerve

Lateral plantar nerve

Medial plantar nerve

A   B

Fig. 20.7 Nerves of the lower limb, an overview: **A**, on the anterior aspect; **B**, on the posterior aspect.

behind medial malleolus, it divides into **medial and lateral plantar nerves**, which together supply all the muscles of the sole.

5. **Common peroneal nerve:** At the lateral side of the neck of fibula, it divides into the deep and superficial peroneal nerves. The **deep peroneal nerve** is present in the anterior compartment of the leg and supplies all the anterior leg muscles.

The **superficial peroneal nerve** is present in the lateral compartment of the leg and supplies all the lateral leg muscles.

In addition to the muscles, all the nerves (vide supra) also supply joints and provide cutaneous innervation to the lower limb.

ARTERIES (Fig. 20.8)

The blood to the lower limb is mostly supplied by the **femoral artery** and its branches.

1. **Femoral artery:** It begins at the midpoint of inguinal ligament as the continuation of the external iliac artery.

It enters the front of thigh and quickly gives off **deep femoral artery (profunda femoris artery)** which supplies all the structures of the thigh.

2. **Popliteal artery:** It is the continuation of femoral artery into the popliteal fossa. The popliteal artery descends through the popliteal fossa and at the head of fibula it divides into the **anterior** and **posterior tibial arteries.**

3. **Anterior tibial artery:** It lies in the anterior compartment of the leg which it supplies and continues into the dorsum of the foot as *dorsalis pedis artery.*

4. **Dorsalis pedis artery:** It lies on the dorsum of the foot which it supplies.

5. **Posterior tibial artery:** It lies in the posterior compartment of the leg which it supplies. At the ankle, behind the medial malleolus it divides into *medial and lateral plantar arteries.*

6. **Medial and lateral plantar arteries:** They are the terminal branches of posterior tibial artery and supply the sole of the foot.

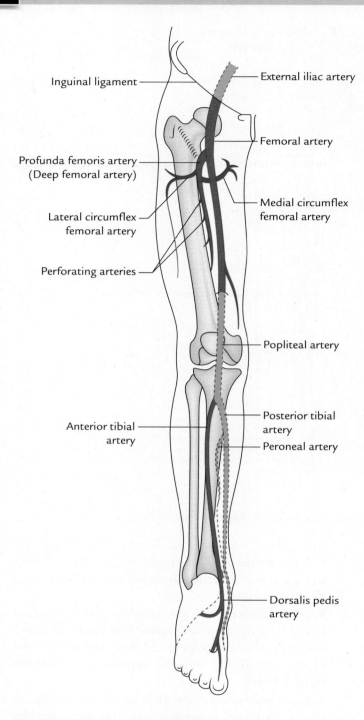

Inguinal ligament

External iliac artery

Femoral artery

Profunda femoris artery
(Deep femoral artery)

Medial circumflex
femoral artery

Lateral circumflex
femoral artery

Perforating arteries

Popliteal artery

Anterior tibial
artery

Posterior tibial
artery

Peroneal artery

Dorsalis pedis
artery

Fig. 20.8 Arteries of the lower limb, an overview.

N.B. In addition to the femoral artery the following arteries also contribute a little to the blood supply of the lower limb:

1. Superior gluteal artery.
2. Inferior gluteal artery.
3. Obturator artery.
   They are all branches of the internal iliac artery.

Clinical correlation

- **Sites where arterial pulse can be palpated/felt in the lower limb:**
  1. **Femoral pulse** can be felt at the midinguinal point (i.e., the point midway to anterior superior iliac spine and pubic symphysis.
  2. **Popliteal pulse** can be felt behind the knee deep in the popliteal fossa with knee flexed.
  3. **Posterior tibial pulse** can be felt behind the medial malleolus midway between it and tendocalcaneus.
  4. **Dorsalis pedis pulse** can be felt on the dorsum of the foot just medial to the tendon of extensor hallucis longus.

- **Acute arterial occlusion:** It is mostly caused by embolism or thrombosis. It usually occurs in the femoral artery where it gives off the profunda femoris artery. The clinical features include five P's: Pain, Paresthesia, Pallor, Paralysis, and Pulselessness.

- **Chronic arterial occlusive disease:** It is mostly caused by the atherosclerosis. It commonly involves femoral or popliteal artery (50% of cases). However, in the diabetic patients, it may also involve anterior tibial, posterior tibial, and peroneal arteries. Clinically, it presents as **intermittent claudication**, i.e., profound leg pain in the leg on walking for some distance which is relieved by taking rest for 5–10 minutes and reoccurs on walking again for the same distance.

VEINS

The veins of the lower limb are classified into three types: **superficial, perforating, and deep veins.** The superficial veins communicate with the deep veins via perforating veins.

1. **Deep veins:** They accompany the arteries of the leg and finally drain into **femoral vein**, which continues as external iliac vein. The named deep veins are: **venae comitantes** of anterior and posterior tibial arteries, **popliteal vein, and femoral vein.** The deep veins are subject to muscle compression (musculovenous pump) to facilitate the venous return.

2. **Superficial veins:** They drain into deep veins through *perforating veins*. The named superficial veins are **great and small saphenous veins,** which originate from dorsal venous arch of the foot. The great saphenous vein ascends anterior to medial malleolus, continues along the medial side of leg and thigh before emptying into the *femoral vein* in the femoral triangle. The small saphenous vein ascends behind the lateral malleolus in the calf and empties into the popliteal vein in the popliteal fossa.

3. **Perforating veins (perforators):** They connect and direct blood of superficial veins into the deep veins. The presence of valves in them prevent the back flow from the deep veins.

N.B. The venous blood of the lower limb is drained against gravity therefore, all the lower limb veins have valves to overcome the effect of gravity.

Clinical correlation

Varicose veins: The superficial veins (great and small saphenous veins) draining skin continuously shunt their blood into the deep veins by perforating veins.

The incompetence of valves of perforating veins allows backflow of blood into superficial veins. This backflow causes dilatation **of the superficial veins** and their tributaries called **varicose veins**.

LYMPHATICS

The lymphatics of the lower limb are classified into two types—superficial and deep.

1. **Superficial lymphatics:** They lie superficial to deep fascia and drain into the **superficial inguinal lymph nodes** present just below the inguinal ligament and near the terminal part of great saphenous vein. The lymph from buttock, perineum, and lower abdomen also drain into these lymph nodes.
2. **Deep lymphatics:** They accompany the arteries and drain into **deep inguinal lymph nodes** present within the femoral sheath, which in turn drain into **iliac lymph nodes** within the pelvis and **aortic lymph nodes** in the lower posterior abdominal wall.

N.B. Lymph from glans penis/glans clitoris drain into deep inguinal lymph nodes located in the femoral canal which is termed **lymph node of Cloquet /Rosenmüller.**

Golden Facts to Remember

► Most important function of the lower limb	Transmission of the body weight and locomotion
► Most important digit of the foot	Great toe
► Commonest fracture in the lower limb	Fracture neck of femur
► Most commonly dislocated bone in the lower limb	Patella
► Most common peripheral neuropathy in the lower limb	Compression of the common peroneal nerve (against the neck of fibula)
► Most commonly used nerve in the body for grafting	Sural nerve
► Most commonly used vein in the body for grafting	Great saphenous vein
► Commonest site of venous thrombosis in the body	Deep veins of the lower limb
► Most common lower limb injuries	Injuries of the knee, leg, and foot
► Longest muscle in the body	Sartorius
► Thickest nerve in the body	Sciatic nerve
► Largest bone in the body	Femur
► Largest sesamoid bone in the body	Patella
► Strongest ligament in the body	Iliofemoral ligament
► Strongest tendon in the body	Tendocalcaneus
► Largest synovial cavity in the body	Synovial cavity of the knee joint

Bones of the Lower Limb

Each lower limb contains 31 bones:

- **Hip bone/innominate bone** the bone of gluteal region (1).
- **Femur**, the bone of thigh (1).
- **Patella** or **knee cap** (1).
- **Tibia and fibula**, the bones of leg (2).
- **Tarsal bones** (7).
- **Metatarsals**, (5). } Bones of foot
- **Phalanges**, (14).

HIP BONE (OS COXAE, OS INNOMINATUM)

The hip bone is a large irregular flat bone in the region of hip. It is formed by the fusion of three primary bones—the **ilium**, the **ischium**, and the **pubis**.

PARTS

The hip bone presents upper and lower expanded parts and a middle constricted part which carries *a cup-shaped hollow (acetabulum)* on the outer aspect. The upper expanded part is called *ilium*. The lower expanded part presents an oval or triangular foramen called *obturator foramen*. The part anteromedial to this foramen is called **pubis**, and the part posteroinferior to it is called **ischium**.

ANATOMICAL POSITION AND SIDE DETERMINATION

The side of the hip bone is determined by holding it in such way that:
- The acetabulum is directed laterally.
- The obturator foramen lies below the acetabulum.
- The flat expanded ilium is directed upward, thin pubis is directed anteromedially, and thick ischium is directed posteroinferiorly.
- The pubic tubercle and anterior superior iliac spine lie in the same coronal plane (Fig. 2.10).
- The ischial tuberosity occupies the lowest position.

FEATURES AND ATTACHMENTS (Figs 21.1 and 21.2)

Ilium

It projects upward from the acetabulum as an expanded fan-shaped plate of bone. It presents the following features:
- Two ends—upper and lower.
- Three borders—anterior, posterior, and medial.
- Three surfaces—iliac fossa, gluteal, and sacropelvic.

Ends

Upper end (Fig. 21.3)
1. It is represented by a curved and thickened border called **iliac crest.** The **highest point of iliac crest** lies at the level of interval between L3 and L4 vertebrae.
2. In the horizontal plane, the iliac crest is concave inward anteriorly and convex inward posteriorly. The anterior and posterior ends of the iliac crest are termed anterior superior iliac spine and posterior superior iliac spine, respectively.
   - **Anterior superior iliac spine** provides attachment to the lateral end of inguinal ligament above and sartorius below.
   - **Posterior superior iliac spine** provides attachment to the sacrotuberous ligament.
3. The iliac crest is divided into a **larger ventral segment** (anterior two-third) and a **smaller dorsal segment** (posterior one-third).
   - **Ventral segment**, presents an outer lip, an intermediate area, and an inner lip.

(a) *Outer lip*
   (i) It presents **tubercle of the iliac crest** 5 cm behind the anterior superior iliac spine.
   (ii) It provides attachment to the following structures:
      - **Tensor fasciae latae**, originates in front of the tubercle of iliac crest.
      - **External oblique muscle**, inserted in its anterior two-third.

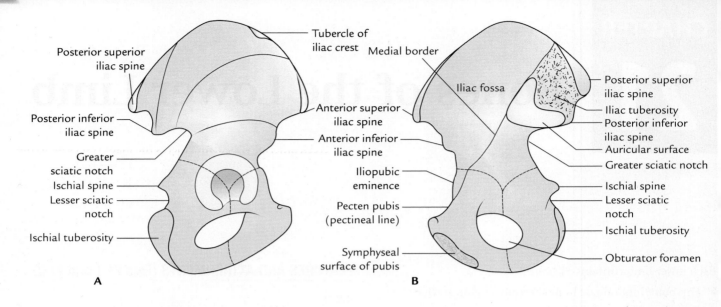

Fig. 21.1 General features of the ilium: **A**, outer surface; **B**, inner surface.

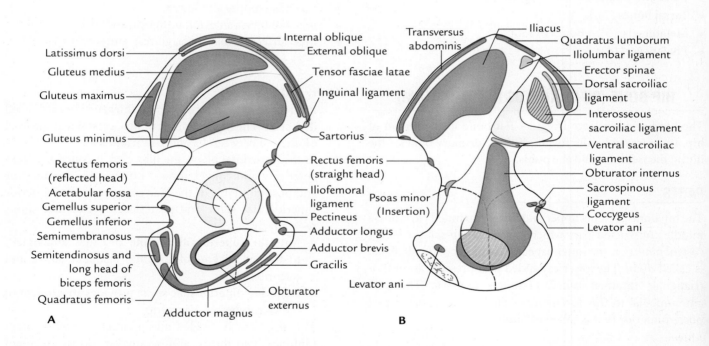

Fig. 21.2 Special features (attachments) of the ilium: **A**, outer surface; **B**, inner surface.

- **Latissimus dorsi,** originates just behind its highest point.
(b) *Intermediate area:* It provides origin to the internal oblique muscle along its whole extent.
(c) *Inner lip*
  (i) Its anterior two-third provides attachment to **transversus abdominis muscle.**
  (ii) Its posterior one-third provides attachment to **quadratus lumborum.**

- **Dorsal segment** is divided by a ridge into inner and outer sloping surfaces:
  - *Outer sloping* surface gives origin to gluteus maximus muscle.
  - *Inner sloping* surface gives origin to erector spinae muscle.

Lower end

The lower end of ilium forms the upper two-fifth of acetabulum.

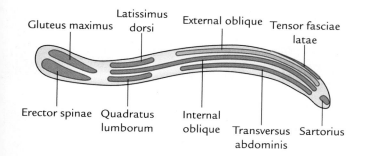

Fig. 21.3 Attachments on the right iliac crest (as seen from above).

Borders of the Ilium

Anterior border

1. It extends from the anterior superior iliac spine to the acetabulum.
2. Its upper half forms a notch and its lower half projects forward as the **anterior inferior iliac spine**, which provides attachment to the straight head of *rectus femoris* in the upper part and *iliofemoral ligament* in the lower part.

Posterior border

1. It extends from the posterior superior iliac spine to the upper end of the posterior border of ischium.
2. It presents from above downward, posterior inferior iliac spine, greater sciatic notch, ischial spine, and lesser sciatic notch.
3. The greater and lesser sciatic notches are converted into greater and lesser sciatic foramina by the sacrospinous and sacrotuberous ligaments (see page 204).

    The structures passing through greater and lesser sciatic foramina are described in Chapter 24, pages 355–356.
4. The dorsal aspect of ischial spine is crossed from lateral to medial side by three structures:
    - Pudendal nerve.
    - Internal pudendal vessels.
    - Nerve to obturator internus.

Mnemonic: **PIN** structures.

Medial border

1. It extends downward, forward, and medially from the iliac crest to the iliopubic eminence.
2. It separates the iliac fossa from the sacropelvic surface.
3. Lower one-third of the medial border forms a rounded **arcuate line**.

Surfaces of the Ilium

Iliac fossa

1. It is a shallow concave surface on the inner aspect of ilium, below the iliac crest, and in front of the medial border.
2. Iliacus muscle arises from its upper two-third.

Gluteal surface

1. It is the outer aspect of the ilium which is convex in front and concave behind.
2. It is divided into four areas by **three gluteal lines:** posterior, anterior, and inferior. All these lines radiate from the upper margin of the greater sciatic notch. *The posterior gluteal* line meets the dorsal segment of the iliac crest, *anterior gluteal* line meets the iliac crest close to the tubercle of the iliac crest, and *inferior gluteal line* meets the upper end of anterior inferior iliac spine.
3. The gluteal surface provides origin to four muscles:
    (a) *Gluteus maximus*, behind the posterior gluteal line.
    (b) *Gluteus medius*, between the anterior and the posterior gluteal lines.
    (c) *Gluteus medius*, between the anterior and the inferior gluteal lines.
    (d) Reflected head of rectus femoris, between the inferior gluteal line and upper margin of acetabulum.

Sacropelvic surface

It is situated behind the medial border, on the inner side of ilium. It is divided into two parts—sacral part dorsally and pelvic part ventrally.

Sacral part of the sacropelvic surface

1. The sacral part presents the **tuberosity of the ilium** behind and the **auricular surface** in front.
2. The **iliac tuberosity** is a rough area below the dorsal part of iliac crest and provides attachment to three ligaments. From behind forward these are:
    (a) iliolumbar, (b) dorsal sacroiliac, and (c) interosseous sacroiliac.
3. The **auricular surface** is an ear-shaped articular surface and articulates with the corresponding surface of the sacrum to form a **sacroiliac joint**.

Pelvic part of the sacropelvic surface

1. It is smooth and continuous with the pelvic surface of the ischium to form the lateral wall of lesser pelvis.
2. It presents **pre-auricular sulcus** just in front of auricular surface, along the lateral border of greater sciatic notch.
3. Most of this surface provides origin to **obturator internus.**

Ischium

It is the thick posteroinferior part of hip bone and consists of a body and a ramus.

Body

It is very thick and lies below and posterior to the acetabulum. It presents two ends—upper and lower; three borders—anterior, posterior, and lateral; and three surfaces—femoral, dorsal, and pelvic.

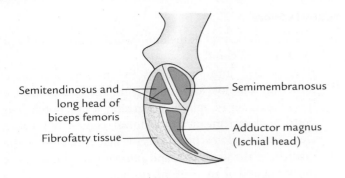

Semitendinosus and long head of biceps femoris

Semimembranosus

Fibrofatty tissue

Adductor magnus (Ischial head)

Fig. 21.4 Attachments on the left ischial tuberosity (posterior aspect).

Ends

Upper end: It forms posteroinferior two-fifth of the acetabulum, where it unites with the ilium and pubis.

Lower end

1. It forms the ischial tuberosity (Fig. 21.4) and gives off ramus which forms an acute angle with body.
2. Ischial tuberosity is rough and divided by a horizontal ridge into an upper quadrilateral area and lower triangular area.
3. The upper quadrilateral area is subdivided by an oblique ridge into upper lateral and lower medial parts.
4. The lower triangular area is subdivided by a longitudinal ridge into outer and inner parts.
5. The ischial tuberosity provides origin to four muscles:
   (a) Semimembranosus arises from the lateral part of the upper quadrangular area.
   (b) Semitendinosus along with long head of biceps femoris arises from the medial part of the upper quadrilateral area.
   (c) Adductor magnus (ischial head), arises from the outer part of lower triangular area.
6. The inner part of the lower triangular area is covered by fibrofatty tissue and transmits the body weight in sitting position.
7. Medial margin of the ischial tuberosity is sharp and provides attachment to the lower end of sacrotuberous ligament.

Borders

Anterior border: It forms the posterior margin of the obturator foramen and gives attachment to the **obturator membrane.**

Posterior border

1. It is continuous above with the posterior border of ilium and ends below the upper end of ischial tuberosity.
2. It presents a triangular projection called **ischial spine.** The tip of spine provides attachment to the sacrospinous ligament, and levator ani and coccygeus muscles arise from its pelvic surface.

3. Ischial spine forms the lower boundary of greater sciatic notch and the lower boundary of lesser sciatic notch.
4. The **gemellus superior** and **gemellus inferior** muscles arise from the upper and lower ends of the lesser sciatic notch, respectively.

Lateral border

1. It forms the lateral margin of the ischial tuberosity.
2. Its upper part is notched close to the lower margin of the acetabulum and lodges the **tendon of obturator externus.**

Surfaces
Femoral surface

1. It is directed forward and laterally, and is situated between the anterior and lateral borders.
2. **Obturator externus** arises from this surface along the obturator foramen.
3. **Quadratus femoris** arises from this surface along the lateral border of the ischial tuberosity.

Dorsal surface

1. It is continuous above with the gluteal surface of ilium.
2. It is divided by a transverse groove into the upper and lower parts.
3. *Tendon of obturator internus* along with *two gemelli* traverses through the groove between the upper and lower parts.

Pelvic surface

It is smooth and lies between the anterior and posterior borders. It gives origin to the **obturator internus.**

Ramus of the Ischium

It arises from the lower part of the body and runs upward, forward, and medially, and meets with the inferior ramus pubis to form **conjoint ischiopubic ramus.**

Conjoint ischiopubic ramus

The conjoint ischiopubic ramus presents two borders, upper and lower, and two surfaces—outer and inner.

1. *Upper border* forms the lower margin of obturator foramen and provides attachment to the *obturator membrane.*
2. *Lower border*
   (a) It forms the lateral boundary of the subpubic angle.
   (b) It is everted. The eversion is more marked in males than females due to attachment of crus of penis.
3. *Outer surface* is concave and provides linear attachment to four muscles. From above downward these are:
   (a) Obturator externus.
   (b) Adductor magnus.
   (c) Adductor brevis.
   (d) Gracilis.

4. *Inner surface* is convex and subdivided by the upper and lower oblique bony ridges into three areas—upper, middle, and lower.
   (a) **Upper ridge** provides attachment to the superior fascia of **urogenital diaphragm**.
   (b) **Lower ridge** provides attachment to the perineal membrane (inferior fascia of urogenital diaphragm) and falciform process of sacrotuberous ligament.
   (c) **Upper area** provides origin to the obturator internus.
   (d) **Middle area** provides attachments to the sphincter urethrae and deep transversus perinei muscles.
   (e) **Lower area** provides attachments from before backward to crus of penis, clitoris, ischiocavernosus, and superficial transversus perinei muscles.

Pubis (Pubic Bone/OS Pubis)

It is the anteroinferior part of the hip bone and consists of three parts—body, superior ramus, and inferior ramus.

Body

It is quadrilateral in outline and flattened anteroposteriorly. It presents the following features: pubic crest, pubic tubercle, and three surfaces (anterior, posterior, and medial).

Pubic crest and pubic tubercle
The pubic crest is the thickened upper border of the body of pubis and its lateral end projects forward to form tubercle called **pubic tubercle**.

Surfaces
Anterior surface

1. It is directed downward, forward, and laterally.
2. It provides attachments to the following four muscles:
   (a) **Adductor longus** arises by a rounded tendon from the angle between the pubic crest and pubic symphysis.
   (b) **Gracilis** arises from its lower part and extends further on the ischiopubic ramus.
   (c) **Adductor brevis** arises lateral to gracilis and extends further on the ischiopubic ramus.
   (d) **Obturator externus** arises from this surface adjacent to the obturator foramen.

Posterior surface

1. It is smooth and forms the anterior wall of bony pelvis, hence also called pelvic surface.
2. It is directed upward and backward, and is related to the urinary bladder.

Medial surface (symphyseal surface): It articulates with the medial surface of the opposite pubic bone to form secondary cartilaginous joint called symphysis pubis.

Superior Ramus of Pubis

It arises from the superolateral angle of the body of pubis and extends laterally above the obturator foramen and ends at **iliopubic eminence** where it unites with the ilium. It is triangular in cross section and presents three borders—posterior (pectineal line), anterior (obturator crest), and inferior; and three surfaces—pectineal, pelvic, and obturator.

Borders
Pectineal line (posterior border)

1. It is also called pecten pubis.
2. It extends laterally as a sharp line from the pubic tubercle to the posterior part of iliopubic eminence where it becomes continuous with arcuate line.
3. Pectineal line provides attachment to a large number of structures:
   (a) **Medial part** from before backward provide attachments to:
      – Lacunar ligament.
      – Reflected part of inguinal ligament.
      – Conjoint tendon.
      – Fascia transversalis.
   (b) **Lateral part** from behind forward provides attachment to:
      – Pectineal ligament (ligament of Cooper).
      – Pectineus muscle.
      – Pectineus fascia.
      – Psoas minor (if present).

Obturator crest (anterior border): It extends from the pubic tubercle to the acetabular margin near the **acetabular notch**.

Inferior border: It forms the upper margin of obturator foramen and provides attachment to the obturator membrane leaving a gap for the *obturator canal*.

Surfaces
Pectineal surface

1. It is a triangular area between the obturator crest and the pectineal line.
2. It extends from the pubic tubercle to iliopubic eminence.
3. Pectineus muscle arises from the upper part of this surface.

Pelvic surface: It lies between the pectineal line and inferior border of the superior ramus and continues medially with the pelvic surface of the body of pubis.
   It is featureless and covered by the peritoneum.

N.B. The pelvic surface of the superior ramus of pubis is crossed subperitoneally by the obliterated umbilical artery.

Obturator surface

1. It is situated between the obturator crest and the inferior border.

2. Obturator nerve and vessels traverse the obturator groove seen on this surface.

Inferior Ramus of Pubis

It extends downward and laterally from the lower part of the body of pubis to join the ramus of ischium and form the conjoint ischiopubic ramus.

OBTURATOR FORAMEN

1. It is a large gap in the lower part of the hip bone situated between the pubis and ischium.
2. It is oval and larger in males and triangular and smaller in females.
3. Obturator membrane is attached along to its margin except where it bridges the obturator groove to convert it into **obturator canal.**

The obturator canal transmits the obturator nerves and vessels.

ACETABULUM (LATIN ACETABULUM: SHALLOW VINEGAR CUP)

1. It is a large cup-shaped cavity on the outer surface of the middle constricted part of the hip bone.
2. It is directed laterally and slightly anteroinferiorly.

3. All the three parts of the hip bone contribute in its formation as follows:
   (a) *Pubis* forms its anterior one-fifth.
   (b) *Ischium* forms its posterior two-fifth.
   (c) *Ilium* forms its superior two-fifth.
4. Its margin is deficient inferiorly to form the **acetabular notch**, which is bridged by the *transverse acetabular ligament*, and the notch is converted into acetabular foramen.
5. The acetabulum receives the head of femur to form the hip joint.
6. The fibrocartilaginous rim, the **acetabular labrum,** is attached to the margins of the acetabulum.
7. The acetabulum presents a horseshoe-shaped articular surface, the **lunate surface,** in its periphery and non-articular area in its central part, the **acetabular fossa.** The acetabular fossa is filled with the pad of fat and the lunate surface is covered by a plate of hyaline cartilage.

The differences between the male and female hip bones are given in Table 21.1.

OSSIFICATION

The hip bone ossifies in cartilage by three primary centres and eight secondary centres (Table 21.2).

Table 21.1 Differences between the male and female hip bones

Features	Female	Male
Greater sciatic notch	Wider (75°)	Narrower (< 50°)
Ischial spine	Not inverted	Inverted
Ischiopubic ramus	Thin and not everted	Thick and everted
Obturator foramen	Triangular	Oval
Acetabular diameter	Less than 5 cm	More than 5 cm
Distance between the pubic tubercle and anterior acetabular margin	Less than transverse diameter of acetabulum	Equal to the transverse diameter of acetabulum
Pre-auricular sulcus	More conspicuous	Less conspicuous
Iliac fossa	Shallower	Deeper

Table 21.2 Ossification of the hip bone

Centres	Age of appearance	Age of fusion
Primary centres • 1 for ilium • 1 for ischium • 1 for pubis	2nd month of IUL 3rd month of IUL 4th month of IUL	18th year
Secondary centres • 2 for iliac crest • 2 for Y-shaped acetabular cartilage • 1 for ischial tuberosity	Puberty	20–25 years (except acetabular cartilage which ossifies at the age of 17 years)

FEMUR

The femur is the longest and strongest bone of the body, present in the thigh (Latin *femur* = thigh). It is about 18 inches (45 long), i.e., about one-fourth of the height of the individual. At the upper end it articulates with the hip bone to form the hip joint, and at the lower end it articulates with the patella and tibia. The femur transmits body weight from the hip bone to the tibia in standing position.

PARTS

The femur is the long bone and consists of three parts: upper end, shaft, and lower end.

The **upper end** consists of the **head, neck,** and **greater and lesser trochanter.**

The **shaft** of the femur is gently convex anteriorly with maximum convexity in the middle third where the shaft is narrowest.

The **lower end** of the femur is enlarged to form **medial and lateral condyles.** Both condyles project backward and are separated by the **intercondylar fossa.** The most prominent points on the condyles are called **epicondyles.**

N.B. The shape of femur departs markedly from other long bones in the sense that the long axis of head and neck projects superomedially at an angle to the long axis of the shaft of bone. This angle allows greater mobility at the hip joint but imposes great strain on the neck during transmission of weight, making it vulnerable to fracture.

ANATOMICAL POSITION AND SIDE DETERMINATION

The side of femur is determined by holding bone vertically in such a way that:

- Its head faces upward, medially, and slightly forward.
- Long axis of the shaft is directed downward and medially with convexity of the shaft facing anteriorly.
- Lower surfaces of both the condyles are in the same horizontal plane.
- **Trick-device:** The anatomical position can be achieved by balancing the neck of femur on your index finger (Fig. 21.5).

N.B.
- *Angle of inclination of femur:* It is an angle between the long axes of neck and shaft of the femur hence also called **neck–shaft angle.** The normal neck–shaft angle is 125° in adults and 160° in children (Fig. 21.6). It is less in female.
- *Angle of femoral torsion:* It is an angle between long axis of the head and neck of femur, and transverse axis of the femoral condyles. It measures about 7° in males and 12° in females (Fig. 21.7).

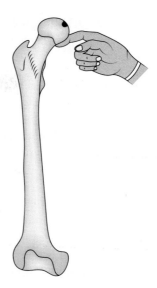

Fig. 21.5 Balancing the femur on the index finger to keep it in the anatomical position.

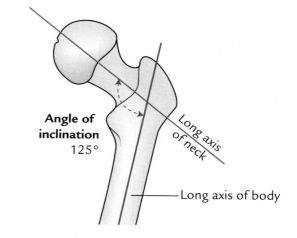

Fig. 21.6 Angle of inclination of the femur.

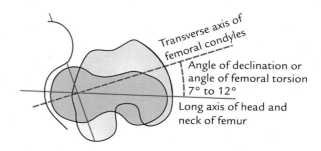

Fig. 21.7 Angle of the femoral torsion (angle of declination of the femur).

FEATURES AND ATTACHMENTS (Figs 21.8 and 21.9)

Upper End

Head

1. It forms about two-third of a sphere and articulates with the acetabulum of the hip bone to form the hip joint.
2. It presents a small pit, the **fovea**, just below and behind the centre, which provides attachment to the ligament of the head of femur (**ligamentum teres femoris**).

Neck

1. It is 5 cm long and connects the head with the shaft.
2. It is directed upward, medially, and slightly forward.
3. The angle between its lower border and the medial border of shaft is called *neck–shaft angle*.
4. The neck presents two borders—upper and lower, and two surfaces—anterior and posterior.

Upper border

1. It is concave and horizontal.

2. It meets the shaft near the greater trochanter.

Lower border

1. It is straight and oblique.
2. It meets the shaft near the lesser trochanter.

Anterior surface

1. It is flat and bears a number of oblique bony ridges.
2. It meets the shaft at **intertrochanteric line**.
3. It is completely intracapsular.

Intertrochanteric line

1. It continues downward and medially below the lesser trochanter on the posterior aspect of femur as **spiral line**.
2. It provides attachment to two ligaments and two muscles:
   (a) Capsule of the hip joint.
   (b) Iliofemoral ligament (strongest ligament in the body).
   (c) Vastus lateralis to its upper end.
   (d) Vastus medialis to its lower end.

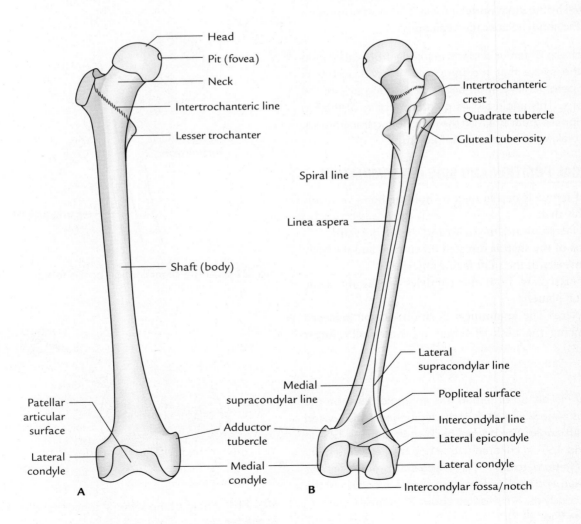

Fig. 21.8 General features of the femur: **A**, anterior view; **B**, posterior view.

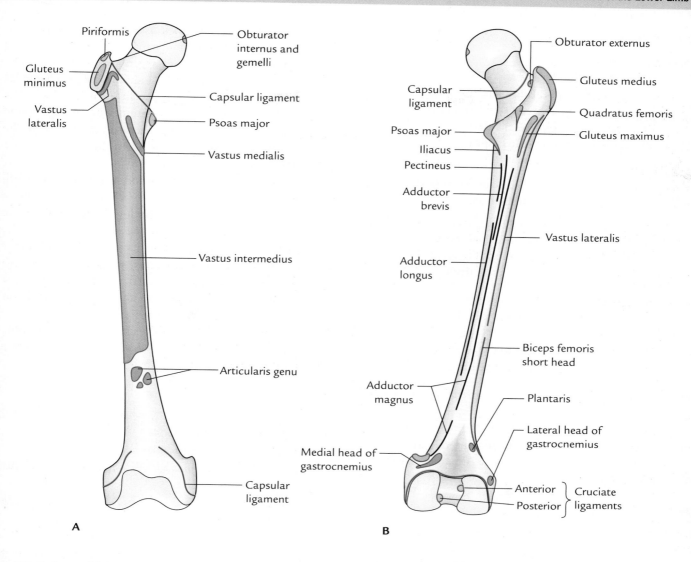

Fig. 21.9 Special features (attachments) of the femur: **A**, anterior view; **B**, posterior view.

Posterior surface
1. It is convex from above downward and concave from side-to-side.
2. It meets the shaft at **intertrochanteric crest**.
3. Its medial half is intracapsular.
4. It presents a faint groove, which lodges the tendon of obturator externus.

Intertrochanteric crest
1. It extends from the posterosuperior angle of greater trochanter to the tip of lesser trochanter.
2. It presents a rounded tubercle near the middle called **quadrate tubercle**, which provides insertion to the quadratus femoris.

N.B. The neck connects the head to the shaft about 5 cm away from the hip joint. This enables the lower limb to swing clear of the pelvis. Thus, the neck of femur is akin to the clavicle in the upper limb.

Greater Trochanter
1. It is a quadrilateral elevation, projecting upward from the lateral aspect of the junction of neck and shaft.
2. It presents one border (upper) and three surfaces (anterior, medial, and lateral).

Upper border

Its posterior part presents the apex or tip of greater trochanter, which provides attachment to the piriformis.

Anterior surface

It provides attachment to the gluteus minimus on a ridge in its lateral part. Its medial part is related to a synovial bursa—trochanteric bursa of gluteus minimus.

Medial surface

It presents two depressions:

1. A depression (**trochanteric fossa**) at its junction with the neck for insertion of obturator externus.
2. A shallow depression above and in front of trochanteric fossa for insertion of obturator internus along with the gemellus superior and gemellus inferior.

Lateral surface

It is quadrilateral and divided diagonally by an oblique ridge into the upper and lower triangular areas.

1. The ridge provides attachment to the *gluteus medius muscle.*
2. The triangular areas—anterior and posterior to the ridge are related to the trochanteric bursae of the gluteus medius and gluteus maximus, respectively.

Lesser Trochanter

1. It is a conical projection arising from the posteromedial surface of the neck–shaft angle. It is directed medially.
2. Its apex provides attachment to the psoas major.
3. Iliacus is attached to its base on the front.

N.B. *Attachment of fibrous capsule at the upper end of femur:* Anteriorly it is attached to the intertrochanteric line but posteriorly it is attached about 1 cm medial to the intertrochanteric crest. Therefore, the lateral part of the posterior surface of the neck of femur is extracapsular and its medial half is intracapsular.

Shaft

Features

Basically the shaft of femur presents three surfaces—anterior, medial, and lateral and three borders—medial, lateral, and posterior.

The middle third of posterior border is represented by a thick ridge called **linea aspera**, which acts as a buttress to resist the compressive forces and prevents the anterior bowing of the shaft. The linea aspera presents inner and outer lips and an intervening intermediate area.

When the upper end of linea aspera is traced upward, its inner and outer lips diverge and enclose a triangular **posterior surface** in the upper one-third of the shaft. The inner (medial) lip becomes continuous with the **spiral line** and the outer (lateral) lip becomes continuous with the **gluteal tuberosity,** which extends up to the root of greater trochanter.

When the lower end of linea aspera is traced downward, its inner and outer lips, diverge below, and enclose a triangular **popliteal surface** in the lower one-third of the shaft. The inner (medial) lip becomes continuous with the **medial supracondylar line,** which ends at the **adductor tubercle.** The outer (lateral) lip becomes continuous with **lateral supra condylar line.** Thus, strictly speaking, the shaft presents five surfaces—anterior, medial, lateral, upper posterior, and lower posterior (popliteal surface).

The borders and surfaces of the shaft of femur in upper one-third, middle one-third, and lower one-third are given in Table 21.3.

Attachments

The shaft of femur provides attachment to the following muscles and intermuscular septa:

1. **Attachments of intermuscular septa:**
   (a) *Medial intermuscular septum* is attached to the medial lip of linea aspera.
   (b) *Lateral intermuscular septum* is attached to the lateral lip of the linea aspera.

2. **Muscular attachments:**
   (a) *Vastus intermedius* arises from the upper three-fourth of anterior surface and adjoining lateral surface.
   (b) *Articularis genu* arises by few small slips from the lower one-fourth of anterior surface immediately below the vastus intermedius.

Table 21.3 Borders and surfaces of the shaft of femur

Part of femur	Borders	Surfaces
Middle 1/3rd of the shaft	• Medial border • Lateral border • Posterior border (linea aspera)	• Anterior surface • Medial surface • Lateral surface
Upper 1/3rd of the shaft	• Medial border • Lateral border • Spiral line • Gluteal tuberosity	• Anterior surface • Medial surface • Lateral surface • Posterior surface
Lower 1/3rd of the shaft	• Medial border • Lateral border • Medial supracondylar line • Lateral supracondylar line	• Anterior surface • Medial surface • Lateral surface • Popliteal surface

(c) *Vastus lateralis* arises in a linear fashion from the upper part of intertrochanteric line, anterior and inferior borders of greater trochanter, lateral margin of gluteal tuberosity, and lateral lip of linea aspera.

(d) *Vastus medialis* arises in a linear fashion from the lower part of intertrochanteric line, spiral line, and the medial lip of linea aspera and the upper one-fourth of medial supracondylar line.

(e) *Gluteus maximus* is inserted into the gluteal tuberosity.

(f) *Adductor longus* is inserted into the medial lip of linea aspera.

(g) *Pectineus* is inserted into a line extending from the lesser trochanter to the upper end of linea aspera.

(h) *Adductor brevis* is inserted into a line extending from the lesser trochanter to the upper part of linea aspera.

(i) *Adductor magnus* is inserted into the medial margin of gluteal tuberosity, linea aspera, medial supracondylar line, and adductor tubercle.

(j) *Gastrocnemius:* The **medial head** arises from the popliteal surface just above the medial condyle. The **lateral head** arises mainly from the lateral condyle but also extends over the lower end of lateral supracondylar line.

(k) *Plantaris* arises from the lower end of lateral supracondylar line just above the lateral head of gastrocnemius.

N.B. *Arrangement of nine structures attached to the linea aspera:* From medial to lateral side, these are (Fig. 21.10):
- Vastus medialis.
- Medial intermuscular septum.
- Adductor brevis (in the upper) and adductor longus (in the lower part).
- Adductor magnus.
- Short head of biceps femoris.
- Posterior intermuscular septum.
- Vastus lateralis.
- Vastus intermedius.

Lower End

Medial Condyle

1. Its most prominent point is called medial epicondyle, which provides attachment to the upper end of medial collateral ligament.
   A projection posterosuperior to the medial epicondyle is called **adductor tubercle,** which provides insertion to the ischial head of adductor magnus.
2. Its lateral surface forms medial boundary of intercondylar fossa.

Lateral Condyle

1. It is stouter and stronger than the medial condyle but less prominent.

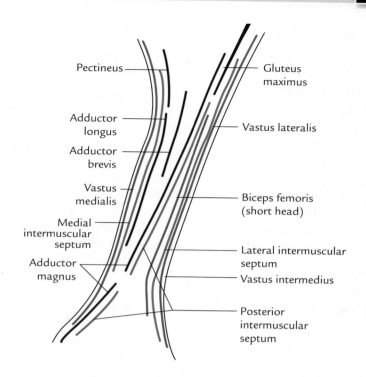

Fig. 21.10 Structures attached to the linea aspera (magnified view).

2. Its lateral surface presents a prominence called **lateral epicondyle** which provides attachment to the fibular collateral ligament of the knee joint.
3. Smooth impression above and behind the lateral epicondyle gives origin to the lateral head of gastrocnemius.
4. A groove below and behind the lateral epicondyle provides attachment to popliteus in its anterior part. Tendon of popliteus occupies the posterior part of this groove during full flexion at the knee joint.
5. Its medial surface forms the lateral boundary of intercondylar fossa.

Intercondylar Fossa (Intercondylar Notch)

1. It is a deep notch, which separates two condyles posteriorly.
2. It is limited posteriorly above by intercondylar line.
3. It presents medial and lateral walls and floor.
4. Medial wall of the fossa provides attachments to the upper end of **posterior cruciate ligament** in its anteroinferior part.
5. Lateral wall of the fossa provides attachment to the upper end of **anterior cruciate ligament** in its posterosuperior part.

Mnemonic: LAMP = Lateral condyle provides attachment to Anterior cruciate ligament and Medial condyle to Posterior cruciate ligament.

Articular Surface

The lower end of femur presents a V-shaped articular surface occupying the anterior, inferior, and posterior surfaces of both condyles.

1. The apex of 'V' is called **patellar surface** which occupies the anterior surfaces of two condyles and articulates with the patella.
2. The two links of 'V' form tibial surfaces which occupy the inferior and posterior surfaces of two condyles to come in contact with corresponding articular surfaces of tibial condyles.
3. The **patellar surface** is saddle-shaped. Its lateral portion is broader and extends to a higher level than the medial portion, corresponding to articular surface of the patella.

N.B. *Attachment of fibrous capsule at the lower end of femur:* Posteriorly, it is attached to the intercondylar line and articular margins. Anteriorly, it is deficient for communication of suprapatellar bursa with the synovial cavity of knee joint. Laterally and medially, it is attached along a line 1 cm above the articular margins. It is important to note that the groove for popliteus is intracapsular.

Clinical correlation

- **Fracture neck of femur:** It is very common in elderly particularly in women due to osteoporotic changes in the neck.
- **Types of fracture:** The fracture may be intracapsular (*subcapital*, *transverse cervical*) or extracapsular (*basal*, *intertrochanteric*, and *subtrochanteric*). In intracapsular fracture, the retinacular vessels—the chief source of blood supply to the head—are injured. This leads to delayed healing or non-union of fracture, or even avascular necrosis of the head of femur (for details, see *Clinical and Surgical Anatomy*, 2nd Edition by Vishram Singh).

  In intracapsular fracture of the neck of femur, the affected limb is shortened and characteristically held in laterally rotated position with the toes pointing laterally.

OSSIFICATION

The femur ossifies from five centres: one primary and four secondary centres. The primary centre appears in the midshaft. Three secondary centres appear in the upper end and one secondary centre in the lower end. The age of appearance and fusion of these centres is given in Table 21.4.

Clinical correlation

Medicolegal significance of ossification centre at the lower end of femur: The secondary centre at the lower end of femur is unique in the sense that it appears during birth/just before birth (ninth month of IUL). It is of medicolegal importance because its appearance in radiograph indicates maturity of the fetus (for details, see *Textbook of Clinical Embryology* by Vishram Singh).

PATELLA (KNEE CAP)

The patella is the largest sesamoid bone, found in the tendon of quadriceps femoris. It is situated in front of the knee joint, hence it is also called knee cap. It is a flattened and triangular bone with the base facing upward, and the apex downward. Its anterior aspect is convex and rough, whereas its posterior surface presents a large articular surface divided into small medial part and large lateral part.

ANATOMICAL POSITION AND SIDE DETERMINATION

Hold the patella in such a way that:

- Its apex faces downward and its base faces upward.
- Its articular surface faces posteriorly. The large lateral part of articular surface determines the side.

Trick-device: Keep the articular surface of patella on the table-top in such a way that its base is directed toward you and its apex away from you. Now observe the tilt of patella. The patella, as a rule, always tilts toward the side it belongs to.

Table 21.4 Ossification of the femur

Centres	Time of appearance	Time of fusion	
Primary centre In mid shaft	7th to 8th week of IUL		
Secondary centres • 1 for head • 1 for greater trochanter • 1 for lesser trochanter	• 1 year • 3 years • 13 years	Three separate epiphysis	18th year
For lower end 1	9 months (at the time of birth)		20 years

FEATURES AND ATTACHMENTS (Figs 21.11 and 21.12)

The patella presents the following features:

- Apex.
- Three borders: Superior, medial, and lateral.
- Two surfaces: Anterior and posterior.

Apex

It is directed downward and provides attachment to the ligamentum patellae, which connects the patella to the tibial tubercle.

Borders

Superior border (also called base)

It provides attachment to rectus femoris in the anterior part and vastus intermedius in its posterior part.

Lateral border

It provides attachment to vastus lateralis in its upper one-third and lateral patellar retinaculum in the lower two-third.

Medial border

It provides attachment to vastus medialis in the upper two-third and medial patellar retinaculum in its lower one-third.

The lateral and medial patellar retinaculum are the expansions of the tendons of vastus lateralis and vastus medialis, respectively.

Surfaces

Anterior surface

1. It is rough, convex, longitudinally striated, and presents numerous vascular foramina.
2. It is subcutaneous and **subcutaneous prepatellar bursa** intervenes between it and skin.

Posterior surface

1. Its lower one-fourth is rough and non-articular, while its upper three-fourth is smooth and articular.
2. Small non-articular part near the apex is divided into two areas: lower and upper.
   (a) *Lower area* provides attachment to **ligamentum patellae.**
   (b) *Upper area* is related to **infrapatellar pad of fat.**

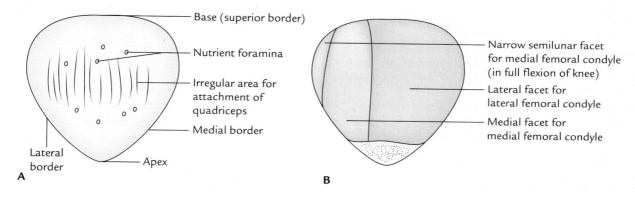

Fig. 21.11 General features of the right patella: A, anterior aspect; B, posterior aspect.

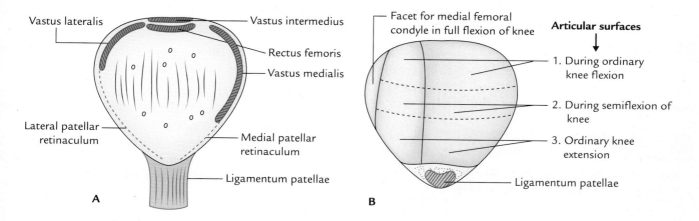

Fig. 21.12 Special features of the right patella: A, anterior aspect; B, posterior aspect.

3. The large articular area is primarily divided by a vertical ridge into a larger lateral and a smaller medial area in order to fit with the reciprocal articular surfaces of the femur. The vertical ridge itself occupies the groove on the patellar surface of femoral lower end in the position of extension.
   (a) Larger lateral articular area lies in contact with the lateral femoral condyle in all positions of the knee.
   (b) Small medial articular area is further divided by another vertical ridge into a large lateral part and a narrow medial part called **medial strip**. The medial strip comes in contact with the under surface of medial femoral condyle during full flexion at the knee.
       Leaving aside this medial strip, whole of articular surface of the patella is subdivided into upper, middle, and lower areas by two faint horizontal lines.

The patellar surface of femur comes in contact with the upper area in ordinary flexion, with the middle area in semiflexion, and with the lower area in ordinary extension.

Clinical correlation

- **Dislocation of the patella:** The patella has natural tendency to dislocate laterally due to upward and lateral pull by the quadriceps. However, it is countered by three factors:
  (a) More forward projection of lateral femoral condyle.
  (b) More prolonged insertion of vastus medialis to the medial border of the patella than that of vastus lateralis on the lateral border.
  (c) Medial pull exerted by medial patellar retinaculum.
- **Fracture of the patella:** (a) A direct blow on the patella fractures it into two or more pieces, and (b) a sudden and forceful contraction of quadriceps femoris causes a transverse fracture of the patella. The patella being a sesamoid bone is devoid of the periosteum, hence when fractured bony union does not take place.

OSSIFICATION

The patella ossifies from several centres which appear during 3–6 years and fuse quickly to form a single centre. The ossification of patella is completed at puberty.

Clinical correlation

Abnormal ossification of the patella. Abnormal ossification centres in the patella may form two or three separate pieces of the patella (called bipartite or tripartite patella). This condition can be differentiated from fracture of the patella as it is bilateral and the pieces have smooth margins.

TIBIA (SYNONYM SHINBONE)

The tibia is the second largest bone in the body situated on the medial side in the leg. The tibia is the pre-axial bone and homologous with the lateral bone of the forearm, the radius. It transmits weight of the body from femur to the foot.

PARTS

The tibia is a long bone and consists of three parts: upper end, lower end, and intervening shaft.

The **upper end** is expanded and bears prominent **medial and lateral condyles** and **tibial tuberosity**. The medial condyle is larger than the lateral condyle. The two condyles articulate with the condyle of the femur.

The **shaft** has three borders—anterior, medial, and lateral; and three surfaces—medial, lateral, and posterior. The anterior border is the sharpest and takes a sinuous course from the tibial tuberosity and becomes continuous below with the anterior border of the medial malleolus.

The **lower end** is small and projects medially and inferiorly as **medial malleolus**.

ANATOMICAL POSITION AND SIDE DETERMINATION

The side of tibia is determined by holding the bone vertically in such a way that:

1. Its expanded end with condyles faces upward.
2. Its tibial tuberosity and sharp sinuous anterior border of the shaft faces anteriorly.
3. Medial malleolus is on the medial side.
4. Superior surface of the upper end (tibial plateau) lies in a horizontal plane.

FEATURES AND ATTACHMENTS (Figs 21.13 and 21.14)

Upper End

It presents two condyles (medial and lateral), an intercondylar area and tibial tuberosity.

Medial Condyle

It is larger than the lateral condyle and presents four surfaces: superior, posterior, anterior, and medial.

Superior surface (Fig. 21.15)
1. It has a smooth oval articular surface which articulates with the femoral condyle.
2. It is slightly concave in the centre and flattened at the periphery. The peripheral flattened part is covered by fibrocartilaginous plate, the **medial meniscus**.

Posterior surface
It presents a deep transverse groove for the insertion of tendon of semimembranosus.

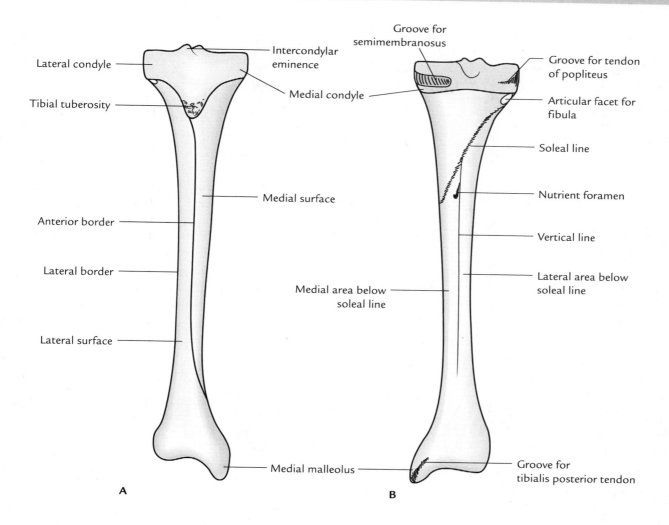

Fig. 21.13 General features of the tibia: **A**, anterior view; **B**, posterior view.

Anterior and medial surfaces
The anterior and medial surfaces are marked by the vascular foramina and adjoining margin provides attachment to the medial patellar retinaculum.

Lateral Condyle
Like medial condyle the lateral condyle also presents four surfaces:

Superior surface
1. It presents a circular articular surface for articulation with the lateral femoral condyle.
2. It is slightly concave in the centre and flattened at the periphery. The flattened peripheral part is covered by a plate of fibrocartilage—the **lateral meniscus**.

Posterior surface
1. Inferolaterally this surface presents a circular smooth *articular facet for the head of fibula.*

2. Between the articular facet for the fibula and the margin of superior surface there is a shallow *groove for the tendon of popliteus.*

Anterior and lateral surfaces
1. The anterior surface has a flat *triangular facet for the attachment of the iliotibial tract.*
2. Anterior and lateral surfaces provide attachment to the lateral patellar retinaculum.

Intercondylar Area
1. It is the rough area on the superior surface of the upper end of tibia between the articular surfaces of two condyles.
2. The middle of intercondylar area is narrow and marked by an elevation called **intercondylar eminence**. The medial and lateral parts of the eminence are more prominent and constitute the medial and lateral **intercondylar tubercles**.

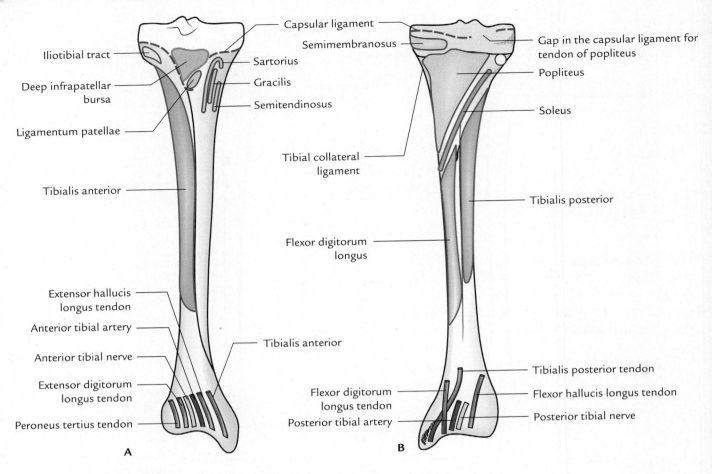

Fig. 21.14 Special features (attachment) of the tibia: **A**, anterior aspect; **B**, posterior aspect.

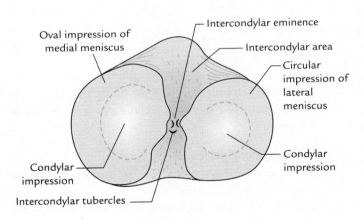

Fig. 21.15 Features on the upper aspect of the tibia.

3. From before backward, the intercondylar area provides attachments to six structures (Fig. 21.16):
    (a) Anterior horn of Medial meniscus.
    (b) Anterior Cruciate ligament.
    (c) Anterior horn of Lateral meniscus.
    (d) Posterior horn of Lateral meniscus.
    (e) Posterior horn of Medial meniscus.
    (f) Posterior Cruciate ligament.

Mnemonic: Medical College Lucknow, Lucknow Medical College.

Tibial Tuberosity

1. It is a projection at the apex of rough triangular area located on the anterior aspect upper end of the tibia.
2. It is divided into an upper smooth and a lower rough part.
3. Upper smooth part provides attachment to the ligamentum patellae.
4. Lower rough part is related to the **subcutaneous infrapatellar bursa** which separates it from the skin.
5. Rough triangular area above the tuberosity is related to the **deep infrapatellar bursa**.

Shaft

It presents three borders—anterior, medial, and lateral; and three surfaces—lateral, medial, and posterior.

Borders

Anterior border (shin of the tibia)

1. It is the sharpest, subcutaneous, and sinuous in course.
2. It extends from the tibial tuberosity to the anterior border of medial malleolus.

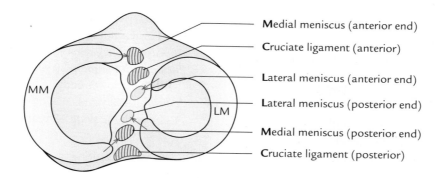

Fig. 21.16 Structures attached in intercondylar area on the superior aspect of the tibia (MM = medial meniscus, LM = lateral meniscus).

Medial border

1. It extends from the medial condyle to the posterior border of medial malleolus.
2. The soleal line joins the medial border at the junction of its upper one-third with the lower two-third.

Lateral (interosseous) border

1. It is sharp and extends from the lateral condyle below the facet for the head of fibula to the anterior border of fibular notch.
2. It provides attachment to the interosseous membrane which unites the tibia and fibula.
3. Its distal part divides to enclose a triangular notch for the attachment of interosseous **inferior tibiofibular ligament**.

Surfaces

Medial surface

1. It faces anteromedially and lies between the anterior and medial borders.
2. It is almost entirely subcutaneous.
3. Its upper part close to the medial border receives insertions of three muscles. From before backward, these are: sartorius, gracilis, and semitendinosus.

Mnemonic: Girl between two surgeons – 'SGS'.

Lateral surface

1. It is directed anterolaterally and lies between anterior and interosseous borders.
2. Its upper two-third provides origin to the **tibialis anterior**.
3. Its lower one-third is crossed by the following structures from medial to lateral sides while passing from the leg to the foot:
   (a) Tibialis anterior.
   (b) Extensor hallucis longus.
   (c) Anterior tibial artery.
   (d) Deep peroneal nerve/anterior tibial nerve.

(e) Extensor digitorum longus.
(f) Peroneus tertius.

Mnemonic: The Himalayas Are Not Dry Plateaus.

Posterior surface

1. It lies between the medial and lateral borders.
2. A rough bony ridge extends from the fibular facet to the junction of upper and middle thirds of the medial border called **soleal line**. This line provides attachments to the following structures from above downward:
   (a) Fascia covering popliteus.
   (b) Fascia covering soleus.
   (c) Soleus (origin).
   (d) Deep transverse fascia.
3. The posterior surface of the tibial shaft is subdivided by the soleal line into an upper small triangular area and a lower large area.
4. A triangular area above the soleal line provides insertion to popliteus.
5. A large area below the soleal line is divided into a medial and a lateral part by a vertical ridge.
6. The **nutrient foramen** of the tibia is located at the upper end of this vertical ridge. Nutrient canal is directed downward. Nutrient artery is a branch of the posterior tibial artery and the **largest nutrient artery of the body**.
7. The flexor digitorum longus arises from the medial area below the soleal line.
8. The tibialis posterior arises from the lateral area below the soleal line.
9. The lower one-fourth of the posterior surface beneath the flexor retinaculum is related to the following structures from medial to lateral:
   (a) Tibialis posterior.
   (b) Flexor digitorum longus.
   (c) Posterior tibial artery.
   (d) Tibial nerve.
   (e) Flexor hallucis longus.

Mnemonic: The Doctors Are Not Hunters.

Lower End

The lower end presents five surfaces (anterior, posterior, medial, lateral, and inferior) and a downward projection from the medial part, the medial malleolus.

Surfaces

1. **Anterior surface** has an upper smooth and featureless part and lower rough and grooved part.
2. **Posterior surface** in its medial part presents a *groove for the tendon of tibialis posterior*.
3. **Medial surface** is subcutaneous and is continuous with the medial surface of the medial malleolus.
4. **Lateral surface** presents a **fibular notch**. Anterior and posterior margins of the fibular notch provide attachment to **anterior and posterior tibiofibular ligaments**. The upper part of the fibular notch is rough and provides attachments to the **interosseous tibiofibular ligament**.
5. **Inferior surface** is smooth and articulates with the body of the talus.

Medial Malleolus

1. Its tip lies at a higher level than that of the lateral malleolus and provides attachment to the *deltoid ligament*.
2. Its lateral surfaces present a comma-shaped articular facet for articulation with the similar facet on the medial surface of the body of the talus.
3. Its posterior surface presents a *vertical groove for the tendon of tibialis posterior*.
4. Medial margin of the groove is prominent and provides attachment to the flexor retinaculum.

CAPSULAR ATTACHMENTS AT THE UPPER AND LOWER ENDS OF TIBIA

1. **At the upper end**, the capsule is attached to the margins of tibial condyles medially, laterally, and posteriorly. Anteriorly it is attached to the sides of triangular area on the anterior aspect of condyles blending with the medial and lateral patellar retinacula and to the tibial tubercle where it blends with the ligamentum patellae.

   Behind the lateral condyle, the capsule is deficient for the passage of tendon of popliteus.
2. **At the lower end**, the capsule is attached to the margins of articular surfaces where it extends on to the lower end of fibula.

OSSIFICATION

The tibia ossifies from three centres—one primary and two secondary.

1. **Primary centre** appears in the middle of shaft at the age of seventh week of IUL.

2. **Secondary centres.**
   (a) For the upper end:
   Appearance: At birth or shortly after birth.
   Fusion with the shaft: 20 years.
   (b) For the lower end:
   Appearance: 2 years.
   Fusion with the shaft: 18 years.

N.B. The upper epiphysis extends anteriorly as a tongue-like process to form the upper part of tibial tuberosity.

Clinical correlation

- **Osteomyelitis of the upper end of tibia:** The upper end of tibia is the commonest site of **acute osteomyelitis**, but knee joint remain unaffected because the capsule of knee joint is attached near to the margins of articular surfaces proximal to the epiphyseal line.
- **Fracture of tibia:** The tibia is commonly fractured at the junction of upper 2/3rd and lower 1/3rd of its shaft. (The tibial shaft is narrowest at the junction of upper two-third and lower one-third, hence the commonest site of fracture.)

   The lower one-third of the tibial shaft is bare area (hence devoid of any muscular attachment) and have low blood supply; for this reason, the fractures in the lower 1/3rd of the shaft of tibia show delayed union or non-union (for details, see *Clinical and Surgical Anatomy*, 2nd Edition by Vishram Singh).

FIBULA

The fibula is the lateral bone of the leg and is homologous with the ulna of forearm. In Latin, the term fibula means "pin"; hence the lateral bone of leg is rightly named fibula because it is a long pin-like bone. It is a long slender post-axial bone of the leg and does not take part in the transmission of the body weight.

It subserves two important functions:

1. It provides attachments—muscles.
2. Its lower end along with the lower end of tibia forms a socket (**tibiofibular mortise**), to hold the talus in place.

PARTS

The fibula is a long bone and consists of three parts: upper end, lower end, and intervening shaft.

- The **upper end** (head) is round and presents a circular articular facet. An upward projection posterolateral to this facet is called styloid process.
- The **shaft** is described to have anterior, interosseous, and posterior borders; and medial, lateral, and posterior surfaces. However, only interosseous border is clear-cut; other borders and surfaces spiral so that it is difficult to

ascertain. None of them remains strictly in the position implied by its name. Therefore, making an attempt to identify them is just wastage of time.

- The **lower end** is flattened and bears a *triangular articular facet* on its medial surface for articulation with the talus. Behind and below this is a roughened fossa called malleolar fossa.

SIDE DETERMINATION AND ANATOMICAL POSITION

The side of fibula can be determined by holding it vertically in such a way that:

- Its round end called head is directed upward.
- Its relatively flattened end is directed downward.
- A triangular articular facet on its lower end faces medially.
- A depression at the lower end (malleolar fossa) lies behind and below the triangular articular facet at this end.

FEATURES AND ATTACHMENTS (Figs 21.17 and 21.18)

Upper End

It presents head and neck.

Head

It is round and presents the following three features:

1. An **oval or circular articular facet** on its superior aspect for articulation with the lateral condyle of the tibia.
2. A **styloid process** posterolateral to the articular facet which provides attachment to the *fibular collateral ligament*.
3. A sloping surface in front of the styloid process for C-shaped insertion of biceps femoris.

Neck

It is a constriction below the head, connecting it with the shaft. The common peroneal nerve is related to the posterolateral aspect of neck and anterior tibial artery on its medial aspect.

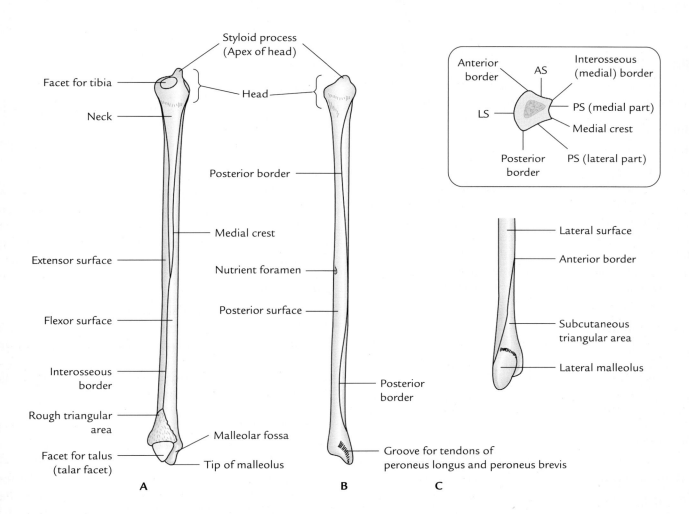

Fig. 21.17 General features of the right fibula: **A**, medial aspect; **B**, posterior aspect; **C**, lateral aspect of lower part. Figure in the inset is the transverse section of the lower part of shaft showing borders and surfaces (AS = anterior surface, PS = posterior surface, LS = lateral surface).

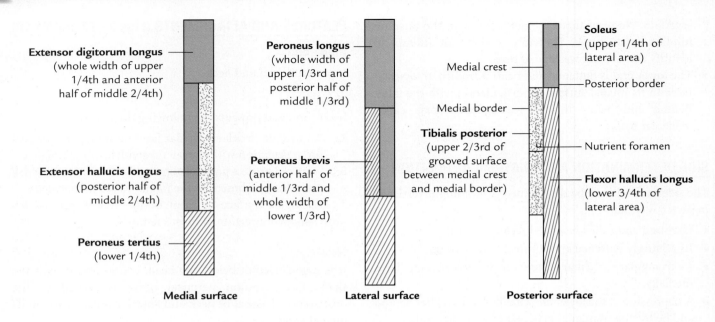

Fig. 21.18 Schematic diagram to show the attachments of muscles on the different surfaces of the fibula.

Shaft

It presents three borders—anterior, posterior, and medial; and three surfaces—medial, lateral, and posterior.

Borders

Anterior border

1. It provides attachment to the anterior intermuscular septum of the leg in its upper three-fourth.
2. It begins just below the anterior aspect of the head. Inferiorly it splits to enclose a triangular area, which continues on the lateral surface of lateral malleolus.
3. Superior extensor retinaculum is attached to the anterior margin of the triangular area and superior peroneal retinaculum to the posterior margin of triangular area.

Posterior border

1. It extends from the posterior aspect of head to the lateral margin of groove on the posterior surface of the lateral malleolus.
2. Posterior intermuscular septum of the leg is attached to its upper three-fourth.

Interosseous medial border

1. It lies close and just medial to the anterior border (separated from it only by 3 mm in the upper part).
2. Inferiorly it ends at the upper end of the roughened area for the interosseous ligament.
3. Interosseous membrane is attached along its whole length except at the upper end to leave a gap for the passage of anterior tibial vessels.

Surfaces

Medial (extensor) surface

1. It is narrow and lies between the anterior and interosseous borders.
2. It gives origin to *extensor digitorum* longus in upper three-fourth (whole width of its upper fourth and anterior half of its middle two-fourth).
3. *Extensor hallucis longus* arises from the posterior half of the middle two-fourth medial to the *extensor digitorum longus.*
4. Its lower one-fourth provides origin to the *peroneus tertius.*

Lateral (peroneal) surface

1. It lies between the anterior and posterior borders.
2. *Peroneus longus* arises from the upper two-third (whole width of upper one-third and the posterior half of the middle one-third).
3. *Peroneus brevis* arises from the anterior half of its middle one-third and whole width of its lower one-third.

Posterior (flexor) surface

1. It is extensive and lies between the interosseous and posterior borders.
2. Its upper two-third is divided into medial concave and flattened lateral parts by a sharp vertical ridge **medial crest.**
3. Fascia covering the tibialis posterior is attached to the medial crest.
4. Medial concave part gives origin to tibialis posterior.

5. Lateral flattened part gives origin to the soleus in upper one-fourth and to the flexor hallucis longus in lower three-fourth.
6. Peroneal artery descends along medial crest.
7. Nutrient artery, a branch of the peroneal artery, enters the nutrient foramen present just above the middle of the posterior surface. Nutrient canal is directed downward.

Lower End (Fig. 21.19)

The lower end of fibula is expanded anteroposteriorly to form **lateral malleolus**, which presents four surfaces—anterior, posterior, medial, and lateral.

1. **Anterior surface** is rough and round. It provides attachment to the anterior talofibular ligament. A notch at its lower border provides attachment to the calcaneofibular ligament.
2. **Posterior surface** presents a groove, which lodges tendons of peroneus brevis and peroneus longus, the latter being superficial to the former.
3. **Medial surface** presents a triangular articular surface in front and a depression (malleolar fossa) below and behind it.
   The upper part of malleolar fossa provides attachment to the posterior tibiofibular ligament and its lower part to the **posterior talofibular ligament.**
4. **Lateral surface** is triangular and subcutaneous.

OSSIFICATION

The fibula ossifies from three centres: one primary and two secondary.

1. Primary centre appears in the middle of the shaft: at the age of eighth week of IUL.

2. Secondary centres:
   (a) For the upper end:
   Appearance: 3–4 years.
   Fusion with the shaft: 20 years.
   (b) For the lower end:
   Appearance: 1–2 years.
   Fusion with the shaft: 18 years.

N.B. In fibula, **law of union of epiphysis** is violated [cf. according to this law, epiphyseal (secondary) centre which appears first unites last with the diaphysis. In fibula, epiphyseal centre for lower end appears first and also unites first]. The explanation to this violation is that epiphyseal centre in the lower end of fibula appears earlier because it is pressure epiphysis and in the upper end later because it is traction epiphysis. Since the growing end fibula is its upper end (as evidenced by the direction of nutrient foramen) it unites with the diaphysis last although its epiphyseal centre also appears last.

> ### Clinical correlation
>
> - **Bone grafts:** Since the fibula does not take part in the transmission of body weight, it is a common source of bone for grafting.
> - **Fibular fracture:** The fibula is commonly fractured, 2 to 5 cm proximal to the distal end of the lateral malleolus. It is often associated with *'fracture dislocation of the ankle joint'.*

SKELETON OF THE FOOT (Figs 21.20 and 21.21)

The skeleton of the foot from behind forward consists of the following bones:

- Tarsals.
- Metatarsals.
- Phalanges.

TARSAL BONES

These are short bones which together form **tarsus**. These are arranged in three rows:

(a) *Proximal row* consists of talus and calcaneus.
(b) *Middle row* consists of navicular.
(c) *Distal row* consists of three cuneiforms (medial, intermediate, and lateral) and cuboid.

N.B. *Identification of bones in the skeleton of the foot:*
- *Calcaneus* (heel bone) is the largest and most proximal bone.
- *Talus* is the second largest bone and lies above the calcaneus like a rider, hence highest bone in the skeleton of foot.

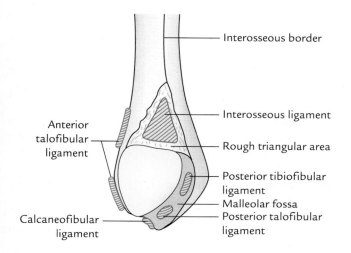

Fig. 21.19 Special features of the lower end of right fibula (medial aspect).

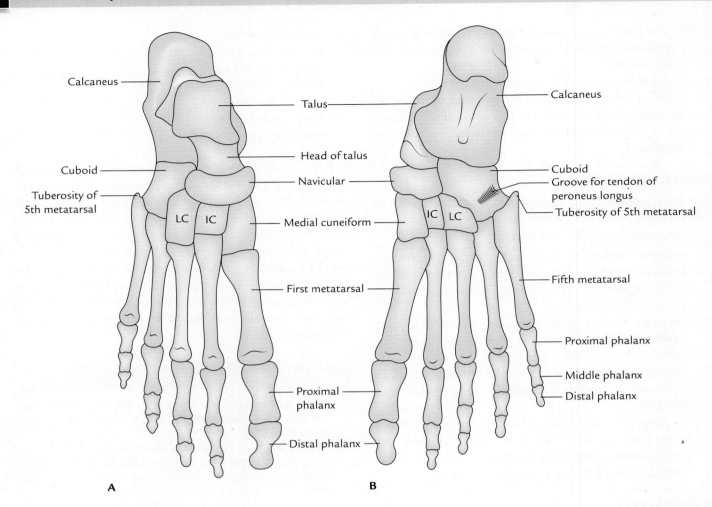

Fig. 21.20 General features of the skeleton of the foot: **A**, dorsal aspect; **B**, plantar aspect (IC = intermediate cuneiform, LC = lateral cuneiform).

- *Navicular* is boat-shaped and lies in front of the head of talus.
- *Cuboid* is cubical in shape in front of the lateral part of calcaneum.
- *Cuneiforms* are small wedge-shaped bones and arranged from side to side in front of navicular.

Talus (Latin Talus = Ankle Bone)

The talus is the second largest bone of the foot situated on the upper surface of the anterior two-third of the calcaneus. It forms the connecting link between the bones of the foot and the leg. It participates in the formation of three joints—ankle (talocrural), talocalcaneal (subtalar), and talocalcaneonavicular (pretalar).

N.B. Talus is the only bone of the foot, which is devoid of any muscular attachment.

Side Determination and Anatomical Position
The side of talus is determined by keeping it on the table-top in such a way that:

1. Its rounded head is directed forward.
2. Its trochlear articular surface (which is convex anteroposteriorly and concave from side to side) faces upward.
3. Triangular articular surface on the side of body faces laterally while the comma-shaped articular surface on the side of body is directed medially.

Features and Attachments (Fig. 21.22)
The talus presents a head, a neck, and a body.

Head
1. It is directed forward, medially, and slightly downward.
2. Its *anterior surface* presents a convex articular surface which articulates with the concavity of navicular bone.

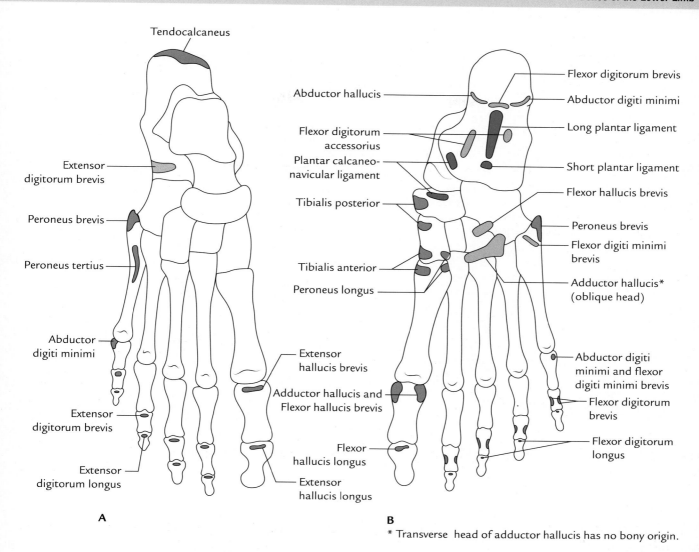

Fig. 21.21 Special features of the skeleton of the foot: **A**, dorsal aspect; **B**, plantar aspect.

* Transverse head of adductor hallucis has no bony origin.

3. Its *inferior surface* presents three articular facets:
   (a) **Posterior facet** is largest and articulates with the middle facet of calcaneus and forms a plane synovial subtalar joint.
   (b) **Middle facet** articulates with a spring ligament.
   (c) **Anterolateral facet** articulates with the anterior facet of calcaneus.

Neck
1. It is a constriction between the head and the body.
2. It projects forward and medially from the body making an angle of 150° with the body (neck–body angle).
3. Distal part of dorsal surface of neck provides attachment to the **dorsal talonavicular ligament**.
4. Lateral surface of the neck provides attachment to the **anterior talofibular ligament**.

5. Plantar surface of the neck presents a narrow deep groove called **sulcus tali** which forms **sinus tarsi** with the corresponding groove of calcaneus.

Body
The body of talus is cuboidal in shape. It presents five surfaces—superior, inferior, medial, lateral, and posterior.

Superior surface: It presents trochlear articular surface being wide anteriorly. It articulates with the distal surface of the tibia.

Inferior surface: It presents a large oval concave facet which articulates with the posterior facet of calcaneus to form the **subtalar joint**.

Medial surface: Its upper part presents a *comma-shaped* articular facet which articulates with the medial malleolus.

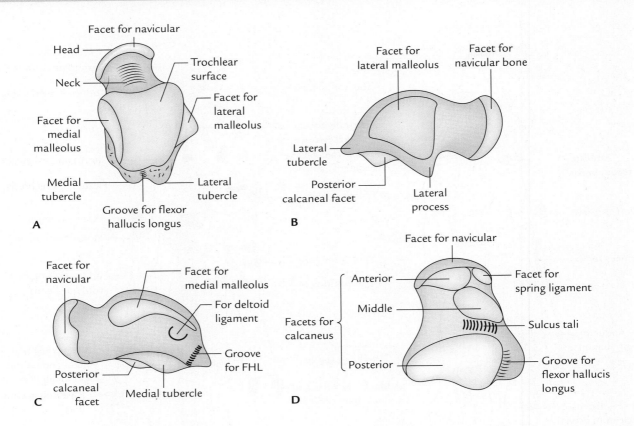

Fig. 21.22 External features of the right talus: A, dorsal aspect; B, lateral aspect; C, medial aspect; D, plantar aspect (FHL = flexor hallucis longus).

Lateral surface: It presents a *triangular articular facet* to articulate with lateral malleolus.

Posterior surface: It is narrow and projects backward as the **posterior process of talus**. It presents an oblique groove bounded by a small medial and large lateral tubercles. The groove lodges the tendon of flexor hallucis longus.

Clinical correlation

Fracture neck of talus: It sometimes occurs due to forceful dorsiflexion of foot. The arteries supplying the talus enter through the front part of the neck and pass backward. These arteries are damaged in the fracture neck of talus and cause delayed union or necrosis of the posterior segment.

Ossification
The talus ossifies from one centre which appears during the sixth month of intrauterine life.

Calcaneus (Latin Calcaneus = Heel)
The calcaneus is the largest and strongest bone of the foot. It is situated below the talus and extends behind it. It is directed forward and laterally with an upward inclination.

Side Determination and Anatomical Position
The side of calcaneus is determined by holding it in its anteroposterior axis in such a way that:

1. Its narrow end bearing concavo-convex facet faces anteriorly.
2. Its concave surface bearing shelf-like projection faces medially.
3. Surface bearing large convex articular facet faces dorsally.

Features and Attachments (Fig. 21.23)
The calcaneum presents six surfaces—anterior, posterior, superior, plantar, lateral, and medial.

Anterior surface
It is the smallest and bears a concavo-convex articular facet to articulate with cuboid.

Posterior surface
It is divided into the following three parts:

(a) *Upper one-third* is smooth and related to a synovial bursa.
(b) *Middle one-third* provides attachment to tendocalcaneus and plantaris.
(c) *Lower one-third* is subcutaneous and weight bearing during standing posture.

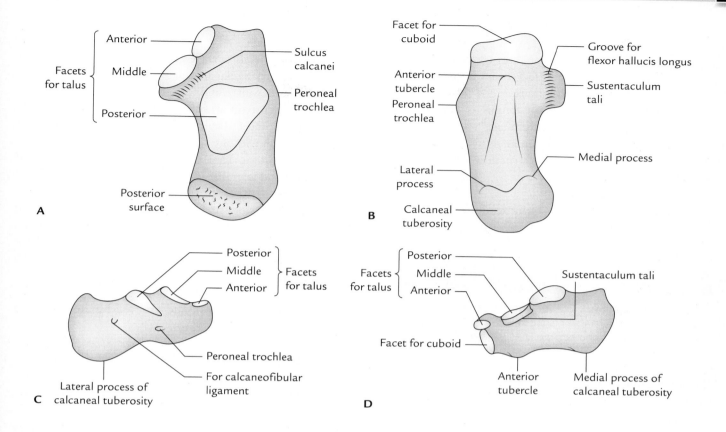

Fig. 21.23 General features of the right calcaneus: A, dorsal aspect; B, plantar aspect; C, lateral aspect; D, medial aspect.

Superior (dorsal) surface

1. It is divided into the following three areas:
   (a) Posterior one-third (non-articular).
   (b) Middle one-third (articular).
   (c) Anterior one-third (partly articular and partly non-articular).
2. *Posterior one-third* is rough and covered with pad of fibrofatty tissue deep to tendocalcaneus.
3. *Middle one-third* bears a large oval facet—the posterior facet for talus.
4. *Anterior one-third* more anteriorly presents two articular facets called middle and anterior facets for talus.
5. Non-articular part of anterior one-third behind the articular facets is divided into medial narrow and lateral wide parts:
   (a) Medial narrow part is grooved and called sulcus calcanei, which provides attachment to the interosseous talocalcanean ligament.
   (b) Lateral part is large and provides attachments to:
       (i) Extensor digitorum brevis.
       (ii) Inferior extensor retinaculum.
       (iii) Stem of bifurcate ligament.

Plantar (inferior) surface

It is rough and marked by three tubercles.

1. A small tubercle at the anterior end called *anterior tubercle*.
2. An elevation at its posterior end called *calcaneal tuberosity* presenting a **large medial and small lateral tubercles**.
3. Triangular area between the three tubercles provides attachment to the **long plantar ligament**.

A groove in front of the anterior tubercle gives attachment to **short plantar ligament**.

Lateral surface

1. It is almost flat and subcutaneous.
2. It presents a small elevation in its anterior part called **peroneal trochlea (tubercle)** which lies 2 cm below the tip of lateral malleolus.
3. Peroneal trochlea lies between the groove for the tendon of peroneus brevis above and the groove for the tendon of peroneus longus below.

Medial surface

1. It is concave from above downward.

2. A shelf-like projection called **sustentaculum tali** projects from its upper anterior part.
3. Superior surface of sustentaculum tali bears a facet for talus while its inferior surface bears a groove for the tendon of flexor hallucis longus.
4. Tendon of flexor digitorum longus is related to the medial surface of sustentaculum tali.
5. Medial surface of sustentaculum tali provides attachments to the following structures from anterior to posterior:
   (a) Spring ligament.
   (b) A slip from tibialis posterior tendon.
   (c) Deltoid ligament (superficial fibres).
   (d) Medial talocalcaneal ligament.

Clinical correlation

Calcanean fracture: It occurs when a person falls on his heals from a considerable height. The calcaneum breaks into a number of pieces and fracture lines usually run vertically.

Navicular Bone (Latin Navicular = A Little Ship)

The navicular bone is boat-shaped. It is flattened anteroposteriorly and presents six surfaces—anterior, posterior, dorsal, plantar, medial, and lateral.

1. **Anterior surface** is convex and possesses three articular facets for three cuneiforms. The medial facet is the largest.
2. **Posterior surface** is deeply concave and articulates with the head of talus.
3. **Dorsal surface** is convex and rough, and provides attachment to the dorsal talonavicular ligament.
4. **Plantar surface** presents a groove in its medial part through which passes the tendon of tibialis posterior. Its lateral part provides attachment to the **spring ligament.**
5. **Medial surface** projects downward to form **tuberosity of navicular bone**, which provides insertion to the major part of the tendon of tibialis posterior.
6. **Lateral surface** is rough and may present a facet for cuboid.

Side Determination and Anatomical Position

The side of navicular bone is determined by holding it in such a way that:

1. Its deep concave surface faces posteriorly.
2. A prominent projection, the navicular tuberosity, is directed medially.
3. A groove adjacent to tuberosity faces inferiorly.

Cuboid Bone

The cuboid bone as the name implies is cuboid in shape. It is situated in front of calcaneum and behind the fourth and fifth metatarsals.

It presents six surfaces: anterior, posterior, dorsal, plantar, medial, and lateral.

1. **Anterior (distal) surface** presents medial quadrangular and lateral triangular articular facets, which articulate with the bases of fourth and fifth metatarsals, respectively.
2. **Posterior (proximal) surface** presents a concavo-convex articulate facet (saddle-shaped articular facet) for articulation with the anterior surface of the calcaneum.
3. **Dorsal (superior) surface** is rough and flat. It is directed upward and laterally, and provides attachment to dorsal ligaments of the foot.
4. **Plantar (inferior) surface** presents an oblique groove in its distal part for the passage of tendon of peroneus longus.
5. **Medial surface** presents two articular facets—a large distal oval facet and a small proximal oval facet which articulate with the navicular and lateral cuneiform bones, respectively.
6. **Lateral surface** is small and grooved by the tendon of peroneus longus.

Cuneiform Bones (Latin Cuneiform = Wedge-Shaped)

These bones are wedge-shaped and three in number—medial (first cuneiform), intermediate (second cuneiform), and lateral (third cuneiform).

The medial cuneiform is the largest and the intermediate cuneiform is the smallest.

1. Proximal surfaces of cuneiforms articulate with the navicular bone.
2. Distal surface of medial cuneiform articulates with the base of first metatarsal.
3. Distal surface of intermediate cuneiform articulates with the base of second metatarsal.
4. Distal surface of lateral cuneiform articulates with the base of third metatarsal.

N.B. The base of second metatarsal is most fixed/secured because it fits into the **mortise** formed by three cuneiforms. For this reason, the **axial line of foot** passes through the second toe and movements of abduction or adduction of toes are mentioned with reference to the second toe.

METATARSAL BONES

These are five miniature long bones. The five metatarsal bones together constitute the **metatarsus.**

They are numbered from medial to lateral sides as first, second, third, fourth, and fifth.

Identification

First metatarsal

1. It is the shortest, thickest, and strongest, and is adapted for weight transmission.

2. Proximal surface of its base presents a kidney-shaped articular surface.

Second metatarsal

1. It is the longest metatarsal bone.
2. Proximal surface of its base has a triangular concave articular surface.

Third metatarsal

1. Proximal surface of its base has a flat triangular articular facet.
2. The lateral side of its base has two facets while the medial side has one facet.

Fourth metatarsal

1. The proximal surface of its base has a quadrilateral facet, which articulates with the cuboid.
2. The lateral side of base has one facet while its medial side has one facet divided into two parts—proximal and distal.

Fifth metatarsal

The lateral side of its base projects proximally and slightly laterally to form a large tuberosity (styloid process).

Features and Attachments

Each metatarsal consists of three parts: distal end (head), shaft (body), and proximal end (base).

Head

1. It articulates with the base of corresponding proximal phalanx to form the metatarso-phalangeal (MP) joint.
2. Each side of the head presents a tubercle dorsally to provide attachment to the collateral ligament of MP joint.

Shaft

1. Its plantar aspect is concave from before backward.
2. Sides of the shaft provide attachments to the *interossei muscles*.
3. Plantar aspect of the fifth metatarsal gives origin to the **flexor digiti minimi**.

Base

The shapes of articular surfaces on the proximal surfaces of bases of metatarsals and their articulations are given in Table 21.5.

1. Base of the first metatarsal provides insertion to:
   (a) Tendon of *tibialis anterior* inferomedially.
   (b) Tendon of *peroneus longus* inferolaterally.
2. Plantar aspects of bases of middle three (second to fourth) metatarsals provide insertion to slips of *tibialis posterior* and origin to the oblique head of *adductor hallucis*.

Table 21.5 Shapes of the proximal surfaces of the bases of the metatarsals and their articulations

Metatarsal	Shape of the articular surface	Articulation
1st	Kidney-shaped	Medial cuneiform
2nd	Triangular	Intermediate cuneiform
3rd	Triangular	Lateral cuneiform
4th	Quadrangular	Cuboid
5th	Triangular	Cuboid

3. Base of the fifth metatarsal provides the following attachments:
   (a) *Peroneus brevis* is inserted on the styloid process of base.
   (b) *Peroneus tertius* is inserted on the dorsal aspect of the base.
   (c) *Flexor digiti minimi brevis* originates from the plantar aspect of the base.

Ossification

Each metatarsal ossifies from two centres—**one primary** and **one secondary**.

1. **Primary centre** for shafts of all the metatarsals appears during 9th week of IUL except for the shaft of first metatarsal which appears during 10th week of IUL.
2. **Secondary centre** appears during 3rd to 4th year in the heads of all the metatarsals except in the first metatarsal where it appears in the base. All of them join with the shaft during 17–20 years.

The differences between the metatarsals and metacarpals are given in Table 21.6.

Clinical correlation

- **Fracture of the tuberosity (styloid process) of the fifth metatarsal:** It usually occurs due to forced inversion of the forefoot, when the tendon of peroneus brevis pulls off the styloid process leading to its avulsion. This fracture is also called **Jones' fracture** after the name of an orthopaedic surgeon Sir Robert Jones, who himself sustained this injury.
- **March fracture:** It typically occurs in the shaft or neck of second and third metatarsals due to aggressive prolonged march past by the soldiers.

PHALANGEAL BONES

The phalangeal bones are miniature long bones. They are 14 in number in each foot—two for the great toe and three for each of the other four toes.

Table 21.6 Differences between metatarsals and metacarpals

Metatarsals	Metacarpals
More massive and more strong	Less massive and less strong
Head is smaller than base (except first)	Head is larger or equal to the base (except first)
Dorsal surface of the shaft presents no flattening	Dorsal surface presents triangular flattening
Shaft narrows from the base to the head	Shaft thickens from the base to the head
Concave surface of the shaft faces downward	Concave surface of the shaft faces forward
Numbered (1 to 5) from medial to lateral side	Numbered (1 to 5) from lateral to medial side

The phalanges in the great toe are proximal and distal, and phalanges in other toes are proximal, middle, and distal.

1. The base of the proximal phalanx presents a concave facet which articulate with the head of metatarsal bone to form the metacarpophalangeal joint.
2. The distal end of the proximal phalanx presents a pulley-like articular surface and articulates with the middle phalanx in the lateral four toes and with terminal phalanx of first toe. Thus, lateral four toes possess two interphalangeal (IP) joints, proximal and distal, and the great toe possesses only one IP joint.
3. Both, proximal and distal articular surfaces of the middle phalanx are pulley-shaped.
4. The distal phalanx of each toe bears a rough tuberosity on plantar aspect of its distal end.

Ossification

1. Each phalanx ossifies from two centres: a primary centre for the shaft and a secondary centre for the base.
2. The time of appearance of **primary centres** is as follows:
   (a) For proximal phalanges: 12th week of IUL.
   (b) For middle phalanges: 15th week of IUL.
   (c) For distal phalanges: 9th week of IUL.
3. The time of appearance of **secondary centres** is as follows.
   (a) For proximal phalanges: 2 years.
   (b) For middle phalanges: 4 years.
   (c) For distal phalanges: 8 years.

The fusion of epiphysis (base) with diaphysis (shaft) occurs in about the 18th year.

Golden Facts to Remember

➤ Longest and strongest bone in the body	Femur
➤ Largest sesamoid bone in the body	Patella
➤ Third trochanter	Prominent gluteal tuberosity
➤ Commonest site of the fracture femur	Neck of femur
➤ Commonest site of the fracture tibia	Shaft of tibia at the junction of middle one-third and lower one-third
➤ Largest nutrient artery in the body	Nutrient artery of tibia
➤ Largest and strongest bone of the foot	Calcaneum
➤ First tarsal bone to ossify	Calcaneum
➤ Most common accessory bone of the foot	Accessory navicular bone (navicular secundarium)
➤ Shortest and strongest metatarsal bone	First metatarsal
➤ Longest metatarsal bone	Second metatarsal

Clinical Case Study

A 71-year-old woman fell in her bathroom. After the fall, she could not get up or even move her right leg. She was taken to the orthopedic surgeon who on examination noted that toes of the patient's right foot were pointing laterally. On measuring the length, the right lower limb was found shorter as compared to the left limb. The X-ray revealed **subcapital fracture of the neck of right femur.**

Questions

1. What is the commonest cause of the fracture neck of femur in elderly women following a trivial fall?
2. How is the length of the lower limb measured?
3. Give the reason of shortening of the lower limb in this case.
4. Give the anatomical basis of the lateral rotation of the thigh in fracture neck of femur.

Answers

1. Osteoporosis due to old age and deficiency of estrogen.
2. It is measured from the anterior superior iliac spine to the medial malleolus.
3. Following fracture neck, the shaft of femur is pulled up by the contraction of hamstring and adductor muscles.
4. The thigh is laterally rotated by the contraction of gluteus maximus and short lateral rotators of the thigh (e.g., piriformis, obturator internus, gemelli, and quadratus femoris). Further, in the fracture neck of femur, the psoas major becomes lateral rotator due to shift in its axis of action.

CHAPTER 22

Front of the Thigh

The thigh is the part of the lower limb between the hip and knee joints. For descriptive purposes, the thigh is divided into three regions—front of the thigh, medial side of the thigh, and back of the thigh.

The front of the thigh corresponds to the back of arm.

The study of the front of thigh is of immense clinical and surgical importance.

SURFACE LANDMARKS (Fig. 22.1)

1. **Fold of the groin** is a shallow curved groove extending from the pubic tubercle to the anterior superior iliac spine. It corresponds to the underlying inguinal ligament and separates the anterior abdominal wall from the front of the thigh.
2. **Anterior superior iliac spine** is palpated at the lateral end of the fold of the groin.
3. **Pubic tubercle** is a small bony projection felt at the medial end of the fold of groin.
4. **Greater trochanter** lies a hand's breadth below the tubercle of the iliac crest and forms a prominence in front of the hollow on the side of the hip.
5. **Midinguinal point** is a point midway between the anterior superior iliac spine and the pubic symphysis.
6. **Midpoint of inguinal ligament** is a point midway between the anterior superior iliac spine and the pubic tubercle.
7. **Medial and lateral condyles of femur and tibia** form large bony masses on the medial and lateral sides of the knee, respectively. The most prominent points on the condyles are called epicondyles.
8. **Fleshy swelling above the medial condyle of the femur** is formed by the lower part of the vastus medialis muscle.
9. **Patella (knee cap)** is easily felt as a triangular bone in front of the knee. It is freely mobile when the knee is extended but becomes rigid when the knee is flexed.
10. **Tibial tuberosity** is easily felt as a bony prominence on the front of the upper end of the tibia.

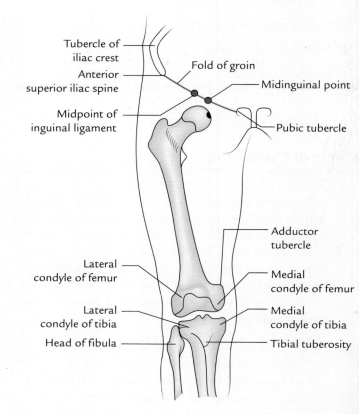

Fig. 22.1 Bony landmarks of the thigh.

11. **Ligamentum patellae** can be felt as a strong fibrous band stretching between patella and tibial tuberosity.
12. **Adductor tubercle** can be felt just above the medial condyle of the femur and on deep pressure a cord-like tendon of adductor magnus is felt above the tubercle.

SUPERFICIAL FASCIA

The superficial fascia on the front of the thigh near the inguinal region consists of two layers: thick superficial fatty layer and thin deep membranous layer, which are continuous above with the corresponding layers of the anterior abdominal wall.

The membranous layer of the superficial fascia is attached in a linear fashion to the deep fascia of thigh (fascia lata) along a horizontal line which extends laterally from the pubic tubercle for about 8 cm. The line of fusion of the membranous layer of superficial fascia to the fascia lata in front of the thigh corresponds to the flexion crease of the hip joint called **Holden's line**.

The superficial fascia on the front of the thigh contains:

1. Cutaneous nerves.
2. Cutaneous arteries.
3. Termination of saphenous vein and its tributaries.
4. Superficial inguinal lymph nodes.

Cutaneous Nerves (Fig. 22.2)

The skin on the front of the thigh is supplied by seven cutaneous nerves which are derived from the lumbar plexus (described in Chapter 12, p. 196). These are:

1. Ilioinguinal nerve (L1).
2. Femoral branch of the genitofemoral nerve (L1, L2).
3. Lateral cutaneous nerve of the thigh (L2, L3).
4. Intermediate cutaneous nerve of the thigh (L2, L3).
5. Medial cutaneous nerve of the thigh (L2, L3).
6. Saphenous nerve (L3, L4).
7. Cutaneous branch of the obturator nerve (L2, L3).

The **ilioinguinal nerve** (L1) is the collateral branch of the iliohypogastric nerve. It emerges through the superficial inguinal ring and supplies the skin at the root of the penis, and the anterior one-third of the scrotum in male; and mons pubis and anterior one-third of labium majus in female; and the skin of the upper medial aspect of the thigh.

The **femoral branch of the genitofemoral nerve** (L1) pierces the femoral sheath and the overlying deep fascia 2 cm below the midinguinal point, and supplies the skin over the femoral triangle.

The **lateral cutaneous nerve of the thigh** (L2, L3) is a direct branch of the lumbar plexus. It enters the thigh by passing behind or through the lateral end of the inguinal ligament, a centimeter medial to the anterior superior iliac spine, and divides into anterior and posterior branches. It supplies the skin on the anterolateral side of the upper thigh.

Clinical correlation

The lateral cutaneous nerve of the thigh is sometimes compressed as it passes through the inguinal ligament, causing pain and paresthesia (altered sensations) in the upper lateral aspect of the thigh leading to a clinical condition called 'meralgia paresthetica'. The surgical treatment of this condition requires division of the inguinal ligament and releasing the nerve from the compression.

The **intermediate cutaneous nerve of the thigh** (L2, L3) is a branch of the anterior division of the femoral nerve. It passes vertically downward and pierces the deep fascia at the junction of the upper one-third and middle one-third of the thigh. It divides into two or more branches and supplies the skin on the front of the thigh as far down as the knee.

The **medial cutaneous nerve of the thigh** (L2, L3) is a branch of the anterior division of the femoral nerve. It divides into anterior and posterior branches, which run medially across the femoral vessels, pierce the fascia lata at the mid-thigh, and supply the skin on the medial side of the thigh.

The **saphenous nerve** (L3, L4) is a branch of the posterior division of the femoral nerve. It pierces deep fascia on the medial side of the knee and runs downward in front of the great saphenous vein. It gives *infrapatellar branch* before piercing the deep fascia, which runs downward and laterally to supply skin over the ligamentum patella.

The **cutaneous branch of the obturator nerve** (L2, L3) is a small twig which arises from the anterior division of the obturator nerve and supplies the lower one-third of the medial aspect of the thigh.

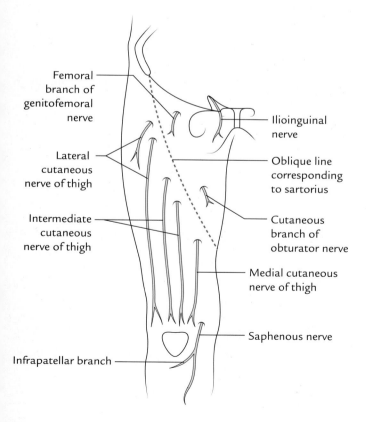

Fig. 22.2 Cutaneous nerves on the front of the thigh.

N.B. The lateral, intermediate, and medial cutaneous nerves of the thigh pierce the deep fascia of thigh (fascia lata) along an oblique line that roughly corresponds to the course of the sartorius muscle.

Patellar Plexus

It is a plexus of nerves present in front of the patella, ligamentum patellae, and the upper end of the tibia, and supplies the skin over these structures. It is formed by the branches from (a) the lateral cutaneous nerve of thigh, (b) the intermediate cutaneous nerve of thigh, (c) medial cutaneous nerve of thigh, and (d) infrapatellar branch of the saphenous nerve.

Cutaneous Arteries

These are three small arteries arising from the femoral artery, a little below the inguinal ligament (Fig. 22.3).

1. The **superficial external pudendal artery** arises medially from the femoral artery, pierces the cribriform fascia, runs medially in front of the spermatic cord, and supplies the external genitalia.
2. The **superficial epigastric artery** arises anteriorly from the femoral artery, pierces the cribriform fascia, to ascend anterior to the inguinal ligament and runs towards the umbilicus. It supplies the lower part of the anterior abdominal wall.
3. The **superficial circumflex iliac artery** (smallest branch) arises near the superficial epigastric artery, pierces the fascia lata lateral to the saphenous opening, to run upward and laterally below the inguinal ligament.

Long (Great) Saphenous Vein (Fig. 22.3)

It is the largest and longest superficial vein of the lower limb.

It begins on the dorsum of the foot from the medial end of the dorsal venous arch, runs upward in front of the medial malleolus, and ascends on the medial side of the leg. It enters the medial aspect of the thigh by passing behind the knee (posterior to the medial condyle). In the thigh, it inclines forward to reach the saphenous opening where it pierces the cribriform fascia and opens into the femoral vein by hooking the inferior crescentic margin of the saphenous opening.

Before piercing the cribriform fascia, it receives three tributaries: superficial epigastric vein, superficial external pudendal vein, and superficial circumflex iliac vein (Fig. 22.3).

The saphenous vein is described in detail in Chapter 33.

Superficial Inguinal Lymph Nodes

The superficial inguinal lymph nodes are variable in their number and size. They are divided into two sets—horizontal and vertical. The two sets are arranged in a T-shaped manner (Fig. 22.4).

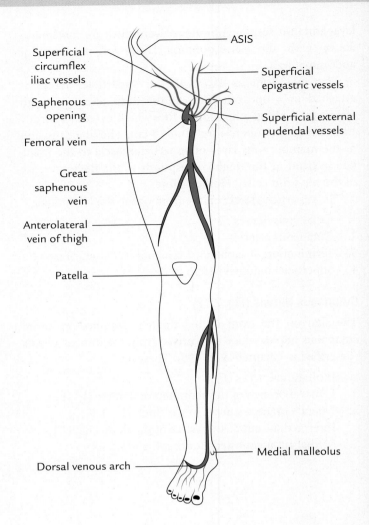

Fig. 22.3 Superficial vessels on the front of the thigh (ASIS = anterior superior iliac spine).

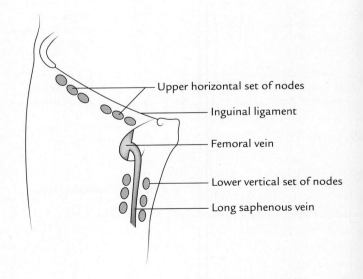

Fig. 22.4 Superficial inguinal lymph nodes.

The nodes of the upper horizontal set (five or six in number) are located a short distance below the inguinal ligament. The nodes of this set can be subdivided into the upper lateral and upper medial groups. The nodes of the lower vertical set (four or five in number) lie along the upper part of the long saphenous vein.

The efferent lymph vessels from the superficial inguinal nodes pass through the saphenous opening and drain into the deep inguinal nodes.

DEEP FASCIA OF THE THIGH

The deep fascia of the thigh is very strong and envelops the thigh like a sleeve. It is called **fascia lata** because it encloses a wide area of the thigh (Latin *Latus*: broad). Its attachments are as follows:

1. *Superiorly,* on the front of the thigh, it is attached to the anterior superior iliac spine, inguinal ligament, and pubic tubercle. Laterally it is attached to the iliac crest; posteriorly (through the gluteal fascia) to the sacrum, coccyx, and sacrotuberous ligament; and medially it is attached to the pubis, pubic arch, and ischial tuberosity.
2. *Inferiorly* on the front and sides of the knee, it is attached to subcutaneous bony prominences and the capsule of the knee joint.

MODIFICATIONS OF DEEP FASCIA OF THE THIGH

The deep fascia of the thigh presents two modifications—**iliotibial tract** and **saphenous opening**.

Iliotibial Tract (Fig. 22.5)

The fascia lata is thickened on the lateral aspect of the thigh to form about 2 inches wide band called **iliotibial tract**. Superiorly along the iliac crest, this tract splits into two layers to enclose the two muscles (tensor fasciae latae and gluteus maximus) and forms a single thickened sheet, the **gluteal aponeurosis** between them which covers the gluteus medius. The superficial lamina is attached to the tubercle of the iliac crest and the deep lamina to the capsule of the hip joint. Inferiorly, the tract is attached to a smooth area on the anterior surface of the lateral condyle of the tibia.

The upper part of iliotibial tract provides insertion to two muscles: the gluteus maximus (except deep fibres of its lower half) and the tensor fasciae latae.

Functional Significance

The iliotibial tract stabilizes the knee both in extension and in partial flexion; hence it is used constantly during walking and running. On leaning forward with slightly flexed knees the iliotibial tract is the main support of the knee against gravity and prevents the individuals from falling forward.

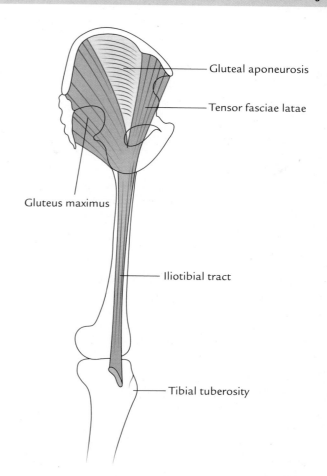

Gluteal aponeurosis

Tensor fasciae latae

Gluteus maximus

Iliotibial tract

Tibial tuberosity

Fig. 22.5 Attachment of the iliotibial tract. Note superficial portion of gluteus maximus and tensor fasciae latae insert into the iliotibial tract from opposite directions.

Saphenous Opening (Fig. 22.6)

This is an oval opening in the fascia lata in the upper medial part of the front of the thigh. The centre of the opening is about 4 cm below and lateral to the pubic tubercle. Its vertical length measures about 3–4 cm. The opening is bounded inferolaterally by a sharp crescentic (falciform) margin. It is formed by the superficial stratum of the fascia lata, which lies in front of the femoral sheath. The medial margin of the opening is ill-defined and formed by the deep stratum which lies at a deeper level and becomes continuous with the fascia overlying the pectineus (pectineal fascia). It lies behind the femoral sheath.

The saphenous opening is closed by a membrane of areolar tissue—the cribriform fascia which is pierced by number of structures making it sieve-like, hence the name cribriform.

N.B. In the region of saphenous opening, the fascia lata is twisted to form an oval opening and presents two strata, superficial and deep.

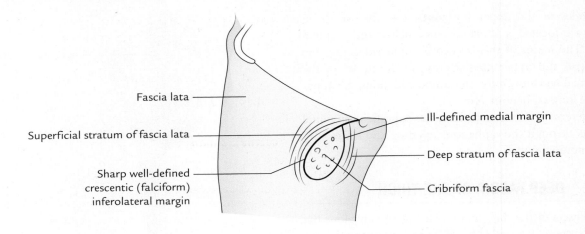

Fig. 22.6 The saphenous opening. Note the saphenous opening resembles a double-breasted jacket.

Structures passing through the saphenous opening are as follows:

1. Great saphenous vein.
2. Superficial epigastric and superficial external pudendal vessels.
3. Few lymph vessels connecting superficial and deep inguinal lymph nodes.

Clinical correlation

The fascia lata is attached to the under surface of the inguinal ligament. When the thigh is extended, it pulls the abdominal wall downward and makes it tense. Therefore, in order to relax the abdomen (for palpation of abdominal contents) the patient is asked to draw the legs up to overcome the pull of the fascia lata on the abdominal wall.

FASCIAL COMPARTMENTS OF THE THIGH (Fig. 22.7)

The fascia lata encloses the entire thigh like a sleeve/stocking. Three intermuscular fascial septa (lateral, medial, and posterior) pass from the inner aspect of the deep fascial sheath of the thigh to the linea aspera of the femur and divide the thigh into three compartments—anterior, medial, and posterior.

The *anterior (extensor) compartment*, lies between lateral and medial intermuscular septa; the *Medial (adductor) compartment*, lies between medial and posterior septa; and the *posterior (flexor) compartment*, lies between posterior and lateral septa.

Each compartment contains muscles, nerves, and arteries.

N.B. The lateral intermuscular septum is the strongest and extends from the iliotibial tract to the lateral lip of linear

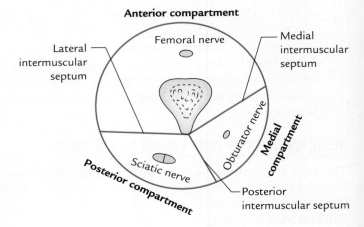

Fig. 22.7 Fascial compartments of the thigh.

aspera. The medial intermuscular septum is attached to the medial lip of the linear aspera. The posterior intermuscular septum is poorly defined.

ANTERIOR COMPARTMENT OF THE THIGH

The extensor compartment of the thigh is bounded laterally by lateral intermuscular septum and medially by medial intermuscular septum.

CONTENTS

1. **Muscles:** Quadriceps femoris, articularis genu, sartorius, and tensor fasciae latae.
2. **Nerve:** Femoral nerve.
3. **Artery:** Femoral artery.

MUSCLES

Quadriceps Femoris

This muscle is so named because it consists of four parts: rectus femoris, vastus lateralis, vastus medialis, and vastus intermedius. It is supplied by the femoral nerve. It forms most of the bulk on the anterior aspect of the thigh and is the most powerful extensor of the knee joint.

N.B. All the parts of quadriceps cross only one joint, i.e., knee joint, except rectus femoris which crosses two joints, i.e., hip and knee joints.

The origin, insertion, and nerve supply of various parts of quadriceps femoris are described in the following text.

Rectus Femoris (Fig. 22.8)

It is a long straight muscle with fusiform bipinnate belly in the upper two-third and flat tendon in the lower one-third (Latin *rectus* = straight).

Origin

It arises from the ilium by two heads:
(a) *Straight head* arises from the upper part of the anterior inferior iliac spine.
(b) *Reflected head* arises from a groove above the acetabulum.

Insertion

The two heads meet at an acute angle and form a fusiform belly, which occupies the front of the thigh. In the lower one-third of the thigh, the muscle ends in a flat tendon which descends vertically downward to be inserted into the base of the patella.

Nerve supply

It is by posterior division of the femoral nerve.

Actions

It extends the knee and flexes the hip.

N.B. The rectus femoris is also called the *"kicking muscle"* because it extends the knee and flexes the hip—the actions required during kicking.

Vastus Lateralis (Fig. 22.8)

Origin

It takes a linear and aponeurotic origin from the upper part of the intertrochanteric line, anterior and inferior borders of the greater trochanter, lateral lip of gluteal tuberosity, and upper half of the lateral lip of linea aspera. It also arises from the lateral intermuscular septum.

Insertion

It is inserted (a) by a broad aponeurosis into the tendon of rectus femoris, lateral part of the base of patella, upper one-third of the lateral border of the patella, and (b) retinacular fibres to the front of the lateral condyle of tibia which replaces the anterolateral aspect of the capsule of the knee joint.

Nerve supply

It is by the posterior division of the femoral nerve.

Actions

Extension of the knee joint.

Vastus Medialis

It covers the medial surface of the shaft of femur.

Origin

It takes a linear origin from the lower part of intertrochanteric line, spiral line, medial lip of linea aspera, and upper two-third of the medial supra condylar line. It also arises from the medial intermuscular septum.

Insertion

It is inserted by a broad aponeurosis into the tendon of rectus femoris, medial part of the base, and upper two-third of the medial border of the patella. From its lower attachment it sends a fibrous expansion, the medial **patellar retinaculum**, to the front of the medial condyle of the tibia which replaces the anteromedial part of the capsule of the knee joint.

Nerve supply

It is by the nerve to vastus medialis, which is the thickest muscular branch of the posterior division of the femoral nerve.

Actions

Extension of the knee joint.

N.B. The lower fibres of vastus medialis are attached far more down on the medial border of patella than those of the vastus lateralis on the lateral border. Therefore, they prevent the natural tendency of patella to dislocate laterally during the extension of the knee joint.

The role of vastus medialis is indispensable for the stability of the patella.

Vastus Intermedius (Fig. 22.8)

Origin

It arises from the anterior and lateral aspects of the upper three-fourth of the shaft of femur.

Insertion

Into the base of patella deep to the tendon of rectus femoris.

Nerve supply

It is by the posterior division of the femoral nerve.

Action

Extension of the knee joint.

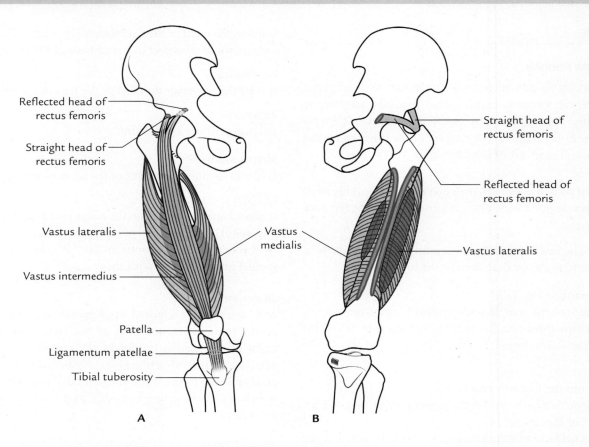

Fig. 22.8 Origin and insertion of quadriceps femoris: **A**, anterior view; **B**, posterior view.

Articularis Genu

It consists of three or four muscular slips which are considered to be a detached part of the vastus intermedius.

Origin

It arises from the anterior surface of the lower part of the shaft of the femur, few centimeters above the patellar articular margin.

Insertion

Into the upper part of the synovial membrane of the knee joint.

Nerve supply

It is by a twig from the nerve to vastus intermedius.

Actions

The articularis genu pulls up the synovial membrane upward to prevent its damage when the knee is extended.

Sartorius (Fig. 22.9)

It is the longest muscle in the body, which crosses the front of the thigh obliquely from the lateral to the medial side.

Origin

It arises from the anterior superior iliac spine and upper half of the notch immediately below it.

Insertion

The muscle spirals obliquely across the thigh from lateral to medial side to reach the posterior aspect of the medial condyle of femur, where its tendon runs forward to be inserted into the upper part of the medial surface of the shaft of tibia in front of the insertions of gracilis and semitendinosus. The insertion of sartorius is inverted hockey-stick-shaped.

Nerve supply

It is by the anterior division of the femoral nerve.

Actions

It flexes both the hip and the knee joints, and adducts and rotates the thigh laterally to bring the lower limb into the sitting position of a tailor (Latin *sartor*: tailor)/"palthi-position" adopted by Indian Hindus during meal.

Tensor Fasciae Latae (Fig. 22.9)

It is a short thick muscle, which lies at the junction of the gluteal region and the upper part of the front of the thigh.

Origin

It arises from the outer lip of the iliac crest extending from the anterior superior iliac spine to the tubercle of the crest.

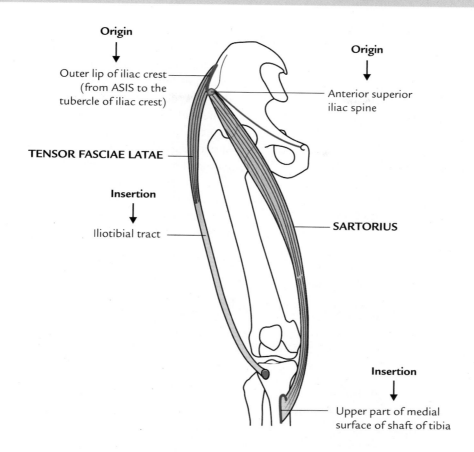

Fig. 22.9 Origin and insertion of the tensor fasciae latae and sartorius (ASIS = anterior superior iliac spine).

Insertion

The muscle passes downward and slightly backward and inserted into the iliotibial tract 3–5 cm below the level of the greater trochanter.

Nerve supply

It is by the superior gluteal nerve.

Actions

It abducts the hip joint and maintains the extended position of the knee joint through the iliotibial tract.

N.B. Morphologically, the *tensor fasciae latae* is a muscle of the gluteal region which has migrated on the lateral aspect of the thigh during the course of evolution but retains its nerve supply. It is supplied by the superior gluteal nerve—the nerve of gluteal region.

The origin, insertion, nerves supply, and actions of the muscles of the front of the thigh are summarized in Table 22.1.

FEMORAL TRIANGLE

It is a triangular depression on the front of the upper one-third of the thigh below the inguinal ligament. Its apex is directed downward.

Boundaries

These are as follows (Fig. 22.10):

Lateral: Medial border of sartorius.
Medial: Medial border of adductor longus.
Base: Inguinal ligament.

Apex: It is formed by the meeting point of the medial borders of adductor longs and sartorius.

Floor: It is gutter-shaped and muscular. From lateral to medial side it is formed by the following muscles (Fig. 22.11):

1. Iliacus.
2. Psoas major (tendon).
3. Pectineus.
4. Adductor longus.

Roof: It is formed by the fascia lata having saphenous opening (Fig. 22.12). The superficial fascia overlying the roof contains superficial branches of the femoral artery and accompanying veins, upper part of great saphenous vein, superficial inguinal lymph nodes, femoral branch of the genitofemoral nerve, and branches of ilioinguinal nerve.

Contents

The main contents of the femoral triangle are as follows (Fig. 22.13):

1. Femoral artery and its branches.
2. Femoral vein and its tributaries.
3. Femoral nerve.
4. Deep inguinal lymph nodes.
5. Lateral cutaneous nerve of the thigh.

In addition to above structures, it also contains:

1. Femoral branch of the genitofemoral nerve.
2. Fibrofatty tissue.

A brief account of some contents of the femoral triangle is given in the following text.

The **femoral artery** traverses the femoral triangle from the midpoint of its base to the apex. The artery passes downward and medially. As a result, at the base of triangle, it lies lateral to the femoral vein but at its apex it lies anterior to the vein. The femoral artery gives three superficial branches (superficial epigastric, superficial circumflex iliac, and superficial external pudendal) and two deep branches (profunda femoris and deep external pudendal). The profunda femoris is the largest branch of the femoral artery. It arises from the lateral side of the femoral artery about 3.5 cm below the inguinal ligament

Table 22.1 Origin, insertion, nerve supply, and actions of the muscles of the front of the thigh

Muscle	Origin	Insertion	Nerve supply	Actions
1. Quadriceps femoris (a) Rectus femoris	• Straight head: from the upper half of the anterior inferior iliac spine • Reflected head: from the groove above the acetabulum	Base of patella	Femoral nerve	Flexion of the hip joint and extension of the knee joint
(b) Vastus lateralis	• Upper part of the intertrochanteric line • Anterior and inferior borders of greater trochanter • Lateral lip of the gluteal tuberosity • Upper half of lateral lip of linea aspera	• Base and upper 1/3rd of the lateral border of the patella • Expansion to the capsule of the knee joint and iliotibial tract	Femoral nerve	Extension of the knee joint
(c) Vastus medialis	• Lower part of the intertrochanteric line • Spiral line • Medial lip of the linea aspera • Upper 2/3rd of medial supracondylar line	• Base and upper 2/3rd of the medial border of the patella • Expansion to the capsule of the knee joint	Femoral nerve	Extension of the knee joint
(d) Vastus intermedius	Upper 3/4th of the anterior and lateral surfaces of the shaft of femur	Base of patella	Femoral nerve	Extension of the knee joint
2. Articularis genu	• Anterior surface of the lower part of the shaft of femur	Synovial membrane of the knee joint	Femoral nerve	Pulls up the synovial membrane of the knee joint during its extension
3. Sartorius	• Anterior superior iliac spine and upper half of the notch below it	Upper part of the medial surface of the shaft of the tibia	Femoral nerve	• Flexion of the hip and knee joints • Lateral rotation of the thigh
4. Tensor fasciae latae	• Outer lip of the iliac crest from anterior superior iliac spine to the tubercle of iliac crest	Iliotibial tract 3–5 cm below the greater trochanter	Superior gluteal nerve	Abduction of the hip joint

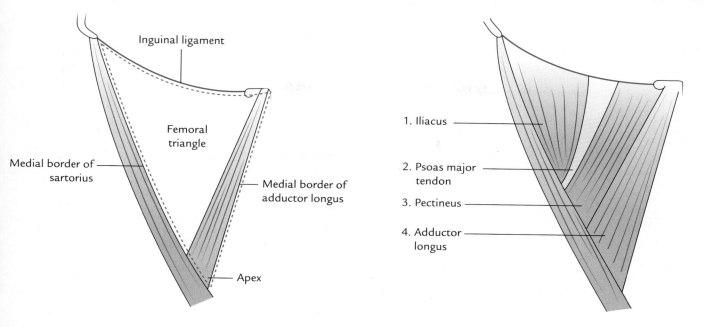

Fig. 22.10 Boundaries of the femoral triangle.

Fig. 22.11 Muscles forming the floor of the femoral triangle.

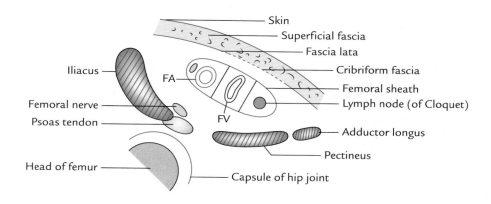

Fig. 22.12 Sagittal section through the upper part of femoral triangle showing structures forming its roof and floor (FV = femoral vein, FA = femoral artery).

and spirals medially behind the femoral vessels. It gives rise to medial and lateral circumflex femoral arteries. The medial circumflex artery disappears by passing between the psoas major and pectineus. The lateral circumflex femoral artery passes laterally between the anterior and posterior divisions of the femoral nerve.

The **deep external pudendal artery** pierces the fascia lata and passes medially behind the spermatic cord.

The **femoral vein** accompanies the femoral artery. The vein is posterior to the femoral artery at the apex and medial to it at the base of the triangle. It receives the great saphenous vein and profunda femoris vein and veins corresponding to the superficial branches of femoral artery.

The **femoral nerve** lies lateral to the femoral artery, outside the femoral sheath, in the groove between the iliacus and the psoas major. About 2.5 cm below the inguinal ligament it divides into anterior and posterior divisions which enclose lateral circumflex femoral artery between them. The anterior division gives off two cutaneous branches—intermediate and medial cutaneous nerves of the thigh. The medial cutaneous branch accompanies the lateral side of the artery; at the apex of the triangle it crosses the front of the artery from lateral to medial side. The posterior division gives rise to one cutaneous nerve—the saphenous nerve. It extends downward along the lateral side of the artery.

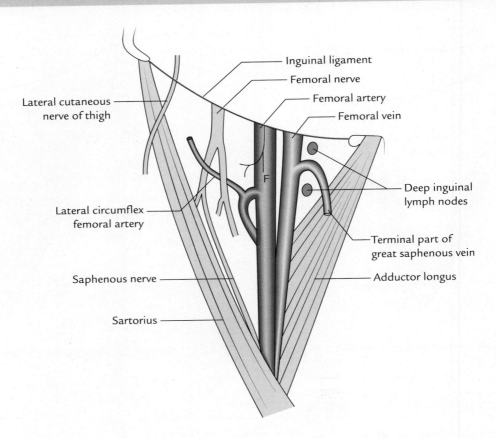

Fig. 22.13 Boundaries and contents of the femoral triangle (F = femoral branch of the genitofemoral nerve).

The **lateral cutaneous nerve of the thigh** is already described on p. 329.

The **deep inguinal lymph nodes** are usually three in number and lie medial to the upper part of the femoral vein. The lowest one is situated below the junction of great saphenous and femoral veins, the middle one in the femoral canal (the gland of Cloquet/Rosenmüller), and the highest one in the femoral ring.

Femoral Sheath (Fig. 22.14)

It is a funnel-shaped fascial sheath enclosing the upper 3–4 cm of the femoral vessels.

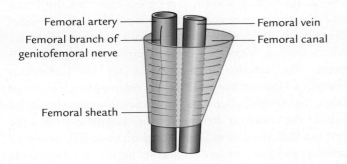

Fig. 22.14 Femoral sheath. Note the asymmetry of the femoral sheath.

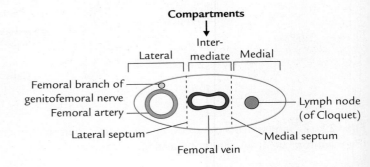

Fig. 22.15 Compartments of the femoral sheath.

The femoral sheath is divided into three compartments, *viz.* lateral, intermediate, and medial by two anteroposterior septa (Fig. 22.15).

1. The *lateral compartment* contains the femoral artery and the femoral branch of the genitofemoral nerve.
2. The *intermediate compartment* contains the femoral vein.
3. The *medial compartment* is small and known as the femoral canal.

The femoral sheath, femoral canal, and femoral hernia are described in Chapter 4, pp. 47–48.

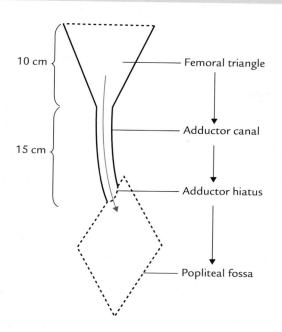

Fig. 22.16 Femoral triangle and adductor canal. (The red arrow indicates the passage of femoral artery.) Note the adductor canal is a narrow passage for the femoral vessels.

ADDUCTOR CANAL (SUBSARTORIAL CANAL/HUNTER'S CANAL)

The adductor canal is an intermuscular tunnel situated on the medial side of the middle one-third of the thigh (Fig. 22.16).

It extends from the apex of the femoral triangle, above, to the tendinous opening in the adductor magnus, below. It provides passage to the femoral vessels from femoral triangle to the popliteal fossa (Fig. 22.16).

Boundaries (Fig. 22.17)

The adductor canal is triangular in cross section. Its boundaries are as follows:

Anterolateral wall: It is formed by vastus medialis.
Posterior (floor): It is formed by adductor longus above and adductor magnus below.
Medial (roof): It if formed by a strong fibrous membrane stretching across the anterolateral and posterior boundaries. The roof is overlapped by the sartorius muscle.

N.B. The *subsartorial plexus* of nerves lies on the roof underneath the sartorius. The plexus is formed by branches from the medial cutaneous nerve of the thigh, the saphenous nerve, and the anterior division of the obturator nerve. It supplies the overlying fascia lata and the skin.

Contents (Fig. 22.18)

These are as follows:

1. Femoral artery.
2. Femoral vein.
3. Saphenous nerve.
4. Nerve to vastus medialis.

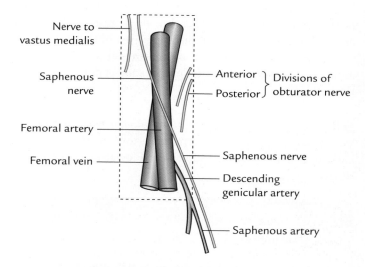

Fig. 22.18 Contents of the adductor canal.

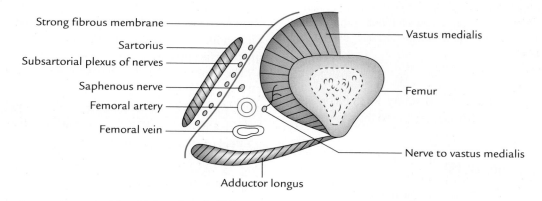

Fig. 22.17 Boundaries and contents of the adductor canal as seen in the transverse section through middle one-third of the thigh.

5. Anterior and posterior divisions of the obturator nerve (occasional).
6. Descending genicular artery, a branch of the femoral artery.

A brief account of contents is given in the following text.

The **femoral artery** enters the canal at the apex of the femoral triangle, traverses the whole length of the adductor canal, and leaves it by passing through the tendinous opening in the adductor magnus (adductor hiatus). Within the canal it gives off muscular branches and a descending genicular branch. The descending genicular artery arises before the femoral artery leaves the canal.

The **femoral vein** lies posterior to the femoral artery in the upper part and lateral to the artery in the lower part.

The **saphenous nerve** (longest cutaneous nerve of the body) crosses the femoral artery anteriorly from lateral to medial side. It leaves the canal by piercing the fibrous roof.

Just before leaving the canal it gives off **infrapatellar branch** which pierces the sartorius, and joins the patellar plexus and supplies the prepatellar skin.

The **nerve to vastus medialis** (thickest muscular branch of the femoral nerve) lies lateral to the femoral artery, and enters the vastus medialis in the upper part of the canal.

The **posterior division of obturator nerve** runs on the anterior surface of the adductor magnus and ends by supplying the knee joint.

N.B. The spiral course of the femoral vein and saphenous nerve with respect to the femoral artery in the adductor canal is due to medial rotation of the lower limb during its development.

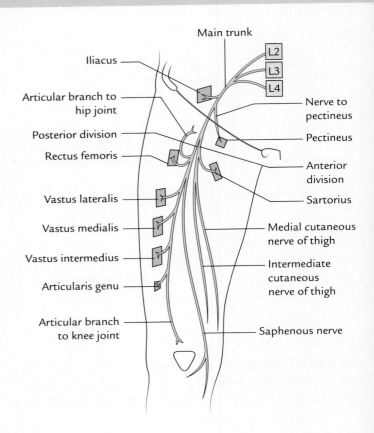

Fig. 22.19 Course, branches, and distribution of the femoral nerve.

Clinical correlation

Clinical significance of adductor canal: The femoral artery is exposed and ligated in the adductor canal during surgery for **aneurysm of the popliteal artery**. This is because the artery at this side is healthy and does not tear when tied, which may occur if the artery is tied in the popliteal fossa immediately above the popliteal aneurysm. This procedure was first performed by a famous surgeon, Dr John Hunter. The adductor canal was named after his name as **Hunter's canal**.

N.B. After ligation of the femoral artery in the adductor canal, the collateral circulation is established through arterial anastomosis around the knee joint.

FEMORAL NERVE (Fig. 22.19)

It is the chief nerve of the anterior compartment of the thigh. It is the largest branch of the lumbar plexus and arises from the dorsal divisions of the anterior primary rami of L2, L3, L4

nerves. It enters the thigh posterior to the inguinal ligament just lateral to the femoral sheath. About 2 cm below the inguinal ligament it divides into **anterior** and **posterior divisions** which are separated by the lateral circumflex femoral artery.

Anterior division: It gives off two cutaneous branches and one muscular branch:

(a) The *cutaneous nerves* are: (a) medial cutaneous nerve of the thigh and (b) intermediate cutaneous nerve of the thigh.
(b) The *muscular branch* supplies the sartorius.

Posterior division: It gives off one cutaneous branch, the saphenous nerve, and four muscular branches to supply the quadriceps femoris.

The femoral nerve is described in detail on p. 468.

Clinical correlation

Effect of injury to femoral nerve: If femoral nerve is injured (very rare) by penetrating wound in the groin, the effects will be as follows:
Motor: Paralysis of the quadriceps femoris.
Sensory: Loss of sensations on the anterior and medial aspects of the thigh.

FEMORAL ARTERY

It is the chief artery of the lower limb. It is the continuation of external iliac artery and enters the femoral triangle behind the inguinal ligament at the midinguinal point. It runs downward and medially successively through the femoral triangle and adductor canal. At the lower end of the adductor canal (i.e., at the junction of middle one-third and lower one-third of the thigh), it leaves the thigh through the adductor hiatus (a tendinous opening in the adductor magnus) to enter the popliteal fossa where it continues as the **popliteal artery** (Fig. 22.20).

Surface Marking (Fig. 22.21)

When the thigh is in a position of slight flexion, abduction, and lateral rotation, the upper two-third of a line drawn from the midinguinal point to the adductor tubercle represents the femoral artery.

Branches (Fig. 22.22)

In the femoral triangle:

1. *Three superficial branches:* Superficial epigastric artery, superficial external pudendal artery, and superficial circumflex iliac artery.
2. *Three deep branches:* Profunda femoris artery, deep external pudendal artery, and muscular branches.

In the adductor canal:

1. Muscular branches.
2. Descending genicular artery.

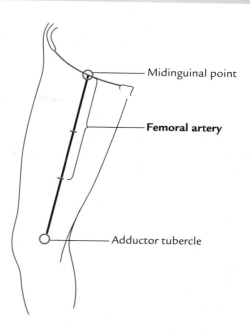

Fig. 22.21 Surface marking of the femoral artery.

The three superficial branches are already described on page 31 and profunda femoris artery is described on page 350.

The **deep external pudendal artery** arises just below the superficial external pudendal artery and passes medially deep to the spermatic cord or round ligament of the uterus and supplies the scrotum or labium majus.

The **descending genicular artery** leaves the canal by descending within the substance of vastus medialis and divides into articular and saphenous branches. The saphenous branch, also called **saphenous artery**, accompanies the saphenous nerve as it emerges through the roof of adductor canal.

N.B. *Alternative names of femoral artery:* Some vascular surgeons, call the initial part of femoral artery, proximal to the origin of profunda femoris artery as 'common femoral artery' and its continuation distally as 'superficial femoral artery.'

Clinical correlation

Compression, palpation and cannulation of femoral artery:

- The femoral artery can be compressed against the femoral head at the midinguinal point to control the bleeding in the distal part of the limb.
- The pulsations of the femoral artery are felt by the clinicians in the femoral triangle just below the midinguinal point.
- Since the femoral artery is quite superficial in the femoral triangle, it is the preferred artery for cannulation and injecting dye to perform procedures like angiography. It is also the preferred vessel for performing the coronary angiography and angioplasty.

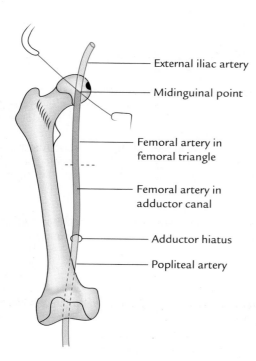

Fig. 22.20 Course and extent of the femoral artery.

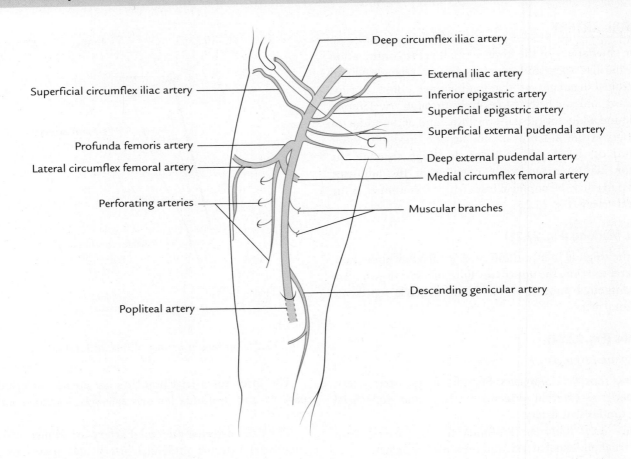

Superficial circumflex iliac artery

Profunda femoris artery
Lateral circumflex femoral artery

Perforating arteries

Popliteal artery

Deep circumflex iliac artery
External iliac artery
Inferior epigastric artery
Superficial epigastric artery
Superficial external pudendal artery
Deep external pudendal artery
Medial circumflex femoral artery
Muscular branches

Descending genicular artery

Fig. 22.22 Branches of the femoral artery.

FEMORAL VEIN

The femoral vein is the upward continuation of the popliteal vein at the adductor hiatus. Thus, it begins at the lower end of the adductor canal, ascends in adductor canal, and enters the femoral triangle, where after traversing the intermediate compartment of the femoral sheath it continues as the external iliac vein behind the inguinal ligament medial to the midinguinal point.

Tributaries

1. Great saphenous vein (longest tributary).
2. Profunda femoris vein.
3. Medial and lateral circumflex femoral veins.
4. Deep external pudendal vein.
5. Direct muscular tributaries.

Clinical correlation

Puncture and cannulation of femoral vein:
- The femoral vein is the preferred vein for intravenous infusions in infants and children and in patients with peripheral circulatory failure.
- The femoral vein is also used for inserting a catheter into the right atrial chamber and right ventricle to collect blood sample or to record pressure or to reach the pulmonary arteries.

Route to right ventricle:
Femoral vein → external iliac vein → common iliac vein → inferior vena cava → right atrium → right ventricle.

Golden Facts to Remember

▶ Largest muscle of the extensor compartment of the thigh	Quadriceps femoris
▶ Longest muscle in the body	Sartorius
▶ Tailor's muscle	Sartorius
▶ Largest branch of the femoral artery	Profunda femoris artery
▶ All the parts of quadriceps act on the knee joint only *except*	Rectus femoris which acts on both hip joint and knee joint
▶ Kicking muscle	Rectus femoris
▶ Commonest site of intramuscular injection in the thigh	Anterolateral aspect of the thigh into the vastus lateralis muscle
▶ Longest cutaneous nerve in the body	Saphenous nerve

Clinical Case Study

A 65-year-old woman visited the emergency department of a hospital and complained of abdominal pain and repeated vomiting. On questioning the patient told that the pain was severe and colicky in nature and most severe in the region of umbilicus. On examination, the abdomen was distended and excessive loud bowel sound could be heard with the stethoscope. A small lemon-sized swelling was also noticed on the upper medial aspect of the right thigh. The swelling was located inferolateral to the pubic tubercle. The patient told she is having this swelling for the last 3 or 4 months. A diagnosis of **"acute intestinal obstruction secondary to the right femoral hernia"** was made.

Questions

1. Name the hernia which is located below and lateral to the pubic tubercle. Name the passage through which the hernia has entered into the thigh.
2. What is the cause of strangulation of femoral hernia?
3. What are the boundaries of femoral ring?
4. What is the direction of femoral hernia and its importance to the surgeon?
5. Give the cause of intestinal obstruction.
6. Give the anatomical basis of pain in the umbilical region.

Answers

1. Femoral hernia: femoral ring and femoral canal.
2. Unyielding nature of the femoral ring.
3. See page 48.
4. The direction of femoral hernia is downward, forward, and upward (see pages 48–49). During manual reduction of femoral hernia, the surgeon reverses the order by pushing the hernia downward, backward, and upward.
5. Venous congestion followed by an arterial occlusion of the intestinal loop due to strangulation of hernia.
6. A loop of the small intestine was pushed into the hernial sac and pain from the small intestine was referred in the region of umbilicus.

CHAPTER 23

Medial Side of the Thigh

The adductor compartment of the thigh is well developed. Its counterpart in the arm has undergone degeneration during the course of evolution and is represented only by a weak coracobrachialis muscle of the flexor compartment of the arm.

BOUNDARIES

The medial compartment of the thigh is bounded:

Anteriorly by the anterior intermuscular septum which separates it from the anterior (extensor) compartment of the thigh.

Posteriorly by an ill-defined posterior intermuscular septum which separates it from posterior (flexor) compartment of the thigh. The posterior intermuscular septum is ill-defined and incomplete due to the presence of a composite muscle, the *adductor magnus*, consisting of two components—adductor and flexor (hamstring) belonging to adductor and flexor compartments of the thigh, respectively.

CONTENTS

- **Muscles:** Adductor longus, adductor brevis, adductor magnus, gracilis, pectineus, and obturator externus.
- **Nerve:** Obturator nerve.
- **Arteries:** Profunda femoris artery and obturator artery.

N.B. The *obturator externus* lies deep in this region and is functionally related to the gluteal region. It rotates the thigh laterally; the chief function of others is adduction of the thigh.

MUSCLES

The muscles of the medial compartment of the thigh are arranged into three layers. From superficial to deep these are (Fig. 23.1):

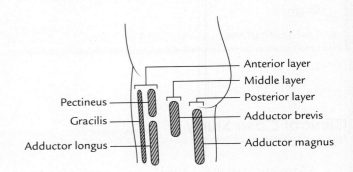

Fig. 23.1 Schematic diagram to show three layers of the adductor muscles of the thigh.

1. **Anterior (first) layer** consists of pectineus, adductor longus, and gracilis.
2. **Middle (second) layer** consists of adductor brevis.
3. **Posterior (third) layer** consists of adductor magnus.

The bony attachments of muscles of medial compartment of the thigh are shown in Figure 23.2.

N.B.
- All the muscles of the adductor compartment of the thigh are supplied by the obturator nerve.
- Two muscles of the adductor compartment of thigh, *viz.,* pectineus and adductor magnus, are composite muscles, hence they have dual innervations. The pectineus is supplied by the femoral and obturator nerves while the adductor magnus is supplied by the obturator nerve (posterior division) and tibial part of sciatic nerve.

Pectineus (Fig. 23.3)

It is a flat quadrilateral muscle which lies in the floor of femoral triangle between psoas major laterally and adductor longus medially.

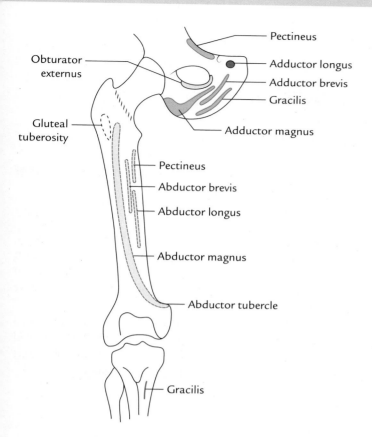

Fig. 23.2 Bony attachments of the muscles of medial compartment of the thigh. Origin is shown by the red colour and insertion is shown by the blue colour.

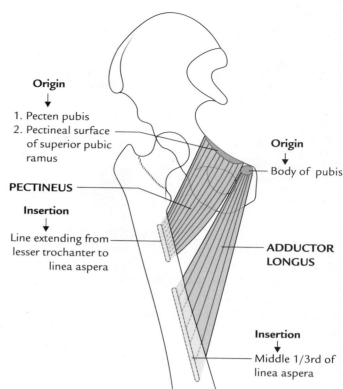

Fig. 23.3 Origin and insertion of the pectineus and adductor longus.

Origin

It arises from the pecten pubis, upper half of the pectineal surface of the superior ramus of pubis and pectineal fascia.

Insertion

The muscle slopes downward, backward, and laterally to be inserted along a line extending from the lesser trochanter to the upper end of the linea aspera.

Nerve supply

It is by two nerves. The anterior fibres are supplied by the *femoral nerve* and the posterior fibres by the *anterior division of the obturator nerve.*

Action

It adducts the thigh at the hip joint.

Adductor Longus (Fig. 23.3)

It is a triangular muscle which lies in the same plane as pectineus. It forms the floor and medial boundary of the femoral triangle.

Origin

It arises by a rounded tendon from the front of the body of pubis in the angle between the pubic crest and the pubic symphysis.

Insertion

The muscles slope downward, backward, and laterally as a broad fleshy belly to be inserted into the middle one-third of the linea aspera.

Nerve supply

The nerve supply is by the anterior division of the obturator nerve.

Action

It is a powerful adductor and medial rotator of the thigh at the hip joint.

N.B. In *horse riders*, the rounded tendon of adductor longus often gets calcified due to its friction with the horseback. This calcified tendon is called **rider's bone**. Some authorities are of view that rider's bone is a sesamoid bone, which occasionally develops in the tendon of adductor longus.

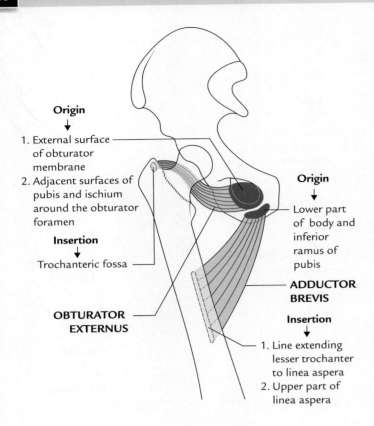

Origin
1. External surface of obturator membrane
2. Adjacent surfaces of pubis and ischium around the obturator foramen

Insertion
Trochanteric fossa

OBTURATOR EXTERNUS

Origin
Lower part of body and inferior ramus of pubis

ADDUCTOR BREVIS

Insertion
1. Line extending lesser trochanter to linea aspera
2. Upper part of linea aspera

Fig. 23.4 Origin and insertion of the adductor brevis and the obturator externus.

Adductor Brevis (Fig. 23.4)

It is a triangular muscle which sometimes peeps in the floor of the femoral triangle between pectineus and adductor longus.

Origin

It arises from the anterior surface of the body of pubis and the outer surface of the inferior ramus of pubis in the interval between the gracilis and the obturator externus.

Insertion

The muscle passes downward, backward, and laterally to be inserted along a line extending from the lesser trochanter to the upper part of linea aspera, behind the pectineus and upper part of the adductor longus.

Nerve supply

It is usually supplied by the anterior division of the obturator nerve but occasionally it may also be supplied by the posterior division of the obturator nerve.

Action

It adducts the thigh at the hip joint.

Adductor Magnus (Fig. 23.5)

It is a large composite muscle consisting of two parts: adductor and hamstring.

Origin

It arises from:

(a) The **adductor part** arises from the outer surface of ischiopubic ramus, mainly from ramus of ischium.
(b) The **hamstring part** arises from the inferolateral part of the ischial tuberosity.

Insertion

(a) The fibres of *adductor part* pass obliquely downward, backward, and laterally to be inserted in linear fashion into the medial margin of gluteal tuberosity, medial lip of linea aspera, and upper part of medial supracondylar line up to the adductor hiatus.
(b) The fibres of the *hamstring part* pass vertically downward to be inserted into the *adductor tubercle* by a rounded tendon, which sends a fibrous expansion to the lower part of medial supracondylar line below the hiatus.

Nerve supply

It is by:

1. *Adductor part* by the posterior division of the obturator nerve.
2. *Hamstring part* by the tibial part of the sciatic nerve.

Actions

(a) Adduction and medial rotation of the thigh at the hip joint.
(b) Hamstring part is a weak extensor of the thigh at the hip joint.

Gracilis (Fig. 23.5)

It is a long slender muscle (G. **gracilis** = slender) which lies on the medial side of the other muscles of the adductor compartment. *It is the only muscle of the adductor compartment which is not attached to the femur.*

Origin

It arises from the medial margin of the lower half of the body pubis and adjoining anterior part of the inferior pubic ramus.

Insertion

It passes downward vertically on the medial side of thigh to the upper part of the medial surface of tibia, where it is inserted between the insertions of sartorius (in front) and semitendinosus (behind).

Nerve supply

By the anterior division of obturator nerve.

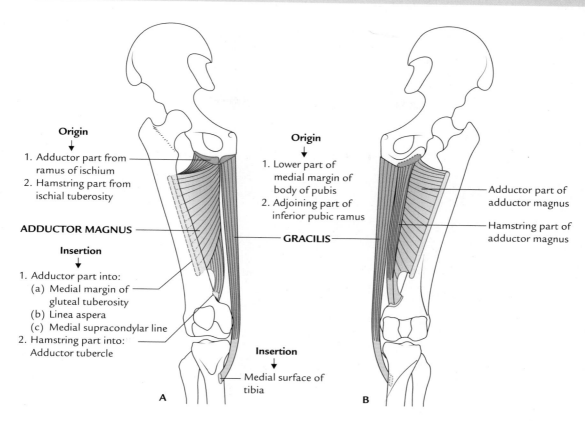

Origin
1. Adductor part from ramus of ischium
2. Hamstring part from ischial tuberosity

ADDUCTOR MAGNUS

Insertion
1. Adductor part into:
   (a) Medial margin of gluteal tuberosity
   (b) Linea aspera
   (c) Medial supracondylar line
2. Hamstring part into: Adductor tubercle

Origin
1. Lower part of medial margin of body of pubis
2. Adjoining part of inferior pubic ramus

GRACILIS

Adductor part of adductor magnus

Hamstring part of adductor magnus

Insertion
Medial surface of tibia

A

B

Fig. 23.5 Origin and insertion of the adductor magnus and gracilis: **A,** anterior view; **B,** posterior view.

Actions
It adducts the thigh. In addition, it is a flexor of the knee joint and a medial rotator of the leg.

N.B. The adductor muscles of the thigh have been known collectively as custodes virginitatis (i.e., **custodian of virginity**).

The origin, insertion, nerve supply, and actions of the adductor muscles of the thigh are summarized in Table 23.1.

Obturator Externus (Fig. 23.4)
It is a fan-shaped muscle lying above and lateral to the pectineus. Strictly speaking, it is not a muscle of adductor compartment but described here because of its close relationship with the structures of the adductor compartment of the thigh.

Origin
It arises from the outer surface of the anterior half of the obturator membrane and adjoining anterior and inferior margins of the obturator foramen.

Insertion
The fibres converge backward and laterally to form a tendon, which spirals upward over the inferior and posterior surfaces of the neck of femur to be inserted into the **trochanteric fossa** of greater trochanter of the femur.

Nerve supply
By the posterior division of the obturator nerve.

Actions
It is the lateral rotator of the thigh.

OBTURATOR NERVE (Fig. 23.6)

It is the chief nerve of the adductor compartment of the thigh. It arises from the lumbar plexus in the abdomen. It is formed by the ventral division of the anterior primary rami of L2, L3, L4 spinal nerves. It enters the thigh by passing through the obturator canal.

Course and Distribution (Fig. 23.6A)
While passing through the obturator canal the obturator nerve divides into anterior and posterior divisions.

1. The *anterior division* passes downwards into the thigh in front of the obturator externus. It then descends behind the pectineus and the adductor longus, and in front of the adductor brevis. The anterior division supplies the following muscles:
   (a) Pectineus.

Table 23.1 Origin, insertion, nerve supply, and actions of muscles of the adductor compartment of the thigh

Muscle	Origin	Insertion	Nerve supply	Actions
Pectineus (flat, quadrilateral muscle, composite muscle)	• Pecten pubis • Upper half of the pectineal surface of the superior ramus of the pubis • Fascia covering the pectineus	Line extending from the lesser trochanter to the linea aspera	Femoral nerve and anterior division of the obturator nerve	Adduction of the thigh
Adductor longus (triangular muscle, forming the medial part of the floor of the femoral triangle)	Body of the pubis in the angle between the pubic crest and the pubic symphysis	Middle 1/3rd of linea aspera	Obturator nerve (anterior division)	Adduction and medial rotation of thigh
Adductor brevis (triangular muscle lying behind the pectineus and adductor longus)	• Anterior surface of the body of pubis • Outer surface of the inferior ramus of the pubis between the gracilis and the obturator externus	Line extending from the lesser trochanter to the linea aspera, and upper part of the linea aspera itself just lateral to pectineus	Obturator nerve (anterior and posterior divisions)	Adduction of thigh
Adductor magnus (large composite)	(a) Hamstring part: inferolateral part of the ischial tuberosity (b) Adductor part: outer part of the ischiopubic ramus	• Medial margin of gluteal tuberosity • Linea aspera • Medial supracondylar line • Adductor tubercle	• Adductor part by the obturator nerve (posterior division) • Hamstring part by the tibial part of sciatic nerve	• Adduction and medial rotation of thigh • Weak extension of hip joint
Gracilis	Medial margin of the lower half of the body of the pubis: adjoining anterior part of inferior ramus of the pubis	Upper part of the medial surface of tibia between the insertions of sartorius (in front) and the semitendinosus (behind)	Obturator nerve (anterior division)	• Adduction of thigh • Flexion and medial rotation of leg

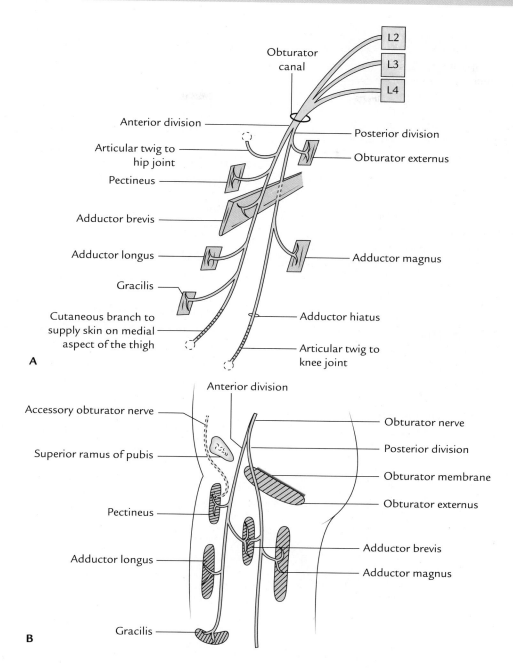

A

B

Fig. 23.6 Obturator nerve: **A**, course and distribution; **B**, accessory obturator nerve.

(b) Adductor longus.

(c) Gracilis.

(d) Adductor brevis.

The anterior division also gives an articular twig to the hip joint. Distal to the adductor longus, it enters the adductor canal where it provides a twig to the subsartorial plexus of nerves and terminates by supplying the femoral artery in the adductor canal.

2. The *posterior division* enters the thigh by piercing the anterior part of the obturator externus muscle which it

supplies. It then descends behind the adductor brevis and in front of the adductor magnus. The posterior division supplies the following muscles:

(a) Obturator externus.

(b) Adductor magnus.

(c) Adductor brevis.

Its terminal part forms an articular branch called **genicular branch,** which pierces the adductor magnus or passes through hiatus for femoral vessels to reach the popliteal fossa where it runs along the popliteal vessels and pierces the oblique popliteal ligament to supply the knee joint.

- **Adductor spasm of the thigh:** Spasm of the adductors of the thigh in spastic paraplegia may be relieved by surgical division of the obturator nerve.
- **Referred pain:** In diseases of the knee joint, the pain may be referred to the hip joint along the obturator nerve (L2, L3, and L4) because it supplies both these joints.

N.B. *Accessory obturator nerve (Fig. 23.6B):* In about 30% individuals, accessory obturator nerve arises from the lumbar plexus. It is formed by the ventral divisions of the anterior primary rami of L3, L4 spinal nerves. It crosses the superior ramus of pubis deep to pectineus, which it supplies. It gives an articular twig to the hip joint and terminates by communicating with the anterior division of the obturator nerve. If small, it supplies only the pectineus muscle (Fig. 23.6A).

ARTERIES

PROFUNDA FEMORIS ARTERY (DEEP FEMORAL ARTERY; Fig. 23.7)

It is the largest branch of the femoral artery and is the chief source of blood supply to the muscles of all the three compartments of the thigh (Fig. 23.7). It arises from the lateral side of the femoral artery in the femoral triangle about 4 cm below the inguinal ligament, behind the femoral vessels, giving off medial and lateral circumflex arteries. It then passes posteriorly between pectineus and adductor longus then descends close to femur successively between adductor longus and adductor brevis, between adductor longus and adductor magnus. Here it gives off **first three perforating arteries**. Its terminal part pierces the adductor magnus as the **fourth perforating artery** to reach the back of the leg.

Branches

The branches of profunda femoris artery are summarized as follows:

- Muscular branches.
- Medial circumflex femoral artery.
- Lateral circumflex femoral artery.
- Four perforating arteries.
  1. The **muscular branches** as the name implies, supply the muscles.
  2. The **medial circumflex femoral artery** leaves the femoral triangle by passing posteriorly, between the pectineus and the psoas major muscles.

     Then it passes successively between the obturator externus and adductor brevis and between the

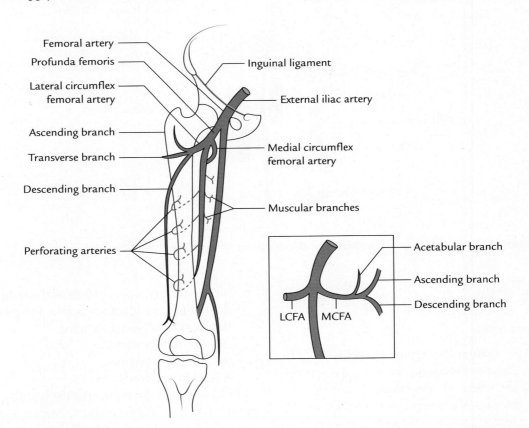

Fig. 23.7 Profunda (deep femoral) femoris artery: Figure in the inset shows branches of the medial circumflex femoral artery (LCFA = lateral circumflex femoral artery, MCFA = medial circumflex femoral artery).

quadratus femoris and upper border of the adductor magnus. Here is gives off *transverse* and *ascending branches*. The *transverse branch* takes part in the formation of *cruciate anastomosis*. The *ascending branch* passes to the trochanteric fossa and takes part in the formation of *trochanteric anastomosis*.

The *acetabular branch* of the medial circumflex femoral artery arises before the terminal branches and enters the acetabulum through acetabular notch deep to transverse acetabular ligament.

- The *posterior retinacular branches* of medial circumflex femoral artery pass through capsule of hip joint to supply the head and neck of the femur.

N.B. The medial circumflex femoral artery is especially important because it supplies most of the blood to the head and neck of femur by its posterior retinacular branches.

3. The **lateral circumflex femoral artery** is the largest branch of the profunda femoris artery. It runs laterally between the anterior and posterior divisions of the femoral nerve and divides into ascending, transverse, and descending branches. The *ascending and transverse branches* take part in the cruciate anastomosis on the back of the thigh just below the greater trochanter (Fig. 23.7). The *descending branch* runs down along the anterior border of the vastus lateralis and takes part in the anastomosis around the knee.

4. The **perforating arteries** are four in number. They are numbered from above downward as first, second, third and fourth; the fourth one being the continuation of the profunda femoris artery.

Clinical significance of profunda femoris artery: The profunda femoris artery is of great clinical importance because it is deeply located and lies in close proximity to the femoral shaft; hence, it is prone to injury in fracture of femoral shaft. The artery is also liable to injury during surgical procedure of fixing metallic screws in the femur by an orthopedic surgeon.

OBTURATOR ARTERY

It arises from the anterior division of internal iliac artery in the pelvis. It enters the adductor compartment of the thigh through the obturator canal. Just outside the obturator canal, it divides into medial and lateral branches. The lateral branch gives off an **acetabular twig,** which enters the acetabulum through a gap between acetabular notch and transverse acetabular ligament where it supplies acetabular fat and gives off a slender artery to the femoral head along the ligament of the head of femur.

N.B. *Abnormal obturator artery:* Normally a pubic branch of the obturator artery anastomoses with the pubic branch of the inferior epigastric artery. Sometimes this anastomosis is so large and well developed that the obturator artery appears to be a branch of the inferior epigastric artery.

Golden Facts to Remember

➤ Chief artery for the muscles of thigh	Profunda femoris artery
➤ Largest branch of the profunda femoris artery	Lateral circumflex femoral artery
➤ Largest muscle of the adductor compartment of thigh	Adductor magnus
➤ All the muscles of the adductor compartment of thigh are inserted into the femur *except*	Gracilis (which is inserted into the tibia)
➤ Muscles of the adductor compartment of thigh supplied by two different nerves	(a) Pectineus (by femoral and obturator nerve) (b) Adductor magnus (by obturator and tibial part of sciatic nerve)
➤ Custodes virginitatis	Adductor muscles of the thigh
➤ Rider's bone	Calcified tendon of adductor longus/sesamoid bone in the tendon of adductor longus

Clinical Case Study

A 55-year-old businessman came to the hospital and complained that he could walk only for about 50–60 yards before a cramp-like pain in his right leg forces him to take rest. After taking rest, pain disappears and again he could walk for the same distance. On examination, the femoral pulses were normal in both the limbs. The arteriography revealed a blockage of the right femoral artery just above the level of adductor tubercle. A diagnosis of "**intermittent claudication**" was made.

Questions

1. Which is the chief artery of the lower limb?
2. If the femoral artery is blocked above the adductor tubercle, which artery plays a major role in establishing the collateral circulation in the lower limb?
3. What is the preferred site of ligation of femoral artery?
4. Which artery is likely to be injured in fracture shaft of femur and why?
5. What will be the effects if profunda femoris artery is ruptured?

Answers

1. Femoral artery.
2. Profunda femoris artery.
3. Proximal to the origin of profunda femoris artery.
4. Profunda femoris artery, as this artery lies in close proximity to the shaft of femur.
5. Severe bleeding inside the thigh muscles, which may cause "*thigh compartment syndrome.*"

Gluteal Region

The gluteal region overlies the back and side, of the lateral half of the pelvis. It extends from the iliac crest superiorly to the gluteal fold (at the lower limit of the prominence of buttock) inferiorly. Medially it extends up to mid-dorsal line and natal cleft, and laterally up to an imaginary line joining the anterior superior iliac spine to the anterior edge of the greater trochanter. The gluteal region is one of the commonest sites of intramuscular injections.

SURFACE LANDMARKS (Fig. 24.1)

- **Buttock:** It is a round bulge on the posterior aspect of the gluteal region.
- **Gluteal fold:** It is a transverse skin crease, which forms the lower limit of the gluteal region. It is produced by a linear adherence of the skin to the deep fascia, obliquely across the inferior border of gluteus maximus.
- **Natal cleft:** It is a midline cleft between the two buttocks, which begins at the level of third spine of the sacrum and deepens inferiorly with lower sacral spines and coccyx lying in its floor.
- **Coccyx:** It lies just behind the anal orifice and can be identified by its relative mobility under pressure.

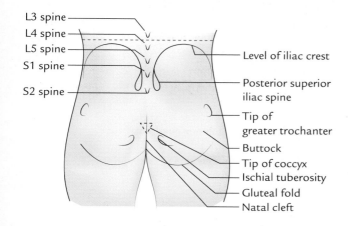

Fig. 24.1 Surface landmarks of the gluteal region.

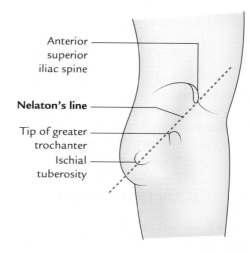

Fig. 24.2 Nelaton's line.

- **Posterior superior iliac spine (PSIS):** It lies in a skin dimple at the level of second sacral (S2) spine.
- **Ischial tuberosity:** It is a rounded bony mass on which one sits. It lies below the PSIS in the same vertical plane at a lower level than the tip of coccyx. It can be felt by pressing your fingers upward into the medial part of the gluteal fold. It is 5 cm above the gluteal fold and about same distance from the midline.
- **Tip of greater trochanter:** It lies just in front of hollow on the side of hip, about one hand's breadth below the tubercle of iliac crest.
- **Iliac crest:** It can be felt as a curved bony ridge in a groove at the lower limit/margin of the waist. The highest point of iliac crest corresponds to the interval between the spines of L3 and L4 vertebrae.

N.B.

- *Nelaton's line (Fig. 24.2):* It is the line joining the anterior superior iliac spine and the most prominent point of ischial tuberosity. It crosses the tip of greater trochanter.

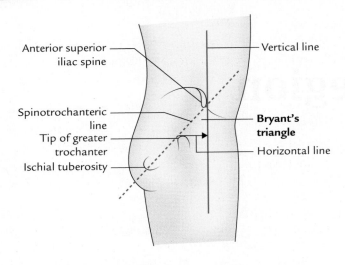

Fig. 24.3 Bryant's triangle.

- *Bryant's triangle (Fig. 24.3):* With the patient in supine position, first draw a vertical line passing downwards from the anterior superior iliac spine (ASIS) and now draw a line extending from ASIS to the tip of greater trochanter (spinotrochanteric line). Lastly draw a horizontal line from the tip of greater trochanter to the first line. The triangle thus formed is called **Bryant's triangle.**

SUPERFICIAL FASCIA

The superficial fascia in the gluteal region is thick and contains abundant subcutaneous fat particularly in adult females, which is responsible for a characteristic round contour of the buttock in them.

CUTANEOUS NERVES (Fig. 24.4)

The cutaneous nerves of the gluteal region are derived from several sources, and converge in this region from all the directions (Fig. 24.4). The cutaneous innervation of the gluteal region is divided into four quadrants—upper anterior, upper posterior, lower anterior, and lower posterior.

1. **Upper anterior quadrant** is supplied by the:
   - lateral cutaneous branch of subcostal nerve (T12), and
   - lateral cutaneous branch of iliohypogastric nerve (L1).
2. **Upper posterior quadrant** is supplied by the:
   - cutaneous branches from dorsal rami of upper three lumbar nerves (L1, L2, L3) and upper three sacral nerves (S1, S2, S3).
3. **Lower anterior quadrant** is supplied by the:
   - posterior division of lateral cutaneous nerves of the thigh (L2, L3).
4. **Lower posterior quadrant** is supplied by the:
   - posterior cutaneous nerves of the thigh (S1, S2, S3), and
   - perforating cutaneous nerves (S2, S3).

CUTANEOUS ARTERIES AND LYMPH VESSELS

The **cutaneous arteries** supplying the gluteal region are derived from the superior and inferior gluteal arteries.

The **lymph vessels** from the gluteal region drain into the lateral group of superficial inguinal lymph nodes.

DEEP FASCIA (Fig. 24.5)

The deep fascia of the gluteal region is attached above to the iliac crest and behind to the sacrum. It splits twice along the iliac crest, first time to enclose the tensor fasciae latae and second time to enclose the gluteus maximus. Between tensor fasciae latae and gluteus maximus is a thick fascial sheet called **gluteal aponeurosis** which covers the gluteus medius.

1. The layers which enclose the gluteus maximus are interconnected by numerous fibrous septa which traverse through this muscle and divide it into numerous

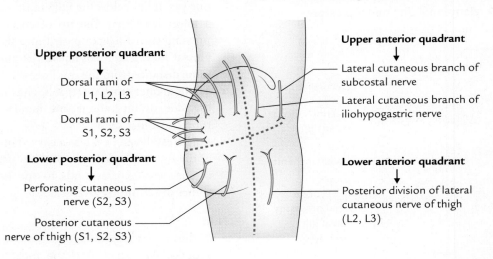

Fig. 24.4 Cutaneous nerves of the gluteal region.

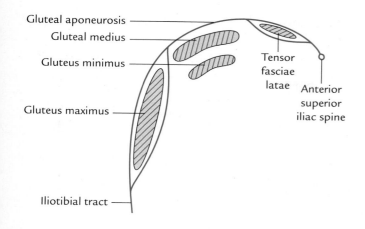

Fig. 24.5 Schematic diagram to show the deep fascia of the gluteal region.

discrete fasciculi. *Note:* Gluteus maximus is the most fasciculated muscle in the body.

2. Traced laterally, the deep fascia is continuous with the *iliotibial tract.*

GLUTEAL LIGAMENTS (Fig. 24.6)

It is of utmost importance for the students to study two important gluteal ligaments (sacrotuberous and sacrospinous ligaments) in the gluteal region before they proceed to study the deep structures in this region.

Sacrotuberous Ligament

It is broad band of fibrous tissue which extends from sides of the sacrum and coccyx to the medial side of the ischial tuberosity.

Sacrospinous Ligament

It is triangular sheet of fibrous tissue which extends from ischial spine to side of the sacrum and coccyx.

The sacrotuberous and sacrospinous ligaments are described in detail in Chapter 13, p. 204.

The sacrotuberous and sacrospinous ligaments convert the greater sciatic notch and lesser sciatic notch into greater sciatic foramen and lesser sciatic foramen, respectively.

1. The **greater sciatic foramen** is a passageway for structures leaving the pelvis and entering the gluteal region (e.g., sciatic nerve, superior and inferior gluteal vessels, etc.).
2. The **lesser sciatic foramen** is a passageway for structures entering the perineum (e.g., pudendal nerve and artery).

N.B. The greater sciatic foramen is considered as the "**door of the gluteal region**" through which all arteries and nerves enter into the gluteal region from the pelvis.

The **structures passing through the greater sciatic foramen** (Fig. 24.7) are as follows:

1. Piriformis: It emerges from the pelvis and almost completely fills the foramen. It is the key muscle of this region.
2. Structures passing below the piriformis:
   (a) Inferior gluteal nerve and vessels.
   (b) Sciatic nerve (most lateral structure).
   (c) Posterior cutaneous nerve of the thigh.
   (d) Nerve to quadratus femoris.
   (e) Pudendal nerve.
   (f) Internal pudendal vessels.
   (g) Nerve to obturator internus.

The last three structures cross the dorsal aspect of ischial spine and adjoining part of sacrospinous ligament

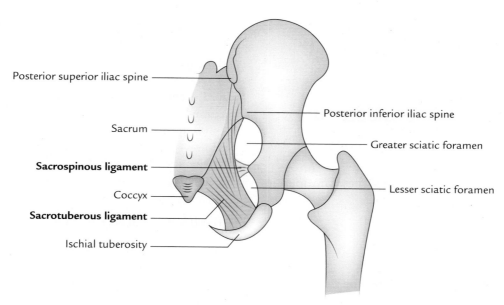

Fig. 24.6 Gluteal ligaments (sacrotuberous and sacrospinous ligaments).

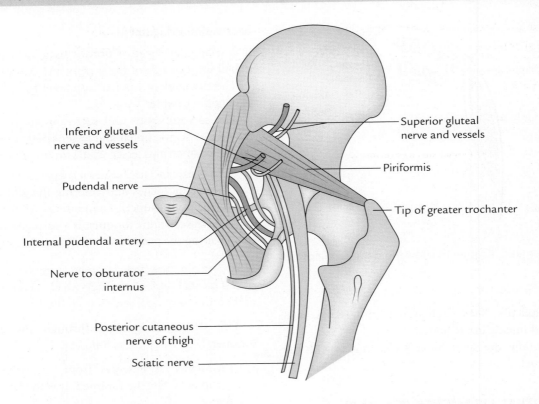

Fig. 24.7 Structures passing through the greater and lesser sciatic foramina.

(with internal pudendal artery between the nerves to obturator internus laterally and pudendal nerve medially), and curves forward to enter the perineum. The pudendal nerve and internal pudendal vessels run in the pudendal canal.

The **structures passing through the lesser sciatic foramen** are as follows:

(a) Tendon of obturator internus.
(b) Nerve to obturator internus.
(c) Internal pudendal vessels.
(d) Pudendal nerve.

MUSCLES OF THE GLUTEAL REGION

The muscles of the gluteal region are divided into two groups—major and minor.

- *Major muscles of the gluteal region:* These are four in number as given below:
  (a) Gluteus maximus.
  (b) Gluteus medius.
  (c) Gluteus minimus.
  (d) Tensor fasciae latae.
- *Minor muscles of the gluteal region:* These are six in number as follows:
  (a) Piriformis.

(b) Superior and inferior gemelli.
(c) Obturator internus.
(d) Quadratus femoris.
(e) Obturator externus.

The obturator externus is the muscle of adductor compartment of thigh but only functionally related to this region. It is described in Chapter 23, p. 347.

The *major muscles of gluteal region* are larger in size and placed superficially. They are mainly extensor, abductors, and medial rotators of the thigh.

The *minor muscles of gluteal region* are smaller in size and placed deeply under cover of the lower part of the gluteus maximus. They are lateral rotators of the thigh and help to stabilize the hip joint.

However, the major muscles are described in detail in the following text. The attachments, nerve supply and actions of muscles of the gluteal region are given in Table 24.1.

GLUTEUS MAXIMUS (Fig. 24.8)

The gluteus maximus is the largest, most coarsely fibred, and most superficial gluteal muscle. It is quadrilateral in shape and covers all of the other gluteal muscles except for the anterosuperior part of the gluteus medius—the common site for intramuscular injections (Fig. 24.9).

Table 24.1 Attachments, nerve supply, and main actions of the muscles of the gluteal region

Muscle (Fig. 24.9)	Origin	Insertion	Nerve supply	Actions
Gluteus maximus (quadrilateral muscle)	• Gluteal surface of the ilium behind posterior gluteal line • Outer slope of the dorsal segment of ilium • Dorsal surfaces of the sacrum and ilium • Sacrotuberous ligament	• 3/4th of the muscle into the iliotibial tract • 1/4th of the muscle into the gluteal tuberosity	• Inferior gluteal nerve (L5; S1, S2)	• Chief extensor of the hip joint • Assists in getting up from sitting position
Gluteus medius (fan-shaped muscle)	Gluteal surface of the ilium between anterior and posterior gluteal lines	Oblique ridge on the lateral surface of the greater trochanter	Superior gluteal nerve (L5; S1)	• Abductor of the hip joint • Prevents the sagging of pelvis on the unsupported side
Gluteus minimus (fan-shaped muscle)	Gluteal surfaces of the ilium between anterior and inferior gluteal lines	Ridge on the lateral part of the anterior and inferior gluteal lines trochanter		
Tensor fasciae latae (fusiform muscle)	Outer lip of the anterior part of iliac crest (from ASIS to tubercle)	Iliotibial tract	Superior gluteal nerve	Supports the femur on tibia during standing position
Piriformis (pear-shaped muscle, Latin *pirum* = pear)	Pelvic surface of the middle three pieces of sacrum by three digitations	Apex/tip of greater trochanter	Ventral rami of S1, S2	Lateral rotator of the thigh at hip joint
Gemellus superior	Posterior surface of the ischial spine	Medial surface of greater trochanter along with tendon of obturator internus	Nerve to obturator internus (L5; S1, S2)	Lateral rotator of the thigh at hip joint
Gemellus inferior	• Upper part of the ischial tuberosity • Lower part of greater sciatic notch	Same as that of gemellus superior	Nerve to quadratus femoris (L4; L5, S1)	Lateral rotator of the thigh at hip joint
Obturator internus (fan-shaped muscle)	Pelvic surface of the obturator membrane and surrounding bones	Medial surface of greater trochanter of femur in front of trochanteric fossa	Nerve to obturator internus (L5; S1)	Lateral rotator of the thigh at hip joint
Quadratus femoris (quadrilateral muscle)	Lateral border of the ischial tuberosity	Quadrate tubercle on the intertrochanteric crest and area below it	Nerve to quadratus femoris (L5; S1)	Lateral rotator of the thigh at hip joint

Origin

It arises from:

(a) Posterior part of the gluteal surface of ilium above and behind the posterior gluteal line.

(b) Outer sloping surface of the dorsal segment of iliac crest.

(c) Aponeurosis of erector spinae muscle.

(d) Dorsal surfaces of the lower part of sacrum and adjoining part of the coccyx.

(e) Sacrotuberous ligament.

Insertion

The insertion occurs as follows:

(a) One-fourth of the muscle (deep fibres of the lower part) is inserted into the gluteal tuberosity of femur.

(b) Three-fourth of the muscle (superficial and deep fibres of the upper part) is inserted into the iliotibial tract, which in turn inserts itself on the lateral condyle of the tibia.

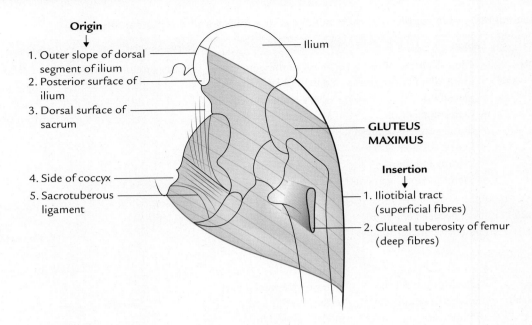

Origin

1. Outer slope of dorsal segment of ilium
2. Posterior surface of ilium
3. Dorsal surface of sacrum
4. Side of coccyx
5. Sacrotuberous ligament

Ilium

GLUTEUS MAXIMUS

Insertion

1. Iliotibial tract (superficial fibres)
2. Gluteal tuberosity of femur (deep fibres)

Fig. 24.8 Origin and insertion of the gluteus maximus.

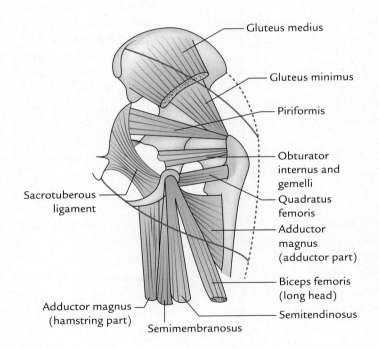

Gluteus medius

Gluteus minimus

Piriformis

Obturator internus and gemelli

Quadratus femoris

Adductor magnus (adductor part)

Biceps femoris (long head)

Semitendinosus

Sacrotuberous ligament

Adductor magnus (hamstring part)

Semimembranosus

Fig. 24.9 Muscles under cover of the gluteus maximus. The upper and lower borders of gluteus maximus muscle are indicated by thick red lines.

Nerve supply

The gluteus maximus is supplied by the inferior gluteal nerve (L5; S1, S2).

Actions

1. The gluteus maximus is the chief extensor of the hip joint during standing-up from sitting position and climbing upstairs.
2. It plays a very important role in rising from a sitting position and maintaining the erect posture.

The **structures under cover of gluteus maximus** are given in Figure 24.10 and Table 24.2.

GLUTEUS MEDIUS (Fig. 24.11)

The gluteus medius is a fan-shaped muscle. Its posterior one-third is deep and covered by the gluteus maximus while its anterior two-third is superficial and not covered by the gluteus maximus. Hence, the intramuscular injection should be ideally given in this part.

Origin

Gluteus medius arises from the gluteal surface of ilium between the anterior and posterior gluteal lines and gluteal aponeurosis.

Insertion

The muscle fibres converge downward, forward, and laterally to form a flat tendon which is inserted on to the oblique ridge on the lateral surface of the greater trochanter. The oblique ridge runs downward and forward from the tip of the greater trochanter.

Between the tendon of gluteus medius and lateral surface of greater trochanter lies a bursa—the **trochanteric bursa of gluteus medius**.

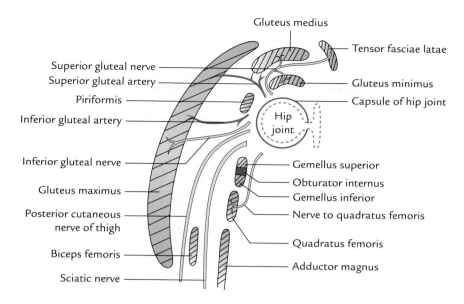

Gluteus medius
Tensor fasciae latae
Superior gluteal nerve
Superior gluteal artery
Gluteus minimus
Piriformis
Capsule of hip joint
Inferior gluteal artery
Hip joint
Inferior gluteal nerve
Gemellus superior
Obturator internus
Gluteus maximus
Gemellus inferior
Nerve to quadratus femoris
Posterior cutaneous nerve of thigh
Quadratus femoris
Biceps femoris
Adductor magnus
Sciatic nerve

Fig. 24.10 Structures under cover of the gluteus maximus.

Table 24.2 Structures under cover of the gluteus maximus muscle

Muscles	Vessels	Nerves	Joints and ligaments	Bursae
All the muscles of the gluteal region except tensor fasciae latae	Superior and inferior gluteal vessels	Superior and inferior gluteal nerves	Hip joint	Trochanteric bursa
Reflected head of the rectus femoris	Internal pudendal vessels	Sciatic nerve	Sacroiliac joint	Ischial bursa (occasional)
Origin of hamstrings	Trochanteric arterial anastomosis	Posterior cutaneous nerve of the thigh	Sacrotuberous ligament	Gluteo-femoral bursa
Insertion of the upper fibres of the adductor magnus	Cruciate arterial anastomosis	• Nerve to quadratus femoris • Pudendal nerve • Nerve to obturator internus • Perforating cutaneous nerve	• Sacrospinous ligament • Ischiofemoral ligament	

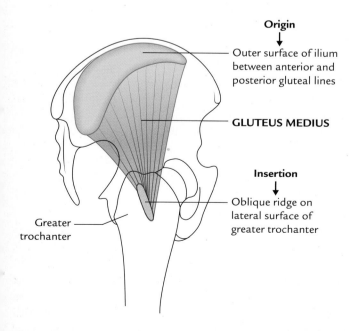

Fig. 24.11 Origin and insertion of the gluteus medius.

Origin
Outer surface of ilium between anterior and posterior gluteal lines
GLUTEUS MEDIUS
Insertion
Oblique ridge on lateral surface of greater trochanter
Greater trochanter

Nerve supply
The nerve supply is by the superior gluteal nerve.

Action
It is the main abductor of the hip joint.

GLUTEUS MINIMUS (Fig. 24.12)

The gluteus minimus is also a fan-shaped muscle and lies beneath the gluteus medius.

Origin
It arises from the gluteal surface of ilium between the anterior and inferior gluteal lines.

Insertion
The muscle fibres converge downward and slightly laterally to form a tendon, which is inserted on to the ridge in the lateral part of the anterior surface of the greater trochanter.

Between the tendon of gluteus minimus and the anterior surface of greater trochanter lies a bursa—the **trochanteric bursa of gluteus minimus**.

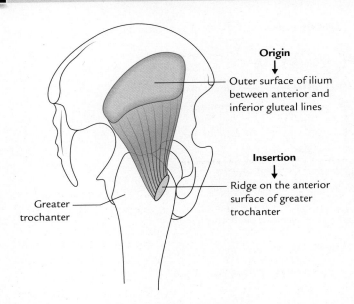

Origin
↓
Outer surface of ilium between anterior and inferior gluteal lines

Insertion
↓
Ridge on the anterior surface of greater trochanter

Greater trochanter

Fig. 24.12 Origin and insertion of the gluteus minimus.

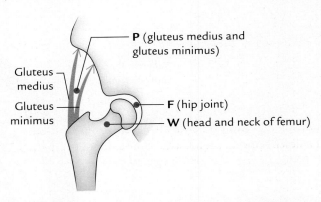

P (gluteus medius and gluteus minimus)

Gluteus medius

Gluteus minimus

F (hip joint)

W (head and neck of femur)

Fig. 24.13 Abductor mechanism of the hip joint (F = fulcrum, W = weight, P = power).

femur (Fig. 24.13). If any of these components is deranged, the **gluteal-limp** occurs.

Nerve supply
The gluteus minimus is supplied by the superior gluteal nerve.

Action
It is the abductor of the hip joint.

N.B. *Abductor mechanism of the hip joint:* This mechanism consists of three components: (a) power (**P**) provided by the gluteus medius and minimus, (b) fulcrum (**F**) provided by the hip joint, and (c) weight (**W**) by the head and neck of the

Clinical correlation

Trendelenburg's sign: Acting from below, both the gluteus medius and minimus prevent the unsupported side of the pelvis from sagging during walking and thus maintain the horizontal level of the pelvis provided the hip joint and neck-shaft angle of the femur are normal.

When the gluteus medius and minimus of one side are paralyzed due to injury of the superior gluteal nerve. The pelvis sags on the healthy side if that foot is off the ground. As a result, the person walks with a **lurching gait**. This is clinically known as **Trendelenburg's sign (Fig. 24.14).**

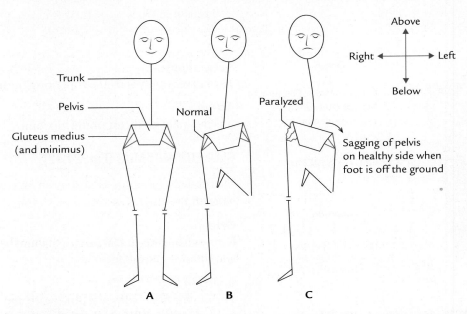

Trunk

Pelvis

Gluteus medius (and minimus)

Normal

Paralyzed

Above

Right ← → Left

Below

Sagging of pelvis on healthy side when foot is off the ground

A   B   C

Fig. 24.14 Trendelenburg's sign: **A,** when both feet are supporting the body weight, horizontal level of pelvis is maintained (i.e., anterior superior iliac spines lie in the same horizontal plane); **B,** when only one foot (e.g., right in this figure) is supporting the body weight, the unsupported side of the pelvis is normally raised or prevented from sagging by the opposite gluteus medius and minimus muscles; **C,** if the gluteus medius and minimus muscles are paralyzed on one side (e.g., right side in this case), the unsupported left side of pelvis sags (this is positive Trendelenburg's sign).

TENSOR FASCIAE LATAE

This is a muscle of the gluteal region but during evolution the tensor fasciae latae muscle had migrated to the upper lateral aspect of the thigh but retains its nerve supply (e.g., superior gluteal nerve).

It tenses the fascia lata and iliotibial tract, thereby supporting the femur on tibia during standing position.

It is described with the muscles of the anterior compartment of the thigh in Chapter 22, p. 334–335.

ARTERIES OF THE GLUTEAL REGION

The arteries of the gluteal region are as follows:

1. Superior gluteal artery.
2. Inferior gluteal artery.
3. Internal pudendal artery.

SUPERIOR GLUTEAL ARTERY

The superior gluteal artery is a branch of the posterior division of internal iliac artery. It enters the gluteal region through greater sciatic foramen above the piriformis along with the superior gluteal nerve. Here it divides into the superficial and deep branches. The **superficial branch** passes between gluteus medius and maximus, and supplies both of them. The **deep branch** passes laterally between gluteus medius and minimus, and subdivides into upper and lower branches. The upper branch takes part in the formation of **spinous anastomosis** close to the anterior superior iliac spine and the lower branch takes part in the formation of **trochanteric anastomosis** (p. 370).

INFERIOR GLUTEAL ARTERY

The inferior gluteal artery is a branch of anterior division of the internal iliac artery and enters in the gluteal region below the piriformis along with the inferior gluteal nerve and continues with the posterior cutaneous nerve of the thigh. It gives off three sets of branches:

1. **Muscular branches** to the adjacent muscles.
2. **Anastomotic branches** to cruciate and trochanteric anastomoses.
3. Artery to sciatic nerve (Latin *arteria nervi ischiadici*) accompanies the sciatic nerve and sinks into its substance to supply it. It is the remnant of the **axis artery of the lower limb.**

NERVES OF THE GLUTEAL REGION

The nerves of the gluteal region are as follows:

1. Superior gluteal nerve.
2. Inferior gluteal nerve.

The other nerves in the gluteal region are:

1. Sciatic nerve.
2. Posterior cutaneous nerve of thigh.
3. Nerve to quadratus femoris.
4. Pudendal nerve.
5. Nerve to obturator internus.
6. Perforating cutaneous nerve.

SUPERIOR GLUTEAL NERVE

The superior gluteal nerve arises from the sacral plexus in the pelvis and is formed by the dorsal branches of the ventral rami of L4, L5; S1. It enters the gluteal region through the greater sciatic notch above the piriformis in company with superior gluteal artery. Here it curves upward and forward, runs between the gluteus medius and the minimus, and supplies both of them. It then comes out by passing between the anterior borders of these muscles and supplies the tensor fasciae latae from its deep surface. It also provides an articular twig to the hip joint.

INFERIOR GLUTEAL NERVE

The inferior gluteal nerve arises from the sacral plexus in the pelvis and is formed by the dorsal branches of the ventral rami of L5; S1, S2. It enters the gluteal region through the greater sciatic notch in company with inferior gluteal artery and posterior cutaneous nerve of the thigh. Here it curves upward to supply the gluteus maximus from its deep surface.

SCIATIC NERVE

It enters the gluteal region through the greater sciatic foramen below the piriformis (Fig. 24.7). (It is the most lateral structure emerging through the greater sciatic foramen below the piriformis.) It runs downward and slightly laterally under cover of gluteus maximus midway between the greater trochanter and the ischial tuberosity, and enters the back of the thigh at the lower border of the gluteus maximus. The sciatic nerve is described in detail in Chapter 25, p. 367.

Surface Marking of Sciatic Nerve in the Gluteal Region (Fig. 24.15)

To represent the course of sciatic nerve in the gluteal region, two points are located—upper and lower.

1. The **upper point** is located about 2.5 cm lateral to the midpoint of a line joining the PSIS and ischial tuberosity.
2. The **lower point** is located midway between the greater trochanter and the ischial tuberosity.

A thick (about 2 cm wide) curved line (with outward convexity) joining these two points represents the sciatic nerve.

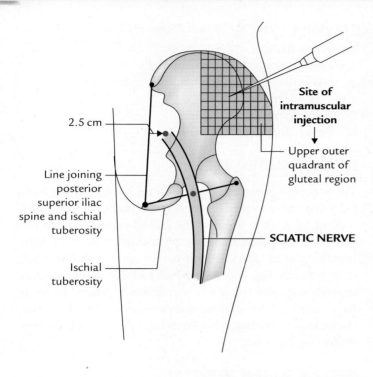

Fig. 24.15 Surface marking of the sciatic nerve in the gluteal region.

POSTERIOR CUTANEOUS NERVE OF THE THIGH

The posterior cutaneous nerve of thigh arises from the sacral plexus in the pelvis from dorsal divisions of the ventral rami of S1, S2, S3 of sacral plexus, and enters the gluteal region through the greater sciatic foramen below the piriformis and medial to the sciatic nerve. It runs downward and medially superficial to the sciatic nerve. It is continuous on the back of the thigh deep to the fascia lata.

It gives the following branches:

1. A peroneal branch to supply the skin of posterior two-third of scrotum or labium majus.
2. Gluteal branches to supply the skin of the posteroinferior quadrant of the gluteal region.

N.B. The unique feature of posterior cutaneous nerve of the thigh is that the most part of this nerve lies deep to deep fascia.

NERVE TO QUADRATUS FEMORIS

The nerve to quadratus femoris arises from ventral divisions of ventral rami of L4, L5; S1 of sacral plexus. It enters the thigh through the greater sciatic foramen below the piriformis and runs downward deep to sciatic nerve. It runs downwards deep to the tendon of obturator internus and two gemelli and supplies inferior gemellus and quadratus femoris. It also gives an articular twig to the hip joint.

PUDENDAL NERVE

The pudendal nerve arises from ventral divisions of the ventral rami of S2, S3, S4 of sacral plexus. It enters the gluteal region just to leave it. It enters the gluteal region through the greater sciatic foramen below the piriformis. It crosses the dorsal aspect of apex of the sacrospinous ligament medial to internal pudendal vessels and leaves the gluteal region by passing through the lesser sciatic foramen to enter the pudendal canal (for details see Chapter 15, page 235).

NERVE TO OBTURATOR INTERNUS

The nerve to obturator internus arises from ventral divisions of the ventral rami of L5; S1, S2 of sacral plexus. It enters the gluteal region through greater sciatic foramen below the piriformis. It crosses the dorsal aspect of ischial spine lateral to internal pudendal vessels and then passes forward through the lesser sciatic foramen deep to the fascia covering the obturator internus. It supplies obturator internus and gemellus superior.

PERFORATING CUTANEOUS NERVE

The perforating cutaneous nerve arises from the sacral plexus (S2, S3). It pierces the lower part of sacrotuberous ligament and then winds around the lower border of gluteus maximus to supply the skin of the posteroinferior quadrant of the gluteal region.

Clinical correlation

- **Intramuscular injection in gluteal region:** The gluteal region is one of the commonest sites of intramuscular injection of drugs. It is given in the **gluteus medius muscle** at this site. If given randomly it may damage the sciatic nerve. It is safe only when it is given in the upper lateral quadrant of the gluteal region or above the line extending PSIS to the upper border of greater trochanter. This line approximately corresponds to the upper border of the gluteus maximus (for details, see *Clinical and Surgical Anatomy*, 2nd Edition by Vishram Singh).
- **Sciatic nerve block:** The sciatic nerve is blocked by injecting an anesthetic agent a few centimeters below the midpoint of the line joining the PSIS and the upper border of the greater trochanter.
- **Piriformis syndrome:** It is a clinical condition characterized by pain in buttock due to compression of the sciatic nerve by the piriformis. It commonly occurs in sports that require excessive use of gluteal muscles (e.g., ice skaters, cyclists, etc.), causing hypertrophy or spasm of piriformis.

Golden Facts to Remember

▶ All the structures enter the gluteal region through greater sciatic foramen *except*

Tendon of obturator internus which enters the gluteal region through lesser sciatic foramen

▶ Largest muscle of the body

Gluteus maximus

▶ Key muscle of the gluteal region

Piriformis

▶ All the major muscles of the gluteal region are supplied by the superior gluteal nerve *except*

Gluteus maximus (which is supplied by the inferior gluteal nerve)

▶ Most coarsely fibred muscle of the body

Gluteus maximus

▶ All the gluteal muscles are covered by the gluteus maximus *except*

Anterosuperior part of the gluteus medius

▶ Main extensors of the hip during walking

Hamstring muscles

Clinical Case Study

A 27-year-old political party worker sustained a bullet shot injury in his right buttock in police firing during a rally for price hike.

He was admitted in the hospital and fully recovered. He was discharged from the hospital but he developed a characteristic limp during walking. There was a sagging of the left hip while taking step on the right foot. On examination the **Trendelenburg's sign** was positive.

Questions

1. Name the nerve which was injured by the bullet shot.
2. Enumerate the muscles supplied by the injured nerve.
3. What is Trendelenburg's sign?
4. Name the characteristic gait in unilateral injury and in bilateral injury of the superior gluteal nerve.

Answers

1. Superior gluteal nerve.
2. Gluteus medius, gluteus minimus, and tensor fasciae latae.
3. When one foot is off the ground, the tilting of the pelvis on that side is prevented by the contraction of gluteus medius and minimus of the opposite side. If these muscles are paralyzed due to injury of the superior gluteal nerve the pelvis will tilt or sag on the opposite healthy side if that foot is off the ground.
4. (a) Lurching gait if injury is unilateral and (b) waddling gait if injury is bilateral.

Back of the Thigh and Popliteal Fossa

BACK OF THE THIGH

The back of the thigh extends from the gluteal fold above to the back of the knee below.

CUTANEOUS INNERVATION

The skin over the back of the thigh is supplied by the following nerves (Fig. 25.1):

1. *Posterior cutaneous nerve of the thigh* runs downward in the midline on the back of thigh deep to fascia lata and superficially to the long head of biceps femoris. On reaching the popliteal fossa, it pierces the fascial roof of the fossa and accompanies the short saphenous vein down to the middle of the calf. Its branches supply the skin on the back of thigh and proximal part of the back of leg.

2. *Cutaneous branches of the obturator nerve* supply the medial part of the back of thigh in the upper part.

3. *Medial branches of the anterior cutaneous nerve of the thigh* supply the medial part of the back of thigh in the lower part.

4. *Lateral cutaneous nerve of the thigh* sends twigs to the posterior aspect of thigh in the upper part.

CONTENTS OF POSTERIOR COMPARTMENT OF THE THIGH

The posterior compartment of the thigh is also called flexor compartment. It is completely separated from the anterior compartment by the lateral intermuscular septum, but it is incompletely separated from the medial compartment of thigh by the ill-defined posterior intermuscular septum.

The contents of posterior compartment of the thigh are as follows:

- **Muscles:** Hamstring muscles and short head of the biceps femoris.
- **Nerve:** Sciatic nerve.
- **Arteries:** Arterial anastomoses on the back of the thigh.

MUSCLES ON THE BACK OF THE THIGH

These muscles on the back of the thigh are called the ***hamstring muscles*** (Latin *ham* = back of thigh). However conventionally the short head of the biceps femoris is not included in the hamstring group.

The hamstring muscles are:

1. Semitendinosus.
2. Semimembranosus.
3. Biceps femoris (long head).
4. Ischial head of adductor magnus.

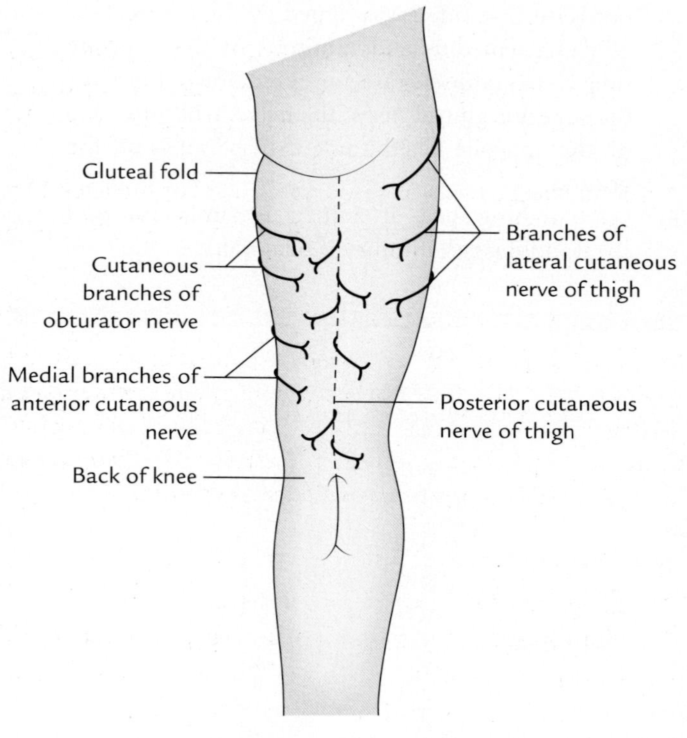

Fig. 25.1 Cutaneous nerves on the back of the thigh.

Gluteal fold

Cutaneous branches of obturator nerve

Medial branches of anterior cutaneous nerve

Back of knee

Branches of lateral cutaneous nerve of thigh

Posterior cutaneous nerve of thigh

The **characteristic features of hamstring muscles** are:

1. All arise from the ischial tuberosity.
2. All are inserted into one of the bones of the leg.
3. All are supplied by tibial part of the sciatic nerve.
4. All are flexors of the knee and extensors of the hip joint.

The bony attachments of the hamstring muscles are shown in Figure 25.2.

N.B.

• The posterior thigh muscles were named "hamstrings" because their tendons on the back of knee are used to hang up hams (hip and thigh regions of animals viz., pigs.)

• The adductor magnus reaches only up to the adductor tubercle of the femur, but is included amongst the hamstrings group of muscles because the **tibial collateral ligament** of the knee joint morphologically represents the degenerated tendon of this muscle, which is attached below on the tibia.

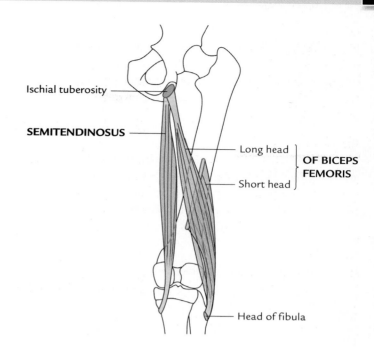

Fig. 25.3 Origin and insertion of biceps femoris and semitendinosus muscles.

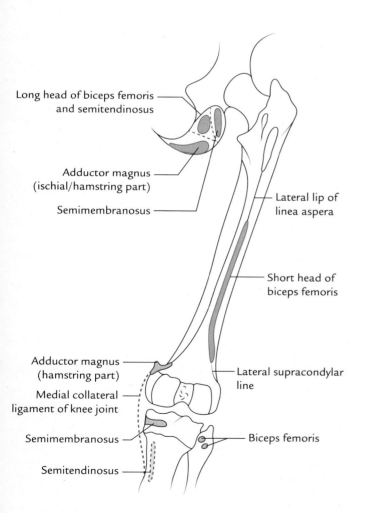

Fig. 25.2 Bony attachments of the muscles of the back.

Biceps Femoris (Fig. 25.3)

The biceps femoris muscle as its name implies consists of two heads—long head and short head.

Origin

1. **Long head,** arises from lower medial part of the upper quadrilateral area of the ischial tuberosity in common with the semitendinosus and also from the lower part of the sacrotuberous ligament.
2. **Short head,** arises from the lower part of the lateral lip of the linea aspera and upper two-third of the lateral supracondylar line.

Insertion

The two heads unite in the lower third of the thigh to form a conjoint tendon, which slopes downward and laterally to be inserted on to the head of fibula in front of the styloid process. Just before insertion the tendon is either folded around or split by the fibular collateral ligament.

Nerve supply

1. **Long head,** by the tibial part of the sciatic nerve.
2. **Short head,** by the common peroneal part of the sciatic nerve.

Semitendinosus (Fig. 25.3)

It is so named because its lower half is tendinous.

Origin

It arises along with the long head of biceps femoris from lower medial part of the upper quadrilateral area of the ischial tuberosity. It is fleshy in the upper part and forms a cord-like tendon in the lower part, which lies on the semimembranosus muscle.

Insertion

In the lower part of the back of thigh, it diverges medially and passes behind the medial condyle of the femur and then curves downward and forward to be inserted into the upper part of the medial surfaces of the tibia behind the insertion of sartorius and gracilis muscles.

Nerve supply

It is by tibial part of the sciatic nerve.

Semimembranosus (Fig. 25.4)

It is so called because this broad muscle is half membranous.

Origin

It arises from the upper lateral part of the quadrilateral area of the ischial tuberosity. It is membranous in the upper half and fleshy in the lower half. It lies deep to semitendinosus.

Insertion

The fleshy part converges below to form a tendon, which is inserted into a horizontal groove on the back of the medial condyle of tibia.

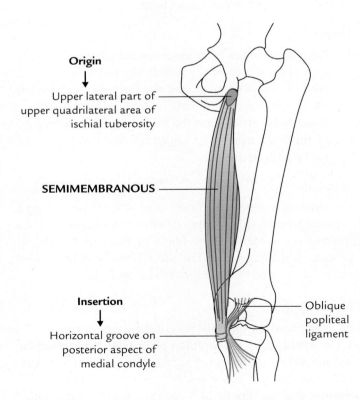

Fig. 25.4 Origin and insertion of semimembranosus muscle.

Origin
↓
Upper lateral part of upper quadrilateral area of ischial tuberosity

SEMIMEMBRANOUS

Insertion
↓
Horizontal groove on posterior aspect of medial condyle

Oblique popliteal ligament

N.B.

- The tendon of insertion gives rise to the following three expansions:
  1. A fibrous band extends upward and laterally behind the posterior aspect of the capsule of knee joint to form *oblique popliteal ligament of the knee.*
  2. A fibrous expansion extends downward and laterally across the fascia covering the popliteus to be attached to the soleal line.
  3. Some fibres descend downward for attachment on the medial border of the upper part of tibia behind the tibial collateral ligament.
- A synovial bursa lines deep to the tendon of insertion of semimembranosus which may communicate with the synovial cavity of the knee joint.

Nerve supply

It is by tibial part of the sciatic nerve.

Ischial Head of the Adductor Magnus (Fig. 25.2)

Origin

It arises from the inferolateral part of the ischial tuberosity.

Insertion

It descends almost vertically downward to be inserted on the adductor tubercle.

Nerve supply

It is by tibial part of the sciatic nerve.

The origin, insertion, and nerve supply of muscles of the back of the thigh are summarized in Table 25.1.

Actions of the Hamstring Muscles

1. They are the chief flexors of the knee joint and weak extensor of the hip joint (Fig. 25.5); however, the two actions cannot be performed maximally at the same time.
2. The hamstrings are the hip extensors during walking on the flat ground when the gluteus maximus exercise minimal activity.
3. The action of hamstring muscles restricts the range of motion (ROM) of the hip flexion when the knee is extended, viz., during toe touching (Fig. 25.6).

Clinical correlation

Clinical significance of hamstring muscles:
- If hamstring muscles are paralyzed, the patient tends to fall forward because the gluteus maximus muscle cannot maintain the necessary tone to stand upright.
- In ancient times, the soldiers used to slash the back of the knees of horses of their opponents in order to cut the tendons of hamstring muscles, to bring the horse and its rider down. They also used to cut the hamstring tendons of soldiers so that they could not run. This was termed "hamstringing" the enemy.

Table 25.1 Origin, insertion, and nerve supply of the muscles on the back of thigh

Muscle	Origin	Insertion	Nerve supply
Biceps femoris (a) Long head	(a) *Long head*: From lower medial part of upper quadrilateral area of ischial tuberosity	Into the head of the fibula in front of its styloid process	(a) Long head, by the tibial part of the sciatic nerve (L5; S1, S2)
(b) Short head	(b) *Short head*: From lateral lip of the linea aspera and from the upper two-third of the lateral supracondylar line		(b) Short head by the common peroneal part of the sciatic nerve (L5; S1, S2)
Semitendinosus	From the lower medial part of upper quadrilateral area of the ischial tuberosity,	Into the upper part of the medial surface of the tibia	Tibial part of the sciatic nerve (L5; S1, S2)
Semimembranosus	From the upper lateral part of upper quadrilateral area of ischial tuberosity	Into the horizontal groove on the posterior aspect of the medial condyle of the tibia	Tibial part of the sciatic nerve (L5; S1, S2)
Ischial part of adductor magnus	From inferolateral aspect of the ischial tuberosity	Into the adductor tubercle	Tibial part of the sciatic nerve (L5; S1, S2)

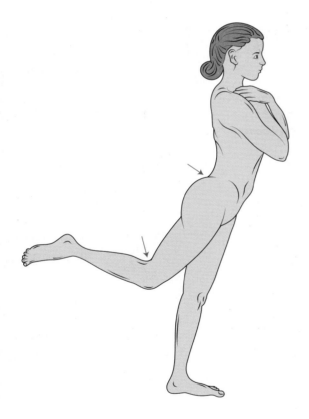

Fig. 25.5 Extension of the hip joint and flexion of the knee joint by the hamstring muscles.

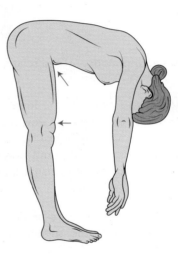

Fig. 25.6 Restriction of range of motion of hip flexion when the knee is extended (e.g., toe-touching action).

SCIATIC NERVE

The sciatic nerve is the thickest nerve in the body. It is about 1.5 to 2 cm wide at the beginning. It arises from sacral plexus in the pelvis and consists of two parts—tibial part and common peroneal part (Fig. 25.7).

The **tibial part** is formed by the ventral divisions of anterior primary rami of L4, L5; S1, S2, S3.

The **common part** is formed by the dorsal divisions of anterior primary rami of L4, L5; S1, S2.

The two parts are usually enclosed in a common sheath of the connective tissue.

Extent

It begins in the pelvis and terminates at or just above the superior angle of the popliteal fossa by dividing into tibial and common peroneal nerve.

Course

In the pelvis, it lies in front of piriformis under cover of its fascia. It enters the gluteal region through greater sciatic foramen below the piriformis. Here it runs downward with slight lateral convexity and passes between the ischial tuberosity and greater trochanter.

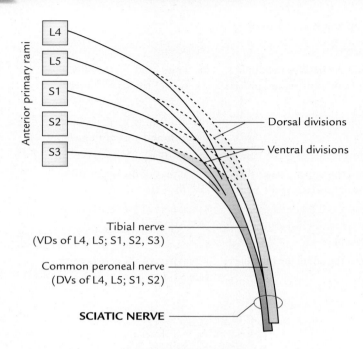

Fig. 25.7 Origin and formation of the sciatic nerve.

It enters the back of thigh at the lower border of the gluteus maximus and runs vertically downward. Just above or at the superior angle of the popliteal fossa (approximately at the junction of upper two-third and lower one-third of the back of thigh) it divides into two terminal branches—tibial and common peroneal nerves.

N.B. *Variations in the mode of exit of the sciatic nerve from pelvis (Fig. 25.8):* Normally the sciatic nerve enters the gluteal region through greater sciatic foramen below the piriformis. Sometimes sciatic nerve divides into tibial and common peroneal components within the pelvis. In such cases, the mode of exit from pelvis occurs as follows:

(a) The common peroneal nerve passes through the piriformis and tibial nerve passes below the piriformis (12%).

(b) The common peroneal nerve passes above the piriformis and tibial nerve passes below the piriformis (0.5%).

Surface Markings (Fig. 25.9)

The sciatic nerve is marked on the back of thigh by joining the following three points:

1. **First point** is marked 2.5 cm lateral to the midpoint of the line joining the anterior superior iliac spine and ischial tuberosity.
2. **Second point** is marked midway between the ischial tuberosity and greater trochanter.
3. **Third point** is marked at the junction of the upper two-third and lower one-third of the back of the thigh.

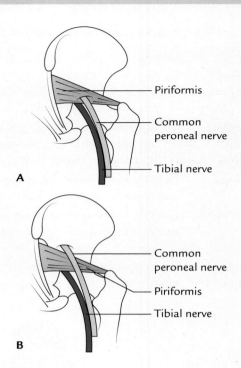

Fig. 25.8 The variations in the mode of exit of the sciatic nerve from pelvis: **A**, common peroneal nerve passing through the piriformis (12%); **B**, common peroneal nerve passing above the piriformis (0.5%).

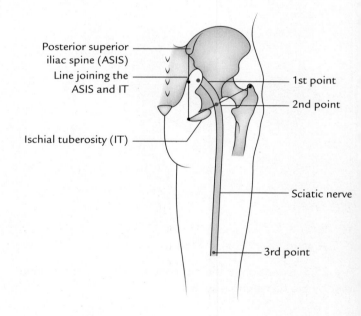

Fig. 25.9 Surface marking of the sciatic nerve.

A thick curved line (about 2 cm wide) with outward convexity joining the first and second points represents the sciatic nerve in the gluteal region and a thick straight line of the same width joining the second and third points represents the sciatic nerve in the thigh.

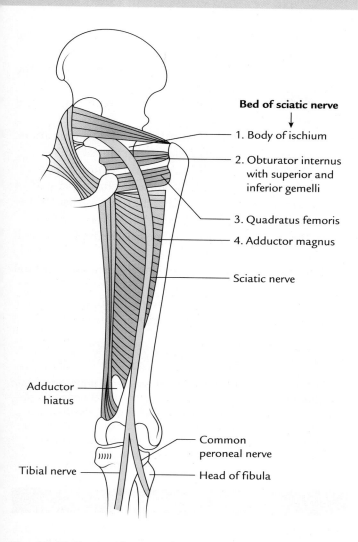

Bed of sciatic nerve
↓
1. Body of ischium
2. Obturator internus with superior and inferior gemelli
3. Quadratus femoris
4. Adductor magnus

Sciatic nerve

Adductor hiatus

Tibial nerve

Common peroneal nerve

Head of fibula

Fig. 25.10 Deep relations of the sciatic nerve (sciatic-bed).

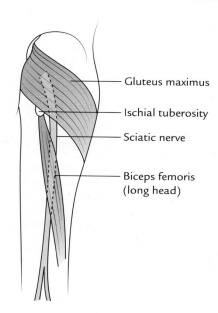

Gluteus maximus

Ischial tuberosity

Sciatic nerve

Biceps femoris (long head)

Fig. 25.11 Superficial relations of the sciatic nerve.

Branches

1. Articular branches to the hip joint arise in the gluteal region.
2. Muscular branches to the hamstring muscles arise in the lower part of the gluteal region or in the upper part of the thigh from the medial side of the nerve (Fig. 25.12).
3. Muscular branch to the short head of biceps femoris arises in the lower part of the thigh from the lateral side of the nerve (Fig. 25.12).

Relations

Deep Relations (Bed of the Sciatic Nerve)

From above downward the sciatic nerve is related to (Fig. 25.10):

(a) Body of ischium (posterior surface).
(b) Tendon of obturator internus and associated gemellus superior and gemellus inferior muscles.
(c) Quadratus femoris.
(d) Adductor magnus.

Superficial Relations

From above downward, the sciatic nerve is related to:

(a) Gluteus maximus (in the gluteal region).
(b) Long head of biceps femoris (in thigh).

The sciatic nerve is accessible on the back of thigh, only in the angle between the gluteus maximus and long head of biceps femoris (Fig. 25.11).

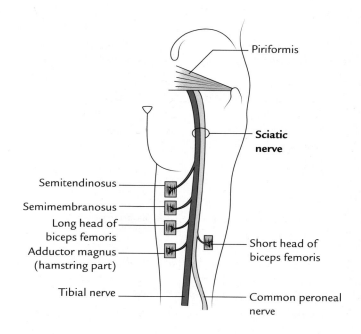

Piriformis

Sciatic nerve

Semitendinosus

Semimembranosus

Long head of biceps femoris

Adductor magnus (hamstring part)

Short head of biceps femoris

Tibial nerve

Common peroneal nerve

Fig. 25.12 Branches of the sciatic nerves to the muscles of the back of the thigh.

N.B.

All the muscular branches of the sciatic nerve arise from the medial side except nerve to short head of biceps femoris, which arises from the lateral side.

Therefore, the side lateral to the sciatic nerve is safe side and the side medial to it is dangerous side/unsafe side.

Clinical correlation

Sleeping foot: The sciatic nerve is uncovered on the back of thigh in the angle between the lower border of gluteus maximus and long head of biceps femoris. The temporary compression of the sciatic nerve against femur at the lower border of gluteus maximus causes paresthesia in the lower limb. It is called "**sleeping foot**", e.g., when a person sits on the hard edge of the chair for a long time.

ARTERIAL ANASTOMOSES ON THE BACK OF THE THIGH (Fig. 25.13)

The arterial anastomoses on the back of thigh are as follows:

1. **Longitudinal arterial anastomosis:** The main arterial supply to the back of the thigh is derived from the perforating branches of the profunda femoris artery. The perforating arteries pierce the adductor magnus and divide into ascending and descending branches. Close to the posterior aspect of the insertion of adductor magnus a chain of **longitudinal arterial anastomosis** is formed by the ascending and descending branches of four perforating arteries. The ascending branch of first perforating artery takes part in the formation of **cruciate anastomosis** and lowest branch anastomose with the superior muscular branch of the popliteal artery.

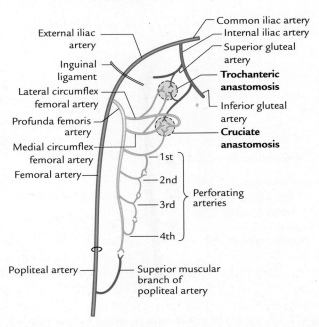

Fig. 25.13 Arterial anastomoses on the back of the thigh.

2. **Trochanteric anastomosis:** It is situated in the trochanteric fossa.

The trochanteric anastomosis is formed by the following arteries:
1. Ascending branch of the medial circumflex femoral artery.
2. Ascending branch of lateral circumflex femoral artery.
3. Descending branch of the inferior gluteal artery.
4. Descending branch of the superior gluteal artery.

3. **Cruciate anastomosis:** It is situated at the upper part of the back of femur at the level of the lesser trochanter. The *cruciate anastomosis* is formed by the following arteries:
1. Transverse branch of the medial circumflex femoral artery.
2. Transverse branch of the lateral circumflex femoral artery.
3. Ascending branch of the first perforating artery.
4. Descending branch of the inferior gluteal artery.

Clinical correlation

Clinical significance of longitudinal arterial anastomosis on the back of thigh: It provides a collateral channels of blood supply to the lower limb bypassing the external iliac and femoral arteries, e.g., in ligation of femoral artery above the origin of profunda femoris artery it maintains an efficient blood supply through collateral circulation.

POPLITEAL FOSSA

The popliteal fossa is a diamond-shaped hollow on the back of the knee joint. It becomes prominent when the knee is flexed. This fossa is an important anatomical region because it provides passage for main vessels and nerves from the thigh to the leg.

BOUNDARIES (Fig. 25.14)

The fossa is bounded:
Superomedially: Semitendinosus and semimembranosus.

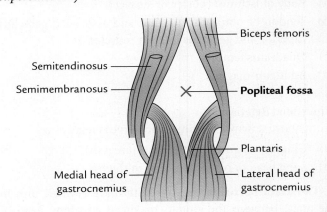

Fig. 25.14 Boundaries of the popliteal fossa.

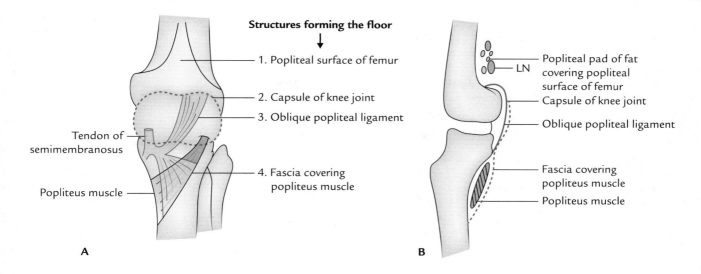

Structures forming the floor
↓
1. Popliteal surface of femur
2. Capsule of knee joint
3. Oblique popliteal ligament
4. Fascia covering popliteus muscle

Tendon of semimembranosus

Popliteus muscle

A

Popliteal pad of fat covering popliteal surface of femur
LN
Capsule of knee joint
Oblique popliteal ligament
Fascia covering popliteus muscle
Popliteus muscle

B

Fig. 25.15 Floor of the popliteal fossa: **A**, surface view; **B**, diagrammatic medial view (LN = popliteal lymph nodes).

Superolaterally: Biceps femoris.
Inferomedially: Medial head of gastrocnemius.
Inferolaterally: Lateral head of gastrocnemius supplemented by the plantaris.
Floor (or anterior wall; Fig. 25.15): It is formed from above downward by:

(a) The popliteal surface of the femur.
(b) The capsule of the knee joint and oblique popliteal ligament.
(c) The popliteal fascia covering the popliteus muscle.

Roof (or posterior wall): It is formed from the strong popliteal fascia. The superficial fascia over the roof contains:

(a) Short saphenous vein.
(b) Three cutaneous nerves: (i) terminal part of the posterior cutaneous nerve of the thigh, (ii) posterior division of the medial cutaneous nerve of the thigh, and (iii) sural communicating nerve). The roof is pierced by all these structures except the posterior division of medial cutaneous nerve of the thigh (Fig. 25.16).

CONTENTS (Fig. 25.17)

The main contents of the popliteal fossa are:

1. Popliteal artery and its branches.
2. Popliteal vein and its tributaries.
3. Tibial nerve and its branches.
4. Common peroneal nerve and its branches.
5. Popliteal lymph nodes.
6. Popliteal pad of fat.

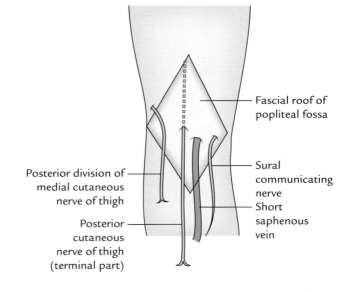

Fascial roof of popliteal fossa

Posterior division of medial cutaneous nerve of thigh

Sural communicating nerve

Short saphenous vein

Posterior cutaneous nerve of thigh (terminal part)

Fig. 25.16 Structures piercing the roof of the popliteal fossa.

In addition to the above-mentioned structures, the popliteal fossa also contains the following structures:

1. Posterior cutaneous nerve of the thigh (terminal part).
2. Descending genicular branch of the obturator nerve.
3. Terminal part of short saphenous vein.

N.B. *The relationship of tibial nerve, popliteal vein, and popliteal artery in the popliteal fossa:* The popliteal artery is crossed superficially by popliteal vein from the lateral to medial side; which in turn is crossed superficially by the tibial nerve from the lateral to medial side. As a result, the relative relationship of these structures differs in the upper, middle, and lower parts of the fossa as follows (Fig. 25.18):

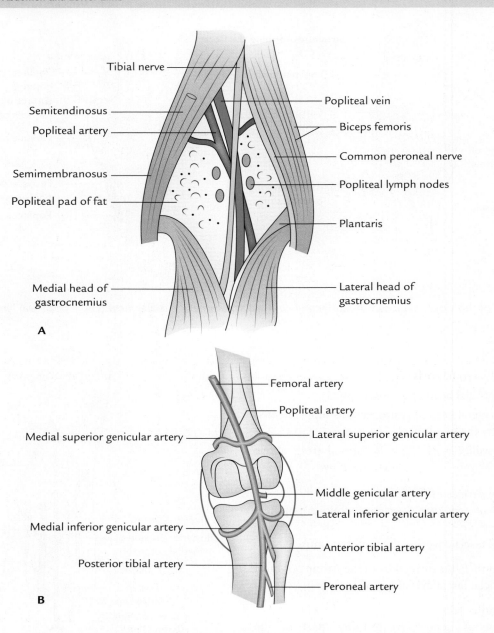

Fig. 25.17 **A,** Boundaries and contents of the popliteal fossa; **B,** genicular branches of the popliteal artery.

(a) *In the upper part of the fossa* from the lateral to medial side, the order is Nerve, Vein, and Artery (NVA).
(b) *In the middle part of the fossa* from superficial to deep, the order of arrangement is Nerve, Vein, and Artery (NVA).
(c) *In the lower part of the fossa* from the lateral to medial side, the order of arrangement is Artery, Vein, and Nerve (AVN).

SALIENT FEATURES OF THE PRINCIPAL CONTENTS

Popliteal Artery

It is the continuation of femoral artery. It begins at the adductor hiatus (an osseo-aponeurotic opening in the adductor magnus at the junction of middle one-third and lower one-third of the thigh), crosses the floor of popliteal fossa from the medial to lateral side to reach the lower border of the popliteus where it terminates by dividing into **anterior and posterior tibial arteries**.

Relations

These are as follows:

Anterior (deep): Floor of the popliteal fossa (i.e., popliteal surface of femur, posterior aspect of the knee joint, and fascia covering the popliteus muscle; Fig. 25.19).

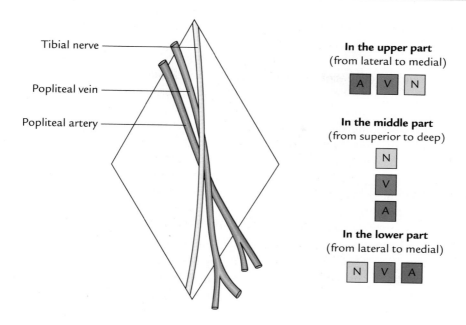

Fig. 25.18 Highly schematic diagram to show relationship of the tibial nerve, popliteal vein, and popliteal artery in the popliteal fossa. Relations of neurovascular structures at three levels (viz., upper, middle, and lower parts) are depicted on the right side.

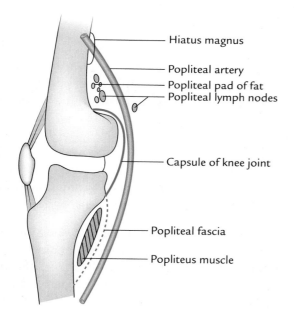

Fig. 25.19 Anterior (deep) relations of the popliteal artery.

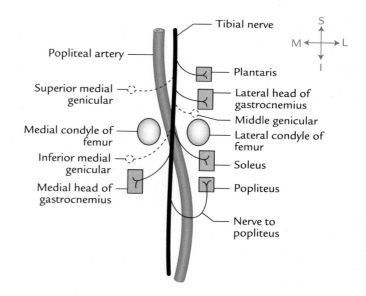

Fig. 25.20 Branches of the tibial nerve in the popliteal fossa.

Posterior (superficial): Popliteal vein, tibial nerve, fascial roof, superficial fascia, and skin (from deep to superficial).

Branches

These are divided into three groups—cutaneous, muscular, and articular (genicular).

1. **Cutaneous branches:** They pierce the roof and supply the overlying skin.
2. **Muscular branches:** They are large and several in number. The upper branches (two or three in number) supply adductor magnus and hamstring muscles. One or two of them anastomose with the fourth perforating artery.

The lower muscular branches supply the triceps surae muscles (i.e., two heads of gastrocnemius and soleus) and plantaris.

3. **Genicular (articular) branches (Fig. 25.20):** They are five in number and supply the knee joint.
   (a) *Superior medial and lateral genicular arteries:* They wind around the corresponding side of the femur immediately above the corresponding femoral condyles and take part in the formation of **genicular anastomosis.**
   (b) *Inferior medial and lateral genicular arteries:* They wind around the corresponding tibial condyles and pass deep to the corresponding collateral ligaments of the knee joint to take part in the formation of **genicular anastomosis.**
   (c) *Middle genicular artery:* It pierces the oblique popliteal ligament of the knee to supply the cruciate ligaments and synovial membrane of the knee joints.

N.B. *Genicular anastomosis* (Fig. 25.21): It is an arterial anastomosis around the knee joint formed by the branches of popliteal, anterior tibial and posterior tibial, femoral, and profunda femoris arteries.

This anastomosis maintains adequate blood supply to the knee joint and leg during flexion of the knee joint, when the popliteal artery is compressed (kinked) and blood flow in it becomes sluggish.

The anastomosis takes place as follows (Fig. 25.21):

1. *Superior medial genicular artery* anastomosis with the descending genicular branch of the femoral artery and inferior medial genicular artery.

2. *Inferior medial genicular artery* anastomosis with the superior medial genicular artery and saphenous artery—a branch of the descending genicular artery (a branch of femoral artery).

3. *Superior lateral genicular artery* anastomosis with the descending branch of the lateral circumflex femoral artery and inferior lateral genicular artery.

4. *Inferior lateral genicular artery* anastomosis with the superior lateral genicular artery, anterior and posterior recurrent branches of the anterior tibial artery, and circumflex fibular branch of posterior tibial artery.

Popliteal Vein

The popliteal vein is formed at the lower border of the popliteus by the union of veins (venae comitantes) accompanying the anterior and posterior tibial arteries. It ascends superficial to popliteal artery and crosses it from the medial to lateral side in the popliteal fossa. The popliteal vein continues as **femoral vein** at adductor hiatus.

Tributaries

The tributaries of popliteal vein are as follows:

1. Small saphenous vein.
2. Veins corresponding to the branches of popliteal artery.

Tibial Nerve (L4, L5; S1, S2, S3)

It is the *larger terminal branch of the sciatic nerve.* It extends vertically downward from the superior angle to the inferior angle of the popliteal fossa. It crosses popliteal artery superficially from the lateral to medial side with popliteal vein intervening between the artery and nerve.

Branches (Fig. 25.20)

These are as follows:

1. **Muscular branches:** They supply gastrocnemius (both heads), soleus, plantaris, and popliteus.

N.B. All the muscular branches of the tibial nerve arise from its lateral side except the nerve to medial head of gastrocnemius, which arises from its medial side. Therefore, lateral side of the tibial nerve is termed **dangerous side** and medial side as the **safe side**.

The *nerve to popliteus* crosses superficially to the popliteal artery, runs downward and laterally, and then winds around the lower border of popliteus, which it supplies from its deep surface. In addition to the popliteus, it also supplies many other structures.

Structures supplied by the nerve popliteus are:
(a) Popliteus muscle.
(b) Tibialis posterior muscle.
(c) Superior tibiofibular joint.
(d) Tibia.

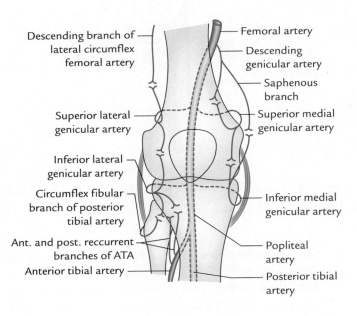

Fig. 25.21 Arterial anastomosis (genicular anastomosis) around the knee joint (ATA = anterior tibial artery).

Descending branch of lateral circumflex femoral artery

Femoral artery

Descending genicular artery

Saphenous branch

Superior lateral genicular artery

Superior medial genicular artery

Inferior lateral genicular artery

Circumflex fibular branch of posterior tibial artery

Inferior medial genicular artery

Ant. and post. reccurrent branches of ATA

Popliteal artery

Anterior tibial artery

Posterior tibial artery

(e) Interosseous membrane.

(f) Inferior tibiofibular joint.

2. **Genicular branches:** They are three in number (superior medial genicular, inferior medial genicular, and middle genicular) and accompany the arteries of the same name.

The **middle genicular nerve** pierces the oblique popliteal ligament and supplies the interior of the knee joint.

3. **Cutaneous branch:** It is called the **sural nerve** and arises about the middle of the popliteal fossa. It runs vertically downward underneath the deep fascial roof of fossa and leaves the fossa by piercing the roof near its inferior angle.

4. **Vascular branches:** They supply the vasomotor fibres (T10–L2) to the popliteal vessels.

Common Peroneal Nerve (L4, L5; S1, S2)

It is the *smaller terminal branch of the sciatic nerve.* It appears in the popliteal fossa beneath the long head of the biceps femoris and slopes downward and laterally along the medial side of the tendon of biceps femoris up to the lateral angle of the fossa. Here it crosses superficial to the plantaris, lateral head of gastrocnemius to reach the back of the head of fibula. Finally, it winds around the posterolateral aspect of the neck of fibula, pierces the peroneus longus muscle, and terminates by dividing into **deep** and **superficial peroneal nerves.**

Branches

In the popliteal fossa, the common peroneal nerve gives rise to two cutaneous branches and three genicular branches.

Cutaneous branches

These are as follows:

1. **Sural communicating nerve:** It arises opposite to the head of the fibula, and crosses superficially to the lateral head of gastrocnemius to join the **sural nerve.**

2. **Lateral cutaneous nerve (lateral sural nerve):** It arises lower down and pierces the deep fascia to supply the skin on the upper part of the lateral side of the leg.

Genicular (articular) branches

These are superior lateral genicular, inferior lateral genicular, and recurrent genicular nerves. The first two supply the knee joint and the last one supplies the superior tibiofibular joint.

N.B.

- The common peroneal nerve can be palpated against the neck of fibula.
- The common peroneal nerve gives no muscular branch in the popliteal fossa.

Popliteal Lymph Nodes

They are usually five to six in number and embedded in the popliteal pad of fat. They are found at the following three sites:

1. One node lies at the junction of small saphenous vein and popliteal vein.

2. Few nodes lie deep to the popliteal artery.

3. Remaining nodes are situated on both sides of the popliteal artery.

The popliteal lymph nodes drain:

(a) Back and lateral side of calf of the leg.

(b) Lateral side of heel and foot.

Posterior Cutaneous Nerve of the Thigh

It pierces the fascial roof about the middle of the popliteal fossa and provides cutaneous innervation up to the middle of the back of leg.

Genicular Branch of the Obturator Nerve

It is the continuation of the posterior division of the obturator nerve. It first runs on the posterior surface of the popliteal artery and then pierces oblique popliteal ligament to supply the capsule of the knee joint.

Clinical correlation

- **Popliteal pulse:** To feel the popliteal pulse, first flex the knee to relax the popliteal fascia. Then place the fingertips of both hands in the popliteal fossa with thumbs resting on patient's patella.

  Popliteal pulse is the most difficult pulse to feel amongst all the peripheral pulses.

- **Popliteal aneurysm:** The popliteal artery is more prone to aneurysm than any other artery in the body. Clinically, popliteal aneurysm presents as a pulsatile midline swelling in the popliteal fossa.

- **Baker's cyst:** It is cystic swelling which occurs in the popliteal fossa due to inflammation of synovial bursa underneath the tendon of semimembranosus or protrusion of synovial membrane of the cavity of knee joint through the fibrous capsule of the joint.

Golden Facts of Remember

▶ Thickest nerve in the body	Sciatic nerve
▶ All the muscles on the back of the thigh are supplied by tibial part of the sciatic nerve *except*	Short head of biceps femoris being supplied by the common peroneal part of the sciatic nerve
▶ Most difficult peripheral pulse to feel	Popliteal pulse
▶ Artery most prone to aneurysm in the body	Popliteal artery

Clinical Case Study

A 55-year-old man complaining of swelling on the back of his knee joint visited the hospital. He stated that he noticed this swelling about one month back. On examination the doctor found a midline pulsatile swelling in the popliteal fossa. The diagnosis of "popliteal aneurysm" was made.

Questions

1. Name the structures from which the swelling on the back of the knee can originate.
2. How doctors differentiate swelling of the popliteal aneurysm from swelling due to Baker's cyst?
3. Give the relationship of popliteal artery, popliteal vein, and tibial nerve in the posteroanterior direction.
4. What is the most deeply located neurovascular structure in the popliteal fossa?

Answers

1. Swellings on the back of the knee can originate from the structures within and around the popliteal fossa as given in the following box.

Structure	Swelling (pathological condition)
• Skin and soft tissues	• Lipoma, sebaceous cyst
• Short saphenous vein	• Varicosity of this vein in the roof
• Popliteal artery	• Popliteal aneurysm
• Popliteal lymph nodes	• Lymphadenopathy (enlargement of lymph nodes due to inflammation)
• Bursa beneath the	• Baker's cyst semimembranosus
• Synovial cavity of the knee	• Effusion in the joint and protrusion of the synovial membrane through the capsule of the joint

2. Swelling due to popliteal aneurysm is pulsatile and located in the midline whereas swelling due to Baker's cyst is cystic and located laterally on the medial side.
3. From posterior to anterior, the relationship is as follows: tibial nerve, popliteal vein, and popliteal artery.
4. Popliteal artery.

Hip Joint

The hip joint is a ball and socket type of synovial joint between the head of the femur and the acetabulum of the hip bone (Fig. 26.1). It is the largest **ball** and **socket type of joint** in the body. Its main functions are: (a) to support the body weight during standing and (b) to transmit the forces generated by movements of trunk femur during walking. It is multiaxial and permits same movements as shoulder joint in the upper limb because the long and narrow neck of femur acts as strut and makes an angle with the shaft (neck–shaft angle). However, its range of movements is restricted due to its role in weight bearing.

TYPE

Synovial joint of ball and socket variety

ARTICULAR SURFACES

The head of the femur articulates with the horse-shoe-shaped acetabulum of the hip bone to form the hip joint. (Fig. 26.2):

1. The *head of femur* forms more than half of a sphere. It is covered by the articular hyaline cartilage except for a small pit—the *fovea capitis* for ligamentum teres.

2. The *acetabulum* (Latin *acetabulum* = vinegar cup) presents three features: a horseshoe-shaped lunate surface, acetabular notch, and acetabular fossa. Out of these, only lunate surface is articular and covered by an articular cartilage. The depth of the acetabulum is increased by the acetabular labrum.

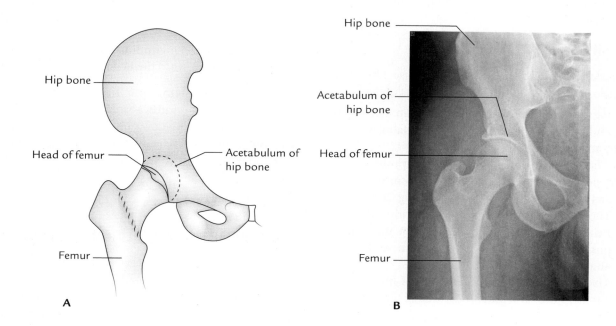

A

B

Fig. 26.1 Hip joint: A, line diagram of the right hip joint; B, radiograph of the right hip joint.

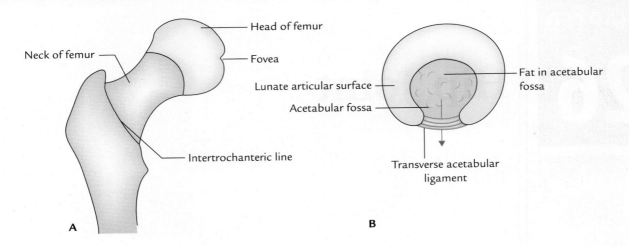

Fig. 26.2 Articular surfaces of the hip joint: **A**, head of femur; **B**, acetabulum of the hip bone. Note arrow passing through the acetabular foramen.

Though proximal and distal articular surfaces are reciprocally curved but they are not co-extensive.

LIGAMENTS

The ligaments of the hip joint are as follows:

1. Capsular ligament (joint capsule).
2. Iliofemoral ligament (strongest).
3. Pubofemoral ligament.
4. Ischiofemoral ligament.
5. Transverse acetabular ligament.
6. Acetabular labrum.
7. Ligamentum teres femoris (round ligament of the head of femur).

CAPSULAR LIGAMENT

The capsular ligament is a strong and dense fibrous sac which encloses the joint. Its attachments are as under:

1. *On the hip bone*, it is attached 5–6 mm beyond the acetabular margin, outer aspect of the acetabular labrum and transverse acetabular ligament.
2. *On the femur*, it is attached anteriorly to the intertrochanteric line and posteriorly 1 cm in front of (medial to) the intertrochanteric crest (Fig. 26.3).
   (a) The capsule is thicker anterosuperiorly, where the maximal stress occurs, particularly in the standing position. Posteroinferiorly it is thin and loosely attached.
   (b) The capsule is made up two types of fibres—inner circular fibres and outer longitudinal fibres.
   (c) The inner circular fibres form collar around the femoral neck (*zona orbicularis*). These fibres are not directly attached to the bones.

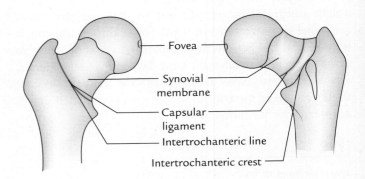

Fig. 26.3 Attachment of the capsular ligament of hip joint on the femur.

(d) The outer longitudinal fibres are reflected along the neck toward the head to form the **retinacula**.

The **synovial membrane** lines inner aspect of the fibrous capsule, the intracapsular portion of the femoral neck, glenoid labrum (both surfaces), transverse acetabular ligament, ligamentum teres, and fat in the acetabular fossa. It is thin on the deep surface of the iliofemoral ligament where it is compressed against the head (Fig. 26.4).

ILIOFEMORAL LIGAMENT (LIGAMENT OF BIGELOW)

The iliofemoral ligament is inverted Y-shaped ligament, which lies anteriorly and intimately blended with the capsule. Its apex is attached to the lower half of the anterior inferior iliac spine and area between it and above acetabular margin. Its base is attached to the intertrochanteric line. This ligament consists of three parts—a lateral thick band of oblique fibres,

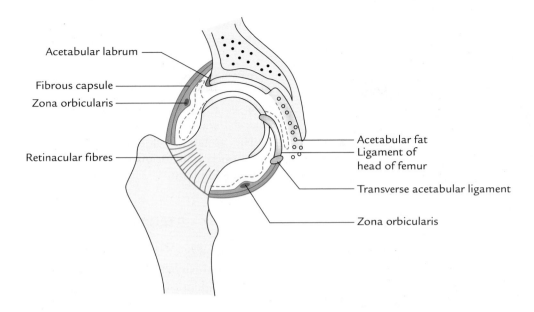

Fig. 26.4 Coronal section of the right hip joint showing the fibrous capsule and the lining of synovial membrane.

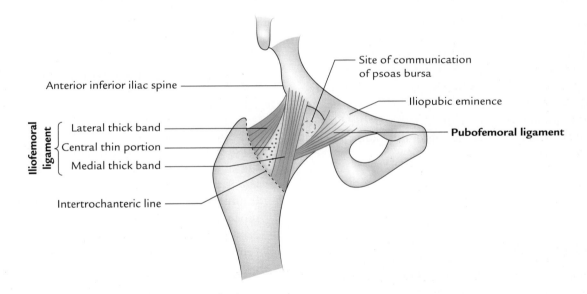

Fig. 26.5 Iliofemoral and pubofemoral ligaments.

a medial thick band of vertical fibres, and a large central thin portion (Fig. 26.5).

N.B. **Iliofemoral ligament** is the strongest ligament of body and prevents the trunk from falling backward in the standing posture.

PUBOFEMORAL LIGAMENT

The pubofemoral ligament is a triangular ligament with base above and apex below. It lies inferomedially and

supports the joint on this aspect. Its base is attached to the iliopubic eminence, superior pubic ramus, and obturator crest. Inferiorly it blends with the anteroinferior part of the capsule and medial band of the iliofemoral ligament (Fig. 26.5).

ISCHIOFEMORAL LIGAMENT (Fig. 26.6)

The ischiofemoral ligament is relatively weak and supports the capsule posteriorly. Above it is attached to the ischium posteroinferior to the acetabulum. From ischium its fibres

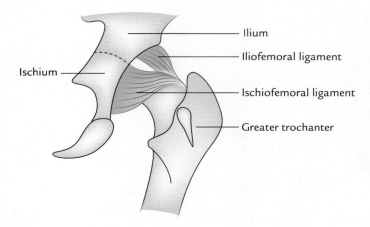

Fig. 26.6 Ischiofemoral and iliofemoral ligaments.

spiral behind the femoral neck to be attached into the greater trochanter deep to the iliofemoral ligament.

ROUND LIGAMENT OF THE HEAD OF FEMUR

This ligament is also called ligamentum teres of the head of femur. It is a flat triangular ligament with apex attached to the fovea of the head, and its base to the transverse acetabular ligament (Fig. 26.7). It is ensheathed by a conical reflection of the synovial membrane. It does not increase the stability of the joint.

It transmits arteries to the head of the femur derived from the acetabular branches of the obturator and medial circumflex femoral arteries.

N.B. Morphologically, the ligament of the head of femur represents the part of capsule that has been included within the joint.

ACETABULAR LABRUM

The acetabular labrum is a fibrocartilaginous rim attached to the acetabular margin. It is triangular in cross section. The

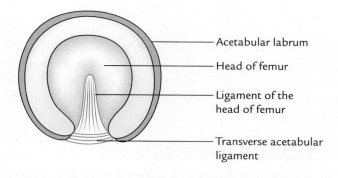

Fig. 26.7 Acetabular (glenoid) labrum, transverse acetabular ligament, and ligament of the head of femur.

labrum not only deepens the acetabulum (socket) but grasps the head of femur lightly to hold it in position.

TRANSVERSE ACETABULAR LIGAMENT

It is a part of acetabular labrum, which bridges the acetabular notch; however, it is devoid of cartilage cells. The acetabular notch thus becomes converted into the foramen which transmits the acetabular vessels and nerves to the hip joint.

STABILITY OF THE HIP JOINT

The stability of the hip joint is provided by the following factors which help to prevent its dislocation:

1. Depth of the acetabulum and narrowing of its mouth by the acetabular labrum.
2. Three strong ligaments (iliofemoral, pubofemoral, and ischiofemoral) strengthening the capsule of the joint.
3. Strength of the surrounding muscles, e.g., gluteus medius, gluteus minimus, etc.
4. Length and obliquity of the neck of femur.

RELATIONS (Fig. 26.8)

The relations of the hip joint are as follows:

Anteriorly:

1. Tendon of iliopsoas separated from joint by a synovial bursa, pectineus (lateral part), straight head of rectus femoris.
2. Femoral nerve in the groove between the iliacus and the psoas.
3. Femoral artery in front of the psoas tendon.
4. Femoral vein in front of the pectineus.

Posteriorly:

1. Piriformis, obturator externus, obturator internus, superior and inferior gemelli, quadratus femoris, and gluteus maximus.
2. Superior gluteal nerve and vessels above the piriformis.
3. Inferior gluteal nerve and vessels below the piriformis.
4. Sciatic nerve, posterior cutaneous nerve of the thigh, and nerve to quadratus femoris.

Superiorly:

1. Reflected head of rectus femoris medially.
2. Gluteus minimus, gluteus medius, and gluteus maximus laterally.

Inferiorly:

1. Pectineus.
2. Obturator externus.

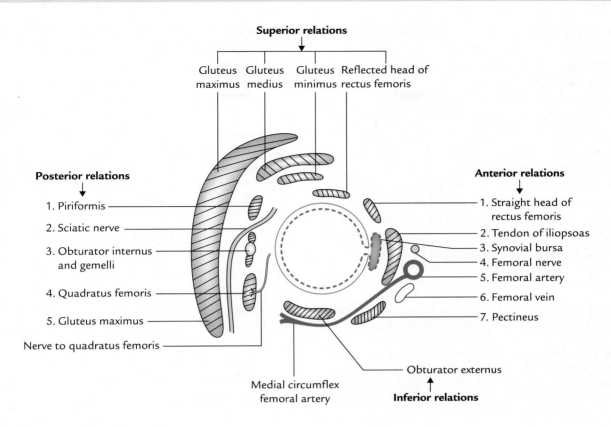

Fig. 26.8 Relations of the hip joint.

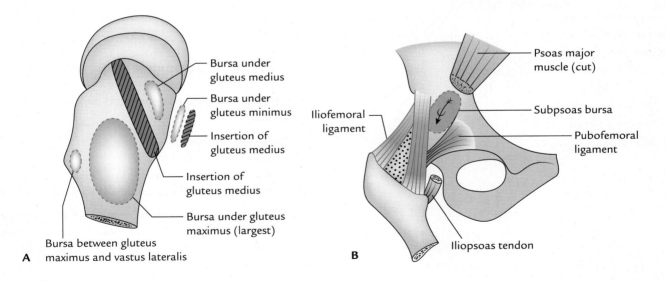

Fig. 26.9 Bursae around the hip joint: A, bursae on greater trochanter; B, subpsoas bursa communicating with the cavity of hip joint (arrow).

BURSAE AROUND THE HIP JOINT (Fig. 26.9)

These are seven in number: four under glutens maximus, one under gluteus medius, one under gluteus minimus, and one under psoas tendon as under:

1. Between gluteus maximus and smooth area of the ilium lying between the posterior curved line and the outer lip of the iliac crest.
2. Between gluteus maximus and lower part of the outer aspect of the greater trochanter (trochanteric bursa).

3. Between gluteus maximus and ischial tuberosity (ischial bursa).
4. Between the tendon of gluteus maximus and vastus lateralis (gluteofemoral bursa).
5. One bursa under the cover of gluteus medius between it and upper part of the lateral aspect of the greater trochanter.
6. One bursa under the gluteus minimus between it and anterior aspect of the greater trochanter.
7. One between the iliopubic eminence and the psoas tendon. It is called **subpsoas bursa.** In 10% individuals the psoas bursa communicates with the synovial cavity of the hip joint through a gap in the thin part of the capsule between the iliofemoral and pubofemoral ligaments.

Clinical correlation

Weaver's bottom: The subgluteal bursa between the gluteus maximus and ischial tuberosity is frequently inflamed and enlarged in people whose profession requires long periods of sitting, e.g., weavers, leading to a clinical condition called **weaver's bottom**.

ARTERIAL SUPPLY

The hip joint is supplied by the branches of the following arteries:

1. Medial circumflex femoral artery.
2. Lateral circumflex femoral artery.
3. Obturator artery.
4. Superior gluteal artery.
5. Inferior gluteal artery.

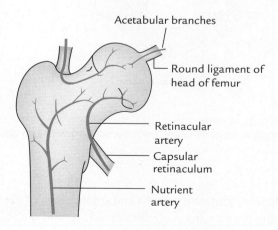

Acetabular branches

Round ligament of head of femur

Retinacular artery

Capsular retinaculum

Nutrient artery

Fig. 26.10 Arterial supply of the head of femur.

N.B. The arterial supply of the head and neck of the femur is clinically very important. It is derived from the following three sources (Fig. 26.10):

(a) **Acetabular branches** of the obturator artery and the medial circumflex femoral arteries. These arteries reach the head through the round ligament of the head.
(b) **Retinacular vessels** (the **chief source**) arise from the medial circumflex femoral artery, run along the neck of the femur through the retinaculum of the capsule.
(c) **Nutrient artery** of the femur gives few branches to the neck and head of femur.

NERVE SUPPLY

The hip joint is supplied by the following nerves:

1. Femoral nerve via nerve to rectus femoris.
2. A branch from anterior division of obturator nerve.
3. A branch from accessory obturator nerve (if present).
4. A branch from nerve to quadratus femoris.
5. A branch from superior gluteal nerve.
6. A twig from sciatic nerve (occasional).

N.B. Four consecutive spinal segments (L2, L3, L4, L5) control the movements of the hip joints as under:
- L2 and L3 regulate flexion, adduction, and medial rotation.
- L4 and L5 regulate extension, abduction, and lateral rotation.

MOVEMENTS

The hip joint is a multiaxial joint and permits the following movements:

- Flexion and extension.
- Abduction and adduction.
- Medial and lateral rotation.
- Circumduction (combination of the above movements).

The flexion and extension movements occur around the transverse axis, medial and lateral rotation occur around the vertical axis, and abductor and adduction movements occur around the anteroposterior axis.

Range of Movements

The flexion is 110°–120°. It is limited by contact of the thigh with the abdomen and adduction is limited by contact with the opposite thigh. The range of other movements is as under:

- Extension = 15°
- Abduction = 50°

Table 26.1 Muscles producing the movements of the hip joint

Movements	Muscles producing movements
Flexion	• Psoas major and iliacus (chief flexor) • Sartorius, rectus femoris, and pectineus
Extension	• Gluteus maximus (chief extensor) • Hamstring muscles
Abduction	• Gluteus medius and minimus (chief abductors) • Tensor fasciae latae and sartorius
Adduction	• Adductor longus, adductor brevis, and adductor magnus (chief adductors) • Pectineus and gracilis
Medial rotation	• Anterior fibres of gluteus minimus and medius (chief medial rotators) • Tensor fasciae latae
Lateral rotation	Piriformis, obturator externus, obturator internus and associated gemelli, quadratus femoris (These muscles are generally termed short rotators)

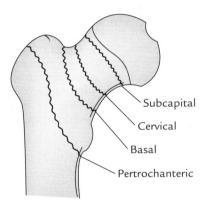

Fig 26.11 Types of fracture of the neck of femur.

- Medial rotation = 25°
- Lateral rotation = 60°

The muscles producing the various movements of the hip joint are given in Table 26.1.

Clinical correlation

- **Dislocation of the hip joint:**
(a) **Congenital dislocation:** The congenital dislocation of the hip joint is more common than any other joint in the body. It occurs due to two reasons:

(i) The joint capsule is loose at birth.
(ii) Hypoplasia of the acetabulum and femoral head: In this condition, the head of femur slips upward into the gluteal region because the upper margin of the acetabulum is developmentally deficient.
Clinically, it presents as:
   - Inability of the newborn to abduct the thigh.
   - Affected limb is shorter in length and externally rotated.
   - Asymmetry of skin folds of the thighs.
   - Lurching gait with positive Trendelenburg's sign.
(b) **Acquired dislocation:** The acquired dislocation of the hip joint is uncommon because this joint is very strong and stable. However, it may occur during an automobile accident when the hip joint is flexed, adducted, and medially rotated from the usual position of the lower limb when one is riding in a car. In this position, the joint is unstable because the femoral head is covered posteriorly by a joint capsule and not by the bone. During head on collision, the knee strikes the dashboard and dislocates the hip joint. The head of the femur is forced out of the acetabulum by tearing the capsule posteroinferiorly and lies on the lateral surface of the ilium. This causes shortening and medial rotation of the affected limb.
   The dislocation of the hip may be posterior (most common), anterior (less common), or central (least common). The sciatic nerve is injured in posterior dislocation.

- **Perthes' disease (pseudocoxalgia):** It is a clinical condition characterized by destruction and flattening of the head of femur with an increased joint space in the radiograph.
- **Coxa vara and coxa valga:** The normal neck–shaft angle is about 120° in adults and 160° in children. If the neck shaft angle of the femur is reduced (e.g., fracture neck of femur, Perthes disease), it is called *coxa vara*. If the angle is increased (e.g., congenital dislocation of the hip joint), it is called **coxa valga**. This may result from Perthes disease, softening the neck due to rickets.
- **Osteoarthritis:** It is a disease of the old age. It is characterized by the growth of *osteophytes* at the articular ends which not only limits the movements but makes them grating and painful.
- **Referred pain of the hip joint:** In diseases of the hip joint such as tuberculosis, the pain is referred to the knee joint because of the common nerve supply of these two joints.
- **Aspiration of the knee joint:** It is usually done by putting a needle 5 cm below the anterior superior iliac spine, upward, backward, and medially.
- **Fractures of the neck of the femur:** Unfortunately, it is referred as **fractured hip** implying that the hip bone is broken. These fractures are usually common in individuals of more than 60 years of age especially in females because their femoral necks become weak and brittle due to **osteoporosis.**

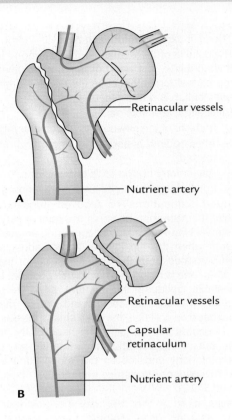

Fig. 26.12 Involvement of arteries supplying the head of femur: A, non-involvement of retinacular vessels in extracapsular pretrochanteric fracture of the neck of femur; B, involvement of retinacular vessels in intracapsular subcapital fracture of the neck of femur.

Types

The fractures of the neck of femur are of four types (Fig. 26.11):

(a) Subcapital (near the head).

(b) Cervical (in the middle).

(c) Basal (near the trochanters).

(d) Pretrochanteric fracture (just distal to two trochanters).

The retinacular vessels derived from the medial circumflex femoral artery supply most of the blood to the head and neck of the femur. A pretrochanteric fracture (extracapsular fracture) does not damage retinacular vessels, hence avascular bone necrosis of head of femur does not occur (Fig. 26.12A). Their damage in intracapsular fracture of the neck (i.e., subcapital and cervical) often lead to aseptic bone necrosis of the head of the femur (Fig. 26.12B).

The fracture of the neck of the femur often occurs due to indirect violence of the trivial nature. The person falls down and cannot get up. The affected limb is much shortened and rotated laterally. The diagnosis is generally confirmed by X-ray by observing following two lines:

(a) **Shenton's line:** In a radiograph of the hip region, the Shenton's line is represented by a continuous curved line formed by the upper border of the obturator foramen and lower margin of the neck of the femur. This curve is disrupted in fracture neck of the femur or dislocation of the hip joint.

(b) **Schoemaker's line:** It is a straight line that extends from the tip of the greater trochanter to the anterior superior iliac spine and continues upward over the anterior abdominal wall to reach the umbilicus. If greater trochanter is elevated (e.g., fracture of the neck of femur) this line passes below the umbilicus.

Golden Facts to Remember

- Strongest and most important ligament of the hip joint — Iliofemoral ligament

- Most common dislocation of the hip joint — Posterior

- Weaver's bottom — Inflamed and enlarged synovial bursa between the gluteus maximus and ischial tuberosity

- Most important source of blood supply to the head of the femur — Retinacular arteries

- Normal neck shaft angle of femur (angle of inclination) — 120° in adults and 160° in children

- Unique feature of the hip joint — High degree of stability as well as mobility

Clinical Case Study

A 75-year-old woman could not stand and move her right leg after a minor fall in bathroom. On examination, it was found that her right limb was shortened and held in characteristic laterally rotated position. The X-ray revealed subcapital intracapsular fracture of the neck of femur.

Questions

1. Classify the types of fracture of the neck of the femur.
2. Give the anatomical basis of the lateral rotation and the shortening of the lower limb.
3. How is the length of the femur measured?
4. What is the possible complication of this type of fracture?
5. What are the clinical implications of the neck shaft angle?

Answers

1. The fractures of the neck of the femur are of two types: intracapsular and extracapsular. The intracapsular fractures are further divided into three subtypes: (a) subcapital, (b) transverse cervical, and (c) basal.

2. (a) The lateral rotation results from the change in the axis of the limb due to the separation of the shaft from the head of the femur. As a result of change in the axis, the psoas major becomes the lateral rotator of the thigh.

   (b) The shortening of the limb results due to upward pull of the muscles connecting the femur with the hip bone. The sudden involuntary muscular contraction causes the upward pull.

3. It is from anterior superior iliac spine to the medial malleolus.

4. Avascular necrosis of the proximal segment (e.g., head of femur) due to damage of the retinacular vessels.

5. The clinical implications of the neck–shaft angle (angle of inclination) are:

   (a) Increase in the angle causes **coxa valga**, e.g., in congenital dislocation of the hip joint. It limits the adduction movement of the hip joint.

   (b) Decrease in the angle causes **coxa vara**, e.g., in fracture neck of femur. It limits the abduction of the hip joint.

Front of the Leg and Dorsum of the Foot

FRONT OF THE LEG

The leg is part of the lower limb that lies between the knee and ankle. In general, the structure on the front of the leg extends on to the dorsum of the foot; hence, they are studied together.

SURFACE LANDMARKS (Fig. 27.1)

Bony Landmarks

1. **Medial and lateral condyles of tibia:** These are visible and palpable landmarks at the sides of the ligamentum patellae. They are easily felt in a flexed knee with the thigh flexed and laterally rotated.
2. **Tibial tuberosity:** It is a bony prominence on the front of the upper part of tibia, 2.5 cm distal to the knee joint.
3. **Anterior border (shin) of the tibia:** It is distinct in most of its extent except in the lower part. It is easily felt as a sharp sinuously curved bony crest extending downward from the tibial tuberosity to the anterior margin of the medial malleolus.
4. **Head of the fibula:** It lies posterolaterally at the level of the tibial tuberosity. It serves as a guide to locate common peroneal nerve which winds around the posterolateral aspect of the neck of fibula where it can be rolled.
5. **Medial surface of tibia:** It is subcutaneous throughout except in the uppermost part where it provides attachment to the tendons of sartorius, gracilis, and semitendinosus. The great saphenous vein crosses the lower one-third of this surface, running obliquely upward and backward from the anterior border of medial malleolus.
6. **Medial malleolus:** It is the bony prominence on the medial side of the ankle.
7. **Lateral malleolus:** It is the bony prominence on the lateral side of the ankle. It is longer but narrower than the medial malleolus, and its tip lies about 0.5 cm below that of the medial malleolus and placed on a more posterior plane.
8. **Peroneal trochlea:** It may be felt as a little prominence about a finger breadth below the lateral malleolus.
9. **Sustentaculum tali:** It can be felt about a thumb breadth below the medial malleolus.
10. **Tuberosity of the navicular bone:** It is a bony prominence felt 1 to 1.5 inches anteroinferior to the medial malleolus. The head of the talus lies above the line joining the sustentaculum tali and tuberosity of the navicular bone.
11. **Tuberosity of the base of fifth metatarsal bone:** It is the most prominent landmark on the lateral border of the foot. It lies midway between the point of the heel and the root of the little toe.

Soft Tissue Landmarks

1. **Gastrocnemius and the underlying soleus muscle:** These together form the fleshy prominence of the back of the leg (calf). The *tendocalcaneus*, the strong and thick tendon of these muscles is easily followed downward to its attachment on calcaneus.
2. **Pulsations of posterior tibial artery:** It can be felt about 2 cm below and behind the medial malleolus.
3. **Pulsations of dorsalis pedis artery:** It can be felt on the dorsum of the foot about 5 cm distal to the malleoli and lateral to the tendon of extensor hallucis longus which becomes prominent when the foot is dorsiflexed.
4. **Tendon of tibialis anterior:** It becomes prominent when the foot is inverted. It is seen as passing downward and medially across the medial part of the anterior aspect of the ankle.
5. **Extensor digitorum brevis:** It produces an elevation on the lateral part of the dorsum of the foot when the toes are extended.
6. **First metatarso-phalangeal joint:** It is located a little in front of the centre of the ball of the big toe. The second, third, fourth, and fifth metatarso-phalangeal joints are located about 2.5 cm behind the webs of the toes.

Front of the Leg and Dorsum of the Foot

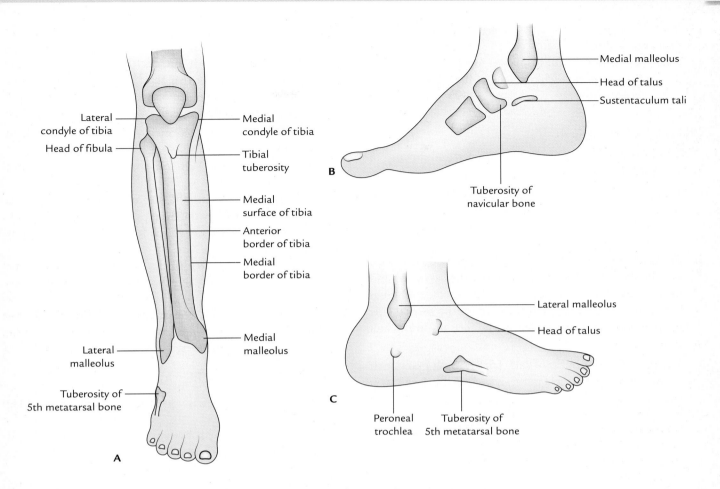

Fig. 27.1 Surface landmarks of the leg and foot: **A**, anterior aspect of the leg and foot; **B**, medial aspect of the foot; **C**, lateral aspect of the foot.

SUPERFICIAL FASCIA

Superficial Veins (Fig. 27.2)

The superficial veins on the dorsum of the leg and foot are as under:

1. **Dorsal venous arch:** It lies on the dorsum of the foot over the proximal parts of the metatarsals.

2. **Dorsal digital veins:** There are two dorsal digital veins in each toe. Each joins the corresponding vein of the adjacent toe to form the dorsal metatarsal vein which terminates in the dorsal venous arch. The *dorsal digital vein* on the medial side of the big toe joins the medial end of the dorsal venous arch to form the *great saphenous vein*. The *dorsal digital vein* on the lateral side of the little toe joins the lateral end of the *dorsal venous arch* to form the *small (short) saphenous vein*.

3. **Great saphenous vein:** It passes upward in front of the medial malleolus, crosses lower one-third of the medial surface of the tibia to reach the medial border of the tibia along which it ascends to reach the back of the

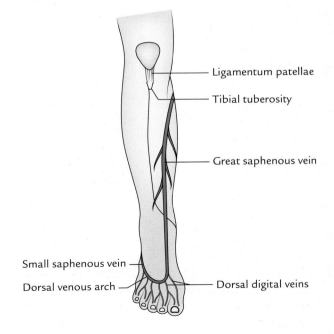

Fig. 27.2 Superficial veins on the front of leg and dorsum of the foot.

knee. The saphenous nerve runs in front of the great saphenous vein.

4. **Small saphenous vein:** It passes upward behind the lateral malleolus to reach the back of the leg where sural nerve accompanies it.

Cutaneous Nerves (Fig. 27.3)

The cutaneous nerves on the front of the leg and dorsum of the foot are as under:

1. **Infrapatellar branch of the saphenous nerve:** It pierces the deep fascia on the medial side of the knee, curves downward and forward to supply the skin over the ligamentum patellae.

2. **Saphenous nerve (L3, L4):** It pierces the deep fascia on the medial side of the knee between the sartorius and gracilis and runs downward in front of the great saphenous vein. It supplies the skin on the medial side of the leg and medial border of the foot up to the ball of the big toe.

3. **Lateral cutaneous nerve of calf (L5; S1,S2):** It is a branch of the common peroneal nerve. It pierces the deep fascia over the lateral head of the gastrocnemius and then descends to supply the skin of the upper two-third of the leg laterally.

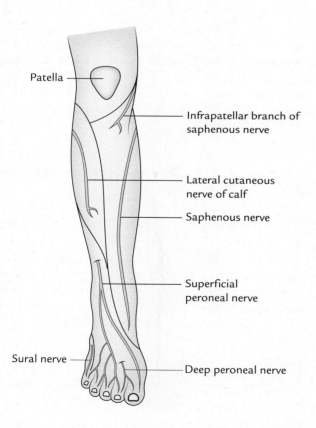

Fig. 27.3 Cutaneous nerves on the front and dorsum of the foot.

4. **Superficial peroneal nerve (L4, L5; S1):** It arises from the common peroneal nerve on the lateral side of the neck of the fibula. It pierces the deep fascia at the junction of the upper two-third and lower one-third of the lateral side of the leg and divides into medial and lateral branches. The superficial peroneal nerve supplies:

   (a) Skin over the lower one-third of the lateral side of the leg.

   (b) Whole of the skin on the dorsum of the foot except for:

      (i) Cleft between the first and second toes which is supplied by the deep peroneal nerve.

      (ii) Lateral border of the foot which is supplied by sural nerve.

      (iii) Medial border of the foot up to the ball of the big toe which is supplied by the saphenous nerve.

5. **Digital branches of the medial and lateral plantar nerves** curve upward and supply the distal parts of the dorsal aspects of the toes.

DEEP FASCIA OF THE LEG

The deep fascia of the leg is very strong and encloses the leg like a tight sleeve.

It does not cover the subcutaneous bony surfaces and is attached to their borders. In other words, it is fused with the periosteum where the bones are subcutaneous.

Two intermuscular septa, anterior and posterior, extend inward from the facial sleeve and get attached to the anterior and posterior borders of the fibula. These together with interosseous membrane divide the leg into three fascial compartments each having its own muscles, arteries, and nerves (Fig. 27.4): anterior, lateral, and posterior. In the posterior compartment, the muscles are divided into three layers by the superficial and deep transverse fascial septa.

RETINACULA

Around the ankle deep fascia is thickened to form strong fibrous bands called retinacula. They are so named because they retain the tendons around ankle in place and prevent their bowstringing during the movements of the foot. The various retinacula around the ankle are:

- **Superior and inferior extensor retinacula,** on the front of ankle
- **Superior and inferior peroneal retinacula,** on the lateral side of ankle.
- **Flexor retinaculum,** on the posteromedial aspect of the ankle.

The retinacula on the front of the ankle are described in the following text. The retinaculae on the lateral and posteromedial sides are described in the lateral and flexor compartments of the leg respectively.

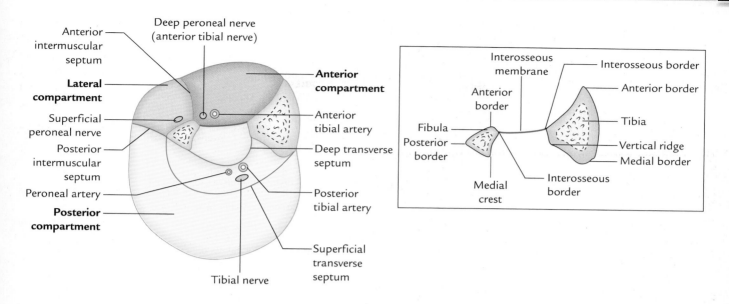

Fig. 27.4 Osseofascial compartments of the leg. Figure in the inset shows transverse section through the tibia and fibula. Note the attachment of interosseous membrane.

Retinacula in Front of the Ankle (Fig. 27.5)

Superior Extensor Retinaculum

It is a broad band of the deep fascia, just above the ankle joint. Vertically it is about 1.5 inches wide.

Attachments

1. *Medially*, it is attached to the lower part of the anterior border of the tibia.
2. *Laterally*, it is attached to the lower part of the anterior border of the fibula.

Relations

1. Medially, it splits to enclose the tendon of tibialis anterior with its synovial sheath.
2. The other structures of the anterior compartment (viz., extensor hallucis longus, deep peroneal nerve, anterior tibial artery, extensor digitorum longus, and peroneus tertius) pass deep to the retinaculum. Here the tendons of these muscles are not surrounded by the synovial sheaths, and deep peroneal nerve and anterior tibial artery lie deep to the tendon of extensor hallucis longus.

Inferior Extensor Retinaculum

It is a Y-shaped band of the deep fascia, situated in front of the ankle joint and the proximal part of the dorsum of the foot. The stem of Y lies laterally, and the upper and lower bands lie medially.

Attachments

1. The *stem* of Y is attached to the anterior nonarticular part of the superior surface of calcaneum in front of the sulcus calcanei, medial to the extensor digitorum brevis.
2. The *upper band* of Y passes upward and medially to be attached to the anterior border of medial malleolus.
3. The *lower band* of Y passes downward and medially over the foot to fuse with the deep fascia of the sole.

Relations

1. The *stem* of Y forms a loop around the tendons of extensor digitorum longus and peroneus tertius with their common synovial sheath.
2. The *upper band* of Y splits to enclose the tendons of tibialis anterior and extensor hallucis longus with their synovial sheaths. The anterior tibial artery and deep peroneal nerve pass deep to it.
3. The *lower band* of Y passes superficially to the tendons of tibialis anterior and extensor hallucis longus with their separate synovial sheaths, and also superficially to the dorsalis pedis artery and deep peroneal nerve.

Functions

1. Keeps the structures of the anterior compartment of the leg at ankle in position.
2. Prevents the tendons from springing medially when the foot is inverted. In this position, there is marked angulation of the tendon of extensor hallucis longus at the ankle.

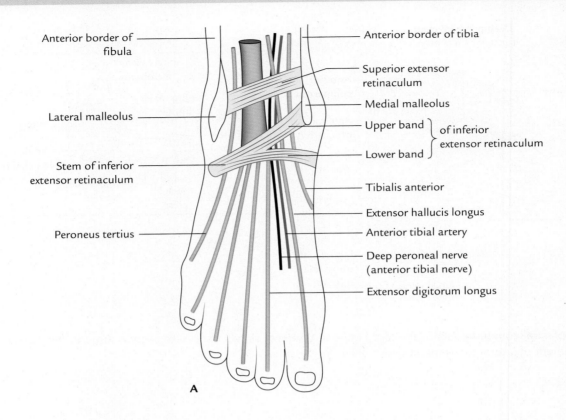

Anterior border of fibula

Anterior border of tibia

Superior extensor retinaculum

Lateral malleolus

Medial malleolus

Upper band ⎫
Lower band ⎭ of inferior extensor retinaculum

Stem of inferior extensor retinaculum

Tibialis anterior

Extensor hallucis longus

Anterior tibial artery

Peroneus tertius

Deep peroneal nerve (anterior tibial nerve)

Extensor digitorum longus

A

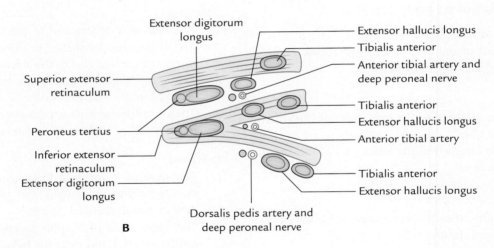

Extensor digitorum longus

Extensor hallucis longus

Tibialis anterior

Anterior tibial artery and deep peroneal nerve

Superior extensor retinaculum

Tibialis anterior

Extensor hallucis longus

Peroneus tertius

Anterior tibial artery

Inferior extensor retinaculum

Extensor digitorum longus

Tibialis anterior

Extensor hallucis longus

Dorsalis pedis artery and deep peroneal nerve

B

Fig. 27.5 Superior and inferior extensor retinacula on the front of the ankle: **A**, surface view showing their attachment; **B**, schematic diagram to show relations of the tendons, vessels, and nerve to these retinacula.

ANTERIOR (EXTENSOR) COMPARTMENT OF THE LEG

Boundaries

Anterior: Deep fascia of the leg.
Medial: Lateral surface of the shaft of the tibia.
Lateral: Anterior intermuscular septum.

Posterior: Interosseous membrane.

Contents (Fig. 27.6)

- **Muscles:** Four muscles (tibialis anterior, extensor hallucis longus, extensor digitorum longus, and peroneus tertius).
- **Artery:** Anterior tibial artery.
- **Nerve:** Deep peroneal nerve (anterior tibial nerve).

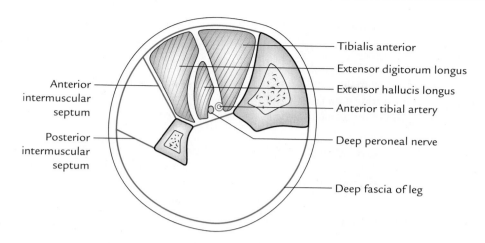

Fig. 27.6 Contents of the anterior compartment of the leg.

MUSCLES OF THE ANTERIOR COMPARTMENT OF THE LEG (Fig. 27.7)

All the muscles of the anterior compartment of the leg arise from the fibula except the tibialis anterior which arises from the tibia (Fig. 27.7). All of them are supplied by the deep peroneal nerve and dorsiflex, the foot at the ankle. The origin and insertion of the muscles of anterior compartment are shown in Figure 27.7 and Table 27.1.

The tibialis anterior being the chief muscle of the anterior compartment is described in detail below.

Tibialis Anterior (Fig. 27.8)

It is a spindle-shaped multipennate muscle. It is the most medial and superficial dorsiflexor of the foot, which lies against the lateral surface of the tibia.

Origin

It arises from:

(a) Upper two-third of the lateral surface of the tibia and adjoining part of the lateral condyle of the tibia.
(b) Adjoining part of the interosseous membrane.
(c) Overlying deep fascia of the leg.

Insertion

The muscle fibres converge below to form a tendon which is related to the lower one-third of the lateral surface of the tibia. It pierces the medial part of superior extensor retinaculum and the upper band of inferior extensor retinaculum. Now it passes medially underneath the inferior band of inferior extensor retinaculum to be inserted *on to the inferomedial side of the base of the first metatarsal bone and adjacent part of the medial cuneiform.*

Nerve supply

By the deep peroneal nerve.

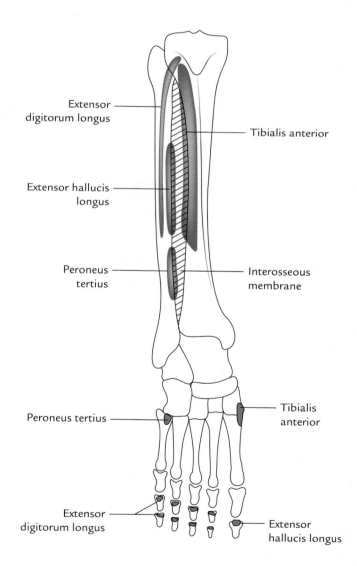

Fig. 27.7 Origin (red colour) and insertion (blue colour) of the muscles of the anterior compartment of leg.

Table 27.1 Origin, insertion, and actions of the muscles of the anterior compartment of the leg

Muscle	Origin from	Insertion into	Actions
Tibialis anterior (it has spindle-shaped multipennate belly)	• Upper 2/3rd of the lateral surface of the tibia • Adjacent part of the interosseous membrane • Its own covering deep fascia • Distal part of the lateral condyle of the tibia	• Medial surface of the medial cuneiform • Adjoining medial surface of the base of the 1st metatarsal	• Dorsiflexion of the ankle • Inversion of the foot • Maintenance of the medial longitudinal arch of the foot
Extensor hallucis longus (Fig. 27.9)	• Middle 2/4th (posterior part) of the medial surface of the shaft of fibula • Adjacent part of the interosseous membrane	Base (dorsal surface) of the distal phalanx of the big toe	• Extension of the phalanges of the big toe • Dorsiflexion of the foot
Extensor digitorum longus (Fig. 27.10)	• Whole of the upper 1/4th and medial part of the middle 2/4th of the anterior surface of the fibula	Middle and distal phalanges of the lateral four toes by four tendons	• Dorsiflexion of the foot • Extension of MP*, PIP**, and DIP*** joints of the lateral four toes
Peroneus tertius	• Lower 1/4th of the anterior surface of the fibula • Adjacent part of the interosseous membrane	Dorsal surface (medial part) of the base of the 5th metatarsal bone	• Dorsiflexion of the foot • Eversion of the foot

*MP: metatarsophalangeal, **PIP = proximal interphalangeal, ***DIP = distal interphalangeal.

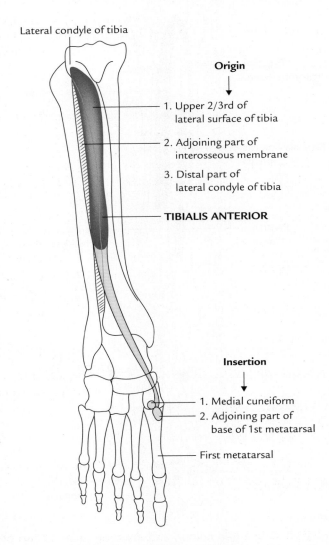

Lateral condyle of tibia

Origin

1. Upper 2/3rd of lateral surface of tibia
2. Adjoining part of interosseous membrane
3. Distal part of lateral condyle of tibia

TIBIALIS ANTERIOR

Insertion

1. Medial cuneiform
2. Adjoining part of base of 1st metatarsal

First metatarsal

Fig. 27.8 Origin and insertion of the tibialis anterior.

Actions

1. It is the chief dorsiflexor of the foot at the ankle joint.
2. It maintains the medial longitudinal arch.
3. It acts as an inverter of the foot at the midtarsal and subtalar joints.

Clinical testing

To test tibialis anterior clinically, ask the patient to stand on heels or dorsiflex the foot against resistance. If normal, its tendon can be seen and palpated.

Clinical correlation

Anterior tibial compartment syndrome/shin splints (Fresher's syndrome): It occurs due to overexertion of the muscles of the anterior compartment especially when the untrained persons who lead a sedentary life are asked to walk or run for long distances. Shin splints also occur in trained runners who do not warm-up.

Muscles of the compartment swell within a tight compartment due to sudden overuse which may impede venous return leading to accumulation of more fluid inside the compartment with unyielding walls. The pressure tends to compress the anterior tibial artery, and reducing the blood supply to the muscles, leading to ischemia and pain. It is frequently seen in freshers (e.g., newly admitted medical students/newly recruited army personnel) who are made to run excessively. Hence, this condition is also referred to as army **fresher's syndrome**.

ANTERIOR TIBIAL ARTERY (Fig. 27.11)

The anterior tibial artery is the main artery of the anterior compartment of the leg. It corresponds to the posterior interosseous artery of the forearm. The blood supply to the

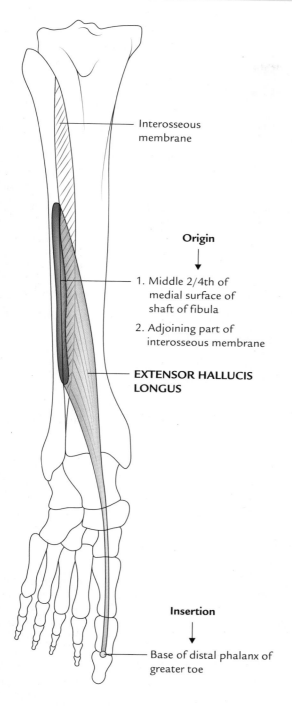

Interosseous membrane

Origin

↓

1. Middle 2/4th of medial surface of shaft of fibula

2. Adjoining part of interosseous membrane

EXTENSOR HALLUCIS LONGUS

Insertion

↓

Base of distal phalanx of greater toe

Fig. 27.9 Origin and insertion of the extensor hallucis longus.

anterior compartment of the leg is reinforced by the perforating branch of peroneal artery. Therefore, the size of peroneal artery is inversely proportional to that of the anterior tibial artery.

The anterior tibial artery is accompanied by two venae comitantes.

Origin

Anterior tibial artery is the smaller terminal branch of popliteal artery given at the lower border of popliteus muscle.

Course

1. It begins in the back of the leg at the lower border of popliteus.
2. It enters the anterior compartment of the leg by passing forward between the two heads of the tibialis posterior, through an opening in the upper part of the interosseous membrane. In the anterior compartment, it runs vertically downward to a point midway between the medial and lateral malleoli, where it enters the foot and changes its name to **dorsalis pedis artery,** which ends near the web between the big and second toes.

Relations (Fig. 27.12)

- In the upper one-third of the leg it lies between the tibialis anterior and extensor digitorum longus.
- In the middle one-third of the leg it lies between the tibialis anterior and extensor hallucis longus.
- In the lower one-third of the leg it lies between extensor hallucis longus and extensor digitorum longus.

It is crossed from the lateral to medial side by the tendon of extensor hallucis longus. As a result, the deep peroneal nerve lies lateral to it in its upper one-third and lower one-third, and anterior to it in its middle one-third.

Branches

1. *Anterior and posterior tibial recurrent arteries:* They take part in the arterial anastomosis around the knee joint.
2. *Muscular branches* to adjacent muscles.
3. *Anterior medial and anterior lateral malleolar arteries:* They take part in the anastomosis around the ankle joint.

N.B. *Variations of the anterior tibial artery:* The anterior tibial artery may fail to grow more than a short way down the leg. In such cases, the dorsalis pedis artery arises from the perforating branch of the peroneal artery or perforating branch of the posterior tibial artery.

DEEP PERONEAL NERVE (ANTERIOR TIBIAL NERVE)

It is the nerve of anterior compartment of the leg and dorsum of the foot. It corresponds to the posterior interosseous nerve of the forearm.

Origin

It is one of the two terminal branches of the common peroneal nerve at the neck of the fibula.

Course and Relations (Fig. 27.12)

- It *begins* on the lateral side of the neck of fibula, under cover of the upper fibres of peroneus longus muscle.

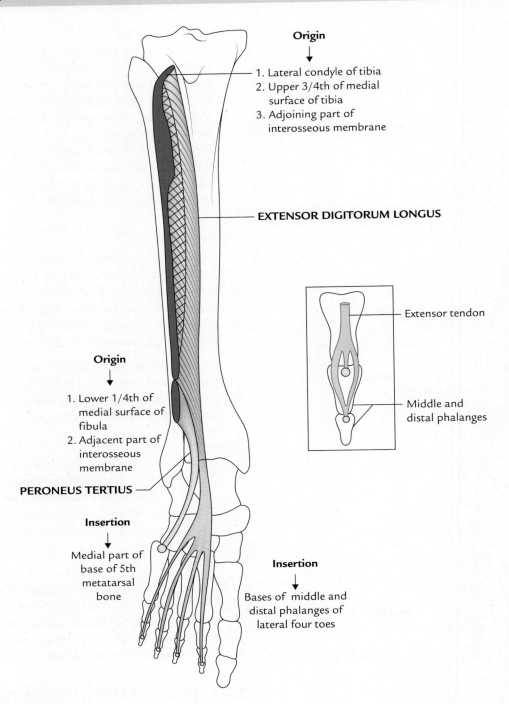

Origin
↓
1. Lateral condyle of tibia
2. Upper 3/4th of medial surface of tibia
3. Adjoining part of interosseous membrane

EXTENSOR DIGITORUM LONGUS

Extensor tendon

Middle and distal phalanges

Origin
↓
1. Lower 1/4th of medial surface of fibula
2. Adjacent part of interosseous membrane

PERONEUS TERTIUS

Insertion
↓
Medial part of base of 5th metatarsal bone

Insertion
↓
Bases of middle and distal phalanges of lateral four toes

Fig. 27.10 Origin and insertion of the extensor digitorum longus and peroneus tertius muscles. Figure in the inset shows the detailed mode of insertion of extensor tendon.

- It *enters the anterior compartment* of the leg by piercing the anterior intermuscular septum. It pierces extensor digitorum longus and descends in this compartment with the anterior tibial artery.
- In the leg, it accompanies the anterior tibial artery. The nerve lies lateral to artery in its upper one-third and lower one-third and anterior to artery in the middle one-third. It is said that in the middle one-third the nerve hesitates to cross the artery from lateral to medial side, so it goes back to the lateral side of the artery. Hence, deep peroneal nerve is also referred to as **nervus hesitans.**
- The nerve ends in front of the ankle by dividing into the lateral and medial terminal branches.

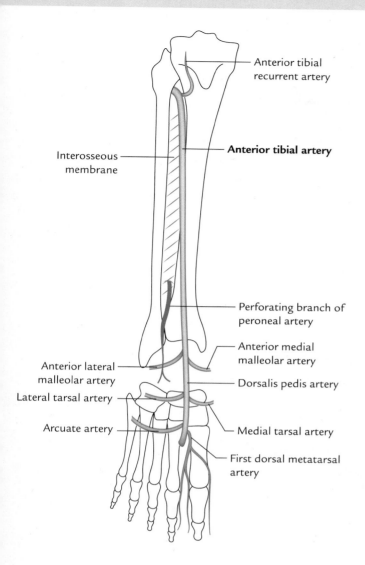

Fig. 27.11 Anterior tibial artery.

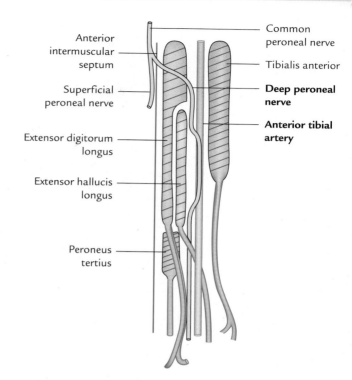

Fig. 27.12 Relation of the anterior tibial artery and deep peroneal nerve.

The *lateral terminal branch* runs laterally and ends in a pseudoganglion deep to the extensor digitorum brevis. Branches from the pseudoganglion supply the extensor digitorum brevis and tarsal and metatarsal joints on the lateral side of the foot.

The *medial terminal branch* runs forward and ends by supplying the skin of the adjacent sides of big and second toes (first interdigital cleft) and the first dorsal interosseous muscle (Fig. 27.13).

Branches

1. *Muscular branches* supply all the four muscles of the anterior compartment of the leg, extensor digitorum brevis on the dorsum of the foot and first dorsal interosseous muscle of the sole of the foot.
2. *Cutaneous branch* supplies the skin of the first interdigital cleft.

DORSUM OF THE FOOT

SENSORY INNERVATION OF THE DORSUM OF THE FOOT (Fig. 27.14)

The sensory innervation to the dorsum of the foot is provided by the following four sets of nerves:

1. **Superficial peroneal (musculocutaneous) nerve:** It provides sensory innervation to most of the dorsum of the foot except the skin of the cleft between the first and second toes. It also supplies medial margin of the great toe.
2. **Deep peroneal nerve:** It provides innervation to the cleft between the first and second toes.
3. **Sural nerve:** It supplies lateral margin of the dorsum of the foot and lateral margin of the little toe.
4. **Saphenous nerve:** It supplies medial margins of the dorsum of the foot up to the head of the first metatarsal.

MUSCLES OF THE DORSUM OF THE FOOT

These are as follows:

(a) *Extrinsic tendons* of the muscles of the anterior compartment of the leg (viz., tibialis anterior, extensor hallucis longus, extensor digitorum longus, and peroneus tertius).

(b) *Intrinsic muscle* on the dorsum of the foot is only one— the extensor digitorum brevis.

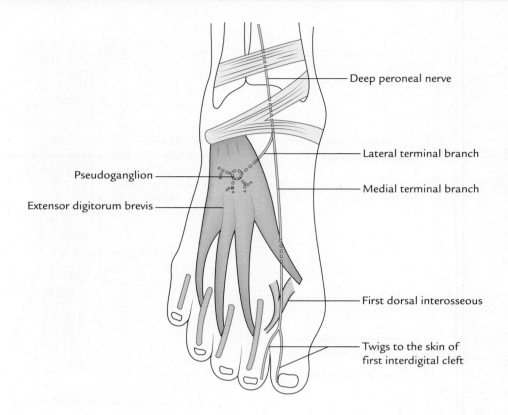

Fig. 27.13 Course and distribution of the deep peroneal nerve on the dorsum of the foot.

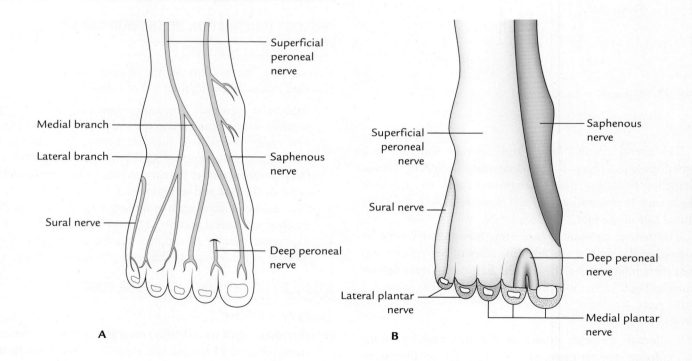

Fig. 27.14 Sensory innervation of the dorsum of the foot: A, cutaneous nerves; B, territories of the cutaneous nerves.

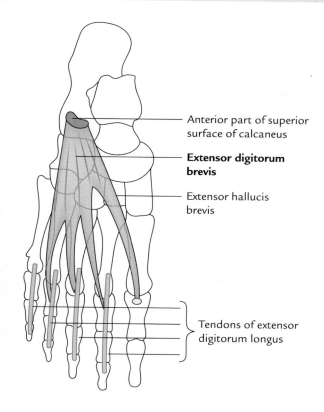

Fig. 27.15 Origin and insertion of extensor digitorum brevis.

Anterior part of superior surface of calcaneus

Extensor digitorum brevis

Extensor hallucis brevis

Tendons of extensor digitorum longus

Extensor Digitorum Brevis (Fig. 27.15)

It is a small muscle situated on the lateral part of the dorsum of the foot, deep to the tendons of extensor digitorum longus. It is the only muscle on the dorsum of the foot and forms a fleshy swelling anterior to the lateral malleolus. **The young novice doctors sometime diagnose it as a contusion.**

Origin

It arises from the anterior part of the superior surface of calcaneum, medial to the attachment of the stem of inferior extensor retinaculum.

Insertion

The muscle divides into four tendons for the medial four toes. The tendon to the big toe crosses in front of dorsalis pedis artery and inserts on the dorsal surface of the proximal phalanx of the big toe. The lateral three tendons join the lateral side of the tendons of the extensor digitorum longus to the second, third, and fourth toes.

N.B. Medial-most part of the extensor digitorum brevis, which forms the tendon for the big toe, separates or becomes distinct early. It is known **as** *extensor hallucis brevis.*

Nerve supply

It is by the lateral terminal branch of the deep peroneal nerve.

Actions

1. Extensor hallucis brevis (EHB) extends the metatarsophalangeal joint of the big toe.
2. The other three tendons extend the metatarsophalangeal and interphalangeal joints of second, third, and fourth toes, particularly when the foot is dorsiflexed.

DORSALIS PEDIS ARTERY

It is the chief artery of the dorsum of the foot.

Origin

The dorsalis pedis artery is the direct continuation of the anterior tibial artery in front of the ankle.

Course (Fig. 27.16)

It passes forward along the medial side of the dorsum of the foot to reach the proximal end of the first intermetatarsal space, where it dips downward between the two heads of the first dorsal interosseous muscle to enter the sole of the foot where it ends by anastomosing with the lateral plantar artery.

Relations
Superficial: Extensor hallucis brevis crosses the artery superficially from the lateral to medial side.
Deep: Ankle joint and tarsal bones.
Medial: Tendon of the extensor hallucis longus (EHL).
Lateral: First tendon of the extensor digitorum longus (EDL).

N.B. *Variations of dorsalis pedis artery:* (a) In about 14% of cases, it may be replaced by the perforating branch of the peroneal artery. (b) It may be too large to compensate for the small *lateral plantar artery* of the sole of foot.

Branches

1. and 2. Lateral and medial tarsal arteries: They take part in the formation of lateral and medial malleolar arterial networks.

3. Arcuate artery: It arises near the base of the second metatarsal, and runs laterally with slight convexity toward the toes, to reach the lateral edge of the foot. It gives **three dorsal metatarsal arteries** (second, third, and fourth), each of which divides into two dorsal arteries for the lateral four toes. The lateral one sends a twig to the lateral side of the little toe.

4. First dorsal metatarsal artery: It arises just before the dorsalis pedis artery dips into the sole of the foot. It divides into dorsal digital arteries for the adjacent sides of the first and second toes. It also gives a dorsal digital artery to the medial side of the big toe.

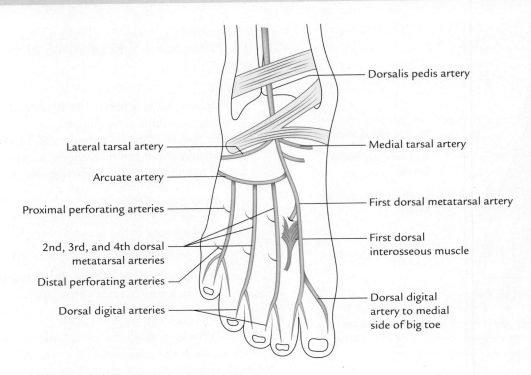

Fig. 27.16 Course and branches of dorsalis pedis artery.

Dorsalis pedis artery pulse: It can be easily felt between the tendons of extensor hallucis longus and first tendon of extensor digitorum longus. It is often palpated in patients suffering from vaso-occlusive diseases of the lower limb, viz., **Buerger's disease**.

The clinicians feeling this pulse should know that the dorsalis pedis artery is congenitally absent in about 14% of the cases. In such cases the absence of dorsalis pedis pulse should be confirmed by the *posterior tibial artery pulse*.

Golden Facts to Remember

► Chief muscle of the anterior compartment of the leg	Tibialis anterior
► Most recent muscle of the anterior compartment of the leg from evolutionary point of view	Peroneus tertius
► Only intrinsic muscle on the dorsum of the foot	Extensor digitorum brevis
► All the muscles of the anterior compartment of the leg arise from the fibula *except*	Tibialis anterior which arises from tibia
► Nervus hesitans	Deep peroneal nerve
► Cutaneous innervation of the whole of the dorsum of the foot is from superficial peroneal nerve *except*	Cleft between the first and second toes which is innervated by the deep peroneal nerve
► Most superficial and strongest dorsiflexor of the foot	Tibialis anterior

Clinical Case Study

A 27-year-old healthy individual was recruited in the army. Few days later he was made to run for a long distance as a part of his training. In the night when he was going to sleep he felt severe pain in his legs which was aggravated by movements. He was given a painkiller by the doctor to relieve the pain. Next day morning he could not dorsiflex his feet. He was taken to the army hospital where the doctors found that both of his legs were swollen and tender to pressure. They also noted foot drop on both the sides. He was diagnosed as a case of *"anterior tibial compartment syndrome"/"shin splints."*

Questions

1. What is meant by the anterior tibial compartment syndrome?
2. What is the cause of this syndrome?
3. Why is the anterior compartment of the leg susceptible to this syndrome?
4. Name the nerve and artery which course within the anterior compartment of the leg and supply muscles present within it.
5. Give the cause of foot drop in this syndrome.

Answers

1. It is a clinical condition characterized by pain and swelling of the distal two-third of the leg.
2. Due to overexertion the muscles of the anterior compartment of the leg swell and compress the anterior tibial artery leading to ischemia and pain.
3. Because the anterior compartment is confined mostly by unyielding bones and deep fascia.
4. Deep peroneal nerve and anterior tibial artery.
5. Compression of the deep peroneal nerve.

CHAPTER 28
Lateral and Medial Sides of the Leg

LATERAL SIDE OF THE LEG

The lateral side of the leg deals with the lateral fascial compartment of the leg and its contents.

LATERAL COMPARTMENT OF THE LEG

Boundaries (Fig. 28.1).

Anterior: Anterior intermuscular septum.
Posterior: Posterior intermuscular septum.
Medial: Lateral surface of the fibula.
Lateral: Deep fascia of the leg.

Contents

1. *Muscles:* Peroneus longus and peroneus brevis.
2. *Nerve:* Superficial peroneal nerve.
3. *Artery:* The lateral compartment of the leg does not have its own artery.
4. *Veins:* Small unnamed veins mostly drain into the short saphenous vein.

N.B. The contents of lateral compartment of the leg are supplied by the branches of the peroneal artery (a branch of posterior tibial artery) which reaches the lateral compartment by flexor hallucis longus and posterior intermuscular septum.

PERONEAL RETINACULA (Fig. 28.2)

The peroneal retinacula are two thick bands of deep fascia on the lateral side of ankle which keep the long tendons of peroneus longus and peroneus brevis in position and act as a pulley for them.

SUPERIOR PERONEAL RETINACULUM

The superior peroneal retinaculum is a thickened fibrous band of deep fascia situated just behind the lateral malleolus.

Attachments

Anteriorly: It is attached to the back of the lateral malleolus.
Posteriorly: It is attached to the lateral surface of the calcaneum and superficial transverse fascial septum of the leg.

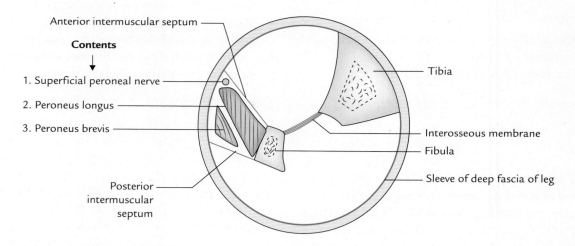

Fig. 28.1 Boundaries and contents of the lateral compartment of the leg.

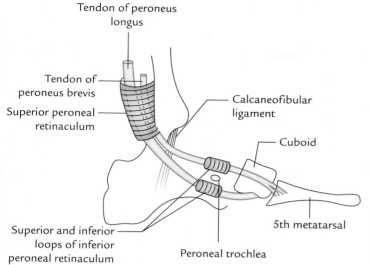

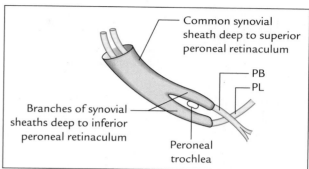

Fig. 28.2 Peroneal trochlea. Figure in the inset shows synovial sheaths around the peroneal tendons (PL = peroneus longus; PB = peroneus brevis).

Relations

The tendons of both peroneus longus and peroneus brevis lie deep to this retinaculum in a single compartment. The tendon of peroneus longus lies superficial to the tendon of peroneus brevis. Both these tendons are enclosed in a common synovial sheath.

INFERIOR PERONEAL RETINACULUM

The inferior peroneal retinaculum is a thickened fibrous band of deep fascia situated anteroinferior to the lateral malleolus.

Attachments

Superiorly: It is attached to the anterior part of superior surface of calcaneum, close to the stem of inferior extensor retinaculum.

Inferiorly: It is attached to the lateral surface of calcaneum.

In between: It is attached to the peroneal trochlea, thus forming two loops, one for the tendon of peroneus brevis and other for the tendon of peroneus longus (Fig. 28.2).

Relations

The tendon of peroneus brevis passes through the superior loop and that of peroneus longus through the inferior loop of the inferior retinaculum. Each tendon is enclosed in a separate synovial sheath, which are the prolongations of the common synovial sheath above, underneath the superior peroneal retinaculum.

Clinical correlation

The synovial sheaths enclosing the tendons of peroneus longus and peroneus brevis are subject to friction and inflammation in athletes who wear tight shoes.

PERONEAL MUSCLES

PERONEUS LONGUS (Fig. 28.3)

The peroneus longus is the longer, larger, and more superficial of the two muscles of the lateral compartment. It is bipennate in the upper part and unipennate in the lower part.

Origin

It arises from:

(a) upper two-third of the lateral surface of the shaft of fibula and adjacent surface of the head of the tibia.

(b) anterior and posterior intermuscular septa of the leg and deep fascia overlying it.

Insertion

The muscle converges below to form a long tendon which lies superficial to the tendon of the peroneus brevis and lodges itself along with the tendon of peroneus brevis into a groove behind the lateral malleolus underneath the superior peroneal retinaculum. After emerging from underneath this retinaculum, the tendon of peroneus longus passes downward and forward through the inferior pulley of the inferior peroneal retinaculum below the peroneal trochlea of the calcaneus.

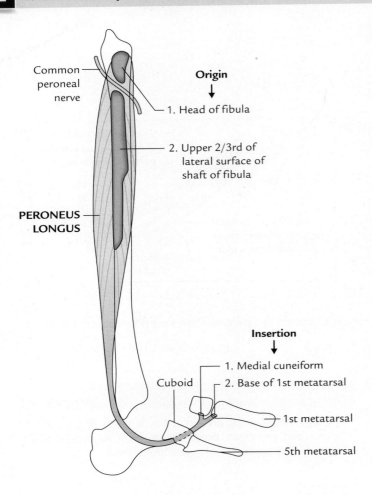

Fig. 28.3 Origin and insertion of the peroneus longus muscle.

On reaching the cuboid bone, the tendon longus changes its direction for the second time to pass through the osseofibrous tunnel on the plantar surface of the cuboid. It then crosses the sole of the foot obliquely from lateral to medial side to be inserted **into the inferolateral surface of the base of the first metatarsal bone and the adjacent part of the medial cuneiform.** The tendon contains a sesamoid bone where it binds around the calcaneus.

Nerve Supply

The peroneus longus is supplied by the superficial peroneal nerve.

Actions

1. It is the chief evertor of the foot.
2. It maintains the lateral longitudinal arch.
3. It also maintains the transverse arches of the foot.

PERONEUS BREVIS (Fig. 28.4)

It is a fusiform bipennate muscle and lies deep to the peroneus longus. As its name indicates, it is shorter than its partner (peroneus longus) in the lateral compartment.

Origin

It arises from:

(a) Lower two-third of the lateral surface of the shaft of the fibula.
(b) Anterior and posterior intermuscular septa of the leg.

Insertion

The muscle converges to form a tendon which passes behind the lateral malleolus underneath the superior peroneal

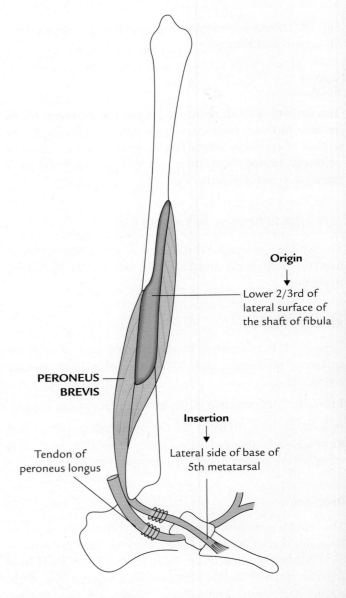

Fig. 28.4 Origin and insertion of the peroneus brevis muscle.

retinaculum. Here it lies in front of the peroneus longus in a common synovial sheath. Then it passes downward and forward above the *peroneal trochlea* of the calcaneus underneath the superior pulley of the inferior peroneal retinaculum. Here it is enclosed in a separate synovial sheath. Finally it passes forward and laterally to be inserted on to the tubercle on the lateral side of the base of the fifth metatarsal.

Nerve Supply

The peroneus brevis muscle is supplied by the superficial peroneal nerve.

Actions

1. It is the evertor of the foot.
2. It maintains the lateral longitudinal arch.

Clinical testing of peroneus longus and brevis

Strongly evert the foot of patient, against resisting; if normal, the tendons of those muscles can be seen and palpated inferior to the lateral malleolus.

The origin, insertion, nerve supply, and actions of the muscles of the lateral compartment of the leg are summarized in Table 28.1.

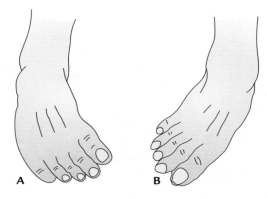

Fig. 28.5 Deformity of foot: **A**, talipes varus; **B**, talipes valgus.

Clinical correlation

Deformity foot due to overactivity of invertor and evertor muscles of the foot (Fig. 28.5)

- Following an injury to the superficial peroneal nerve, the paralysis of the peroneal muscles and associated overactivity of the invertor muscles of the foot produces a deformity of foot called **talipes varus**.
- The overactivity of peroneal muscles following paralysis of the anterior tibial muscles (invertors of foot) produces a deformity of foot called **talipes valgus**.

SUPERFICIAL PERONEAL NERVE (MUSCULOCUTANEOUS NERVE OF THE LEG)

It is the nerve of the lateral compartment of the leg.

Origin

It is one of the two terminal branches of the common peroneal nerve given at the neck of the fibula (Fig. 28.5). It arises in the substance of peroneus longus on the lateral side of the neck of fibula.

Course and Relations (Fig. 28.6)

It begins on the lateral side of the neck of the fibula and descends for a short distance between the peroneus longus and peroneus brevis, and then lies in a groove between the peroneus brevis and extensor digitorum longus.

At the junction of the upper two-third and lower one-third of the leg, it pierces the deep fascia, and soon divides into a medial and a lateral terminal branches which reach the dorsum of the foot.

Table 28.1 Origin, insertion, nerve supply, and actions of the muscles of the lateral compartment of the leg

Muscles	Origin	Insertion	Nerve supply	Actions
Peroneus longus (larger and lies superficial to the peroneus brevis)	• Upper 2/3rd of the lateral surface of the fibula • Adjoining surface of the lateral condyle of the tibia • Anterior and posterior intermuscular septa	• Lateral side of the base of the 1st metatarsal • Adjoining part of the medial cuneiform	Superficial peroneal nerve (L5; S1, S2)	• Eversion of the foot • Weak plantar flexion of the ankle • Maintains the lateral longitudinal arch
Peroneus brevis (smaller and lies deep to the peroneus longus)	• Lower 2/3rd of the lateral surface of the fibula • Anterior and posterior intermuscular septa	Lateral side of the base of the 5th metatarsal bone	Superficial peroneal nerve (L5; S1, S2)	• Eversion of the foot • Weak plantar flexion of the ankle • Maintains the lateral longitudinal arch

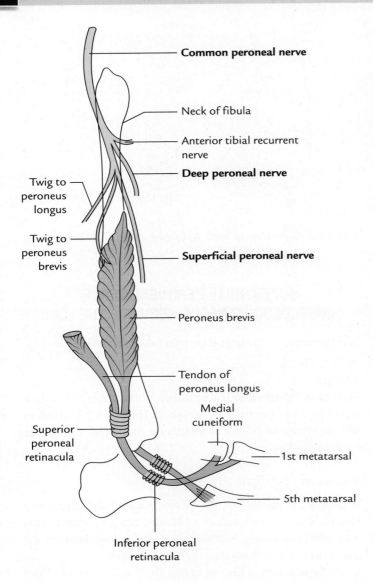

Fig. 28.6 Origin of superficial peroneal nerve from common peroneal nerve on the lateral side of the neck of fibula.

N.B. The distribution of the superficial peroneal nerve corresponds to the distribution of radial nerve in the forearm.

MEDIAL SIDE OF THE LEG

The medial side of the leg consists of the medial surface of the tibia. The greater part of this surface is subcutaneous except for a small upper part, which provides the attachment

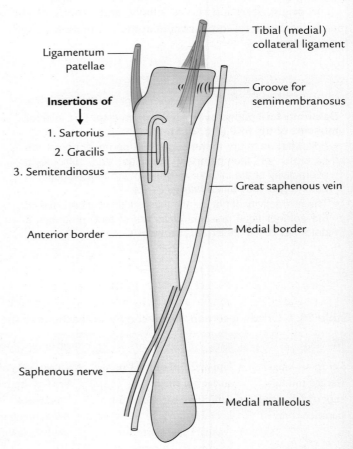

Fig. 28.7 Subcutaneous medial surface of the tibia showing attachment of three tendons of sartorius, gracilis, and semitendinosus; medial collateral ligament and its relation with the great saphenous vein.

Branches and Distribution

1. **Muscular branches** to peroneus longus and peroneus brevis.
2. **Cutaneous branches** supply the skin of the lower one-third of the lateral side of the leg and dorsum of the foot, except for the territories supplied by the saphenous, sural, and deep peroneal nerves.

The *medial terminal branch* of the superficial peroneal nerve crosses the ankle and divides into two dorsal digital nerves, one for the medial side of the big toe and the other for the second interdigital cleft.

The *lateral terminal branch* of the superficial peroneal nerve also divides into two dorsal digital nerves for the third and fourth interdigital clefts.

to tibial collateral ligament and tendons of sartorius, gracilis, and semitendinosus (Fig. 28.7). All these structures are covered by the deep fascia. The great saphenous vein and the saphenous nerve lie in the superficial fascia as they cross the lower one-third of this surface.

1. *Saphenous nerve:* It supplies the skin, fasciae, and periosteum on this surface.

2. *Tibial collateral ligament:* Morphologically, it represents the degenerated part of the tendon of hamstring part of adductor magnus. It partly covers the insertion of semimembranosus and is itself crossed superficially by the tendons of sartorius, gracilis, and semitendinosus.

3. *Tendons of sartorius, gracilis, and semitendinosus:* The three muscles inserted into the upper part of the medial surface of the tibia represent one muscle from each of the three compartments of the thigh. *Sartorius* belongs to the anterior compartment of the thigh and is supplied by the nerve of that compartment—femoral nerve; *gracilis* belongs to the medial compartment of the thigh and is supplied by the nerve of that compartment—obturator nerve; and *semitendinosus* belongs to the posterior compartment of the thigh and is supplied by the nerve of that compartment—sciatic nerve.

N.B. *Guy ropes:* The lower ends of sartorius, gracilis, and semitendinosus are attached together on the upper part of the medial surface of the tibia but above they are attached wide apart from each other on the hip bone; viz., **sartorius** is attached on the ilium (anterior superior iliac spine), **gracilis** on the pubis (body and inferior ramus), and **semitendinosus** on the ischium (ischial tuberosity). The lower end of these muscles is attached at one point. From this arrangement, it seems that these muscles act as 'guy ropes' to stabilize the bony pelvis on the femur (Fig. 28.8).

4. *Bursa anserinus (Fig. 28.9):* It is a large complicated synovial bursa with several diverticula present on the upper part of the medial surface of the tibia. It not only separates the tendons of sartorius, gracilis, and semitendinosus from each other near their insertion but also from the tibial collateral ligament.

5. *Great saphenous vein and saphenous nerve:* The great saphenous vein ascends in front of the medial malleolus and crosses lower one-third of the medial surface of the

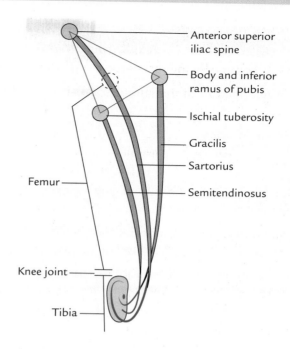

Fig. 28.8 Guy ropes.

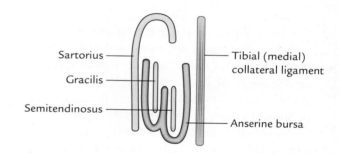

Fig. 28.9 Bursa anserinus.

tibia obliquely with a backward inclination. The saphenous nerve runs downward immediately in front of the great saphenous vein.

Clinical correlation

Anserine bursitis: Repeated trauma on the upper part of the medial aspect causes inflammation of anserine bursa (anserine bursitis) which causes pain and swelling at this site.

Golden Facts to Remember

▶ Most commonly injured nerve in the lower limb	Common peroneal nerve
▶ Unique feature of the lateral compartment of the leg	It does not have its own artery
▶ Bursa anserine	Loculated synovial bursa related to tendons of sartorius, gracilis, and semitendinosus at their insertions
▶ Muscles playing the role of guy ropes in steadying the pelvis	Sartorius, gracilis, and semitendinosus
▶ Inadvertent inversion of the foot is prevented during the "toe off" of the stance phase by	Eversion of the foot by peroneal muscles
▶ Grasping muscle of the foot in apes	Peroneus longus

Clinical Case Study

A few days after the removal of the plaster cast for fracture of the upper end of the right fibula, the patient complained of loss of sensation on the lateral aspect of the lower part of the leg and dorsum of the foot. On examination, the doctor found a loss of sensation on the lateral aspect of the lower part of the leg and dorsum of the foot except on the lateral side of the little toe, in the interdigital cleft between the first and second toes and medial margin of the foot up to the head of the first metatarsal bone. Patient was also unable to dorsiflex and evert his right foot.

Questions

1. Name the nerve injured in this patient.
2. Name the site, where common peroneal nerve is easily palpated?
3. Name the deformity in which the patient cannot dorsiflex his foot.
4. Name the chief evertors of the foot.
5. Name the nerve, which innervate the skin of the interdigital cleft between the first and second toes.

Answers

1. Common peroneal nerve.
2. Lateral side of the neck of the fibula.
3. Foot drop.
4. Peroneus longus and peroneus brevis.
5. Deep peroneal nerve.

Back of the Leg

The back of the leg is also called **calf**. It corresponds to the front of the forearm. It deals with the posterior compartment of the leg. It is bulkiest of the three compartments of the leg because it contains large powerful antigravity muscles (e.g., gastrocnemius and soleus), which raise the heel during walking. The posterior compartment of the leg is continuous superiorly with the popliteal fossa and inferiorly with the sole of the foot.

BONY FRAMEWORK (Fig. 29.1)

The bony framework of the posterior compartment of leg is formed by the posterior aspects of the tibia and fibula, which are joined to each other by the interosseous membrane. When the bony framework of the leg is seen from behind, in addition to the tibia and fibula, posterior aspect of the talus, and posterior one-third of the calcaneus are also seen. The posterior third of calcaneus projects posteriorly to form the heel. It ends in a large medial process, which rests on the ground.

The tibial condyle overhangs the shaft of tibia posteriorly and at the sides. The rounded head of the fibula is quite inferior to the knee joint.

The upper part of the posterior surface of the tibia is crossed obliquely by the **soleal line**. The part below the soleal line is subdivided in its upper three-fourth by a vertical line into medial and lateral areas.

CONTENTS OF SUPERFICIAL FASCIA

The superficial fascia on the back of the leg contains two superficial veins e.g., short and long saphenous veins) and seven cutaneous nerves.

SUPERFICIAL VEINS (Fig. 29.2)

Short (Small) Saphenous Vein

It is formed at the lateral border of the dorsum of the foot by the union of the lateral end of the *dorsal venous arch* and the

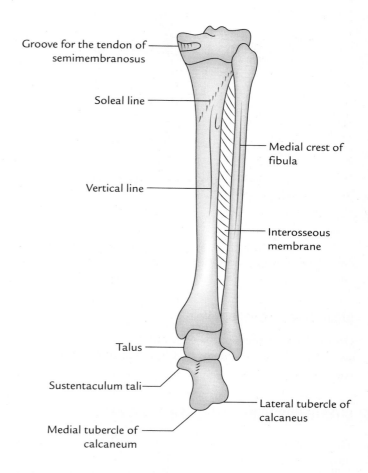

Fig. 29.1 Bony framework of the posterior aspect of the leg.

lateral dorsal digital vein of the little toe. It ascends to reach the back of the leg by passing behind the lateral malleolus. In the leg, it ascends in the mid-line in the lower part of the popliteal fossa; pierces the deep fascia to join the *popliteal vein*. It drains the lateral side of the foot, ankle, and back of the leg. It is connected with the great saphenous veins and the deep veins. It is accompanied by the sural nerve on its lateral side (for details see page 462).

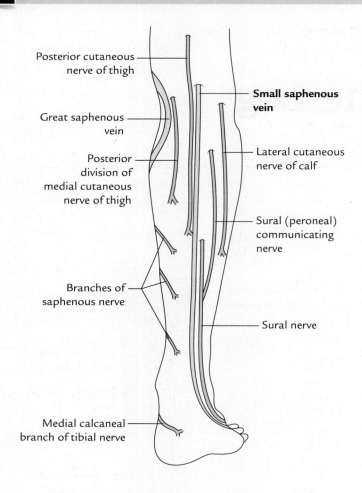

Fig. 29.2 Superficial veins and cutaneous nerves on the back of the leg.

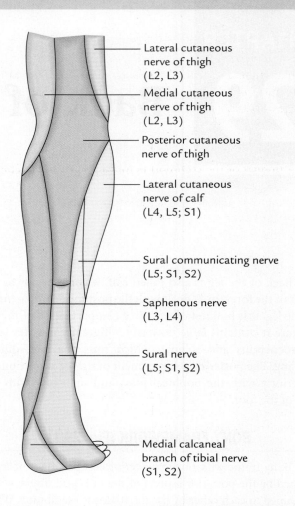

Fig. 29.3 Areas on the back of the leg supplied by different cutaneous nerves.

Great (Long) Saphenous Vein

On the back of the leg it is seen only on the posteromedial side of the knee. It is described in detail in Chapter 33 on pages 458–459.

CUTANEOUS NERVES (Figs 29.2 and 29.3)

The cutaneous nerves as mentioned earlier are seven in number, out of which two supply the skin of the lateral one-third of the back of the leg, two supply the skin of the middle one-third of the leg, two supply the skin of the lateral one-third of the leg, and one nerve supplies the skin of heel.

Saphenous Nerve (L3, L4)

It pierces the deep fascia on the medial side of the knee and accompanies the great saphenous vein, either in front or behind it. It supplies the skin on the medial side of the knee, leg, and medial border of the foot up to the ball of the big toe.

Posterior Division of the Medial Cutaneous Nerve of the Thigh (L2, L3)

It pierces the deep fascia a little above the knee. It supplies the skin of the uppermost part of the medial one-third of the calf.

Posterior Cutaneous Nerve of the Thigh (S1, S2, S3)

It pierces the deep fascia in the middle of the popliteal fossa, and descends with the small saphenous vein to supply the skin of the upper half of the intermediate area of the calf.

Sural Nerve (L5; S1, S2)

It is a branch of the tibial nerve in the popliteal fossa. It pierces deep fascia in the middle of the leg and runs along the short saphenous vein. It is joined by the sural (peroneal) communicating nerve (a branch of common peroneal nerve) about 2 inches above the heel. After passing behind the lateral malleolus, the nerve runs forward along the lateral border of foot, and ends in the skin on the lateral side of the little toe. It supplies the skin of the lower lateral part of the back of the leg, lateral border and adjoining part of the dorsum of the foot, and the lateral side of the little toe.

Lateral Cutaneous Nerve of the Calf (L4, L5; S1)

It is a branch of the common peroneal nerve in the popliteal fossa. It pierces the deep fascia over the lateral head of gastrocnemius and supplies skin of the upper two-third of the lateral area of the leg.

Sural (Peroneal) Communicating Nerve (L5; S1, S2)

It is a branch of the common peroneal nerve. It pierces the deep fascia about 1 inch below the lateral head of gastrocnemius and descends to join the sural nerve about 2 inches above the heel. It supplies skin of the posteromedial part of the lateral area of calf.

Medial Calcaneal Branch (S1, S2)

Medial calcaneal branch of the tibial nerve perforates the flexor retinaculum and supplies the skin of the heel and the adjoining medial side of the sole of the foot.

FLEXOR RETINACULUM

The flexor retinaculum is a thick broad band of the deep fascia (2.5 cm broad) on the medial side of the ankle, behind and below the medial malleolus (Fig. 29.4). It holds the long tendons, vessels, and nerves in position as they curve and pass forward from the back of the leg to the sole of the foot.

Attachments

Anteriorly or *above* : To the posterior border and tip of the medial malleolus.

Posteriorly or *below* : To the medial process of the calcaneal tuberosity.

- *Structures passing deep to flexor retinaculum (Fig. 29.4):*
- From the medial to lateral side, these are: (a) tendon of **t**ibialis posterior, (b) tendon of flexor **d**igitorum longus, (c) posterior tibial **a**rtery and its branches, (d) posterior tibial **n**erve and its terminal branches, and (e) tendon of flexor **h**allucis longus.
- (*Mnemonic:* **T**om, **D**ick, **A**nd **N**ot **H**arry or **T**he **D**octors **A**re **N**ot **H**ere.)

> ### Clinical correlation
>
> **Tarsal tunnel syndrome:** If the tibial nerve is compressed deep to the flexor retinaculum (in the osseofibrous tunnel behind the medial malleolus) it leads to a clinical condition called *tarsal tunnel syndrome*. Clinically, it presents as burning, tingling, and pain in the sole of the foot. These symptoms are relieved by dividing the flexor retinaculum surgically.

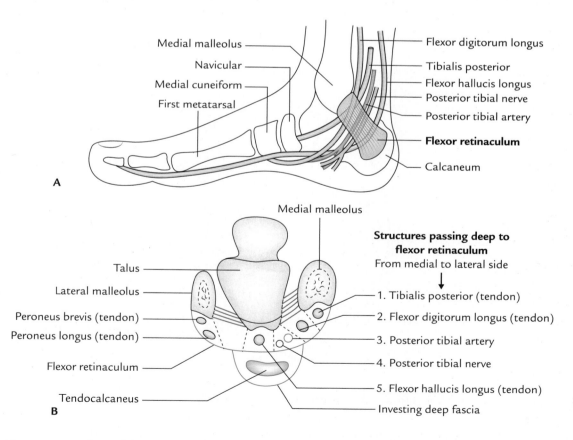

Fig. 29.4 A, Flexor retinaculum of the ankle and the structures passing deep to it; B, transverse section of the ankle showing the flexor retinaculum and the structures passing deep to it.

POSTERIOR COMPARTMENT OF THE LEG

It is the largest osseofascial compartment of the leg.

BOUNDARIES AND SUBDIVISIONS (Fig. 29.5)

Anterior: Posterior surfaces of the tibia, fibula, interosseus membrane, and posterior intermuscular septum.

Posterior: Deep fascia of the leg extending from the medial border of the tibia to the posterior intermuscular septum.

The **posterior compartment of the leg is subdivided** by two strong transverse fascial septa (superficial and deep) into three parts: superficial, middle, and deep.

The **superficial transverse septum** is attached *medially* to the medial border of the tibia and *laterally* to the posterior border of the fibula.

The **deep transverse septum** is attached *medially* to the proximal part of the soleal line and vertical ridge on the posterior surface of the tibia, and *laterally* to the medial crest of the fibula.

- *Superficial part* (between superficial transverse septum and deep fascia) contains gastrocnemius, soleus, and plantaris.

- *Middle part* (between superficial and deep transverse fascial septa) contains flexor digitorum longus, flexor hallucis longus, and posterior tibial nerve and vessels.
- *Deep part* (between deep transverse fascial septum and posterior surfaces of interosseous membrane, tibia, and fibula) contains tibialis posterior.

Contents

- **Muscles:** Superficial and deep groups of the muscles (Table 29.1).
- **Arteries:** Tibial and peroneal arteries.
- **Nerve:** Tibial nerve.

Table 29.1 Superficial and deep muscles of the posterior compartment of the leg

Superficial muscles	Deep muscles
Gastrocnemius	Popliteus
Soleus	Flexor digitorum longus
Plantaris	Flexor hallucis longus
	Tibialis posterior

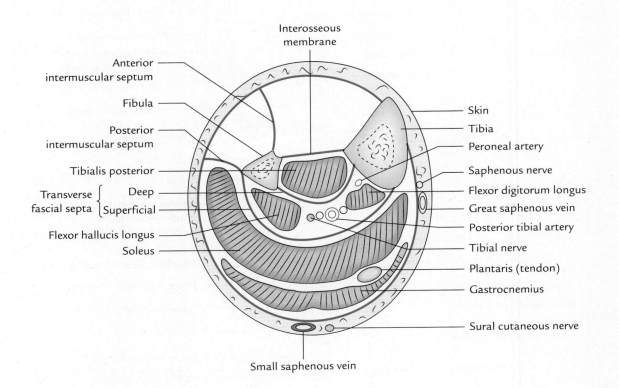

Fig. 29.5 A transverse section of the middle third of the leg showing boundaries and contents of the posterior compartment of the leg.

MUSCLES OF THE POSTERIOR COMPARTMENT OF THE LEG

The bony attachments of the muscles of the back of the leg are shown in Figure 29.6.

Superficial Muscles on the Back of the Leg

These are shown in Figure 29.7.

Gastrocnemius (Fig. 29.8)

It is the largest and most superficial muscle of the posterior compartment. It consists of two heads—medial and lateral.

Origin

1. **Large medial head** arises by a broad flat tendon from the posterosuperior aspect of the medial condyle of the femur behind the adductor tubercle and adjoining part of the posterior (popliteal) surface of the shaft of the femur.
2. **Small lateral head** arises by a broad flat tendon from the lateral surface of the lateral condyle of the femur above

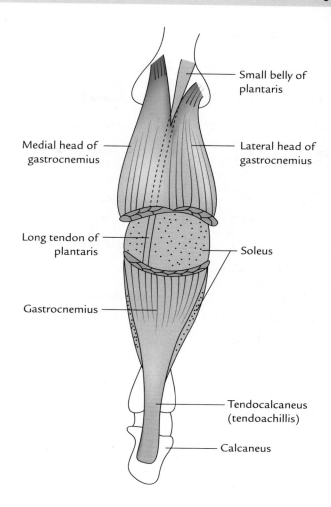

Fig. 29.7 Superficial muscles on the back of the leg (e.g., gastrocnemius, soleus, and plantaris).

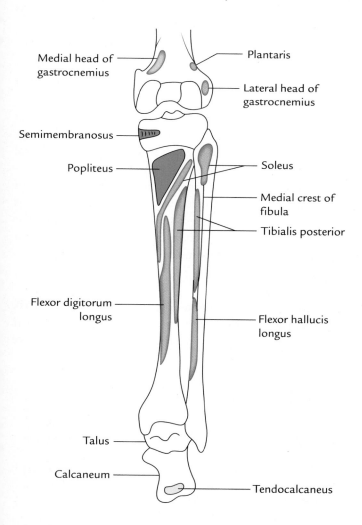

Fig. 29.6 Attachments of the muscles of the back of leg on bony framework of the leg.

the lateral epicondyle and adjoining part of the lateral supracondylar line.

Insertion

The fleshy bellies of the two heads descend and unite at the middle of the leg to form broad thin aponeurotic tendon, which unites with the tendon of soleus, a short distance below the middle of the leg to form a long thick tendon—the tendocalcaneus (tendoachillis), which is inserted into the middle of the posterior surface of calcaneum.

Nerve Supply

Both heads are supplied by the tibial nerve in the popliteal fossa.

Actions

1. It is the chief plantar flexor of the foot at the ankle when the knee is extended.
2. It is also a flexor of the knee.
3. It provides rapid movements of the foot during running and jumping.

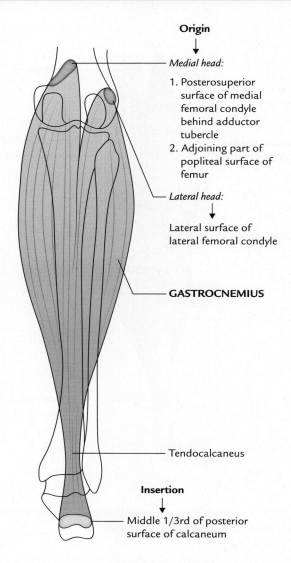

Origin
↓

Medial head:

1. Posterosuperior surface of medial femoral condyle behind adductor tubercle
2. Adjoining part of popliteal surface of femur

Lateral head:

Lateral surface of lateral femoral condyle

GASTROCNEMIUS

Tendocalcaneus

Insertion
↓

Middle 1/3rd of posterior surface of calcaneum

Fig. 29.8 Origin and insertion of the gastrocnemius.

Clinical correlation

Tennis leg: It is painful calf injury in which there is tear or strain of the medial head of gastrocneminus at its musculo-tendinous junction due to overstretching. It commonly occurs in a tennis player who stretches their gastrocnemius too much for a difficult serve.

Soleus (Fig. 29.9)

It is a multipennate muscle lying deep to the gastrocnemius. It is so-named because of its resemblance to a sole/flat fish.

Origin

It has a horseshoe-shaped origin from:

(a) Back of the head and posterior surface of the upper one-fourth of the shaft of the fibula.
(b) Soleal line and middle one-third of the medial border of the tibia.
(c) Tendinous arch between the tibia and fibula.

Insertion

The muscle fibres slope downward to form a massive belly, which gives rise to a tendon. The tendon of soleus fuses with that of gastrocnemius to form **tendocalcaneus,** which is inserted into the middle one-third of the posterior surface of calcaneum.

Nerve Supply

It is supplied by two branches of the tibial nerve:

(a) The first branch supplies the muscle in the popliteal fossa from its superficial surface.
(b) The second branch supplies the muscle in the posterior compartment of the leg from its deep surface.

Actions

1. It is a plantar flexor of the foot at the ankle and steadies the leg on the foot during standing. It is considered as the **"workhorse" of the plantar flexion**.
2. It is slow acting but more powerful than gastrocnemius. It acts as a **bottom gear** during strolling. (*Note:* Gastrocnemius acts as a **top gear** during running and jumping.)

N.B.

- The two heads of gastrocnemius and soleus together form the **triceps surae muscle**.
- A small sesamoid bone is found in the tendon of origin of lateral head of gastrocnemius called **fabella**.
- A small synovial bursa (Brodie's bursa) lies deep to medial head to gastrocnemius.
- **Tendocalcaneus (tendoachillis)** is a conjoint tendon of insertion of gastrocnemius and soleus (**triceps surae**). It is the thickest and strongest tendon in the body and is about 15 cm long. It acts as a prime mover of plantar flexion of the foot at the ankle joint.

Clinical Testing

To test gastrocnemius and soleus together (triceps surae), ask the patient to stand on the toes or plantar flex the foot. If normal the tendocalcaneus can be seen and palpated above the heel.

Clinical correlation

Calf muscle pump and peripheral heart: The gastrocnemius and soleus together make a 'calf muscle pump,' which facilitates the venous return from the lower limb.

The soleus muscle is regarded as the **peripheral heart** because it houses large venous sinuses called soleal sinuses which communicate with the superficial veins by perforating veins and with deep veins directly.

Thus contraction of soleus helps in sucking the blood from superficial veins and propelling it into deep veins.

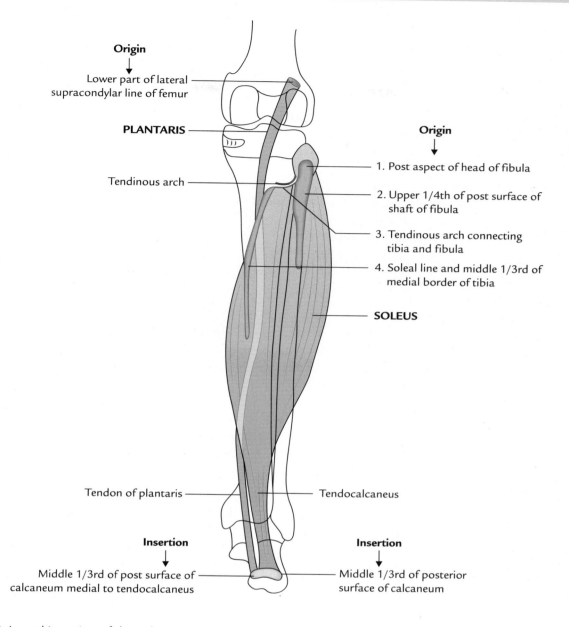

Origin

Lower part of lateral
supracondylar line of femur

PLANTARIS

Tendinous arch

Origin

1. Post aspect of head of fibula

2. Upper 1/4th of post surface of
shaft of fibula

3. Tendinous arch connecting
tibia and fibula

4. Soleal line and middle 1/3rd of
medial border of tibia

SOLEUS

Tendon of plantaris

Tendocalcaneus

Insertion

Middle 1/3rd of post surface of
calcaneum medial to tendocalcaneus

Insertion

Middle 1/3rd of posterior
surface of calcaneum

Fig. 29.9 Origin and insertion of the soleus and plantaris.

Plantaris (Fig. 29.9)

It is a small muscle with a short belly and long slender tendon. It lies between the gastrocnemius and soleus.

Origin

It arises from the lower one-third of the lateral supracondylar line and the adjoining part of the oblique popliteal ligament.

Insertion

Its tendon blends with the medial margin of tendocalcaneus and inserted into the middle one-third of the posterior surface of the calcaneum medial to the attachment of tendocalcaneus.

N.B. The long slender tendon of plantaris is easily mistaken by the first year medical students for a nerve; hence, it is often termed *freshman's nerve*.

Clinical correlation

Tendon grafting: The plantaris is a vestigial muscle in human beings and is absent in 5–10% of people. It has insignificant role either as flexor of the knee or as plantar flexor of the ankle; hence, the tendon of plantaris is used for grafting (e.g., reconstructive surgery of the tendons of the hand).

The origin, insertion, nerve supply, and actions of the superficial muscles of the posterior compartment of the leg are summarized in Table 29.2.

Table 29.2 Origin, insertion, nerve supply, and actions of the superficial muscles of the back of the leg

Muscle	Origin	Insertion	Nerve supply	Actions
Gastrocnemius	• *Lateral head* from the lateral surface of the lateral condyle of the femur • *Medial head* from the popliteal surface of the femur and adjoining posterosuperior aspect of the medial condyle of the femur	Middle one-third of the posterior surface of the calcaneus via tendocalcaneus	Tibial nerve (S1, S2)	• Plantar flexion of the ankle when the knee is extended • Flexes the leg at the knee joint
Soleus	• Posterior aspect of the head and upper one-fourth of the posterior surface of the shaft of fibula • Soleal line and middle one-third of the medial border of the tibia • Tendinous soleal arch between the fibula and tibia	Middle one-third of the posterior surface of the calcaneus via tendocalcaneus	Tibial nerve via two branches (S1, S2)	• Plantar flexion of the ankle independent of position of the knee • Steadies the leg on the foot during standing
Plantaris	• Lower part of the lateral supracondylar line • Oblique popliteal ligament	Middle one-third of the posterior surface of the calcaneus	Tibial nerve	Very weak plantar flexion of the ankle

Deep Muscles on the Back of the Leg

The origin, insertion, nerve supply, and actions of the deep muscles on the back of the leg are given in Table 29.3. Only the popliteus muscle is described in detail.

Popliteus (Fig. 29.10)

It is a thin, flat, triangular muscle, which forms the inferior part of the floor of the popliteal fossa.

Origin

Its origin is intracapsular but extrasynovial. It arises by a tendon from:

(a) The deep anterior part of the groove (popliteal groove) on the lateral surface of the lateral condyle of the femur. (*Note:* The posterior part of the groove is occupied by the tendon of popliteus in full flexion.)
(b) Arcuate popliteal ligament.
(c) Outer margin of the lateral meniscus.

Insertion

The tendon passes downward and medially and flares out to form the fleshy part, which is inserted into:

(a) The medial two-third of the triangular area above the soleal line on the posterior surface of the tibia.
(b) The popliteal fascia.

Nerve Supply

The popliteus is supplied by a branch of tibial nerve. It arises in the popliteal fossa, crosses across the superficial aspect of the muscle, winds round its lower border, and supplies the muscle from its deeper aspect.

Actions

1. It unlocks the locked knee by rotating the femur laterally during initial stages of flexion of the knee.
2. It pulls the lateral meniscus backward and prevents it from being trapped and crushed between the condyles of the femur and tibia.
3. It flexes the knee during couching.

Posterior Tibial Artery (Fig. 29.13)

Origin

It is the larger of the two terminal branches of the popliteal artery because its branches not only supply the posterior compartment but also the lateral compartment of the leg and the sole of the foot.

Course and Relations

1. It begins at the lower border of popliteus, between the tibia and fibula, deep to gastrocnemius and enters the back of the leg by passing deep to the *tendinous arch of soleus*.
2. In the leg, it runs downward and slightly medially to reach the posteromedial side of the ankle, midway between the medial malleolus and the medial tubercle of calcaneum.
3. It terminates deep to the flexor retinaculum by dividing into a **large lateral plantar artery** and a **small medial plantar artery**.

Table 29.3 Origin, insertion, nerve supply, and actions of the deep muscles of the back of the leg

Muscle	Origin	Tendon	Insertion	Nerve supply	Actions
Popliteus	• Anterior part of the popliteal groove on the lateral condyle of the femur	Its tendon of origin is 1 inch long, and intracapsular but extrasynovial	• Medial two-third of the triangular area above the soleal line, on the posterior surface of the tibia	Tibial nerve (L4, L5; S1)	• Unlocks the locked knee by rotating the femur laterally during initial stages of flexion of the knee
Flexor digitorum longus (FDL) (Fig. 29.11)	• Upper two-third of the medial part of the posterior surface of the tibia below the soleal line • Fascia covering the tibialis posterior	Its tendon: • Crosses superficially to the tendon of tibialis posterior in the lower part of the leg and tendon of FHL in the sole • Subdivides into four tendons for lateral four toes, accessorius	Plantar surface of the base of distal phalanges of the lateral four toes	Tibial nerve (S2, S3)	• Plantar flexes lateral four toes • Plantar flexes ankle • Maintains the longitudinal arches of the foot
Flexor hallucis longus (FHL) (Fig. 29.11)	• Lower three-fourth of the posterior surface of the shaft of the fibula, behind the medial crest • Adjoining part of the posterior interosseous membrane	Its tendon: • Grooves two bones, talus between its medial and posterior tubercles and the calcaneum underneath sustentaculum tali • In the sole it is crossed superficially by the tendon of FDL	Plantar surface of the base of distal phalanx of great toe	Tibial nerve (S2, S3)	• Plantar flexes great toe • Plantar flexes the ankle weakly • Supports the medial longitudinal arch of the foot
Tibialis posterior (Fig. 29.12)	• Upper 2/3rd of the lateral part of the posterior surface of tibia below the soleal line • Posterior surface of the fibula in front of the medial crest • Upper two-third of the posterior surface of the interosseous membrane	Its tendon: • Crosses superficially by the tendon of FDL in the lower part of the leg • Grooves back of the medial malleolus • Passes deep to flexor retinaculum and superficially to the deltoid ligament	• Chiefly on tuberosity of the navicular bone • Slips pass to all tarsals, except talus, and bases 2nd to 4th metatarsals	Tibial nerve (L4, L5)	• Invertor of the foot • Maintains the medial and longitudinal arches of the foot

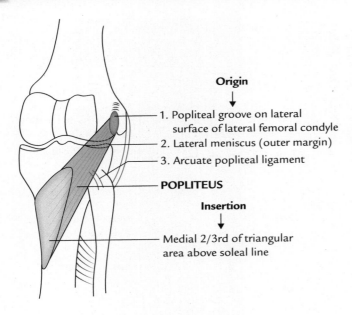

Fig. 29.10 Origin and insertion of the popliteus muscle.

Throughout its course, it is *accompanied* by the tibial nerve, which crosses the artery from the medial to lateral side.

Branches

1. *Peroneal (fibular) artery:* It is the largest and most important branch of the posterior tibial artery. It arises 2.5 cm distal to the inferior border of popliteus.
2. *Muscular branches:* To the muscles of posterior compartment.
3. *Nutrient artery to tibia:* It is the **largest nutrient artery** in the body. It enters the nutrient foramen of tibia below the soleal line.
4. *Circumflex fibular artery:* It encircles the lateral side of the neck of the fibula.
5. *Communicating branch:* It joins with the similar branch of peroneal artery about 5 cm above the ankle.
6. *Medial malleolar branch:* It passes toward the medial malleolus.
7. *Calcaneal branch:* It pierces the flexor retinaculum and supplies soft tissues of the heel.
8. *Terminal branches:* These are medial and lateral plantar arteries of the sole.

Clinical correlation

Posterior tibial pulse: It can be felt against the calcaneum about 2 cm below and behind the medial malleolus, and in front of the medial border of the tendocalcaneus. Since the posterior tibial artery lies deep to the flexor retinaculum, it is important to ask the patient to invert his/her foot to relax the flexor retinaculum. Failure to do so may lead to an erroneous conclusion that this pulse is absent.

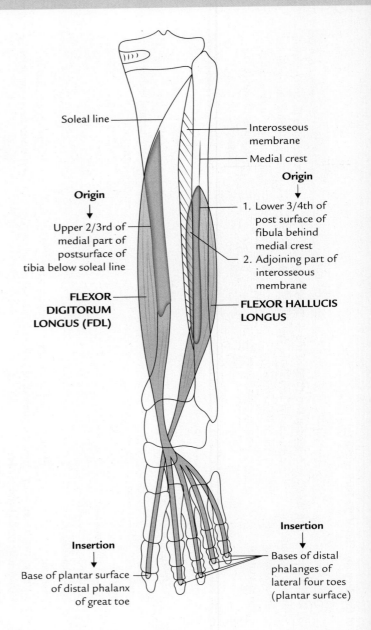

Fig. 29.11 Origin and insertion of the flexor digitorum longus and flexor hallucis longus.

PERONEAL ARTERY (Fig. 29.13)

Origin

It is the largest and most important branch of the posterior tibial artery. It provides blood supply to the posterior and lateral compartments of the leg.

Course and Relations

1. It arises 2.5 cm below the lower border of popliteus.
2. It runs obliquely toward the fibula and then descends along the medial crest of the fibula in a fibrous canal

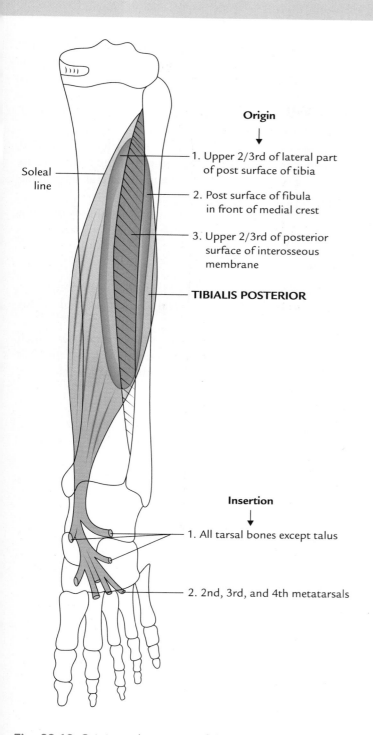

Origin
↓

1. Upper 2/3rd of lateral part of post surface of tibia

2. Post surface of fibula in front of medial crest

3. Upper 2/3rd of posterior surface of interosseous membrane

TIBIALIS POSTERIOR

Soleal line

Insertion
↓

1. All tarsal bones except talus

2. 2nd, 3rd, and 4th metatarsals

Fig. 29.12 Origin and insertion of the tibialis posterior.

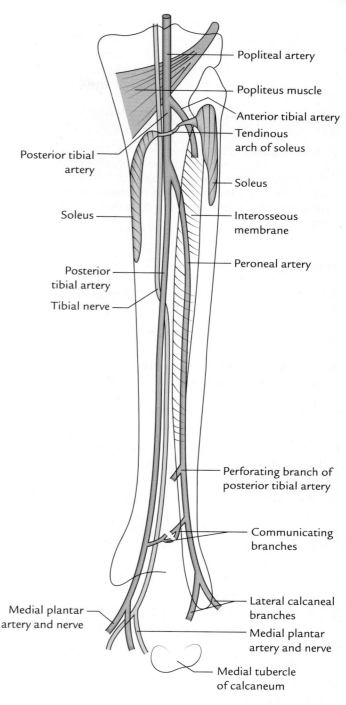

Popliteal artery

Popliteus muscle

Anterior tibial artery

Tendinous arch of soleus

Posterior tibial artery

Soleus

Interosseous membrane

Soleus

Posterior tibial artery

Peroneal artery

Tibial nerve

Perforating branch of posterior tibial artery

Communicating branches

Lateral calcaneal branches

Medial plantar artery and nerve

Medial plantar artery and nerve

Medial tubercle of calcaneum

Fig. 29.13 Courses of the posterior tibial and peroneal arteries, and tibial nerve.

between tibialis posterior and flexor hallucis longus. Now it passes behind the inferior tibiofibular and ankle joints, and ends on the lateral surface of calcaneus and terminates by giving the lateral calcaneal arteries.

N.B. The size of peroneal artery is frequently increased. It may join to reinforce or replace the posterior tibial artery in the lower part of the leg.

Branches

1. *Muscular branches* to the posterior and lateral compartments of the leg.
2. *Nutrient artery* to the fibula.
3. *Communicating branch:* It joins with similar branch of the posterior tibial artery about 5 cm above the ankle.
4. *Perforating branch:* It is large and pierces interosseous membrane about 5 cm above the ankle, appears in the

anterior compartment of the leg, and terminates by anastomosing with the lateral malleolar branches of the anterior tibial and dorsalis pedis arteries.

5. *Lateral calcaneal artery:* It is a terminal branch which takes part in the formation of lateral malleolar plexus.

Clinical correlation

Dorsalis pedis artery pulse: It is felt just lateral to the tendon of extensor hallucis longus against the tarsal bones. The clinicians while taking the pulse of the dorsalis pedis artery must keep in mind that the perforating branch of the peroneal artery may reinforce or even replace the dorsalis pedis artery.

TIBIAL NERVE

The tibial nerve is the larger of the two terminal branches of the sciatic nerve.

Origin and Course

1. It arises on the back of the thigh at the junction of the upper two-third and lower one-third and enters the popliteal fossa (see page 374). From the popliteal fossa it enters into the posterior compartment of the leg, by passing deep to the tendinous arch of origin of the soleus along with the posterior tibial vessels.

2. Its course and relations in the leg are similar to that of the posterior tibial artery.

3. In the leg, the nerve is lateral to the artery at first, and then it crosses posterior to the artery from the medial to lateral side and then runs along the lateral side of the artery.

4. It terminates deep to the flexor retinaculum by dividing into medial and lateral plantar nerves.

Branches

1. *Muscular branches:* Popliteus, tibialis posterior, flexor digitorum longus, flexor hallucis longus, and soleus (from its deep surface).

2. *Cutaneous branches:* Medial calcaneal branches which pierce the flexor retinaculum and supply skin of the back and lower surface of the heel—the weight bearing area of the heel.

3. *Articular branches:* To the ankle joint.

Golden Facts to Remember

▶ Largest compartment of the leg	Posterior compartment
▶ Peripheral heart	Soleus muscle
▶ Most powerful tendon in the body	Tendocalcaneus (Achilles tendon)
▶ Largest nutrient artery in the body	Nutrient artery to tibia (a branch of the posterior tibial artery)
▶ Muscle functioning as organ of proprioception in the leg	Plantaris
▶ "Workhorse" of plantar flexion of the foot	Soleus
▶ Freshman's nerve	Tendon of plantaris
▶ Largest and most important branch of the posterior tibial artery	Peroneal artery
▶ Muscle of the leg having maximum concentration of muscle spindles	Plantaris
▶ All the muscles on the back of the leg are long except	Popliteus which is short

Clinical Case Study

A 55-year-old businessman was advised by his physician to reduce the fatty diet and start regular jogging for half an hour daily in the morning.

On one morning while jogging, he heard a sharp snap and felt a sudden pain in his right lower calf. On examination, the examining doctor found that the upper part of the right calf was swollen and a gap was apparent between the swelling and the heel. Diagnosis of "*ruptured tendocalcaneus*" was made.

Questions

1. What is tendocalcaneus and give its chief action?
2. What is the cause of swelling in the upper part of the calf and an apparent gap between it and the heel?
3. Give the site of insertion of tendocalcaneus.
4. What is the commonest cause of rupture of tendocalcaneus?

Answers

1. It is a conjoint tendon of insertion of gastrocnemius and soleus. Its chief action is the plantar flexion of the foot at the ankle.
2. When tendocalcaneus ruptures, the bellies of gastrocnemius and soleus retract upward causing a swelling in the upper part of the calf, leaving a gap between the divided ends of the tendon.
3. Middle one-third of the posterior surface of the calcaneus.
4. An abrupt take off at the start of a 100 m race.

CHAPTER 30

Sole of the Foot

The region/part of the foot that meets the floor or ground is termed **sole of the foot**. In many ways, the structure of the sole of the foot is similar to that of the palm. The major differences arise due to the functional difference between the hand and the foot. The hand is a prehensile organ whereas the foot is concerned with transmission of body weight and locomotion. Note that parts of the foot are in contact with the ground during various phases of standing, walking, and running positions.

SKIN

The skin of the sole presents the following features:
1. It is thick and hairless.
2. It is firmly bound to the underlying deep fascia (plantar aponeurosis) by the numerous fibrous bands.
3. It is creased at the sites of skin movement.
4. It contains large number of sweat glands.

The above features increase the efficiency of grip of the sole on the ground.

N.B. The skin over the major weight-bearing areas of the sole—the heel, lateral margin, and ball of the foot—is very thick.

SUPERFICIAL FASCIA

The superficial fascia is mostly composed of subcutaneous fat in the meshwork of fibrous septa, which anchor the skin with the underlying deep fascia. The superficial fascia is thick and dense over the weight-bearing points to provide fibrofatty cushions at these sites (e.g., posterior tubercles of the calcaneum, metatarsal heads, and pulps of the digits).

CUTANEOUS NERVES (Fig. 30.1)

The skin of the sole of the foot is supplied by three cutaneous nerves, which arise directly or indirectly from the tibial nerve.

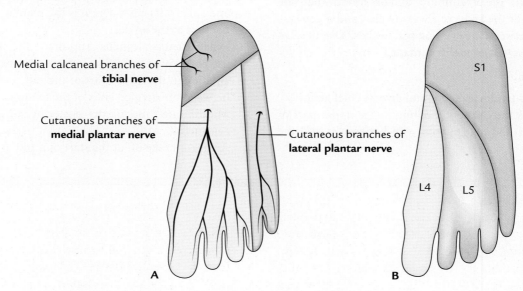

Medial calcaneal branches of **tibial nerve**

Cutaneous branches of **medial plantar nerve**

Cutaneous branches of **lateral plantar nerve**

S1

L4   L5

A   B

Fig. 30.1 Cutaneous innervation of the sole of the foot: **A**, areas supplied by three sets of cutaneous nerves; **B**, the dermatomes.

The areas supplied by the three nerves roughly correspond to the three dermatomes of the sole:

1. **Medial calcaneal branches:** They arise directly from the tibial nerve and supply skin over the posterior and medial portions of the sole—the weight-bearing portion of the heel. The corresponding dermatome is S1.
2. **Cutaneous branches of the medial plantar nerve:** They supply the skin over the larger anteromedial portion of the sole and medial 3½ digits. The corresponding dermatome is L4.
3. **Cutaneous branches of the lateral plantar nerve:** They supply the skin over the smaller anterolateral portion of the sole and lateral 1½ digits. The corresponding dermatome is L5.

DEEP FASCIA

The deep fascia in the region of the sole consists of three parts: central, medial, and lateral. The central part of the deep fascia is very thick and termed *plantar aponeurosis*. The medial and lateral parts are thin and termed medial and lateral plantar fasciae, respectively.

The deep fascia of the sole is composed of compact bundles of collagen fibres which are arranged longitudinally in the plantar aponeurosis and transversely in the medial and lateral plantar fasciae.

The thick central part covers the flexor digitorum brevis. The thin medial and lateral parts cover the abductor hallucis and abductor digiti minimi, respectively.

In the region of toes, the deep fascia forms the *deep transverse metatarsal ligaments* and *fibrous flexor sheaths*.

N.B.

- The deep fascia in the sole is specialized to form three things: (a) plantar aponeurosis, (b) deep transverse metatarsal ligaments, and (c) fibrous flexor sheaths.
- According to some authorities whole of the deep fascia of the sole is termed plantar aponeurosis.

PLANTAR APONEUROSIS (Fig. 30.2)

The plantar aponeurosis is the thickened central part of the deep fascia of the sole.

Features

The plantar aponeurosis is triangular in shape and occupies the central area of the sole. The *apex* of the plantar aponeurosis is attached to the medial tubercle of calcaneum, proximal to the attachment of the flexor digitorum brevis. The *base* of the plantar aponeurosis near the heads of the metatarsals divides into *five bands*, one for each toe. At the point of division, the five processes are bound by the

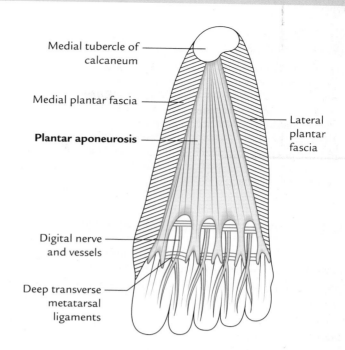

Fig. 30.2 Plantar aponeurosis.

transverse fascial fibres. The digital nerves and vessels pass through the intervals between the processes.

Each band splits opposite the metatarso-phalangeal joints into *a superficial* and *a deep slip*. The superficial slip is attached to the dermis of the skin and blends with the superficial *transverse metatarsal ligaments*. The deep slip divides into two parts, which embrace the flexor tendons, and blend with the *fibrous flexor sheaths* and *deep transverse metatarsal ligaments*.

From the medial and lateral margins of the aponeurosis, the *lateral and medial vertical intermuscular septa* pass deeply, and divide the plantar muscles into three groups—medial, intermediate, and lateral. The thinner *transverse septa* arise from the vertical septa and divide the muscles of the sole into four layers.

N.B. Morphologically the plantar aponeurosis represents the degenerated tendon of plantaris muscle, which has been separated by the enlarging heel during evolution.

Functions

The functions of the plantar aponeurosis are:

1. It firmly fixes the skin of the sole.
2. It provides origin to the muscles of first layer of the sole.
3. It protects the plantar nerve and vessels from compression.
4. It helps to maintain the longitudinal arches of the foot by acting as tie beam.

Plantar fasciitis and calcaneal spur: The plantar aponeurosis is stretched during standing position. Hence, tearing or inflammation (*plantar fasciitis*) often occurs in individuals who do a great deal of standing or walking, viz. traffic police personnel. It causes pain and tenderness in the sole of the foot especially underneath the heel during standing. Repeated attack of the plantar fasciitis leads to calcification in the posterior attachment of the plantar aponeurosis forming a *calcaneal spur*.

DEEP TRANSVERSE METATARSAL LIGAMENTS

These are four short, flat bands of fibrous tissue, which connect the plantar ligaments of the adjoining metatarso-phalangeal joints. They are related dorsally to interossei, and ventrally to lumbricals and digital nerves and vessels.

FIBROUS FLEXOR SHEATHS

The inferior surface of each toe from the head of metatarsal to the base of distal phalanx is provided with a strong fibrous sheath derived from the deep fascia of the toes. It is attached to the sides of the phalanges.

The proximal end of each sheath receives the deeper part of the slip of plantar aponeurosis. The distal end of the sheath is closed and is attached to the base of the distal phalanx.

The sheath along with the inferior surfaces of the phalanges and interphalangeal joints forms a blind tunnel through which pass long flexor tendon/tendons of the toes.

Their structure and arrangement is similar to that of fibrous flexor sheaths of the fingers. They retain flexor tendons in position during flexion of the toes.

MUSCLES OF THE SOLE OF THE FOOT

There are 18 intrinsic muscles and 4 extrinsic tendons in the sole of the foot. The muscles of the sole are described in four layers from superficial to deep (Table 30.1).

The muscles of the sole are chiefly concerned with supporting the arches of the foot. The short and long muscles of the foot act as synergists.

N.B. *Neurovascular planes of the sole:* There are two neurovascular planes between the muscle layers of the sole:

(a) Superficial neurovascular plane between the first and second layers.

(b) Deep neurovascular plane between the third and fourth layers.

In the *superficial neurovascular plane* lies the trunks of medial and lateral plantar nerves, and the arteries.

In the *deep neurovascular plane* lies the deep branches of the lateral plantar nerve and artery.

The origin, insertion, nerve supply, and actions of the muscles of the sole are given in Table 30.2.

To understand the origin and insertion of the muscles of the foot the student must study the layout of the different bones on the plantar aspect of the skeleton of the foot (Fig. 30.3).

Table 30.1 Muscle layers of the sole of the foot

Layer	Muscles	Features
First layer	• Flexor digitorum brevis • Abductor hallucis • Abductor digiti minimi	They cover whole of the sole
Second layer	• Flexor digitorum accessorius • Four lumbricals • Two tendons (tendon of flexor digitorum longus and tendon of flexor hallucis longus)	Flexor digitorum accessorius and lumbricals are attached to the tendon of flexor digitorum longus
Third layer	• Flexor hallucis brevis • Flexor digiti minimi brevis • Adductor hallucis	• They are confined to the metatarsal region of the sole • Two of these muscles act on the big toe and one on the little toe
Fourth layer	• Interossei (3 plantar interossei and 4 dorsal interossei) • Tendon of tibialis posterior • Tendon of peroneus longus	They fill up the intermetatarsal spaces

Table 30.2 Origin, insertion, nerve supply, and actions of the intrinsic muscles of the sole

Muscles	Origin	Belly/Tendon	Insertion	Nerve supply	Actions
First layer (Fig. 30.4)					
• *Flexor digitorum brevis* (resembles flexor digitorum superficialis of the hand)	Medial tubercle of the calcaneum	• It forms 4 tendons for the lateral 4 toes • Each tendon splits into two slips opposite the bases of proximal phalanges to allow passage of the long flexor tendon	Margins of the middle phalanges of lateral 4 toes	Medial plantar nerve (S2, S3)	Flexor of the lateral toes
• *Abductor hallucis* (lies along the medial border of the foot)	• Medial tubercle of the calcaneum • Flexor retinaculum	Its tendon fuses with medial portion of the tendon of flexor hallucis brevis for a common insertion	Medial side of the base of proximal phalanx of the big toe	Medial plantar nerve (S2, S3)	Flexion and abduction of the big toe
• *Abductor digiti minimi* (lies along the lateral border of the foot)	Medial and lateral tubercles of the calcaneum in a continuous line	Its tendon fuses with the tendon of flexor digiti minimi brevis for a common insertion	Lateral side of the base of proximal phalanx of the little toe	Lateral plantar nerve (S2, S3)	Flexion and abduction of the little toe
Second layer (Fig. 30.5)					
• *Flexor digitorum accessorius*	By two heads: • *Medial head* from the medial concave surface of the calcaneum and adjoining part of the medial tubercle • *Lateral head* from the calcaneum in front of the lateral tubercle	The two heads unite at an acute angle	Tendon of the flexor digitorum longus (FDL)	Lateral plantar nerve (S2, S3)	• Straightens the pull of the long flexor tendons • Assists the flexor digitorum longus in flexing the lateral 4 toes
• *Lumbricals* (4 in number and numbered from medial to lateral side) Tendon of flexor digitorum longus (see Table 29.3) Tendon of flexor hallucis longus (see Table 29.3)	From the tendons of the flexor digitorum longus	Tendons pass forwards on the medial sides of the metatarso-phalangeal joints of the lateral four toes	Into the extensor expansions and bases of proximal phalanges of lateral 4 toes	1st by the medial plantar nerve, and 2nd, 3rd, and 4th by the lateral plantar nerve (S2, S3)	Extension of toes at the interphalangeal joints

(Contd.)

(Contd.)

Muscles	Origin	Belly/Tendon	Insertion	Nerve supply	Actions
Third layer (Fig. 30.6)					
• *Flexor hallucis brevis*	It arises by a Y-shaped tendon: • *Lateral limb* from the medial part of the plantar surface of the cuboid bone • *Medial limb* from the lateral cuneiform	Muscle belly splits in two parts. Each part gives rise to a tendon which contains a sesamoid bone near its insertion. The medial tendon blends with the abductor hallucis, and the lateral tendon blends with the adductor hallucis	Each side of the base of proximal phalanx of the big toe (1st digit)	Medial plantar nerve (S2, S3)	Flexion of the proximal phalanx of big toe
• *Flexor digiti minimi brevis*	Base of the 5th metatarsal bone	Forms narrow tendon which blends with the abductor digiti minimi	By a narrow tendon into the lateral side of the base of proximal phalanx of the little toe	Superficial branch of the lateral plantar nerve (S2, S3)	Flexes the proximal phalanx of the little toe
• *Adductor hallucis*	It arises by two heads: • *Large oblique head* from bases of the 2nd, 3rd, and 4th metatarsals • Small *transverse head* from the plantar ligaments of the metatarso-phalangeal joints of 3rd, 4th, and 5th toes	The common tendon of both heads fuses with the lateral tendon of the flexor hallucis brevis	By the composite tendon on the lateral side of the base of proximal phalanx of the big toe	Deep branch of the lateral plantar nerve (S2, S3)	• Adduction of the big toe • Maintains transverse arches of the foot
Fourth layer (Fig. 30.7)					
• *Dorsal interossei* * (4 in number, and lies between the metatarsal bones; Fig. 30.8A)	They are bipennate and arises from the adjacent sides of the metatarsal bones (1–5)	Tendons are arranged on the abductor sides of the toes	• 1st on the medial side of the proximal phalanx of 2nd digit • 2nd–4th on the lateral sides of 2nd–4th digits	Lateral plantar nerve (S2, S3)	• Abducts digits (2nd–4th) • Flexes the metatarso-phalangeal joints
• *Plantar interossei* * (3 in number and lies rather below the metatarsals Fig. 30.8B)	They are unipennate and arises from the medial sides of the metatarsal bones (3rd–5th)	Tendons are arranged on the adductor sides of the toes	Medial sides of bases of the phalanges of 3rd–5th digits	Lateral plantar nerve (S2, S3)	• Adducts the digits (2nd–4th) • Flexes the metatarso-phalangeal joints

*Mnemonic: Plantar interossei ADduct (PAD) the toes and arise from single metatarsal as unipennate muscles; whereas Dorsal interossei ABduct (DAB) the toes and arise from two metatarsals as bipennate muscles.

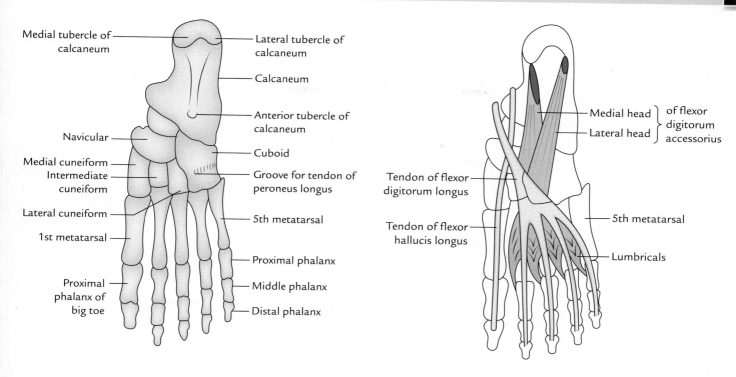

Fig. 30.3 Layout of different bones on the plantar aspect of the skeleton of the foot.

Fig. 30.5 Muscles of the second layer of the sole.

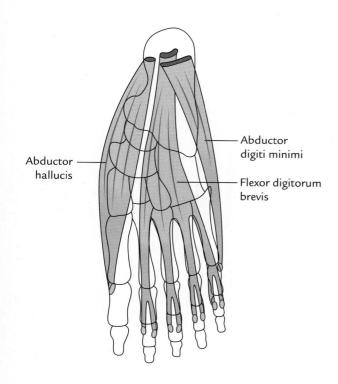

Fig. 30.4 Muscles of the first layer of the sole.

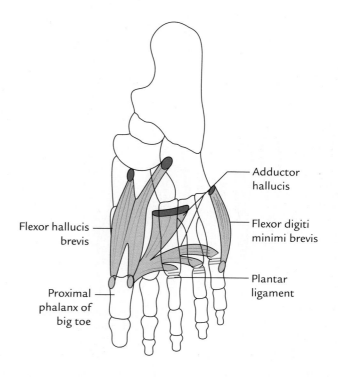

Fig. 30.6 Muscles of the third layer of the sole.

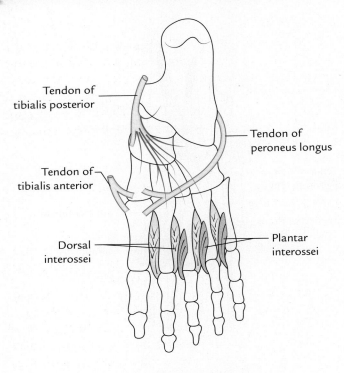

Fig. 30.7 Muscles of the fourth layer of the sole.

PLANTAR NERVES

There are two plantar nerves—medial and lateral.

MEDIAL PLANTAR NERVE

The medial plantar nerve is the *pre-axial nerve* of the foot.

Origin and Course

It is the larger terminal branch of the tibial nerve and begins deep to flexor retinaculum. It passes forward between the abductor hallucis and flexor digitorum brevis. It is accompanied by the medial plantar artery on its medial side.

Branches and Distribution (Fig. 30.9)

It gives rise to the following branches:

1. **Muscular branches to four muscles:**
    (a) Abductor hallucis ⎫
    (b) Flexor digitorum brevis ⎬ by the main trunk.
    (c) Flexor hallucis brevis, by first digital nerve to the medial side of the big toe.
    (d) First lumbrical, by the second digital nerve.

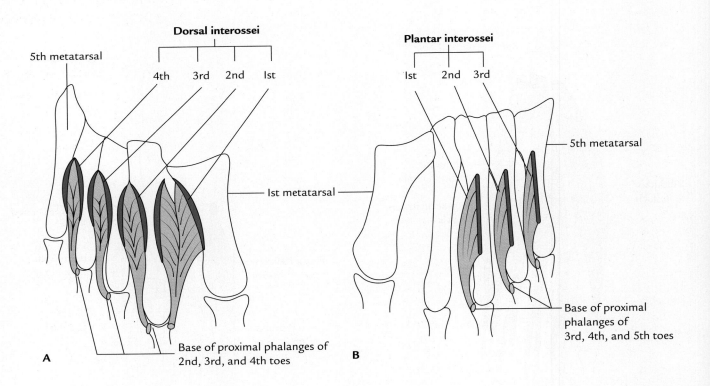

Fig. 30.8 Origin and insertion of interosseous muscles of the foot: A, dorsal interossei; B, plantar interossei.

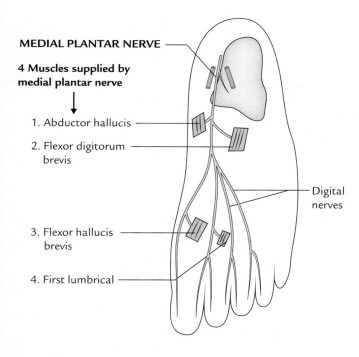

MEDIAL PLANTAR NERVE

4 Muscles supplied by medial plantar nerve

↓

1. Abductor hallucis
2. Flexor digitorum brevis

Digital nerves

3. Flexor hallucis brevis

4. First lumbrical

Fig. 30.9 Course and motor distribution of medial plantar nerves.

2. **Cutaneous branches** (four digital nerves) supply skin of the medial 3½ toes and larger medial part of the sole. Each digital nerve also supplies dorsum of the terminal phalanx.
3. **Articular branches** supply the joints of tarsus and metatarsus.

N.B. The distribution of *medial plantar nerve* in the sole corresponds to the distribution of *median nerve in the hand*.

Clinical correlation

Medial plantar nerve entrapment: The medial plantar nerve may be compressed either deep to flexor retinaculum or deep to abductor hallucis due to the repetitive eversion of the foot (e.g., during gymnastics and running). Clinically, it presents as burning, numbness, and tingling (paraesthesia) on the medial side of the sole and in the region of navicular tuberosity.

Since it commonly occurs in runners, this condition is referred to as **"jogger's foot."**

LATERAL PLANTAR NERVE

The lateral plantar nerve is the *post-axial nerve* of the foot.

Origin and Course

It is the smaller terminal branch of the tibial nerve and begins deep to the flexor retinaculum. It appears in the sole deep to the abductor hallucis. It passes forward and laterally to the base of the fifth metatarsal in between the first and second layers of the muscles. On reaching between flexor digitorum brevis and abductor digiti minimi, it divides into the superficial and deep branches.

Branches and Distribution (Fig. 30.10)

It gives rise to the following branches:

1. **Branches from the main trunk:**
   (a) *Cutaneous* to lateral part of the sole.
   (b) *Muscular* to supply two muscles: abductor digiti minimi and flexor digitorum accessorius.
2. **Branches from the superficial branch:** The *superficial branch* divides into two branches—lateral and medial.
   The *lateral branch* supplies three muscles: flexor digiti minimi brevis, third plantar interosseous, and fourth dorsal interosseous. It also supplies the skin on the lateral side of little toe.
   The *medial branch* communicates with the medial plantar nerve and supplies the skin of the fourth cleft.
3. **Branches of the deep branch:** It courses medially lying between the third and fourth layers of the sole. It supplies

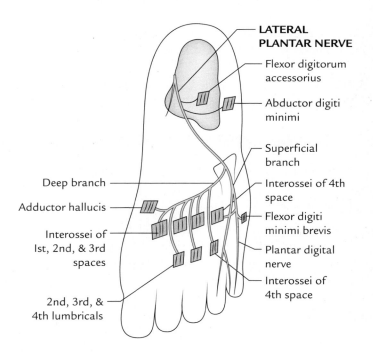

LATERAL PLANTAR NERVE
Flexor digitorum accessorius
Abductor digiti minimi
Superficial branch
Deep branch
Adductor hallucis
Interossei of 4th space
Flexor digiti minimi brevis
Interossei of 1st, 2nd, & 3rd spaces
Plantar digital nerve
Interossei of 4th space
2nd, 3rd, & 4th lumbricals

Fig. 30.10 Course and motor distribution of lateral plantar nerves.

Table 30.3 Motor innervation of the medial and lateral plantar nerves

Medial plantar nerve	Lateral plantar nerve
Four muscles • Abductor hallucis • Flexor digitorum brevis • Flexor hallucis brevis • First lumbrical	• Flexor digitorum accessorius • Abductor digiti minimi • Abductor hallucis • Flexor digiti minimi brevis • All interossei • Second, third, and fourth lumbricals

Table 30.4 Distribution of pre-axial and post-axial nerves in the palm and sole

Pre-axial nerves		Post-axial nerves	
Median nerve	Medial plantar nerve	Ulnar nerve	Lateral plantar nerve
Abductor pollicis	Abductor hallucis	Abductor digiti minimi	Abductor digiti minimi
Flexor pollicis brevis	Flexor hallucis brevis	Flexor digiti minimi	Flexor digiti minimi brevis
Opponens pollicis	No corresponding muscle	Opponens digiti minimi	No corresponding muscle
Flexor digitorum superficialis	Flexor digitorum brevis	Abductor pollicis All interossei	Abductor hallucis All interossei Flexor digitorum accessorius
Lumbricals 1 and 2	Lumbrical 1	Lumbricals 3 and 4	Lumbricals 2, 3, and 4
3½ Digits	3½ Digits	1½ Digit	1½ Digit

nine muscles: abductor hallucis, three lumbricals (second, third, and fourth), and five interossei of the first three intermetatarsal spaces.

The motor innervation of the medial and lateral plantar nerves is summarized in Table 30.3.

N.B. The distribution of pre-axial and post-axial nerves in the palm and sole is given in Table 30.4.

PLANTAR ARTERIES (Figs 30.11 and 30.12)

There are two plantar arteries—medial and lateral.

MEDIAL PLANTAR ARTERY

The medial plantar artery is the smaller terminal branch of the posterior tibial artery. It arises beneath the flexor retinaculum and appears in the sole deep to abductor hallucis accompanied by the medial plantar nerve on its lateral side. It terminates on the medial side of big toe by dividing into following two branches:

1. A small branch, which passes distally along the medial side of the big toe and anastomoses with the digital branch of first plantar metatarsal artery, on the lateral side of the big toe.

2. A large branch, which splits into three *superficial digital branches* and anastomoses with the first to third plantar metatarsal arteries.

Distribution

It gives rise to the following branches:

1. **Muscular branches** to the adjoining muscles.
2. **Cutaneous branches** to the medial side of the sole.
3. **Digital arteries** (vide supra).

LATERAL PLANTAR ARTERY

The lateral plantar artery is the larger terminal branch of the posterior tibial artery. It arises beneath the flexor retinaculum and runs forward towards the base of the fifth metatarsal. The lateral plantar nerve lies on its medial side. At the base of the fifth metatarsal bone, it curves medially with concavity facing proximally and runs towards the first inter-digital space to join the dorsalis pedis artery and thus forms the *plantar arch*.

It gives rise to the following branches:

1. **Muscular branches** to supply the adjoining muscles.
2. **Superficial branches** to supply skin and fasciae laterally.
3. **Anastomotic branch** to anastomose at the lateral border of foot with the lateral tarsal and arcuate arteries.
4. **Calcaneal branch** is occasional to the heel.

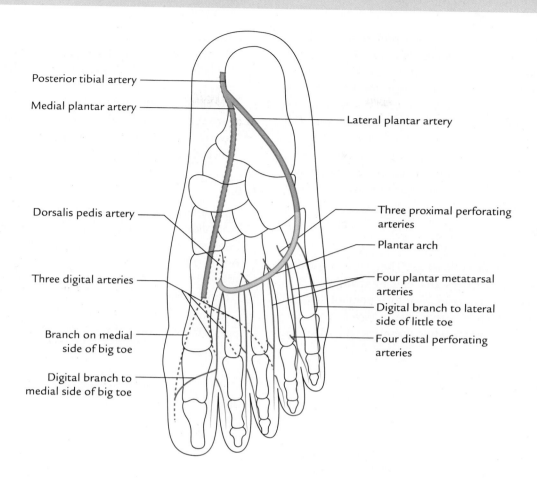

Fig. 30.11 Course and branches of the medial and lateral plantar arteries.

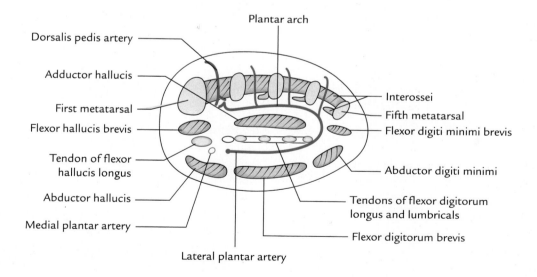

Fig. 30.12 Transverse section of the right foot through the metatarsal showing arrangements of structures in the sole.

N.B. *Plantar arch:* It is an arterial arch formed by the direct continuation of the lateral plantar artery from the base of the fifth metatarsal bone to the first intermetatarsal space. It is completed medially by anastomosing with the terminal part of the dorsalis pedis artery. *It extends from the base of the fifth metatarsal bone to the proximal part of the first intermetatarsal space.* It lies between the third and fourth layers of the sole. It is convex distally across the bases of fourth, third, and second metatarsals. It is accompanied by a deep branch of lateral plantar nerve, which lies in its concavity.

BRANCHES

It gives rise to the following branches:

1. **Four plantar metatarsal arteries:** They pass forward in the intermetatarsal spaces and end by dividing into a pair of plantar digital arteries. Near their point of division, each plantar metatarsal artery gives a *distal perforating branch* to join the corresponding **dorsal metatarsal artery.**

The first plantar metatarsal artery sends a digital branch to the medial side of the big toe. The digital branch to the lateral side of little toe arises from the lateral plantar artery.

2. **Three proximal perforating arteries:** They ascend through the proximal parts of the second, third, and fourth intermetatarsal spaces, and anastomoses with the corresponding dorsal metatarsal arteries.

N.B.

-   All the structures (e.g., main neurovascular bundle and long flexor tendons) enter the sole through a gap between the flexor retinaculum and the calcaneus called **porta pedis** except the tendon of peroneus longus, which enters the sole through a groove beneath the cuboid called **side gate of the sole.**
-   The passages for proximal and distal perforating arteries are called **windows of the sole.**

Golden Facts to Remember

▶ Podiatry	Field that deals with the study and care of the foot
▶ Most common hind foot clinical problem	Plantar fasciitis
▶ All the interossei of sole are supplied by the deep branch of the lateral plantar nerve *except*	Those in the fourth intermetatarsal space, which are supplied by the superficial branch of the lateral plantar nerve
▶ Porta pedis	Osseofibrous tunnel between flexor retinaculum and calcaneus
▶ Policeman's heel	Plantar fasciitis

Clinical Case Study

A 55-year-old woman complained of pain on the plantar surface of her heel and on the medial aspect of the foot. The pain often became severe while beginning to walk in the morning but disappeared after 5–10 minutes of rest after activity. However, it again recurred on walking after rest.

On examination, the doctor located the point of tenderness at the medial tubercle of the calcaneum and on the medial surface of this bone. Pain increased with passive extension of the big toe and was further exacerbated by dorsiflexion of the foot and/or weight bearing. A radiograph of the foot revealed an abnormal bony process protruding from the medial tubercle of the calcaneum. A diagnosis of the plantar fasciitis was made.

Questions

1. What is the meaning of plantar fasciitis? Give its possible cause.
2. What is the plantar fascia? Give its attachments.
3. What is calcaneal spur?
4. Give the cause of tenderness in the region of calcaneal spur.

Answers

1. It is the inflammation of plantar aponeurosis at its proximal attachment to the medial tubercle of the calcaneum due to repeated minor trauma. It occurs in individuals who do a great deal of standing and walking, particularly if inappropriate footwear is worn.
2. See pages 420–421.
3. Repeated attacks of the plantar fasciitis induce ossification in the proximal attachment of the plantar aponeurosis forming a calcaneal spur.
4. Usually a synovial bursa develops at the end of the spur that may become inflamed and tender.

CHAPTER 31

Arches of the Foot

The human foot is described as an architectural marvel of the nature. Its construction is the best example of the structural adaptation to the function.

The foot performs two major functions:

1. It acts as a pliable platform to support the body weight during standing position.
2. It acts as a lever to propel the body forward during walking, running, and jumping.

To fulfill the first function, the foot is designed in the form of elastic arches. These arches are segmented so that they can sustain the stress of weight and thrusts at the optimum level.

To fulfill the second function, the foot is so constructed that it is transformable in a lever. The segmented arched lever converts the foot into a spring, which is ideally suited for its functions.

The foot and its bones are divided into the following three anatomical and functional segments (Fig. 31.1):

1. The *hindfoot* consists of talus and calcaneus.
2. The *midfoot* consists of navicular, cuboid, and cuneiforms.
3. The *forefoot* consists of metatarsals and phalanges.

The skeleton of the foot is arched, both longitudinally and transversely, with the concavity directed towards the plantar surface (i.e., the bones of the foot are arranged to form the **transverse and longitudinal arches**). The presence of arches makes the sole concave both anteroposteriorly and transversely. This is best reflected in the footprint showing the weight-bearing points of the sole (Fig. 31.2).

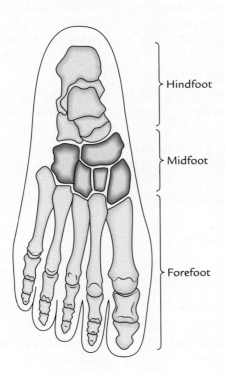

Fig. 31.1 Division of the foot and its bones into three anatomical and functional segments/parts of the skeleton of the foot.

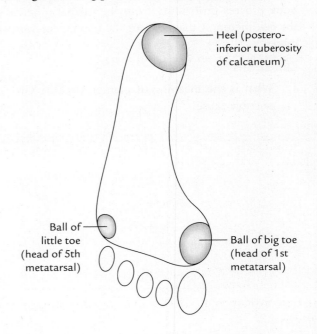

Fig. 31.2 Right foot print showing weight-bearing points.

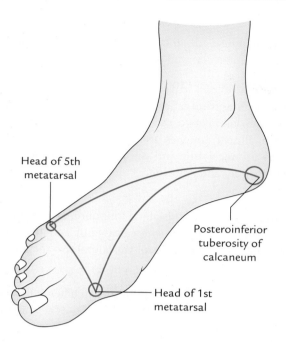

Fig. 31.3 Distribution of the body weight among three points.

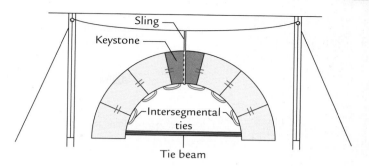

Fig. 31.4 Supports of a stone bridge.

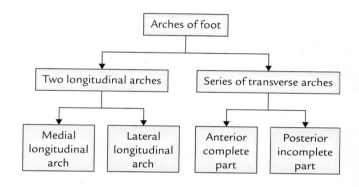

Flowchart 31.1 Classification of the arches of the foot.

During the standing position, the weight of the body is distributed among three points: (a) posteroinferior tuberosity of the calcaneum (heel), (b) head of first metatarsal, and (c) head of fifth metatarsal (Fig. 31.3).

The arches of the foot are present right from birth, but due to the presence of excessive subcutaneous fat in the soles, they are not apparent (i.e., masked) during infancy and childhood.

N.B.

- An arched foot is a distinctive feature of man, which distinguishes him from other primates.

Factors Maintaining the Arches of the Foot

The students can easily appreciate the factors maintaining the arches of the foot by applying the engineering device used to support a stone bridge. The devices used to support a stone bridge are (Fig. 31.4):

1. Shape of stones.
2. Intersegmental ties (staples).
3. Slings.
4. Tie beams.

TYPES OF ARCHES

There are two types of arches of the foot—longitudinal and transverse.

1. There are two longitudinal arches in each foot: (a) medial and (b) lateral.

2. There are a series of transverse arches in each foot. At the heads of metatarsals, the transverse arch is complete but posteriorly it forms a half dome, which is completed by its counterpart in the opposite foot. Thus, in the posterior part of the foot the transverse arch becomes complete when the both feet are held close to each other.

The classification of arches is summarized in Flowchart 31.1.

LONGITUDINAL ARCHES (Fig. 31.5)

Each longitudinal arch has: (a) two pillars, (b) a summit, and (c) joints.

Medial Longitudinal Arch (Fig. 31.5A and B)

The medial longitudinal arch is formed by the calcaneum, talus, navicular, three cuneiforms, and medial three metatarsals.

Pillars

1. The medial half of the calcaneum forms the **posterior pillar** of the medial longitudinal arch.
2. The heads of the medial three metatarsals form the **anterior pillar** of the medial longitudinal arch.

Summit

The talus lies at the summit of this arch. Therefore, the **talus is the keystone of this arch.**

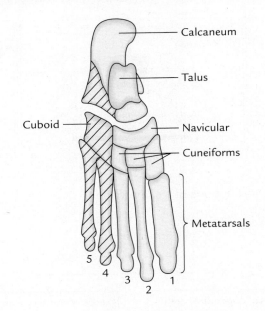

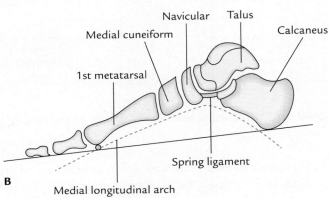

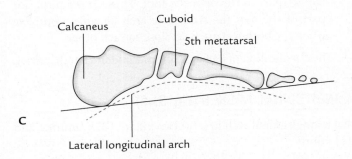

Fig. 31.5 Formation of the longitudinal arches of the foot: **A**, bones forming medial longitudinal arch are unhatched and bones forming lateral longitudinal arch are hatched. Note calcaneum is common to both but primarily it forms the lateral longitudinal arch; **B**, medial longitudinal arch—side view; **C**, lateral longitudinal arch—side view. Note the medial longitudinal arch is higher than the lateral arch. It is more pliant due to the presence of talocalcaneonavicular and subtalar joints. It is more involved in the propulsion, i.e., initiating the next step during walking.

Joints

The main joints of the medial longitudinal arch are talocalcaneonavicular and subtalar joints.

Lateral Longitudinal Arch

The lateral longitudinal arch is formed by the calcaneum cuboid and lateral two metatarsals. It is characteristically low and almost touches the ground (Fig. 31.5C). It is involved in receiving and supporting the body weight during walking and running.

Pillars

The **posterior pillar** of the lateral longitudinal arch is formed by the lateral tubercle of the calcaneum and the **anterior pillar** is formed by the heads of the lateral two metatarsals.

Summit

The summit of the lateral longitudinal arch lies at the level of articular facets on the superior surface of the calcaneum (i.e., at the level of subtalar joint).

Joints

The main joint of the lateral longitudinal arch is **calcaneocuboid joint**.

The lateral longitudinal arch being lower and less mobile than the medial longitudinal arch is adapted for transmission of weight and thrusts.

FACTORS MAINTAINING THE LONGITUDINAL ARCHES

A. Factors Maintaining the Medial Longitudinal Arch (Fig. 31.6)

Bones

The sustentaculum tali partly support the head of talus.

Ligaments

The important ligaments which help to maintain the medial longitudinal arch are: (a) plantar calcaneonavicular ligament (spring ligament) which provides dynamic support to the head of talus, (b) interosseous ligaments connecting the adjacent bones, and (c) interosseous talocalcanean ligament, connecting these bones. These ligaments act as **intersegmental ties**.

Muscles, tendons, and aponeurosis

1. **Acting as slings (i.e., suspending arch from above):** The tendon of **tibialis posterior** lying underneath the spring ligament provides dynamic supports to the head of talus and suspends the arch from above. In this endeavor, it is aptly supported by the tendons of flexor hallucis longus.

    The **flexor hallucis longus** is the bulkiest and strongest muscle to support the medial longitudinal arch. This muscle has three functions with respect to the medial longitudinal arch:

    (a) It stretches the arch like the string of a bow.

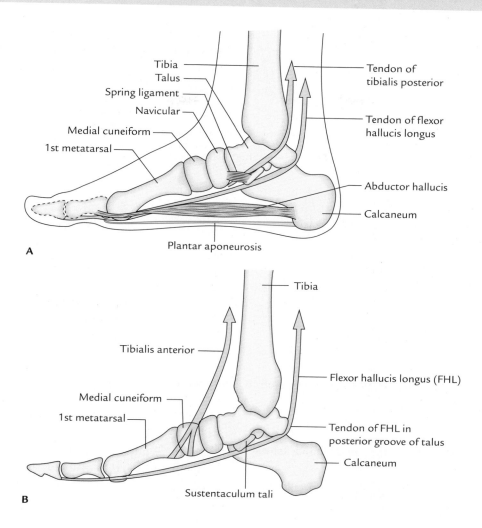

Fig. 31.6 Factors maintaining the medial longitudinal arch: **A**, supports of the head of talus; **B**, slings.

(b) It supports the calcaneus by passing underneath the sustentaculum tali.

(c) It supports the talus by passing along its posterior groove.

   The tendon of **tibialis anterior** also exerts a sling action.

2. **Acting as tie beams (i.e., structures which prevent separation of the pillars):** The medial part of the plantar aponeurosis and abductor hallucis assisted by the flexor hallucis brevis act as tie beam to maintain the height of the medial longitudinal arch.

B. Factors Maintaining the Lateral Longitudinal Arch
(Fig. 31.7)

Bones

The proper shaping of the distal end of calcaneus and proximal end of cuboid. The cuboid is the **keystone of longitudinal arch.**

Ligaments

The important ligaments which help to maintain the lateral longitudinal arch are as follows:

1. **Short plantar ligament:** The short plantar ligament is broad and thick. It lies deep to the long plantar ligament and supports the calcaneocuboid joint from below.

2. **Long plantar ligament:** The long plantar ligament is quite long and supports the joints between the calcaneum, cuboid, and related metatarsals.

   These ligaments act as **intersegmental ties.**

Muscles, tendons, and aponeurosis

1. **Acting as tie beams:** The lateral part of the **plantar aponeurosis** and the intrinsic muscles of the little toe (e.g., lateral part of the flexor digitorum brevis, abductor digiti minimi brevis, and flexor digiti minimi brevis) function as **tie beams** of this arch.

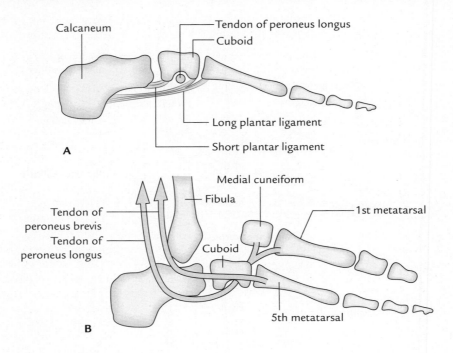

Fig. 31.7 Factors maintaining the lateral longitudinal arch: **A**, short and long plantar ligaments; **B**, tendons of the peroneus brevis and peroneus longus.

Table 31.1 Differences between the medial and lateral longitudinal arches

Medial longitudinal arch	Lateral longitudinal arch
• Formed by more bones and more joints	• Formed by less bones and less joints
• Characteristic feature is **resiliency**	• Characteristic feature is **rigidity**
• Higher and more mobile	• Lower and less mobile
• Involved in propulsion during locomotion (i.e., initiating the next step during walking)	• Involved in receiving and supporting the body weight
• Summit is formed by the talus	• Summit is formed by the calcaneum
• Main joint is talocalcaneonavicular joint (the most vulnerable part of the arch)	• Main joint is calcaneocuboid (the most vulnerable part of the arch)

2. **Acting as slings:** The **tendons of peroneus brevis** and **peroneus tertius**, which are inserted on the base of the fifth metatarsal, act as weak **slings** from above.

The **tendon of peroneus longus**, which grooves the plantar aspect of cuboid and courses transversely across the sole to be inserted on the base of first metatarsal and adjoining part of medial cuneiform, supports the cuboid bone from above through its **pulley-like action.**

The important differences between the medial and lateral longitudinal arches are given in Table 31.1.

TRANSVERSE ARCHES

Anterior Transverse Arch

The heads of the metatarsals form the **anterior transverse arch.** It is a complete arch because during standing position the heads of first and fifth metatarsals come into contact to the ground and form the two ends of the arch.

Posterior Transverse Arch

The posterior transverse arch is formed by greater parts of the tarsus and metatarsus. It is an incomplete arch because only its lateral end comes into contact with the ground during standing position. It forms only half of the dome in one foot. The complete dome is formed when the two feet are brought together (Fig. 31.8).

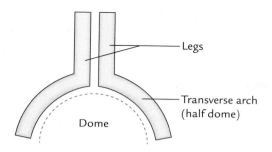

Fig. 31.8 Half dome of the transverse arch is completed when the two feet are kept together.

Factors Maintaining the Transverse Arches

Bones

Most of the tarsal and metatarsal bones have larger dorsal and smaller plantar surfaces (i.e., wedge-shaped), which help to form and maintain the concavity on the plantar aspect of the foot skeleton.

Ligaments

These are small ligaments, which bind together the cuneiform bones and metatarsals. Superficial and deep transverse metatarsal ligaments at the heads of metatarsals function as intersegmental ties to maintain the shallow arch at the heads of metatarsals.

Muscles and tendons

1. **Acting as tie beams:** The tendons of peroneus longus and tibialis posterior support the transverse arch as tie beam.
2. **Acting as slings:** The peroneus tertius and peroneus brevis on the lateral side and tibialis anterior on the medial side support the transverse arch as slings.
3. **Acting as intersegmental ties:** The dorsal interossei act as intersegmental ties.

FUNCTIONS OF THE ARCHES

The functions of the arches of the foot are as follows:

1. Distribute the body weight to the weight-bearing points of the sole (e.g., heel; balls of the toes, mainly those of first and fifth toes and lateral border of the sole).
2. Act as shock absorber during jumping by their spring-like action.
3. The medial longitudinal arch provides a propulsive force during locomotion.
4. The lateral longitudinal arch functions as a static organ of support and weight transmission.
5. The concavity of the arches protects the nerves and vessels of the sole.

- **Flat foot (pes planus):** The flat foot is the commonest of all foot problems. It occurs due to the collapse of medial longitudinal arch. During long periods of standing the plantar aponeurosis and spring ligament are overstretched. As a result, the support of the head of talus is lost and is pushed downward between the calcaneus and the navicular bones. This leads to flattening of the medial longitudinal arch with lateral deviation of the foot.

  The effects of the flat foot are:
  (a) The person usually has clumsy shuffling gait due to the loss of spring in the foot.
  (b) Makes the foot more liable to trauma due to loss of the shock absorbing function.
  (c) The compression of the nerves and vessels of the sole is due to the loss of concavity of the sole.

  The compression of the communication between the medial and lateral plantar nerves leads to neuralgic pain in the forefoot (**metatarsalgia**).

- **High arched foot (pes cavus):** The exaggeration of the longitudinal arch of the foot causes *pes cavus*. This usually occurs because of a contracture (plantar flexion) at the transverse tarsal joint. When the patient walks with a high arched foot there is dorsiflexion of the metatarsophalangeal joints and the plantar flexion of the interphalangeal joints of the toes.

- **Club foot/Talipes:** (Latin *talipes* 5 clubfoot). The club foot may be congenital or acquired. There are five types of clubfoot as under:
  (a) **Talipes equinus (horse like):** In this condition, the foot is plantar flexed and person walks on the toes with heel raised.
  (b) **Talipes calcaneus:** In this condition, the person walks on the heel with forefoot raised.
  (c) **Talipes varus:** In this condition, the foot is inverted and adducted. The person walks on the outer border of the foot.
  (d) **Talipes valgus:** In this condition, the foot is everted and abducted. The person walks on the inner border of his foot.
  (e) **Talipes equinovarus:** It is the commonest deformity of the foot. In this condition, the foot is inverted, adducted, and plantar flexed.

- **Hallux valgus:** In this condition, the big toe is deviated laterally at the metatarsophalangeal joint. It usually occurs due to constant wearing of pointed shoes with high heel. The head of the first metatarsal bone becomes prominent and rubs on the shoe. This leads to the formation of protective **adventitious bursa** called **bunion** on the medial side of the big toe.

- **Hammer toe:** It is a deformity of the toe in which metatarsophalangeal and distal interphalangeal joints are hyper-extended but the proximal interphalangeal joint is acutely flexed. This deformity usually affects the 2nd and 3rd toes.

Golden Facts to Remember

➤ Most important factors in maintaining the transverse arch of the foot	Tendons of peroneus longus and tibialis posterior
➤ Primary weight bearing point of the foot when standing	Posteroinferior tuberosity of the calcaneum
➤ Most vulnerable part of the medial longitudinal arch	Talocalcaneonavicular joint
➤ Most vulnerable part of the lateral longitudinal arch	Calcaneocuboid joint
➤ Keystone of medial longitudinal arch	Talus
➤ Keystone of lateral longitudinal arch	Cuboid
➤ Most pronounced site of the transverse arch	Middle of the metatarsals
➤ Commonest deformity of the foot	Talipes equinovarus
➤ Rocker-bottom foot	Plantar concavity is replaced by plantar convexity (e.g., in trisomy 18, or in Edward syndrome)

Clinical Case Study

A 20-year-old healthy individual went for recruitment in the Army. He fulfilled all the physical requirements except that he was having flat feet. Consequently he was rejected.

Questions

1. What is flat foot (pes planus)?
2. Give the anatomical basis of the collapse of the medial longitudinal arch.
3. What is the keystone of the medial longitudinal arch?
4. What are the effects of flat foot?
5. Define inversion and eversion, and name the joints where these movements take place.

Answers

1. It is a condition in which there is a collapse of the medial longitudinal arch.

2. (a) The loss of support to the head of talus, for details see page 437.
    (b) Overstretching of ligaments supporting the medial longitudinal arch (e.g., spring ligament, short and long plantar ligaments, and plantar aponeurosis).
3. Talus.
4. See page 437.
5. (a) *Inversion* is the movement in which the medial margin of the foot is raised and the sole faces medially.
    Eversion is the movement in which the lateral margin of the foot is raised and the sole faces laterally.
    (b) Movements of inversion and eversion take place at subtalar, talocalcaneonavicular, and midtarsal joints.

Joints of the Lower Limb

The joints of the lower limb include:

1. Hip joint.
2. Knee joint.
3. Tibiofibular joints.
4. Ankle joint.
5. Foot joints.

The hip joint is already described in detail in Chapter 26. The remaining joints are described in this chapter.

KNEE JOINT

The knee joint is the largest and most complicated joint in the body. It is the major weight-bearing joint in the body. It is prone to undergo degenerative changes with advanced age leading to osteoarthritis. Hence it should be studied thoroughly.

TYPE

It is a synovial joint of **modified hinge** variety. It is not a typical hinge joint because it undergoes some degree of automatic (conjunct) rotation during flexion and extension of the knee.

Actually, it is a compound joint consisting of three articulations: right and left *condylar joints* between the condyles of the femur and tibia, and one *saddle joint* between the femur and patella (Figs 32.1 and 32.2).

ARTICULAR SURFACES (Figs 32.1–32.3)

The articular surfaces of the knee joints are:

1. Articular surfaces of medial and lateral condyles of the femur.
2. Trochlear surface of the femur.
3. Articular surface of the patella.
4. Articular surfaces of medial and lateral condyles of the tibia.

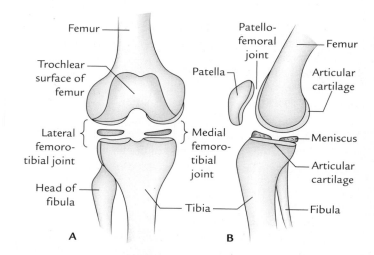

Fig. 32.1 Three primitive joints included in the knee joint: A, condylar type of medial and lateral femorotibial joints; B, saddle type of patellofemoral joint.

The articular surfaces of the knee joints are described in detail in the following text:

1. *Articular surfaces of medial and lateral condyles of the femur occupy the anterior, inferior, and posterior surfaces of these condyles respectively.* They are convex anteroposteriorly and from side to side. The medial condylar surface is longer anteroposteriorly and narrower or mediolaterally than that of lateral condyle. Anteriorly they are continuous with each other through trochlear surface of the femur but posteriorly they are separated from each other by an intercondylar notch.
2. *Trochlear surface of the femur* is located on the anterior aspect of the lower end of the femur. It articulates with the posterior surface of the patella. It is pulley-shaped, consisting of medial and lateral sloping surfaces meeting with each other in a median vertical groove. The lateral sloping surface is longer than that of medial.

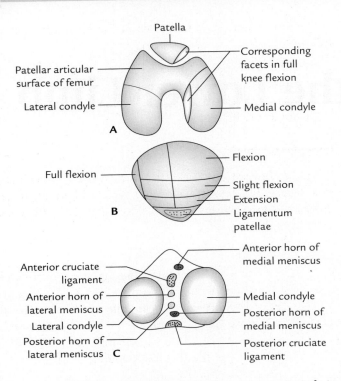

Fig. 32.2 Articular surfaces of the knee joint: **A**, inferior aspect of the patella and lower end of the femur; **B**, posterior aspect of the patella; **C**, superior aspect of the tibia.

3. *Articular surface of the patella is* on the posterior aspect of patella and articulates with the trochlear surface of the femur. It has a larger lateral area and a smaller medial area.

   Near the medial margin of patella, there is a narrow semilunar strip which comes in contact with a similar strip on the medial condyle of femur in full flexion.

4. Articular surfaces of the medial and lateral condyles of tibia are on the upper surfaces of these condyles. They are separated from each other by a rough intercondylar area.

   • The articular surface on medial tibial condyle is oval and larger. Its anteroposterior diameter is more than the transverse diameter.

   • The articular surface on the lateral tibial condyle is circular.

The articular surfaces on the upper surfaces of the medial and lateral condyles of the tibia are slightly concave centrally and flat at the periphery where they are covered by the corresponding menisci.

STABILITY OF THE KNEE JOINT

Structurally, the knee joint is relatively weak because of the incongruence of its articular surfaces. The tibial condyles are

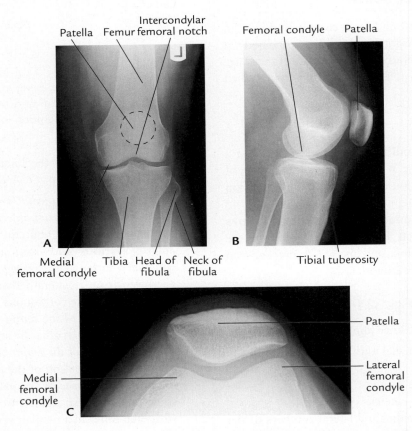

Fig. 32.3 Radiograph of the knee joint: **A**, AP view; **B**, lateral view; **C**, sky view. (*Source:* Fig. 8.2, Page 220, *Integrated Anatomy*, Heylings, David JA; Spence, Roy JA; Kelly, Barry E. Oxford: Churchill Livingstone, 2007, All rights reserved.)

too small and shallow to hold the large convex femoral condyles. The femoropatellar articulation is also not quite stable because of their shallow articular surfaces and due to an outward angulation between the long axes of the femur and tibia.

Factors Maintaining the Stability of the Knee Joint
The stability of the knee joint is maintained by the following factors:

1. Strength and actions of the surrounding muscles and tendons.
2. Medial and lateral collateral ligaments maintain side-to-side stability.
3. Cruciate ligaments maintain anteroposterior stability.
4. Iliotibial tract helps in stabilizing a partly flexed knee.

LIGAMENTS

The important ligaments of the knee joint are as follows (Fig. 32.4):

1. Capsular ligament.
2. Ligamentum patellae.
3. Tibial and fibular collateral ligaments.
4. Anterior and posterior cruciate ligaments.
5. Medial and lateral menisci.

The other secondary ligaments of the knee joint are as follows:

1. Oblique popliteal ligament.
2. Arcuate popliteal ligament.
3. Transverse ligament.
4. Coronary ligaments.

Capsular Ligament

It is a thin **fibrous sac** (Fig. 32.4) which surrounds the joint. It is deficient anteriorly, where it is replaced by the patella, quadriceps femoris, medial and lateral patellar retinacula, and ligamentum patellae.

Femoral attachment
It is attached about 1/2 to 1 cm beyond the articular margins with the following three special features.
Anteriorly it is deficient in the middle where it is pierced by the suprapatellar bursa.
Posteriorly it is attached to the intercondylar line.
Laterally it encloses the origin of popliteus.

Tibial attachment
It is attached about 1/2 to 1 cm beyond the articular margins with the following three special features.

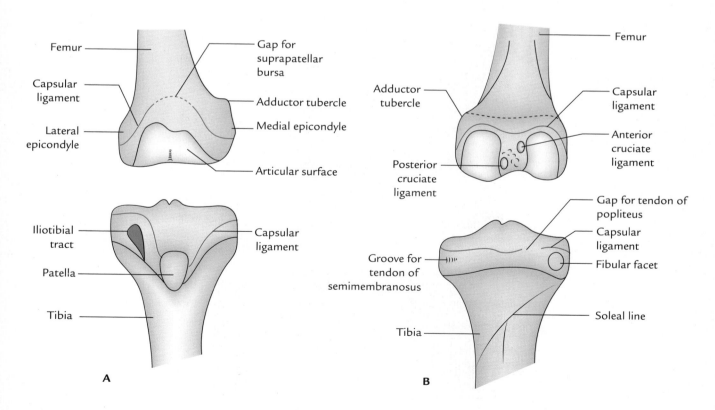

Fig. 32.4 Attachment of capsular ligament of the knee joint: A, anterior aspects of the femur and tibia; B, posterior aspects of the femur and tibia. The arrows indicate gaps in the capsule.

Anteriorly it descends along the margins of the condyles to tibial tuberosity, *where it is deficient* for the attachment of the ligamentum patellae.

Posteriorly it presents a gap behind the lateral condyle for the passage of the tendon of popliteus muscle.

Synovial Membrane

The synovial membrane (Fig. 32.5) lines the inner aspect of the fibrous capsule and the portions of the bones enclosed within it but ceases at the periphery of the articular cartilages the medial and lateral menisci.

In front above the patella, it is prolonged as *suprapatellar bursa,* and below the patella, it covers the deep surface of the infrapatellar pad of fat, which separates it from the ligamentum patellae. The apex of suprapatellar bursa is attached to the *articularis genu muscle.*

A median triangular fold of the synovial membrane called **infrapatellar fold** extends upward and backward from the fat pad to the intercondylar fossa of the femur.

The lateral margins of the infrapatellar synovial fold are free and form the *alar folds,* which contain the fibrofatty tissue.

From the posterior aspect of the fibrous capsule, the synovial membrane projects forward in the intercondylar region as cul-de-sac to envelope the sides of both cruciate ligaments and in front of the anterior cruciate ligament.

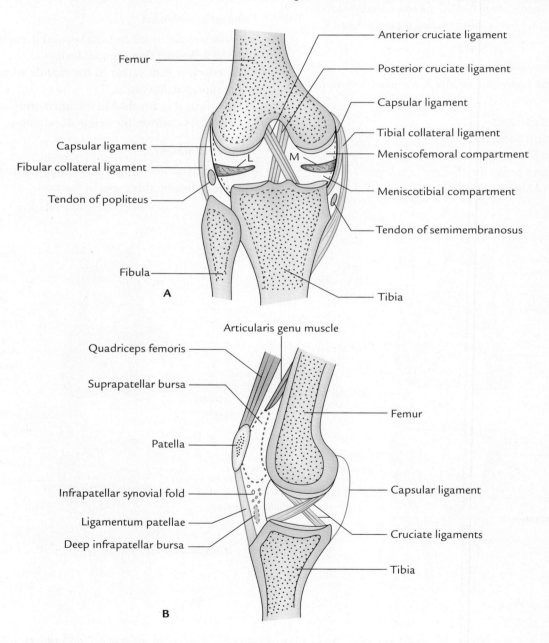

Fig. 32.5 Knee joint: **A**, coronal section; **B**, sagittal section (L = lateral meniscus, M = medial meniscus).

Ligamentum Patellae

It is actually the tendon of insertion of quadriceps femoris, which extends from the apex of the patella to the upper part of the tibial tuberosity.

Ligamentum patellae is about 7.5 cm long and 2.5 cm broad. It is *attached above to the margins and rough posterior surface of the apex of patella, and below it is attached to the smooth, upper part of tibial tuberosity*. It is related to the subcutaneous and deep infrapatellar bursae, and infrapatellar pad of fat.

Tibial (Medial) Collateral Ligament (Fig. 32.6A)

It is a strong, long (about 10 cm), thick, and flat band of fibrous tissue. It consists of **superficial and deep parts**. Both parts are attached above to the medial epicondyle of the femur just below the adductor tubercle.

The **superficial part** of the ligament is long and attached below to the upper part of the medial border and adjoining posterior part of the medial surface of the tibia. It covers the inferior medial genicular nerve and vessels, and anterior part of the tendon of semimembranosus. The tendons of sartorius, gracilis, and semitendinosus cross its lower part superficially.

The deep part of the ligament is short and blends with the fibrous capsule, and with the peripheral margin of the medial meniscus. It is attached below to the medial condyle of the tibia above the groove for the tendon of semimembranosus.

Fibular (Lateral) Collateral Ligament (Fig. 32.6B)

It is short (about 5 cm long) and cord-like ligament. Above it is attached to the lateral epicondyle of the femur just above the popliteal groove. Below it is embraced by the tendon of biceps femoris and attached to the head of fibula in front of its apex. Its deep surface is not adherent to the fibrous capsule. It is separated from the capsule and lateral meniscus by the tendon of popliteus. Its lower part is separated from the capsule by the *inferior lateral genicular nerve and vessels*.

N.B.

- Morphologically, the medial collateral ligament represents the degenerated tendon of insertion of the ischial head of the adductor magnus, and fibular ligament represents the degenerated tendon of the peroneus longus.
- The medial collateral ligament is much thicker and stronger than the lateral collateral ligament because the knee joint gaps more on the medial side, hence the need for stronger stabilization on that side.

Cruciate Ligaments

These are two thick, strong fibrous bands, which act as direct bonds of union between the femur and tibia. They are present inside the knee joint. They represent the collateral ligaments of the primitive femorotibial joints. They maintain anteroposterior stability of the knee joint. They are named anterior and posterior according to their site of attachment to the tibia. The cruciate ligaments are intracapsular but extrasynovial.

The ligaments cross each other like the letter "X" hence the name cruciate.

Anterior Cruciate Ligament

The anterior cruciate ligament is attached below to the anterior part of the intercondylar area of the tibia. It runs upward, backward, and laterally and is attached to the

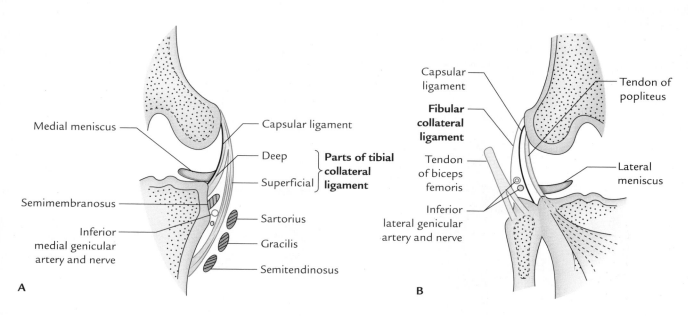

Fig. 32.6 Attachments and relations of collateral ligaments of the knee joint: **A,** tibial (medial) collateral ligament; **B,** fibular (lateral) collateral ligament.

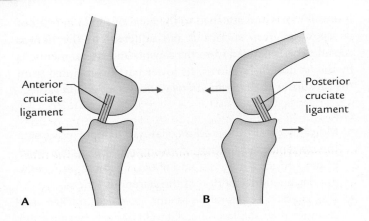

Fig. 32.7 Anterior and posterior cruciate ligaments. Note anterior cruciate ligament is taut during knee extension and posterior cruciate ligament during knee flexion.

posterior part of the medial surface of the lateral condyle of femur. *It is taut during extension of the knee and prevents the posterior dislocation of femur on tibia and anterior dislocation of tibia on femur* (Fig. 32.7A).

Posterior Cruciate Ligament

The posterior cruciate ligament is attached below to the posterior part of the intercondylar area of the tibia. It runs upward, forward, and medially and is attached to the anterior part of the lateral surface of the medial condyle of the femur. *It is taut during flexion of the knee and prevents the anterior dislocation of femur on tibia and posterior dislocation of tibia on femur* (Fig. 32.7B).

Medial and Lateral Menisci (Semilunar Cartilages, Fig. 32.8)

These two crescent-shaped intra-articular discs are made up of fibrocartilage. They have thick peripheral border and thin

inner border. They deepen the articular surfaces of the condyles of tibia, and partially divide the joint cavity into the upper (meniscofemoral) and lower (meniscotibial) compartments. Flexion and extension of the knee take place in the upper compartment, whereas the rotation of the knee occurs in the lower compartment.

Each meniscus has: (a) *two ends* (anterior and posterior), which are attached to tibia; *two borders*—the thick outer border is fixed to the fibrous capsule and the thin inner border which is free; and (b) *two thin surfaces*—the upper surface is concave for the femur; the lower surface is flat for the peripheral 2/3rd of tibial condyles.

Medial Meniscus

It is nearly semilunar in shape and wider behind than in front. It presents anterior posterior ends or horns, which are attached to the intercondylar area of the tibia. It is adherent to the deep part of tibial collateral ligament. It is firmly attached to the tibial plateau by coronary ligaments.

Lateral Meniscus

It is nearly circular in shape with more or less a uniform width. It also presents anterior and posterior horns, which are also attached to the intercondylar area of the tibia.

The posterior horn of the lateral meniscus is attached to the medial condyle of femur by the anterior and posterior **meniscofemoral ligaments**. The anterior meniscofemoral ligament (**ligament of Humphrey**) passes in front of the posterior cruciate ligament whereas the posterior meniscofemoral ligament (**ligament of Wrisberg**) passes behind the posterior cruciate ligament.

These ligaments play an important role in regulating the movements of lateral meniscus during the extension of the knee joint.

The lateral meniscus is attached to the medial part of the tendon of popliteus and thus the mobility of its posterior horn is controlled by the popliteus and two meniscofemoral ligaments.

The differences between medial and lateral menisci are given in Table 32.1.

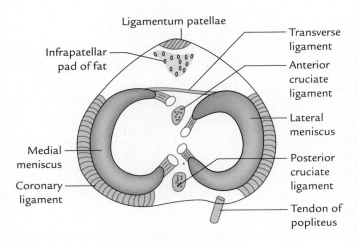

Fig. 32.8 Medial and lateral menisci of the knee joint.

Table 32.1 Differences between the medial and lateral menisci

Medial meniscus	Lateral meniscus
• C-shaped/semilunar in shape	• "O"-shaped/circular in shape
• Attached to the medial collateral ligament	• Attached to the tendon popliteus muscle
• More prone to injury	• Less prone to injury

Functions of the menisci

These are as follows:

1. The menisci increase the concavities of the tibial condyles for better congruence with the femoral condyles.
2. They act as swabs to lubricate the joint cavity.
3. They act as shock absorber to protect the articular cartilage during weight transmission.
4. They adapt to the varying curvatures of the different parts of the femoral condyles.

Clinical correlation

Meniscal tears: The *injuries to menisci* are commonly caused by the twisting strains in a slightly flexed knee, as in kicking a football. The meniscus may get separated from the capsule, or it may be torn longitudinally (**bucket-handle tear**) or transversely.

The medial meniscus is more prone to injury than the lateral because of its firm fixity to tibial collateral ligament, and greater excursion during the rotatory movements. The lateral meniscus is protected by the popliteus muscle because its medial fibres pulls the posterior horn of meniscus backward, so that it is not crushed between the articular surfaces.

Pain on the medial rotation of tibia on the femur indicates injury of the medial meniscus; while pain on the lateral rotation of tibia on the femur indicates injury of the lateral meniscus.

Oblique Popliteal Ligament

It is an expansion from the tendon of semimembranosus muscle. It runs upward and laterally superficial to the capsule to be attached to the intercondylar line of the femur. It blends with and strengthens the capsule of knee joint posteriorly. It

is intimately related to the popliteal artery and pierced by: (a) middle genicular nerve, (b) middle genicular vessels, and (c) posterior division of the obturator nerve.

Arcuate Popliteal Ligament

It is a Y-shaped fibrous band. The stem of the band is attached to the styloid process of the fibula. The large posterior or limb of the band arches over the tendon of popliteus and is attached to the posterior border of the intercondylar area of the tibia. The small anterior limb (often deficient) passes deep to the fibular collateral ligament and is attached to the lateral condyle of the femur.

Transverse Ligament

It extends transversely and connects the anterior ends of the medial and lateral menisci. It is present only in about 40% of the individuals.

Coronary Ligaments

They are parts of the fibrous capsule, which provide attachment to the peripheral margins of the medial and lateral menisci to the tibia.

BURSAE AROUND THE KNEE (Fig. 32.9)

There are about 12 bursae around the knee, four anterior, three lateral, three medial, and two posterior.

Anterior Bursae

These are:

1. **Subcutaneous prepatellar bursa (bursa of housemaid's knee).** It lies deep to the skin in front of lower half of the

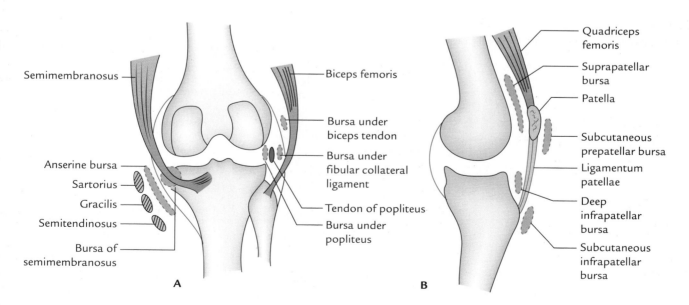

Fig. 32.9 Bursae around the knee joint: A, bursae on the medial and lateral aspects of the knee; B, bursae on the front of the knee.

patella and upper half of the ligamentum patellae and tibial tuberosity.

2. **Subcutaneous infrapatellar bursa** between the skin and smooth lower part of the tibial tuberosity.

3. **Deep infrapatellar bursa**, between ligamentum patellae and tibial tuberosity.

4. **Suprapatellar bursa** between the anterior surface of lower part of the femur and deep surface of the quadriceps femoris.

Lateral Bursae

These are:

1. The bursa between the fibular collateral ligament and tendon of biceps femoris.

2. The bursa between the fibular collateral ligament and tendon of popliteus.

3. The bursa between the tendon of popliteus and lateral condyle of femur. This bursa is really a synovial tube around the tendon of popliteus; hence it communicates with the joint cavity.

Medial Bursae

These are:

1. The bursa, which separates the tendons of sartorius, gracilis, and semitendinosus from each other and from the tibial collateral ligament (**bursa anserine**).

2. The bursa between the tendon of semimembranosus and medial collateral ligament.

3. The bursa between the tendon of semimembranosus and medial condyle of the tibia. It may communicate with the knee joint.

Posterior Bursae

These are:

1. The bursa between the lateral head of gastrocnemius and capsule of the joint.

2. The bursa between the medial head of gastrocnemius and capsule of the joint (**Brodie's bursa**).

RELATIONS OF THE KNEE JOINT (Fig. 32.10)

They are as follows:

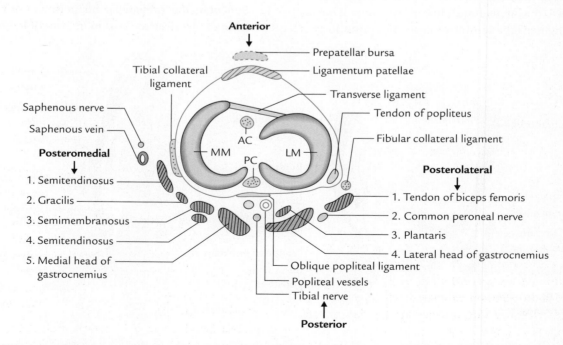

Fig. 32.10 Relations of the knee joint (transverse section of right knee joint) (MM = medial meniscus, LM = lateral meniscus, AC = anterior cruciate ligament, PC = posterior cruciate ligament).

Anteriorly: Tendon of the quadriceps femoris, patella, ligamentum patellae, patellar plexus of the nerves, and prepatellar synovial bursa.
Anteromedially: Medial patellar retinaculum.
Anterolaterally: Lateral patellar retinaculum and iliotibial tract.
Posteriorly: Popliteal vessels, tibial nerve, and oblique popliteal ligament.
Posterolaterally: In the upper part, tendon of biceps femoris and common peroneal nerve; in the lower part, lateral head of gastrocnemius and plantaris.
Posteromedially: In the upper part, sartorius, gracilis, semimembranosus, and semitendinosus.

In the lower part, medial head of gastrocnemius and popliteus.

BLOOD SUPPLY

The knee joint is richly supplied by the blood through the arterial anastomosis around the knee, which is formed by: (a) five genicular branches of popliteal artery, (b) descending genicular branch of femoral artery, (c) descending branch of the lateral circumflex femoral artery, (d) two recurrent branches of the anterior tibial artery, and (e) circumflex fibular branch of the posterior tibial artery.

NERVE SUPPLY

The knee joint has rich nerve supply by:

(a) *Femoral nerve* through its branches to vasti, especially to vastus medialis.
(b) *Tibial and common peroneal nerves* through their genicular branches.
(c) *Obturator nerve* through its posterior division.

MOVEMENTS

The following movements occur at the knee joints:

1. Flexion
2. Extension } Main/active movements.
3. Medial rotation
4. Lateral rotation } Conjunct movements.

Flexion and Extension

These movements occur in the upper meniscofemoral compartment of the joint, i.e., above the menisci.

In flexion the angle between the posterior thigh and leg is decreased whereas in extension the angle between the posterior thigh and leg is increased (i.e., return from the flexion back to the anatomical position).

The movements of the flexion and extension at knee differ from ordinary hinge movements in following two ways:

(a) The *transverse axis* around which these movements takes place is not fixed (e.g., during extension the axis moves forward and upward and during flexion it moves backward and downward).

(b) During these movements, there is an **automatic (conjunct) rotation** of the knee (viz., medial rotation of the femur during last 30° of extension; and lateral rotation of the femur during initial stages of the flexion). When foot is off the ground, tibia rotates instead of femur but in the opposite direction.

Medial and Lateral Rotation

These movements take place in the lower meniscotibial compartment of the joint, i.e., below the menisci. These movements occur around the vertical axis.

The medial and lateral rotations usually occur with flexion and extension (**conjunct rotations**) but may occur independently if the knee is flexed (**adjunct rotations**).

The conjunct rotations play an important role in locking and unlocking of the knee.

N.B. Locking and unlocking of the knee:

(a) **Locking of the knee:** When the foot is on the ground, the locking is defined as the medial rotation of femur on the tibia during the terminal phase of extension of the knee. When the knee is locked it becomes absolutely rigid and all the ligaments of the joint are taut. This is known as "screw home mechanism".

(b) **Unlocking of the knee:** When the foot is on the ground, the unlocking is defined as the lateral rotation of the femur on the tibia during initial phase of the flexion. The unlocking is brought about by the popliteus muscle. When the knee is unlocked, it can be further flexed by the hamstring muscles.

The locking of knee is essential for bearing load during erect posture. The locked joint must be unlocked to facilitate progress of locomotion. Hence, during locomotion locking and unlocking of the knee takes place alternatively and rhythmically.

The differences between the locking and unlocking of the knee are as summarized in the box below:

Locking of the knee joint	Unlocking of the knee joint
• Medial rotation of the femur on tibia during terminal phase of extension	• Lateral rotation of the femur on tibia during initial phase of the flexion
• It is brought about by quadriceps femoris	• It is brought about by the popliteus muscle
• Locked knee becomes absolutely rigid	• Unlocked knee can be further flexed
• All ligaments are taut	• All ligaments are relaxed

Table 32.2 Movements of the knee joint

Movements	Muscles producing movements	
	Chief muscles	**Accessory muscles**
Flexion	• Semimembranosus • Semitendinosus • Biceps femoris	• Popliteus (initiates flexion) • Sartorius • Gracilis • Gastrocnemius • Plantaris
Extension	Quadriceps femoris	Tensor fasciae latae
Medial rotation	• Semitendinosus • Semimembranosus • Popliteus	• Sartorius • Gracilis
Lateral rotation	Biceps femoris	• Gluteus maximus • Tensor fasciae latae

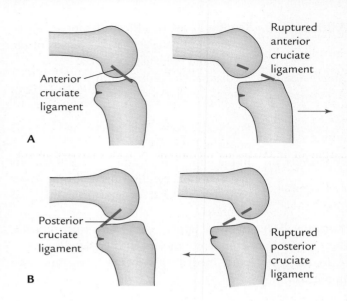

Fig. 32.11 Injury of cruciate ligaments of the knee joint: A, rupture of anterior cruciate ligament (positive anterior Drawer's sign); B, rupture of the posterior cruciate ligament (positive posterior Drawer's sign).

The movements of the knee joint and muscles producing them are given in Table 32.2.

N.B. The range of motion (ROM) of flexion is 130° whereas the range of motion of extension is 0–50°.

The ROM for flexion is greater when the hip joint is fixed. The ROM for extension is greater when the hip is extended and limited when the hip is flexed.

Clinical correlation

• **Osteoarthritis:** Being a weight-bearing joint, the knee joint is commonly involved in *osteoarthritis* (degenerative wear and tear of articular cartilages). The movements may be painful, limited, and produce grating. Radiographs of the knee region reveal osteophytes, i.e., peripheral lipping of the articular ends.

• **Injuries to cruciate ligaments (Fig. 32.11):** *The anterior cruciate ligament is more commonly damaged than the posterior ligament.* The anterior cruciate ligament is injured in the anterior dislocation of the tibia; whereas, the posterior ligament is injured in the posterior dislocation of the tibia. Tear of the cruciate ligaments leads to abnormal anteroposterior mobility.

  If the anterior cruciate ligament is torn the tibia is pulled excessively forward on the femur (**anterior drawer sign**) and if the posterior cruciate ligament is torn the tibia is pulled excessively backward (**posterior drawer sign**; Fig 32.11).

• **Aspiration of the knee joint:** The collections of fluid are common in the knee joint. It gives rise to swelling above and at the sides of the patella. In such cases, patellar tap often demonstrates a floating patella. Aspiration of the fluid can be done on either side of the ligamentum patellae. But the joint is usually approached from its lateral side using three bony points as landmarks for the needle insertion: (a) tibial tuberosity, (b) lateral epicondyle of the femur, and (c) apex of patella. This triangular area is also used for drug injection in treating the knee pathology.

• **Arthroscopy of the knee joint:** It is an endoscopic examination (visualization) of the interior of the knee joint cavity with minimal disruption of the tissues. The ligament repair or replacement can also be performed by using an *arthroscope*.

• **Knee replacement:** If the knee joint is badly damaged by the osteoarthritis, an artificial joint consisting of plastic tibial component and metal femoral component is connected to the tibial and femoral bone ends after removal of the damaged areas.

• **Unhappy triad of the knee joint:** A combination of injury of the (a) tibial collateral ligament, (b) medial meniscus, and (c) anterior cruciate ligament is called "unhappy triad" of the knee joint.

TIBIOFIBULAR JOINTS

There are three joints between the tibia and fibula: (a) superior tibiofibular, (b) middle tibiofibular, and (c) inferior tibiofibular.

SUPERIOR TIBIOFIBULAR JOINT

The **superior tibiofibular joint** is a small plane type of synovial joint between the head of fibula and the lateral condyle of tibia. It may communicate with the knee joint through the popliteal bursa. It permits some gliding or rotatory movements for adjusting the lateral malleolus during movements at the ankle joint (e.g., during dorsiflexion).

MIDDLE TIBIOFIBULAR JOINT

The **middle tibiofibular joint** is a fibrous joint formed by the interosseous membrane connecting the interosseous borders of the shafts of tibia and fibula. Its fibres are directed downward and laterally. It is wide above and narrow below where it blends with the **interosseous ligament of the inferior tibiofibular joint.** A large opening above the upper free margin of interosseous membrane provides passage to the anterior tibial vessels. The interosseous membrane presents a small opening near its lower end for the passage of perforating branch of the peroneal artery.

Functions of the interosseous membrane
These are:

1. Provides additional surface for the attachment of muscles.
2. Binds tibia and fibula.
3. Resists downward movement of fibula by the powerful fibular muscles.

N.B. Most fibres of the interosseous membrane (vide supra) are directed downward and laterally except in the upper part where they are directed downward and medially.

INFERIOR TIBIOFIBULAR JOINT

The **inferior tibiofibular joint** is a *syndesmosis* variety of the fibrous joint. *It is the strongest of all the three tibiofibular joints, because the strength of ankle joint largely depends upon its integrity.*

The roughened opposed surfaces of the lower ends of tibia and fibula are connected by a very strong *interosseous ligament*, which forms the chief bond of union between the lower ends of these bones. The interosseous ligament is covered both in front and behind by the *anterior and posterior tibiofibular ligaments*, respectively. The posterior tibiofibular ligament is stronger than the anterior tibiofibular ligament. Its lower and deep portion forms the *inferior transverse tibiofibular ligament*, which is a strong thick band of yellowish elastic fibres passing transversely from the upper part of malleolar fossa to the posterior border of the articular surface of tibia. It accentuates the concavity of the tibiofibular mortise of the ankle joint.

The inferior tibiofibular joint permits slight movements, to allow the lateral malleolus to rotate laterally during dorsiflexion of the ankle.

A brief comparison of the superior, middle, and inferior tibiofibular joints is given in Table 32.3.

ANKLE JOINT (TALOCRURAL JOINT)

The ankle joint is a strong weight-bearing joint of the lower limb (Fig. 32.12).

TYPE

It is a synovial joint of hinge variety.

ARTICULAR SURFACES (Fig. 32.13)

1. **Proximal articular surface** of the ankle joint is formed by the articular facets of the:
   (a) Lower end of tibia including its medial malleolus.
   (b) Lateral malleolus.
   (c) Inferior transverse tibiofibular ligament.

   These three together form a deep **tibiofibular socket** (also called "**tibiofibular mortise**").

2. **Distal articular surface** of the ankle joint is formed by the: articular facets on the upper, medial, and lateral aspects of the body of the talus.

Table 32.3 Comparison of the superior, middle, and inferior tibiofibular joints

Superior tibiofibular joint	Middle tibiofibular joint	Inferior tibiofibular joint
Plane type of the synovial joint	Fibrous joint	Syndesmosis variety of the fibrous joint
Formed by articulation between the oval articular facet on the lateral condyle of tibia and similar facet on the head of fibula	Formed by the union of interosseous border of tibia and fibula by an interosseous membrane	Formed by the union of rough triangular surface of the lower ends of tibia and fibula by a strong interosseous, and anterior and posterior tibiofibular ligaments
Permits some gliding movements	Permits rotation of fibula during dorsiflexion of the knee	Accentuates the "*tibiofibular mortise*," and allows lateral rotation of the lateral malleolus during dorsiflexion
Innervated by the nerve to popliteus and recurrent genicular nerve	Innervated by the nerve to popliteus	Innervated by the deep peroneal, tibial, and saphenous nerves

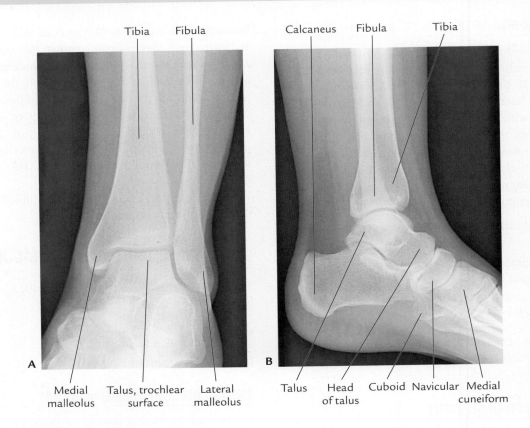

Fig. 32.12 Radiograph of the ankle joint: **A**, AP view; **B**, side view. (*Source:* Fig. 8.4, Page 222, *Integrated Anatomy*, Heylings, David JA; Spence, Roy JA; Kelly, Barry E. Oxford: Churchill Livingstone, 2007, All rights reserved.)

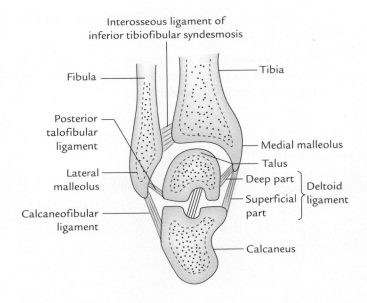

Fig. 32.13 Articular surfaces of the ankle and talocalcanean joints.

The body of talus presents three articular surfaces:

(a) Superior pulley-shaped articular surface (trochlear surface).

(b) Medial comma-shaped articular surface.

(c) Lateral triangular articular surface.

The wedge-shaped body of the talus fits into the socket above.

The articular surface on the inferior aspect of the lower end of tibia articulates with trochlear surface of the talus. The articular surface on the lateral aspect of medial malleolus articulates with the comma-shaped articular surface on the medial side of the talus. The articular surface on the medial aspect of lateral malleolus articulates with the large triangular articular surface on the lateral side of the body of talus.

N.B. The ankle joint resembles a pincer or monkey wrench gripping a section of hemisphere. (cf. tibiofibular mortise gripping the wedge-shaped body of the talus.)

STABILITY OF THE ANKLE JOINT

The trochlear surface on the superior aspect of the body of talus is wider in front than behind.

During dorsiflexion, ankle joint of the anterior wider part of the trochlea moves posteriorly and fits properly into the tibiofibular mortise (pincer), hence joint is stable. During plantar flexion, the narrow posterior part of the trochlea does not fit properly in the tibiofibular mortise (pincer), hence the joint is unstable during plantar flexion.

Factors Maintaining the Stability of the Ankle Joint

1. Close interlocking of its articular surfaces.
2. Strong, medial, and lateral collateral ligaments.
3. Deepening of tibiofibular socket posteriorly by the inferior transverse tibiofibular ligament.
4. Tendons (four in front and five behind) crossing the ankle joint.
5. Other ligaments of this joint.

LIGAMENTS

The important ligaments of ankle joint are:

1. Capsular ligament.
2. Medial and lateral collateral ligaments.

Fibrous Capsule

It surrounds the joint completely. It is attached to the articular margins of the joint all around with two exceptions:

Posterosuperiorly it is attached to the inferior transverse tibiofibular ligament.

Anteroinferiorly it is attached to the dorsum of the neck of talus at some distance from the trochlear surface.

The joint capsule is thin in front and behind to allow hinge movements and thick on either side where it blends with the collateral ligaments.

The **synovial membrane** lines the inner surface of the joint capsule, but ceases at the periphery of the articular cartilages. A small synovial process extends upward into the inferior tibiofibular syndesmosis.

Deltoid or Medial Ligament (Fig. 32.14A)

The deltoid ligament is a very strong triangular ligament on the medial side of the ankle. It is divided into two parts: superficial and deep. Above, both the parts have a common attachment to the apex and margins of the medial malleolus. Below, the attachment of superficial and deep parts differs as under:

Superficial part: Its fibres are divided into three parts: anterior, middle, and posterior.

(a) Anterior fibres (*tibionavicular*) are attached to the tuberosity of navicular bone and the medial margin of spring ligament.
(b) Middle fibres (*tibiocalcanean*) are attached to the whole length of sustentaculum tali.
(c) Posterior fibres (*posterior tibiotalar*) to the medial tubercle and adjoining part of the medial surface of talus.

Deep part (*anterior tibiotalar*) is attached to the anterior part of the medial surface of talus.

Lateral Ligament (Fig. 32.14B)

The lateral ligament consists of three parts: anterior talofibular, posterior talofibular, and calcaneofibular.

1. *Anterior talofibular ligament* is a weak flat band, which extends forward and medially from the anterior margin of lateral malleolus, to the neck of talus just in front of the fibular facet.
2. *Posterior talofibular ligament* is a strong band, which extends backward and medially from the posterior margin of the lateral malleolus to the posterior tubercle of the talus.
3. *Calcaneofibular ligament* is a long rounded cord, which runs downward and backward from the notch on the lower border of lateral malleolus to the tubercle on the lateral surface of the calcaneum.

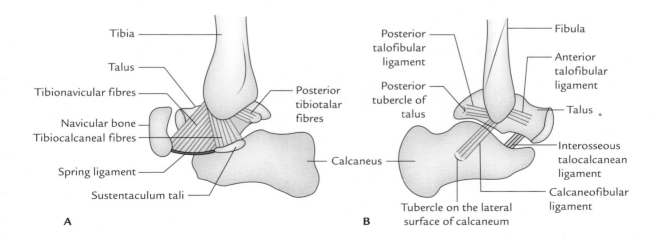

Fig. 32.14 Collateral ligaments of the ankle joint: **A**, deltoid ligament; **B**, lateral ligament.

N.B. Superficially, the *deltoid ligament* is crossed by the tendons of tibialis posterior and flexor digitorum longus whereas *lateral ligament* is crossed superficially by the tendons of peroneus longus and brevis.

RELATIONS OF THE ANKLE JOINT (Fig. 32.15)

Anterior: *Anteriorly* from medial to lateral side the ankle joint is related to the following structures:

1. Tibialis anterior.
2. Extensor Hallucis longus.
3. Anterior tibial Artery.
4. Deep peroneal Nerve.
5. Extensor Digitorum longus.
6. Peroneus tertius.

   Mnemonic: The Himalayas Are Not Dry Plateaus.

Posterior: *Posteriorly* from medial to lateral side the ankle joint is related to the following structures:

1. Tibialis posterior.
2. Flexion Digitorum longus.
3. Posterior tibial Artery.
4. Posterior tibial Nerve.
5. Flexor Hallucis longus.

   Mnemonic: The Doctors Are Not Here.

ARTERIAL SUPPLY

It is by the malleolar branches of anterior tibial, posterior tibial, and peroneal arteries.

NERVE SUPPLY

It is by the branches of deep peroneal and tibial nerves. (The segmental innervations is by L4, L5; S1, S2 spinal segments.)

Movements

The following movements take place at the ankle joint:

1. Dorsiflexion.
2. Plantar flexion.

N.B. When the foot is plantar flexed, the ankle joint also permits some degree of side-to-side gliding, rotation, adduction, and abduction.

Dorsiflexion

In *dorsiflexion,* the forefoot is raised and the angle between front of the leg and dorsum of the foot is diminished. In this movement, the wider anterior part of trochlea is forced posteriorly between the malleoli. It is a **close-packed position of the ankle joint** with maximum congruence of the articular surfaces and tension of ligaments. The ankle joint is most stable in dorsiflexion.

Plantar Flexion

In *plantar flexion,* the forefoot is depressed, and the angle between the leg and foot is increased. In this position, the tibiofibular socket encloses the narrower posterior part of the trochlear surface of talus and some joint space is

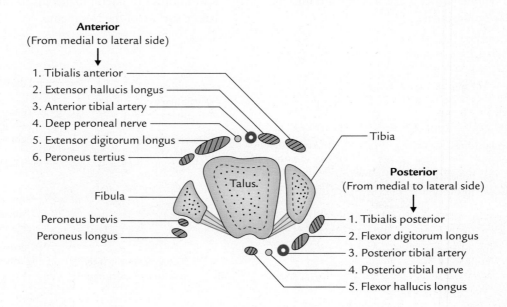

Anterior
(From medial to lateral side)

1. Tibialis anterior
2. Extensor hallucis longus
3. Anterior tibial artery
4. Deep peroneal nerve
5. Extensor digitorum longus
6. Peroneus tertius

Fibula

Peroneus brevis
Peroneus longus

Talus.

Tibia

Posterior
(From medial to lateral side)

1. Tibialis posterior
2. Flexor digitorum longus
3. Posterior tibial artery
4. Posterior tibial nerve
5. Flexor hallucis longus

Fig. 32.15 Relations of the ankle joint (transverse section of the ankle joint).

Table 32.4 Movements of the ankle joint

Movements	Muscles producing movements	
	Principal muscles	Accessory muscles
Dorsiflexion	*Tibialis anterior*	• Extensor digitorum longus • Extensor hallucis longus • Peroneus tertius
Plantar flexion	• Gastrocnemius • Soleus	• Plantaris • Tibialis posterior • Flexor hallucis longus • Flexor digitorum longus

available between the tibiofibular mortise and the narrow posterior part of the trochlea. It is a **loose-packed position** of the ankle joint. The joint is unstable in plantar flexion.

N.B. The ankle joint is stable in dorsiflexion and unstable in plantar flexion.

The range of motion (ROM) for dorsiflexion is 20° and for plantar flexion is 45°.

The dorsiflexion is controlled by the L4, L5 spinal segments and plantar flexion by the S1, S2 spinal segments.

Movements and muscles producing them are given in Table 32.4.

Clinical correlation

- **Ankle sprains (Figs 32.16 and 32.17):** The excessive stretching and/or tearing of ligaments of the ankle joint is called the *ankle sprain*. The ankle sprains are usually caused by the falls from height or twists of ankle.

  When the plantar-flexed foot is excessively inverted, the anterior and posterior talofibular and calcaneofibular ligaments are stretched and torn. The *anterior talofibular ligament is most commonly torn*.

  When the plantar-flexed foot is excessively everted, the deltoid ligament is not torn; instead there is an avulsion fracture of medial malleolus.

  The inversion sprains are more common than eversion sprains.
- **Dislocation of the ankle:** The dislocations of ankle joint are rare because it is a very stable joint due to tibiofibular mortise. However, whenever dislocation occurs it is always accompanied by the fracture of one of the malleoli.
- **Pott's fracture (fracture dislocation of the ankle; Fig. 31.18):** It occurs when the foot is caught in the rabbit hole and everted forcibly. In this condition, the following sequence of events takes place:
  1. *Oblique fracture of the lateral malleolus* due to internal rotation of the tibia.
  2. *Transverse fracture of the medial malleolus* due to pull by strong deltoid ligament.

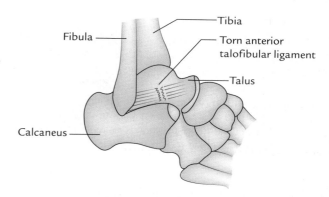

Fig. 32.16 Ankle sprain (note torn fibres of the anterior talofibular ligament).

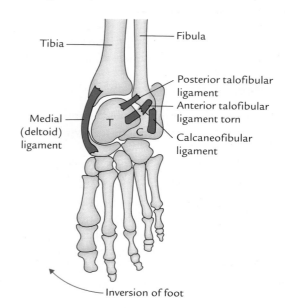

Fig. 32.17 Inversion and eversion injuries of the foot (T = talus, C = calcaneus).

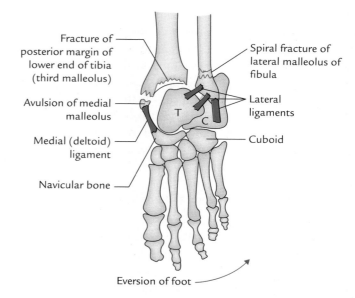

Fig. 32.18 Pott's fracture (T = talus, C = calcaneus).

3. *Fracture of the posterior margin of the lower end of tibia* (**third malleolus**) because it is carried forward.
These stages are also termed **first, second, and third degree of Pott's fracture,** respectively. The third degree of Potts fracture is also called trimalleolar fracture.

- **Optimum position of the ankle:** The optimum position of the ankle is one in which ankle joint is in slight plantar flexion. The knowledge of position is essential for applying plaster cast in the ankle region.

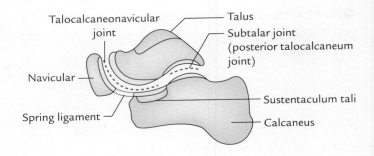

Fig. 32.19 Subtalar and talocalcaneonavicular joints.

JOINTS OF THE FOOT

There are numerous joints in the foot formed between tarsal, metatarsal, and phalangeal bones. The joints of the foot include intertarsal, tarsometatarsal, intermetatarsal, metatarsophalangeal, and interphalangeal joints. Those joints which are of more functional value are discussed.

INTERTARSAL JOINTS

They are of two types: major and minor. Only major intertarsal joints are discussed in the following text.

Subtalar (Talocalcanean) Joints (Fig. 32.19)

There are two joints between the talus and calcanean: posterior talocalcanean joint and anterior talocalcaneonavicular joint. The posterior talocalcanean joint is often designated as **subtalar joint.** It is a plane type of synovial joint. It is formed between the concave facet on the inferior surface of the body of talus and convex facet on the middle one-third of the superior surface of the calcaneum.

Ligaments

These are: (a) fibrous capsule, (b) lateral and medial talocalcanean ligaments, (c) interosseous talocalcanean ligament, and (d) cervical ligament.

The *interosseous talocalcanean ligament* is thick and very strong. It forms the chief bond of union between the talus and calcaneum. It occupies sinus tarsi and separates the *talocalcanean joint* from the *talocalcaneonavicular joint.* It extends obliquely from the sulcus tali to the sulcus calcanei. *It becomes taut in eversion.* The *cervical ligament* is lateral to sinus tarsi. It extends upward and medially from upper surface of the calcaneum to the tubercle on the inferolateral aspect of the neck of talus. It becomes taut in inversion.

Talocalcaneonavicular Joint (Fig. 32.19)

It is a compound articulation consisting of anterior talocalcanean and talonavicular joints. *It is roughly a ball and socket type of synovial joint.* The articular surface on the rounded head of the talus fits into the socket formed by the calcaneum, navicular, and spring ligament.

Ligaments

These are: (a) fibrous capsule, (b) spring ligament, and (c) medial limb (calcaneonavicular part) of *bifurcate ligament.*

The *spring ligament (plantar calcaneonavicular ligament)* is a powerful fibrocartilaginous band, which extends from the anterior margin of the sustentaculum tali to the plantar surface of navicular bone between its tuberosity and articular margin. It takes part in forming the socket for the head of the talus. It is the most important ligament to maintain the medial longitudinal arch. Its upper surface has a triangular fibrocartilagenous facet for the head of the talus. Its plantar surface is supported by the tendon of tibialis posterior medially, and by the tendons of flexor hallucis longus and flexor digitorum longus laterally.

The talocalcaneonavicular joint permits the movements of inversion and eversion.

Calcaneocuboid Joint (Fig. 32.20)

It is a saddle type of synovial joint. The opposed articular surfaces of the calcaneum and cuboid are reciprocally concavoconvex.

Ligaments

The ligaments of the joint are: (a) fibrous capsule, (b) lateral limb (calcaneocuboid part) of bifurcate ligament, (c) long plantar ligament, and (d) short plantar ligament.

The *bifurcate ligament* is Y-shaped. Its stem is attached to the anterolateral part of the sulcus calcanei. Its medial limb (calcaneonavicular part) is attached to the dorsolateral surface of the navicular bone and its lateral limb (calcaneocuboid part) to the dorsomedial surface of the cuboid bone. The two limbs provide support to the joints.

The long planar ligament is the longest ligament. It is strong and its importance in maintaining the arches of foot is surpassed only by the spring ligament. It *extends from triangular plantar surface of the calcaneum to the lips of the groove on cuboid and beyond it to the bases of the middle three metatarsals (second to fourth).* It converts the groove on the plantar surface of cuboid into a tunnel for the passage of tendon of peroneus longus. Morphologically, it represents the divorced tendon of the gastrocnemius.

The *short plantar ligament (plantar calcaneocuboid ligament)* lies deep to long plantar ligament. It is broad and extends from the anterior tubercle of calcaneum to the plantar surface of the cuboid behind its ridge.

Transverse Tarsal (Midtarsal) Joint (Fig. 32.20)

It is a compound joint consisting of calcaneocuboid and talonavicular joints. Talonavicular is also a part of talocalcaneonavicular joint. The calcaneocuboid and talonavicular joints are grouped together because both are placed nearly in the same transverse plane. However, the two joints have different axes of movements. The movements of midtarsal joint help in inversion and eversion of the foot.

INVERSION AND EVERSION OF THE FOOT

The inversion and eversion and rotational movements of the foot on the talus.

The **inversion** is a movement in which the medial border of the foot is raised so that the sole faces medially.

The **eversion** is a movement in which the lateral border of the foot is raised so that the sole faces laterally.

N.B. There is difference in the relational movements associated with inversion and eversion when the foot is off the ground and on the ground as given in Table 32.5.

Joints Taking Part
1. Subtalar joint.
2. Talocalcaneonavicular joint } Main joints.
3. Transverse tarsal/midtarsal joint—Accessory joint.

Axis of Movements (Fig. 32.21)
The movements of *inversion* and *eversion* take place around an **oblique axis** which runs forward, upward, and medially passing from the back of calcaneum through the sinus tarsi to emerge at the superomedial aspect of the neck of talus.

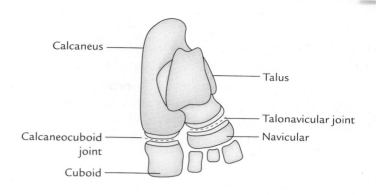

Fig. 32.20 Transverse tarsal (midtarsal) joint.

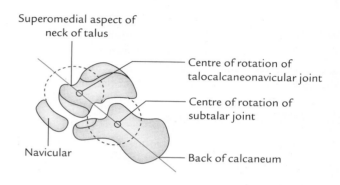

Fig. 32.21 Axis of inversion and eversion (red line).

Range of Movements (ROM)
1. The range of movement of inversion is much more than that of eversion (inversion = 30°, eversion = 20°).
2. The range of these movements is appreciably increased in plantar flexion of the foot because in this position, the narrow posterior part of the trochlear surface of talus occupies the tibiofibular socket (mortise), which permits some degree of side to side movement of the talus.

Table 32.5 Movements of inversion and eversion when the foot is off the ground and when the foot is on the ground

Movement	Inversion	Eversion
When foot is off the ground	• Range of motion is more • Inversion consists of adduction of the forefoot, lateral rotation (supination) of the forefoot, and plantar flexion of the ankle	• Range of motion is more • Eversion consists of abduction of the forefoot, medial rotation (pronation) of the forefoot, and dorsiflexion of the ankle
When foot is on the ground	• Range of motion is less • Inversion consists of only lateral rotation (supination) of the forefoot • Heads of the medial 2 metatarsals are raised	• Range of motion is less • Eversion consists of only medial rotation (pronation) of the forefoot • Heads of the lateral 3 metatarsals are raised

Table 32.6 Movements of inversion and eversion

Movements	Muscles	
	Principal muscles	Accessory muscles
Inversion (ROM = 30°)	• Tibialis anterior • Tibialis posterior	• Flexor hallucis longus • Flexor digitorum longus
Eversion (ROM = 20°)	• Peroneus longus • Peroneus brevis	• Peroneus tertius

Muscles Producing Movements

The movements of inversion and eversion and muscles producing them are given in Table 32.6.

Functional Significance

The movements of inversion and eversion are necessary for walking on uneven and sloping grounds. They greatly help the foot in adjusting it to such grounds. When feet are supporting the body weight, these movements occur in a modified form called supination and pronation.

TARSOMETATARSAL JOINTS

These are **plane type** of synovial joints. They are connected by dorsal, plantar, and interosseous tarsometatarsal ligaments. They are five in number. The first joint possesses a separate cavity, the second and third together have one cavity. These joints permit only limited gliding movements.

METATARSOPHALANGEAL JOINTS

These are **ellipsoidal type** of the synovial joints. They are connected by the capsular, collateral, plantar, and deep transverse metatarsal ligaments. Two collateral ligaments strengthen the sides of each joint. These joints permit the slight gliding movements. The deep transverse ligaments (four in number) connect the plantar ligaments of adjacent metatarsophalangeal joints.

Movements

These joints permit dorsiflexion, plantar flexion, adduction, and abduction.

- The range of dorsiflexion is more (50–60°) than that of plantar flexion (30–40°).
- The *axis of adduction and abduction of the toes passes through the least mobile second metatarsal bone*. (cf. The axis of adduction and abduction of fingers passes through the third metacarpal bone.)

INTERPHALANGEAL JOINTS

These are typical **hinge joints**. They are connected by the capsular and collateral ligaments.

Movements

These joints permit dorsiflexion and plantar flexion of distal phalanges.

Golden Facts to Remember

▶ Most stable position of the knee joint	Erect extended position
▶ Most important muscle to stabilize the knee joint	Quadriceps femoris
▶ Only mammal who does not have menisci and popliteus	Fruit bat
▶ Most frequently injured joint in the lower limb	Ankle joint
▶ Key muscle of the knee joint	Popliteus
▶ Unhappy triad of knee joint	Injury of (a) tibial collateral ligament, (b) medial meniscus, and (c) anterior cruciate ligament
▶ Most commonly injured meniscus of the knee joint	Medial meniscus
▶ Strongest tibiofibular joint	Inferior tibiofibular joint
▶ Most important ligament for maintaining the arches of the foot	Spring ligament

Clinical Case Study

A final year medical student, while playing football received a blow on the lateral side of his right knee and fell on the ground. He felt sharp pain on the medial aspect of the right knee and was not able to extend the leg on the same side. He was taken to the hospital where the examining doctor found that his right knee was swollen especially above the patella. **Drawer's sign** was negative. The radiograph of the knee did not reveal any fracture. He was diagnosed as a case of *torn medial meniscus of the knee joint*.

Questions

1. Enumerate the main intracapsular structures of the knee joint?
2. Why is the injury of medial meniscus more common than that of a lateral meniscus?
3. What is the cause of swelling of the knee especially above the patella in this case?
4. What type of meniscal tear is commonly seen in football players?
5. What is the "*unhappy triad*" of the knee joint?

Answers

1. The main intracapsular structures of the knee joint are: (a) medial and lateral menisci, (b) anterior and posterior cruciate ligaments, and (c) suprapatellar and deep infrapatellar bursae.
2. Because it is firmly attached with the tibial collateral ligament. A sudden blow on the lateral side of a flexed weight-bearing knee can cause rupture of tibial collateral ligament and concomitant tear of the medial meniscus.
3. The accumulation of synovial fluid within the joint due to traumatic synovitis. The distension of suprapatellar bursa led to the large amount of swelling above the patella.
4. Bucket handle tear (longitudinal split of the meniscus).
5. It is a combination of injury to the (a) tibial collateral ligament, (b) medial meniscus, and (c) anterior cruciate ligament.

CHAPTER 33

Venous and Lymphatic Drainage of the Lower Limb

VENOUS DRAINAGE OF THE LOWER LIMB

The **venous drainage of the lower limb** is of immense clinical and surgical importance. The venous blood of the lower limb is drained against gravity. However, a number of factors help to facilitate its drainage (vide infra). If these factors fail to help the drainage, the stagnation of venous blood in the superficial veins cause **varicose veins** and in the deep veins lead to **deep vein thrombosis**.

Factors Helping the Venous Drainage of the Lower Limb

1. The *contraction of the calf muscles* (chief factor) squeezes the blood upward along the deep veins. Note the calf muscles act as "calf pump (peripheral heart)."
2. *Transmitted pulsations from the adjacent arteries.*
3. *Presence of valves in the perforating veins* prevents the reflux of blood into the superficial veins during contraction of the calf muscles.
4. *Presence of valves in the deep veins* supports the column of blood and maintains unidirectional upward flow of the blood.
5. *Negative intrathoracic pressure* becomes more negative during inspiration and yawning.
6. In recumbent position, the "vis-a-tergo" is produced by the contraction of the heart and suction action of the diaphragm.

CLASSIFICATION OF THE VEINS

The veins of the lower limb are classified anatomically and functionally into the following three types (Fig. 33.1):

1. Superficial veins.
2. Deep veins.
3. Perforating veins.

The **superficial veins** essentially include the great and small saphenous veins, which represent pre-axial and post-axial veins of the developing lower limb, respectively. They lie in the superficial fascia on the surface of the deep fascia and are *thick walled* because of the presence of the smooth muscle. They possess valves, which are more numerous in their distal part than in the proximal part. A large proportion of their blood is drained into the deep veins through the perforating veins.

The **deep veins** include the anterior tibial, posterior tibial, peroneal, popliteal, and femoral veins. They are surrounded and supported by the powerful muscles. They possess more valves. They accompany the arteries. Below the knee, they are arranged as a pair of **venae comitantes** along the arteries but above the knee, they form single large vein. All the veins from muscles draining into deep veins also possess valves except those in the soleus where they are arranged in the form of **venous sinuses (soleal sinuses)**.

The **perforating veins (perforators)** pierce the deep fascia and connect the superficial veins with the deep veins. Their valves permit only one-way flow of the blood, from the superficial veins to the deep veins. There are about five perforators along the great saphenous vein, and one perforator along the small saphenous vein.

N.B. The *venous blood* of the thigh and leg flows from the superficial to deep veins (being directed by the valves of perforating veins). However, in foot, the venous blood flows from the deep veins (in the sole) to the superficial veins (on the dorsum of the foot).

SUPERFICIAL VEINS

Great Saphenous Vein

The great saphenous vein lies in the superficial fascia and is easily seen (Greek *saphenous* = easily seen). The great saphenous vein is the **longest vein** of the body and represents the **pre-axial vein** of the lower limb. It is also called long saphenous vein (Fig. 33.2).

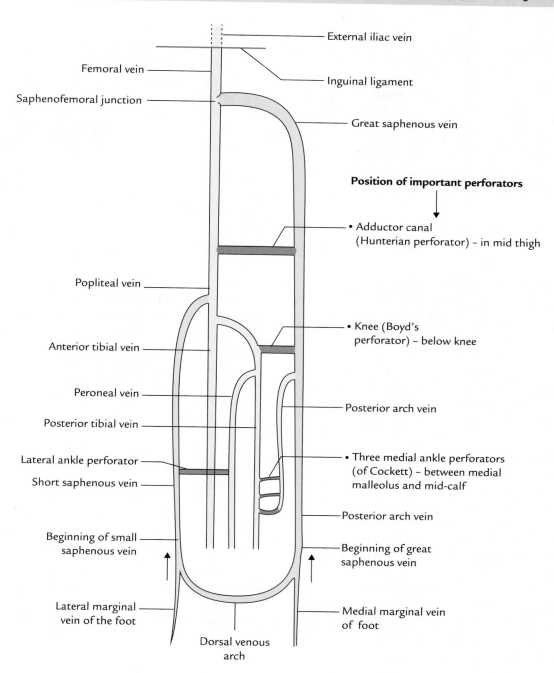

Fig. 33.1 Schematic representation of the veins of the lower limb (deep vein = light blue colour, superficial veins = deep blue colour, perforating vein = violet).

Course

It is formed on the dorsum of foot by the union of the medial end of the **dorsal venous arch of the foot** and **medial marginal vein of the foot**. The vein runs upward about 2.5 cm in front of the medial malleolus, crosses obliquely the medial surface of the lower third of tibia, and then ascends a little behind the medial border of tibia to reach the knee, where it lies on the posteromedial aspect of the knee joint, about one hand-breadth posterior

to the patella; from here it runs upward along the medial side of the thigh to reach the saphenous opening (fossa ovalis).

It passes through the saphenous opening after piercing the cribriform fascia and drains into the **femoral vein** after piercing the femoral sheath.

Tributaries

1. *At the commencement:* Medial marginal vein of the big toe.

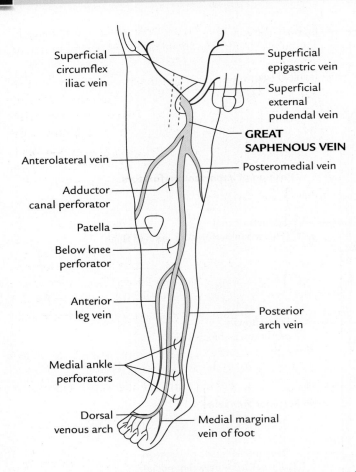

Fig. 33.2 Formation, course, termination, and tributaries of the great saphenous vein.

2. *In the leg:*
   (a) *Communicating veins* between small saphenous and deep veins.
   (b) *Posterior arch vein.* It is fairly large and constant. It collects the blood from the posteromedial aspect of the calf and begins of a series of small venous arches connecting the three medial ankle-perforating veins (perforators).
3. *Just below the knee:*
   (a) *Anterior veins of the leg.* They extend diagonally (upward, forward, and medially) across the shin and join the great saphenous vein.
   (b) *A few veins from the calf* which communicates with the small saphenous vein.
4. *In the thigh:*
   (a) *Anterolateral vein.* It commences in the lower part of the front of thigh, crosses the apex of femoral triangle, and joins the great saphenous vein in the upper part of the thigh.
   (b) *Posteromedial vein (accessory saphenous vein).* It commences from the posteromedial aspects of the thigh and joins with the great saphenous vein; sometimes it may communicate below with the small saphenous vein.

5. *Just before piercing the cribriform fascia:*
   (a) *Superficial epigastric vein.*
   (b) *Superficial circumflex iliac vein.*
   (c) *Superficial external pudendal vein.*
       These veins accompany the corresponding superficial branches of the femoral artery.
6. *Just before the termination in the femoral vein: Deep external pudendal vein* (last tributary) drains the blood from the anterior part of the perineum.

N.B. *Thoraco-epigastric vein:* It runs along the anterolateral wall of the trunk. It connects the superficial epigastric vein with the lateral thoracic vein. Thus, it establishes an important communication between the femoral and axillary veins (i.e., upper and lower limbs).

Valves in the Great Saphenous Vein

There are about 10 to 20 valves in the great saphenous vein, out of which the location of two needs special mention here: (a) one, which lies just before it pierces the cribriform fascia and (b) the other, which lies at its junction with the femoral vein (**saphenofemoral valve**). The saphenofemoral valve is of great functional significance. It lies about 3.5 to 4 cm inferolateral to the pubic tubercle. In about 80% individuals, the external iliac vein possesses a valve, which protects the *saphenofemoral valve* against high venous pressure. The remaining 20% cases who do not have this valve become the victim of high venous pressure and develop **varicose vein**, which commences at the saphenofemoral junction and gradually extends downward.

Surface Marking of the Great Saphenous Vein

1. *At ankle,* it lies 2.5 cm anterior to the medial malleolus.
2. *In leg,* it ascends by crossing the medial surface and medial border of the tibia.
3. *At knee,* it lies about a hand's breadth posterior to the medial margin of the patella.
4. *In thigh,* it ascends obliquely on the medial aspect of the thigh to reach a point 3.5–4 cm inferolateral to the pubic tubercle (saphenofemoral junction).

Clinical correlation

- **Venesection of the great saphenous vein:** The great saphenous vein in front of medial malleolus at ankle is the most preferred site of venesection (cut-down) in emergency situation when the superficial veins elsewhere in the body are collapsed and invisible, to insert the canula for prolonged administration of intravenous fluids.
  Note that, in front of medial malleolus, saphenous nerve lies in front of the vein. Hence, during cut-down procedure, the saphenous nerve should be recognized to avoid its injury.

- **Great saphenous vein graft:** In coronary by pass surgery to relieve the ischemia of the heart, a segment of great saphenous vein is removed and used for aortocoronary grafting to by pass an arterial obstruction. Due to the presence of valves, the vein has to be reversed so that its valves do not obstruct the blood flow.

Small (Short) Saphenous Vein (Fig. 33.3)

It is formed below and behind the lateral malleolus by the union of the lateral end of the dorsal venous arch, and the lateral dorsal digital vein of the little toe. It runs upward behind the lateral malleolus, along the lateral edge of tendocalcaneus, and is accompanied by the *sural nerve* on its lateral side. Thereafter it runs in the middle of the back of the leg, pierces the deep fascia, and undergoes a subfascial course between the two heads of the gastrocnemius until it reaches the middle of the popliteal fossa. Here it turns inward to terminate into the popliteal vein. The *posterior femoral cutaneous nerve* accompanies the upper part of the vein, while passing from deep to superficial (see Fig. 29.2B).

The small saphenous vein contains 7–13 valves.

N.B.

- *Variations of small saphenous vein at its termination:*
  1. Just before piercing the popliteal fascia, it may give rise to a communicating branch to the *accessory saphenous vein.*
  2. Occasionally, it ends below the knee and terminates in the great saphenous vein or in the deep muscular veins of the leg.
  3. It may bifurcate, with one limb terminating in the great saphenous vein and other in the popliteal vein.
- *Pseudo-short saphenous veins:* These large muscular veins drain venous blood from two heads of gastrocnemius into the popliteal vein. The varicosity of these veins may mimic the varicosity of short saphenous vein; hence, they are often termed **pseudo-short saphenous veins**.

PERFORATING VEINS (PERFORATORS)

As described earlier they are communicating venous channels between the superficial and deep veins. These veins are called perforators because they perforate the deep fascia. The perforators are classified into two types: indirect and direct (Fig. 33.4).

1. *Indirect perforators:* They connect the superficial veins with the deep veins through muscular veins.
2. *Direct perforators:* They connect the superficial veins with the deep veins directly.

Location of Perforators

The position of five or six perforators is fairly constant, as mentioned below (Fig. 33.1):

1. **An adductor canal (Hunterian) perforator:** It connects the great saphenous vein with the femoral vein in the lower part of the adductor (Hunter's) canal.
2. **A knee perforator (Boyd's perforator):** It connects the great saphenous vein with the posterior tibial vein just below the knee and close to the medial border of tibia.
3. **A lateral ankle perforator:** It communicates the short saphenous vein with the peroneal vein. It is situated at the junction of middle and lower third of the leg.
4. **Three medial ankle perforators (of Cockett):** These are situated close to the medial border of the lower third of tibia between the medial malleolus and mid-calf and connect the great saphenous vein with the posterior tibial veins.
   (a) *Upper medial ankle perforator:* It lies at the junction of the middle and lower third of the leg.
   (b) *Middle medial ankle perforator:* It lies about 4 cm above the medial malleolus.
   (c) *Lower medial ankle perforator:* It lies posteroinferior to the medial malleolus.

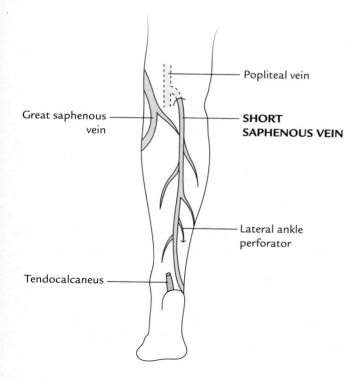

Fig. 33.3 Small (short saphenous) veins.

Labels: Popliteal vein; Great saphenous vein; **SHORT SAPHENOUS VEIN**; Lateral ankle perforator; Tendocalcaneus

N.B. The three medial ankle perforators join with one another (by a series of venous arcades) to form the *posterior arch vein.*

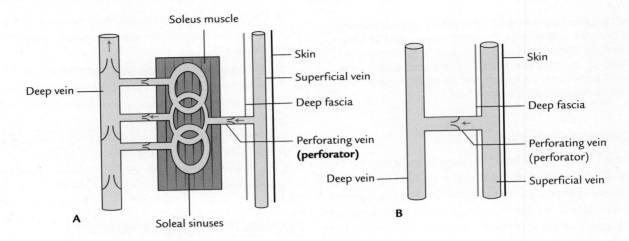

Fig. 33.4 Perforators: **A**, indirect perforators; **B**, direct perforators.

Calf pump and peripheral heart: In upright position, the venous return from the lower limb occurs against gravity and depends largely on the contraction of calf muscles. Therefore, these muscles are termed **calf pump**.

The soleus muscle contains venous sinuses filled with blood. When soleus muscle contracts, it pumps the blood from its large venous sinuses into the deep veins, and when it is relaxed it sucks the blood from the superficial veins, and the venous sinuses within it are refilled. The unidirectional blood flow is maintained by the valves in the perforating veins. Hence, the soleus is sometimes termed **peripheral heart**.

The soleal sinuses are common site for *thrombosis* and source of pulmonary embolism in sedentary individuals. The *phlebitis* of soleal sinus may be dangerous because the spread of infection from here may damage the valves in the perforators.

Deep vein thrombosis: The veins of the lower limb possess **valves**, which direct the blood flow to the heart particularly against gravity in upright posture. The valves are more numerous in the deep veins than in the superficial veins. The veins from the muscles draining into the deep veins have valves except those in the **soleus**, which are arranged in the form of **venous sinuses**. The blood flow is sluggish in the soleal sinuses particularly when the muscles are put to rest. Prolonged rest in bed by some patients after surgery is unwise because it may develop **deep vein thrombosis**, which may culminate into life-threatening complication of the **pulmonary embolism**.

VARICOSE VEINS AND VARICOSE ULCERS OF THE LOWER LIMB

When the veins become dilated and tortuous they are called **varicose veins** (Fig. 33.5). The superficial veins of the lower limbs commonly become varicosed due to incompetency of the valves, following prolonged standing (e.g., bus conductors, traffic police personnel, nurses).

1. *Incompetency of valves in the perforating veins:* If the valves in the perforating veins become incompetent, the defective veins become **"high pressure leaks"** during muscular contraction, whereby the high pressure of the deep veins is transmitted to the superficial veins. As a result, the superficial veins become dilated and tortuous.

2. *Incompetency of valves at the termination of the superficial veins:* For example, if *saphenofemoral valve* becomes incompetent, the great saphenous vein becomes dilated and tortuous. The varicosity commences from the

DEEP VEINS

The deep veins of the leg lie in the tight fascial compartment along the arteries.

The major deep veins of the lower limb are as follows:

1. Deep veins of the sole (e.g., medial and lateral plantar veins).

2. Venae comitantes accompanying the dorsalis pedis, anterior tibial, and posterior tibial arteries.

3. Popliteal vein.

4. Femoral vein.

The features of the deep veins are already described on page 458.

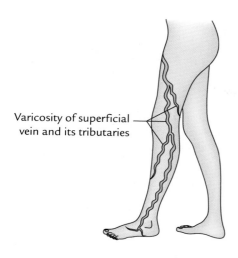

Fig. 33.5 Varicose veins in the left lower limb.

saphenofemoral junction and extends gradually downward.

The dilatation of superficial veins and gradual degeneration of their walls may lead to *varicose ulcers*.

Recognition of Sites of Incompetent Valves

The clinicians recognize the sites of incompetent valves by the following two tests: Trendelenburg test and Perthes' test (tourniquet test). Note, by these tests only superficial veins and perforators can be tested, but not the deep veins.

1. *Trendelenburg test:* The patient is asked to lie down, and the veins are emptied by raising the lower limb and stroking the varicose veins proximally. Now pressure is applied with the thumb at the saphenofemoral junction, and the patient is asked to stand up quickly.

    To test the superficial veins, the pressure is released. If the varicose veins are filled quickly from above, it indicates incompetency of the superficial veins, and test is positive. If the veins are not filled, the test is negative.

    To test the perforating veins, the pressure at the saphenofemoral junction is not released, but maintained for about a minute. Gradual filling of the superficial veins indicates incompetency of valves of the perforating veins, allowing the blood from deep to superficial veins and test is positive.

2. *Perthes' test* (tourniquet test): It is employed to test the incompetence of the deep veins. A tourniquet is tied around the upper part of thigh, tight enough to occlude the saphenous vein but not the femoral vein. The patient is asked to do gentle exercise, i.e., walk quickly for a while, with tourniquet in place. If the perforating and deep veins are normal, the varicose veins will shrink, whereas if they are blocked, the varicose veins become more distended.

N.B. The identification of exact sites of the defective perforators is essential before ligating such perforators. When numerous perforators are involved, the entire length of great saphenous vein is removed by **stripping operation**.

LYMPHATIC DRAINAGE OF THE LOWER LIMB

The knowledge of lymphatic drainage of the lower limb is of great clinical importance because inflammatory lesions of limb cause painful enlargement of the lymph nodes whereas blockage of lymphatics by microfilarial parasites leads to massive edema of the lower limb.

Most of the lymph from lower limb is drained into the inguinal lymph nodes, either directly (mostly) or indirectly (partly) through the popliteal and anterior tibial nodes. However, the deep structures of the gluteal region and upper part of the back of thigh are drained into the internal iliac nodes.

LYMPH NODES

The lymph nodes are classified into two types: superficial and deep.

1. *Superficial lymph nodes* include the superficial inguinal nodes.
2. *Deep lymph nodes* include the deep inguinal nodes, popliteal nodes, and anterior tibial nodes.

SUPERFICIAL LYMPH NODES (Fig. 33.6A)

Superficial Inguinal Nodes

These are present in the superficial fascia of the inguinal region. They are arranged in two groups: upper and lower, resembling the letter "T."

The **upper horizontal group** contains five or six nodes, which lie below the inguinal ligament. The **lateral members of upper group** (2 or 3 nodes) receive **afferent** from:

(a) Gluteal region.
(b) Upper part of the lateral side of the thigh.
(c) Flank and back of the abdominal wall below the umbilical plane.

The **medial members of the upper group** receive **afferent** from:

(a) Subcutaneous tissue of the anterior abdominal wall below the umbilicus.
(b) Penis including prepuce and scrotum in male, vulva and vagina below the hymen in female.

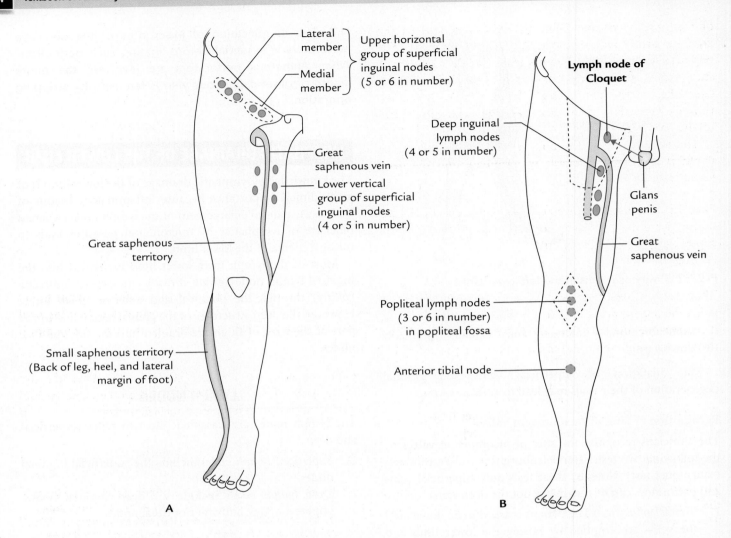

Fig. 33.6 Lymph node groups of the lower limb: **A**, superficial inguinal lymph nodes; **B**, deep inguinal lymph nodes.

(c) Perineum and lower part of the anal canal below the pectinate line.

(d) Few lymphatics from the superolateral angle of uterus which accompany the round ligament of uterus.

The **lower vertical group** consists of four or five nodes. They are placed along both sides of the terminal part of great saphenous vein. They receive afferent from the skin and fasciae of the most of the lower limb (great saphenous territory), except from buttock, which drain into upper lateral group and the short saphenous territory, which drain into popliteal nodes.

N.B.

• The efferents from all the superficial inguinal nodes pierce the cribriform fascia and terminate into the deep inguinal nodes.

DEEP LYMPH NODES (Fig. 33.6B)

Deep Inguinal Lymph Nodes

These are about four to five in number, and lie on the medial side of the upper part of the femoral vein in the femoral triangle. The most proximal node of this group (**gland of Cloquet or Rosenmüller**) lies in the femoral canal. These nodes receive afferents from: (a) the superficial inguinal nodes, (b) popliteal nodes, (c) glans of penis/clitoris, and (d) deep lymphatics of the lower limb accompanying femoral vessels.

Their efferent vessels from the deep inguinal lymph nodes drain into the external iliac nodes after piercing the femoral septum, which closes the femoral ring.

Popliteal Lymph Nodes

The **popliteal lymph nodes** (about three to six in number) lie embedded in the popliteal pad of fat near the termination of the small saphenous vein; one node lies between the popliteal artery and the oblique popliteal ligament. The popliteal nodes receive **afferents** from: (a) the territory of small saphenous vein (i.e., lateral side of the foot, heel, and lateral half of the back of leg), (b) deep parts of the leg, running along the anterior and posterior tibial vessels, and (c) the knee joint.

The efferents from the popliteal nodes run along the popliteal and femoral vessels to terminate into the deep inguinal nodes.

N.B. The **popliteal lymph nodes** are unique in the sense that they are the only deep nodes, which receive both the superficial and deep lymph vessels.

Anterior Tibial Lymph Node

The **anterior tibial lymph node** is an inconstant node found along the upper part of anterior tibial artery. When present, it receives the afferents from the anterior compartment of the leg, and its efferents pass into the popliteal nodes.

LYMPHATICS

Like lymph nodes, the lymph vessels of lower limb are also classified into two groups: superficial and deep.

SUPERFICIAL LYMPHATICS

The superficial lymphatics are larger and more numerous than the deep lymphatics. They run in the superficial fascia. They form two main streams: (a) most of them *(the main stream)* follow the great saphenous vein, and drain into the lower vertical group of superficial inguinal lymph nodes, and (b) the remaining one *(accessory stream)* follows the small saphenous vein, and drains into the popliteal lymph nodes.

DEEP LYMPHATICS

The deep lymphatics are smaller and fewer than the superficial lymphatics. They drain all the structures lying

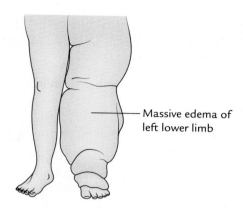

Massive edema of left lower limb

Fig. 33.7 Elephantiasis of the left lower limb.

deep to the deep fascia. They run along the main blood vessels of the lower limb and drain into the deep inguinal nodes, either directly or indirectly through the popliteal nodes.

N.B. The deep lymphatics from the gluteal region and upper part of the back of thigh accompany the gluteal vessels and drain into the internal iliac nodes.

Clinical correlation

- **Elephantiasis (Fig. 33.7):** The lymph vessels of the lower limb are often blocked, particularly in the endemic areas, by the microfilarial parasites (*Wuchereria bancrofti*). This causes massive edema of the lower limb producing a clinical condition called **elephantiasis**. In this condition, there is hypertrophy of the skin and subcutaneous tissue to an unusual proportion.
- **Enlargement of the inguinal lymph nodes:** It is the commonest cause of swelling in the subinguinal region. The common causes of enlargement of these lymph nodes is infection, boil or abscess in the drainage area. The other causes are filariasis, Hodgkin's disease, etc.

  The enlarged inguinal nodes should be differentiated from *ectopic testis, femoral hernia,* and *psoas abscess.*

Golden Facts to Remember

► Longest vein in the body	Great saphenous vein
► Most preferred site of venesection (cut-down)	Great saphenous vein in front of medial malleolus
► Varicose vein	Dilated tortuous vein
► Commonest cause of swelling in the subinguinal area	Enlargement of inguinal lymph nodes
► Lymph node of Cloquet or Rosenmüller	Deep inguinal lymph node present in the femoral canal
► Most of the lymph from the lower limb is drained into	Lower vertical group of superficial inguinal lymph nodes
► Elephantiasis	Massive edema (lymph edema) of lower limb due to blockage of its lymphatics by microfilarial parasites
► Vein of Leonardo da Vinci	Posterior arch vein, a tributary of great saphenous vein
► Commonest cause of varicosities of veins in the lower limb	Incompetency of valves in perforating veins, or superficial veins, or both

Clinical Case Study

A 42-year-old man visited hospital with complaints of chronic dull pain in his both legs. On examination, the doctor found dilated tortuous veins on the medial sides of both lower limbs. The skin in front of medial malleolus was discoloured, dry, and scaly. He was diagnosed as a case of "**varicose veins.**"

Questions

1. Define varicose veins.
2. Which is the vein commonly involved in varicosity?
3. Give two important causes of varicosity of great saphenous vein.
4. Give the cause for discoloured, dry, and scaly skin in front of medial malleolus.
5. What are the complications of varicose veins?
6. Give the anatomical basis of varicose ulcers.
7. What will be the effects if valves in perforating veins, and saphenofemoral valve become incompetent?

Answers

1. Dilated tortuous veins.
2. Great saphenous veins.
3. (a) Incompetency of valves in the perforating veins (perforators), and (b) incompetency of valve at the saphenofemoral junction.
4. Due to less oxygen supply to the skin. The venous stasis in the varicose veins in front of medial malleolus, lowers the oxygen supply to the skin.
5. Thrombophlebitis and venous (varicose) ulcers.
6. The venous stasis affects the oxygen supply of the skin, which initially becomes dry, discoloured, and later sloughs off producing a varicose ulcer.
7. If valves in perforating veins become incompetent, there will be reversal of blood flow from deep to superficial veins leading to the dilatation and tortuosity of these veins and if saphenofemoral valve becomes incompetent, the blood will flow from femoral vein into the great saphenous vein making it dilated and tortuous.

CHAPTER
34
Innervation of the Lower Limb

In view of high incidence of neurological disorders of the lower limb, the innervation of the lower limb is discussed in a separate chapter for easy comprehension by the students and clinicians. This includes the description of major nerves, cutaneous innervation, segmental innervation, and sympathetic innervation of the lower limb.

NERVES OF THE LOWER LIMB

The nerves of the lower limb are derived from the ventral (anterior primary) rami of the lumbar and sacral nerves forming the **lumbar plexus** (L1–L4) in the posterior abdominal wall and the **sacral plexus** (L4–S4) in the pelvis.

The main nerves of the lower limb are as follows:

1. Femoral nerve.
2. Obturator nerve.
3. Sciatic nerve.
4. Tibial nerve.
5. Common peroneal nerve.
6. Superficial peroneal nerve.
7. Deep peroneal nerve.

The last four nerves are actually direct or indirect branches of the sciatic nerve.

The study of these nerves is important because of their frequent involvement in various injuries and peripheral neuropathies.

FEMORAL NERVE (Fig. 34.1)

The **femoral nerve** is the nerve of anterior compartment of the thigh. It arises within the psoas major muscle from the posterior divisions of the L2–L4 ventral rami in the abdomen. It descends through the psoas major and emerges on its lateral border to pass between the psoas and iliacus to enter the thigh behind the inguinal ligament and lateral to the femoral sheath. In femoral triangle, it splits into anterior and posterior divisions, 2 cm distal to the inguinal

ligament. The two divisions straddle the lateral circumflex femoral artery. Its motor branches supply iliacus in the abdomen and all the muscles of anterior compartment of the thigh. Its cutaneous branches supply the large cutaneous area on the anterior and medial aspect of the thigh, medial side of leg, and foot. It also gives articular branches to the hip and knee joints. The femoral nerve is described in detail in Chapter 22, p. 340.

Clinical correlation

- **Injury of the femoral nerve:** It is rare but may be injured by a stab, gunshot wounds, or a pelvic fracture. The following are the characteristic clinical features:
  (a) *Motor loss*
     – Weak flexion of the thigh, due to paralysis of the iliacus and sartorius muscles.
     – Inability to extend the knee, due to paralysis of the quadriceps femoris.
  (b) *Sensory loss*
     – Sensory loss over the anterior and medial aspects of the thigh, due to involvement of the intermediate and lateral cutaneous nerves of the thigh.
     – Sensory loss on the medial side of the leg and foot up to the ball of the great toe (first metatarsophalangeal joint), due to involvement of the saphenous nerve.
- **Femoral nerve neuropathy:** The main trunk of the femoral nerve is not subject to an *entrapment neuropathy* but it may be compressed by the retroperitoneal tumors. A localized neuropathy of the femoral nerve may occur in diabetes mellitus. The following are the characteristic clinical features:
  (a) Wasting and weakness of quadriceps leading to considerable difficulty in walking.
  (b) Pain and paraesthesia on the anterior and medial aspects of the thigh extending down along the medial aspect of the leg and foot along the distribution of the saphenous nerve.

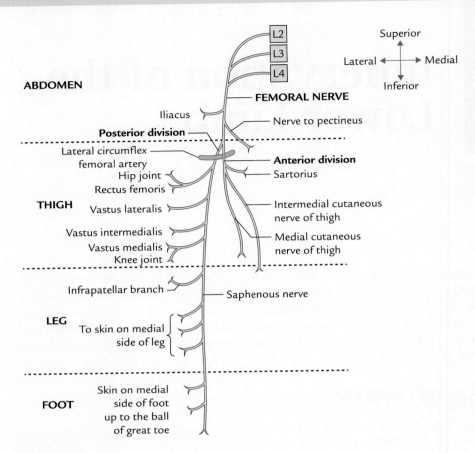

Fig. 34.1 Summary of branches of the femoral nerve. Note all the muscles on the front of thigh are supplied by posterior division except sartorius which is supplied by the anterior division.

OBTURATOR NERVE

The obturator nerve is the nerve of adductor compartment of the thigh. It arises within the psoas major from anterior divisions of the ventral rami of L2–L4 spinal nerves (Fig. 34.2). The nerve descends in the psoas major and emerges from its medial border on the ala of sacrum. It then descends along the lateral wall of the lesser pelvis on the obturator internus and passes through the upper anterior part of the obturator foramen to enter the adductor (medial) compartment of the thigh. Near the obturator foramen it divides into anterior and posterior divisions which straddle the adductor brevis muscle. Its motor branches supply all the muscles of the adductor compartment of the thigh. Its sensory branches supply cutaneous area on the lower-half of the medial aspect of the thigh. It also gives the articular branches to the hip and knee joints. The obturator nerve is described in detail in Chapter 23, p. 347.

Clinical correlation

- **Injury of the obturator nerve:** The obturator nerve may be injured in the anterior dislocation of the hip joint, or during radical retropubic prostatectomy. The following are the characteristic clinical features:
  - (a) *Motor loss:* Loss of adduction of the thigh, due to paralysis of adductor muscles of the thigh.
  - (b) *Sensory loss:* Sensory loss on the medial aspect of thigh, due to involvement of the cutaneous branch of the anterior division of the obturator nerve.
- **Obturator nerve neuropathy:** The syndrome of an obturator nerve entrapment causing the medial thigh pain is described in athletes with large adductor muscles.
- **Surgical division of the obturator nerve:** It is sometimes done to relieve the spasm of adductor muscles in the *spastic paralysis.*
- **Irritation of the obturator nerve:** The inflammation of the ovary causes localized peritonitis in the region of ovarian fossa which may cause irritation of the obturator nerve. In such a case, the pain may be referred to the hip, knee, and medial side of the thigh.
- **Referred pain:** In diseases of the hip joint, the pain may be referred to the medial side of the thigh.

SCIATIC NERVE (Fig. 34.3)

The sciatic nerve (thickest nerve in the body) is the nerve of posterior compartment of the thigh. It arises in the pelvis

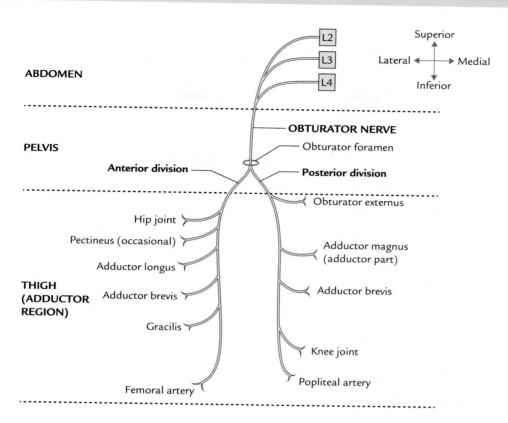

Fig. 34.2 Summary of main branches of the obturator nerve.

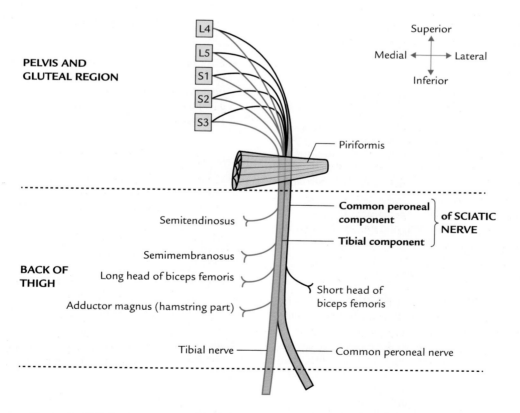

Fig. 34.3 Summary of branches of the sciatic nerve in the thigh. Ventral divisions of ventral rami are shown by green colour and dorsal division of ventral rami by grey colour. Note all the muscles on the back of thigh are supplied by tibial component of sciatic nerve except short head of biceps femoris which is supplied by its common peroneal component.

from ventral rami of L4–S3 spinal nerves. It leaves the pelvis through greater sciatic foramen below piriformis to enter the gluteal region. Here it descends between the greater trochanter and ischial tuberosity along the back of the thigh. A little above the popliteal fossa (junction of middle and lower thirds of the thigh), it divides into terminal tibial and common peroneal nerves.

Distribution

The distribution of sciatic nerves is as follows:

1. **Motor**
   (a) The motor branches from undivided trunk supply all the muscles of the back of thigh, which extend the hip and flex the knee.
   (b) The motor branches of the tibial nerve supply the muscles of the leg, which flex the leg and muscles of the foot, which plantar flex the foot.
   (c) The motor branches of the common peroneal nerve supply muscles of the leg which dorsiflex the foot.
2. **Sensory**
   (a) The sensory branches of the tibial nerves supply the skin on the back of the calf, medial and lateral sides of the heel, lateral border of the foot, and whole of the sole.
   (b) The sensory branches of the common peroneal nerve supply the skin on the anterolateral and lateral surfaces of the leg and whole of dorsum of the foot except the area which is supplied by the deep peroneal nerve.

Clinical correlation

- **Injury of the sciatic nerve:** The sciatic nerve may be injured by penetrating wounds, posterior dislocation of the hip, fracture of the pelvis, total hip replacement surgery (1%), or misplaced therapeutic injection in the gluteal region (most common cause). The following are the characteristic clinical features:
  (a) *Motor loss*
    - Inability to extend the thigh and flex the knee, due to paralysis of the hamstring muscles.
    - Loss of all movements below the knee with foot drop, due to paralysis of all the muscles of the leg and foot.
      The motor loss leads to flail foot which leads to great difficulty in walking. The patient walks with high stepping gait.
  (b) *Sensory loss:* The sensory loss on the back of the thigh and whole of the leg and foot except the area innervated by the saphenous nerve, due to involvement of the cutaneous nerves derived from the tibial and common peroneal nerves.
- **Sciatic nerve neuropathy:** As the sciatic nerve leaves the pelvis, sometimes, it passes through the piriformis muscle and at that point, it may become entrapped leading

to **piriformis syndrome** (see page 362). It is a common anatomical variant but an extremely rare entrapment neuropathy.
- **Sciatica:** It is a term applied to a clinical condition characterized by shooting pain felt along the course of distribution of the sciatic nerve (e.g., buttock, posterior aspect of thigh, lateral aspect of leg, and dorsum of the foot). It occurs due to compression and irritation of L4–S3 spinal nerve roots by herniated intervertebral disc of the lumbar vertebrae.

TIBIAL NERVE (Fig. 34.4)

The **tibial nerve** is the larger terminal branch of the sciatic nerve. It arises above the popliteal fossa and passes downward successively through the middle of popliteal fossa and posterior compartment of the leg, and then enters the sole of the foot by passing deep to the flexor retinaculum where it divides into the **medial enters the side of the foot by passing and lateral plantar nerves**. Its motor branches supply all the muscles of the posterior compartment of the leg directly and all the muscles of the sole through its terminal branches—the medial and lateral plantar nerves. Its sensory branches through the medial and lateral plantar nerves supply whole of the skin of the sole of foot and toes including dorsal aspects of their last phalanges.

Clinical correlation

- **Effects of injury of the tibial nerve:** The tibial nerve may be injured by a lacerated wound in the popliteal fossa or posterior dislocation of the knee joint. The characteristic clinical features are as follows:
  (a) *Motor loss:*
    - Foot is held dorsiflexed and everted, due to paralysis of the muscles of posterior compartment of the leg.
    - Loss of prominence of calf and tendocalcaneus, due to paralysis of the triceps surae muscle (gastrocnemius and soleus).
    - Loss of plantar flexion of foot, due to paralysis of the flexors of ankle.
    - Inability to stand on the toes, due to loss of plantarflexion of foot.
  (b) *Sensory loss:* The loss of sensation in the sole and plantar aspects of the toes including the dorsal aspects of their distal phalanges, due to involvement of the cutaneous branches.
- **Tarsal tunnel syndrome:** It occurs due to compression of the tibial nerve in the osseofibrous tunnel under the flexor retinaculum of the ankle. It clinically presents as pain and paresthesia in the sole of the foot, which often becomes worse at night.
- **Morton's metatarsalgia (also called plantar digital neuroma):** It occurs due to the formation of a neuroma following pressure on one of the plantar digital nerves just

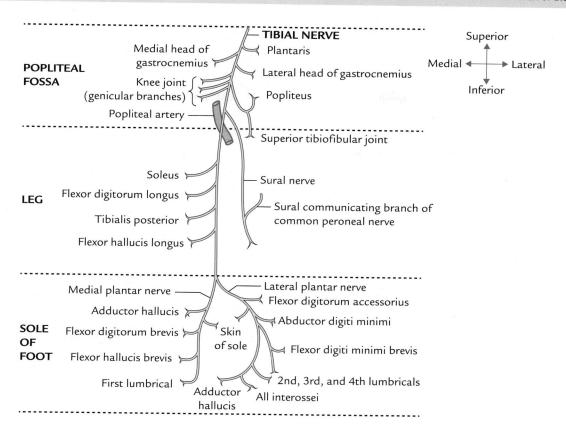

Fig. 34.4 Summary of main branches of the *tibial nerve*. Note all the muscular branches in the popliteal fossa arise from lateral side except for the medial head of gastrocnemius.

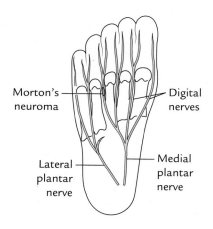

Fig. 34.5 Morton's neuroma leading to Morton's neuralgia.

prior to its bifurcation at one of the toe clefts. It most commonly affects the plantar digital nerve running between the third and fourth metatarsal heads to the third web-space (Fig. 34.5). Clinically, it presents as intermittent pain on the plantar aspect of the forefoot usually between the third and fourth metatarsals.

COMMON PERONEAL NERVE (Fig. 34.6)

The **common peroneal nerve** is the smaller terminal branch of the sciatic nerve. It arises in the lower third of the thigh just above the popliteal fossa. It passes into the popliteal fossa along its upper lateral boundary just beneath the edge of the biceps tendon. Now, it runs over plantaris and the lateral head of gastrocnemius. It runs over the fibular attachment of the soleus to wind around the lateral aspect of the neck of fibula to reach deep to peroneus longus where it divides into two terminal branches—**deep** and **superficial peroneal nerves**.

The **motor branches of the deep peroneal nerve** supply all the muscles of the anterior compartment of the leg including extensor digitorum brevis on the dorsum of the foot.

The **motor branches of the superficial peroneal nerve** supply all the muscles of the lateral compartment of the leg.

The sensory branches of the deep peroneal nerve supply the skin of cleft between the great and second toes.

The sensory branches of the superficial peroneal nerve supply most of the skin on the dorsum of foot except in the cleft between the great and second toes being supplied by the deep peroneal nerve. The lateral margin of the dorsum of foot including the lateral margin of little toe is supplied by the sural nerve. The medial margin of the dorsum of foot up

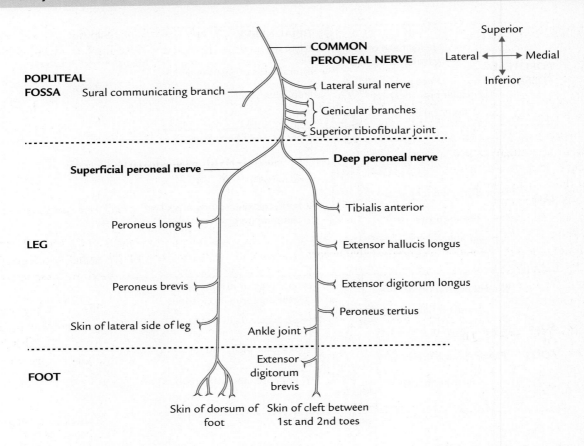

Fig. 34.6 Summary of main branches of the common peroneal nerve.

to the ball of the great toe is being supplied by the saphenous nerve.

- **Effects of injury to the common peroneal nerve:** The common peroneal nerve is extremely vulnerable to injury as it winds around the posterolateral aspect of the neck of the fibula. At this site it may be injured by the direct trauma, fracture neck of fibula, or tightly applied plaster cast. The characteristic clinical features are as follows (Fig. 34.7):
  (a) *Motor loss:*
    – **Foot drop**, due to the paralysis of muscles of the anterior compartment of the leg (dorsiflexors of the foot).
    – **Loss of extension of toes**, due to the paralysis of extensor digitorum longus and extensor hallucis longus.
    – **Loss of eversion of foot,** due to the paralysis of peroneus longus and peroneus brevis (evertors of the foot).
  (b) *Sensory loss:* The sensory loss due to involvement of the cutaneous branches, on the anterolateral aspect of the leg, and whole of dorsum foot except the areas supplied by the saphenous and sural nerves.

N.B. Due to paralysis of the dorsiflexors and evertors of the foot, the patient cannot stand on the heel. He has *high stepping gait*, in which foot is raised higher than the normal so that the toes do not hit the ground. In addition, if the foot is put down on the ground suddenly, it produces a slapping sound called *foot slap*.

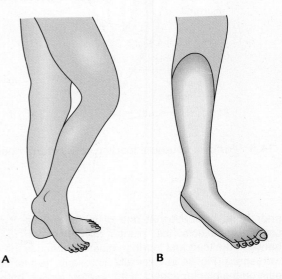

Fig. 34.7 Effects of injury of the common peroneal nerve: A, foot drop; B, sensory loss.

CUTANEOUS INNERVATION OF THE LOWER LIMB
(Figs 34.8 and 34.9)

The cutaneous nerves supplying the lower limb are derived from the branches of nerves of lumbar and sacral plexuses except for some proximal unisegmental nerves arising from T12 or L1 spinal nerves. The most of the cutaneous innervation of the thigh is provided by the lateral and posterior cutaneous nerves of the thigh and cutaneous branches of the femoral nerve, the names of which describe their distribution. The anterior cutaneous nerves from the femoral nerve in addition to the anterior aspect of the thigh also supply the most of the medial aspect of the thigh. The cutaneous innervation of the leg on its anteromedial aspect is provided by the saphenous nerve, the posterolateral aspect by the sural nerve, and the anterolateral aspect by the superficial peroneal nerve. The cutaneous innervation of dorsum of the foot is mostly provided by the superficial peroneal nerves (Fig. 34.9A). The cutaneous innervation of the sole of the foot is provided by the cutaneous branches of

the medial and lateral plantar nerves (Fig. 34.9B). The cutaneous nerves are described in detail with different regions of the lower limb.

SEGMENTAL INNERVATION OF THE LOWER LIMB
(Figs 34.10 and 34.11)

SEGMENTAL INNERVATION OF THE SKIN (DERMATOMES)

The area of the skin supplied by a spinal nerve is termed **dermatome**.

The lower limb bud develops on the ventrolateral aspect of the body wall opposite L1–S3 spinal segments; hence, the skin of the lower limb is innervated by these segments of the spinal cord.

Since the lower limb develops from the ventrolateral aspect of the body wall, it is innervated only by the ventral rami of spinal nerves. The exception to this rule is the superomedial quadrant of the gluteal region, which is

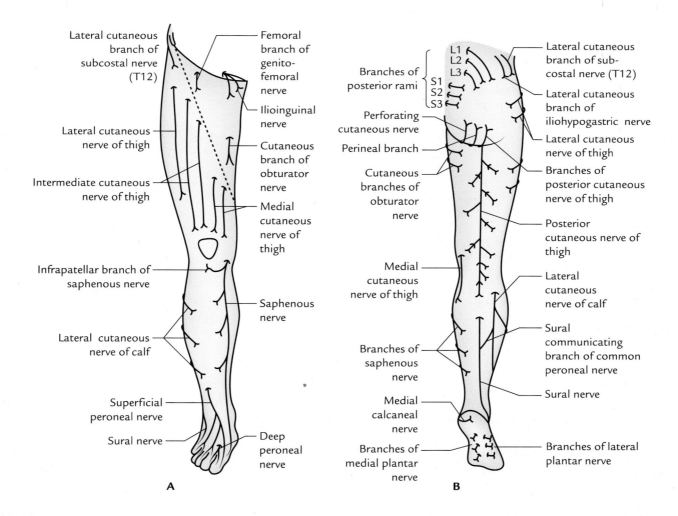

Fig. 34.8 Cutaneous nerves of the lower limb: **A**, on the anterior aspect; **B**, on the posterior aspect.

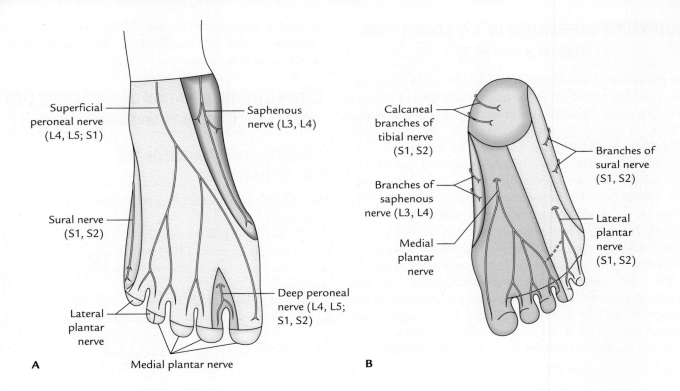

Fig. 34.9 Cutaneous nerves of the foot and their areas of distribution: **A**, dorsum of the foot; **B**, sole of the foot.

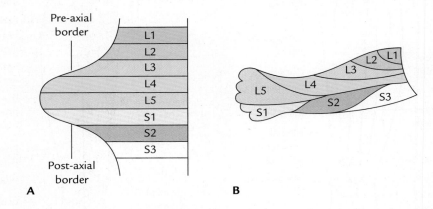

Fig. 34.10 Arrangement of dermatomes in the developing lower limb: **A**, simple dermatomal pattern, L1 spinal nerve supplying the pre-axial strip and S3 spinal nerve supplying the posterior strip; **B**, definitive dermatomal pattern of the lower limb bud.

innervated by the dorsal rami of L1–L3 and S1–S3 spinal nerves.

Initially the limb bud has **cephalic** and **caudal borders** called **pre-axial** and **post-axial borders,** respectively. The great toe is along the pre-axial border and the little toe is along the post-axial border. The arrangement of the dermatome pattern is simple at this stage; L1 spinal nerve supplies pre-axial strip of the skin and S3 spinal nerve supplies the post-axial strip of the skin (Fig. 34.10A).

Later the lower limb bud rotates medially by 90°. Therefore, the great toe comes to lie medially and the little toe lies laterally. As a result, the dermatomes are arranged in a sequence, above downward (L1–L4) along the *pre-axial border,* and below upward (S1–S3) along the *post-axial border* (Fig. 34.10B).

The middle three toes and adjoining area of the dorsum of foot and lateral side of the leg are supplied by L5 segment.

As the limb elongates the central dermatomes (L4, L5; S1) are pulled in such a way that they are represented only in the

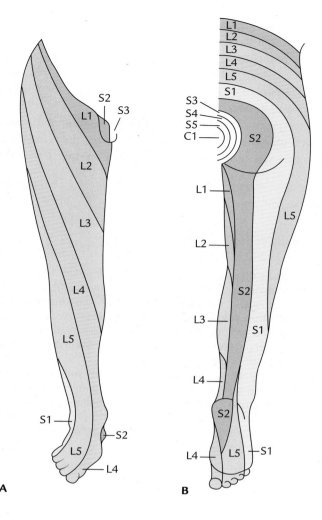

Fig. 34.11 Dermatomes of the lower limb: A, anterior aspect; B, posterior aspect.

In cases of the **paraplegia** (paralysis of lower limbs) clinicians can determine the site of lesion in the spinal cord (segments L1–S3) by performing the sensory examination for pain, touch, and temperature. This is so because sensory loss of the skin following injury to the spinal cord conforms to the dermatome. The upper limit of the sensory loss (dermatome) indicates the level of lesion.

SEGMENTAL INNERVATION OF THE MUSCLES

Most of the muscles are supplied by more than one segment of the spinal cord but only a few segments innervate the muscle predominantly. The damage of the predominant segment causes maximum paralysis. The segmental innervation of the muscles of the lower limb is given in Table 34.2.

The knowledge of these segmental values is of clinical importance in diagnosis of injuries of the nerves or to the spinal cord segments from which they arise.

SEGMENTAL INNERVATION OF THE JOINT MOVEMENTS

The four consecutive spinal segments regulate the movements of a particular joint in the limb. The upper two segments regulate the one movement and the lower two segments regulate the opposite movement, for a joint one segment distal in the limb, the centre (four consecutive spinal segments) lies in block one segment lower in the spinal cord.

The segmental innervation of the joints of lower limb is given in Table 34.3.

distal part of the limb and are buried proximally. The line along which the central dermatomes are buried is called an **axial line**.

The segmental innervation of the skin in adults is shown in Figure 34.11 and is given in Table 34.1.

Table 34.1 Segmental innervation of the skin of the lower limb

Segments	Area supplied
L1, L2, L3	Anterior aspect of the thigh in sequence from above downward
L4	Medial aspect of the leg
L5	Lateral aspect of the leg and medial side of the foot
S1	Lateral side of the foot and sole
S2	Middle of back of the thigh and leg
S3, S4	Buttocks

Table 34.2 Segmental innervation of the muscles of the lower limb

Segments	Muscles innervated
L1	Psoas major
L2, L3	Gracilis, pectineus, sartorius
L3, L4	Quadriceps femoris, adductors of the thigh
L4, L5	Tensor fasciae latae, tibialis anterior, tibialis posterior
L5; S1	Gluteus medius, gluteus minimus, extensor hallucis longus, extensor digitorum longus, peroneus longus, peroneus brevis, semitendinosus, semimembranosus
S1, S2	Gluteus maximus, biceps femoris, gastrocnemius, soleus
S2, S3	Flexor digitorum longus, flexor hallucis longus, interossei

Table 34.3 Segmental innervation of the joints of the lower limb

Joint	Four consecutive spinal segments (centre)	Movements
Hip joint	L2, L3, L4, L5	• Flexion, adduction, and medial rotation (L2, L3) • Extension, abduction, and lateral rotation (L4, L5)
Knee joint	L3, L4, L5; S1	• Extension (L3, L4) • Flexion (L5; S1)
Ankle joint	L4, L5; S1, S2	• Dorsiflexion (L4, L5) • Plantar flexion (S1, S2)

SYMPATHETIC INNERVATION OF THE LOWER LIMB

The sympathetic innervation of the lower limb is derived from the lower three thoracic and upper two lumbar (T10–L2) segments of the spinal cord.

The **preganglionic fibres** arising from the lateral horn cells pass out through ventral roots. Then they pass down in the sympathetic chain to relay in the lumbar and upper two or three sacral ganglia.

The **postganglionic fibres** arising from the lumbar ganglia pass through the femoral nerve to supply the femoral artery and its branches.

The postganglionic fibres arising from the sacral ganglia (S2–S3) pass through the tibial nerve to supply the popliteal artery and its branches.

The sympathetic stimulation causes dilatation of the blood vessels supplying skeletal muscles. However, the sympathetic fibres are vasomotor, sudomotor, and pilomotor to the skin.

N.B. The lower limbs do not have parasympathetic innervation.

Clinical correlation

Buerger's disease: It is an obliterative disorder of the lower limb arteries distal to the knee. It typically occurs in young male smokers. Clinically, it presents as **intermittent claudication**, digital ischaemia, and loss of the ankle pulses. The progressive ischaemia of digits may eventually require amputation of the foot. The treatment includes stopping smoking and sympathectomy.

The sympathetic denervation of the lower limb is achieved by removing second, third, and fourth lumbar ganglia with the intermediate chain (lumbar sympathectomy). It is important to note that the first lumbar ganglion is preserved because it controls the internal urethral sphincter. Its inadvertent removal leads to dry coitus.

Golden Facts to Remember

➤ Thickest nerve in the body	Sciatic nerve
➤ Commonest cause of the sciatic nerve injury	Iatrogenic (i.e., wrongly given injection in the gluteal region by the health professionals)
➤ Most commonly injured nerve in the lower limb	Common peroneal nerve
➤ Commonest site of the injury of common peroneal nerve	Neck of the fibula

Clinical Case Study

A 57-year-old patient was given a course of antibiotics by the intramuscular injections in his left gluteal region during his admission in the hospital. A week after discharge from the hospital, he experienced numbness and tingling sensations in his left lower limb down along the posterior aspect of the thigh and along the lateral sides of the leg and dorsum of the foot. On examination, the doctors found impaired skin sensation along the lateral side of the leg and the dorsum of the foot. When asked to walk his left foot tended to catch on steps. While sitting on the chair with feet off the ground his left foot assumed a plantar-flexed position (**foot drop**).

Questions

1. Name the nerve that is injured in this patient.
2. What is the commonest cause of injury to the sciatic nerve?
3. What are the two components of the sciatic nerve and tell which component is mostly affected by injury and why?
4. Give the anatomical basis of foot drop following the sciatic nerve injury?
5. What is sciatica? Give its common cause?

Answers

1. Sciatic nerve.
2. Misplaced intramuscular injection in the gluteal region.
3. The tibial and common peroneal components. The common peroneal component is most affected probably because its fibres lie most superficial in the sciatic nerve.
4. In sciatic nerve injury, all the muscles below the knee are paralyzed and the weight of foot causes it to assume the plantar-flexed position (foot drop).
5. Sciatica is a clinical condition in which patient complains of pain on the posterior aspect of the thigh, posterior and lateral sides of the leg, and lateral part of the dorsum of foot. It commonly occurs due to prolapse of an intervertebral disc pressing one or more roots of the sciatic nerve.

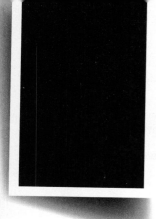

Multiple Choice Questions

CHAPTER 1

1. Select the *incorrect statement* about the boundaries of the abdominal cavity proper:
    (a) It is bounded superiorly by the diaphragm
    (b) It is bounded inferiorly by the perineum
    (c) It is bounded posteriorly by the posterior abdominal wall
    (d) It is open inferiorly

2. All of the following abdominal viscera are protected by the thoracic cage *except*:
    (a) Liver
    (b) Spleen
    (c) Pancreas
    (d) Stomach

3. Select the *incorrect statement* about the abdominal cavity proper:
    (a) It is under cover of the thoracic cage superiorly
    (b) It is continuous inferiorly with the pelvic cavity
    (c) It is partially protected inferiorly by the false pelvis
    (d) It is located between the diaphragm and pelvic outlet

4. All of the following abdominal viscera are partly protected by greater pelvis *except*:
    (a) Ileum
    (b) Caecum
    (c) Sigmoid colon
    (d) Rectum

5. The abdominal cavity extends superiorly into the osseocartilaginous thoracic cage up to:
    (a) 3rd intercostal space
    (b) 4th intercostal space
    (c) 5th intercostal space
    (d) 6th intercostal space

Answers
1. *b*, 2. *c*, 3. *d*, 4. *d*, 5. *b*

CHAPTER 2

1. The angle between the anterior surface of L5 vertebra and pelvic surface of S1 vertebra (lumbosacral angle) is:
    (a) 90°
    (b) 120°
    (c) 180°
    (d) 210°

2. The smooth medial part of ala of sacrum is related to all *except*:
    (a) Lumbosacral trunk
    (b) Femoral nerve
    (c) Iliolumbar artery
    (d) Sympathetic chain

3. Regarding anatomical position of hip bone all are correct *except*:
    (a) Symphyseal surfaces of pubic bones lie in the coronal plane
    (b) Pubic tubercle and anterior superior iliac spine lie in the same coronal plane
    (c) Linea terminalis of pelvis lies at an angle of about 70° to the horizontal plane
    (d) Anterior superior iliac spine lies at the level of the sacral promontory

4. All are the components of linea terminalis *except*:
    (a) Pubic crest
    (b) Pubic tubercle
    (c) Arcuate line of ilium
    (d) Promontory of sacrum

5. The median relations of pelvic surface of the sacrum include all *except*:
    (a) Median sacral vessels

(b) Sympathetic trunks

(c) Middle rectal artery

(d) Rectum

6. **All are contents of sacral canal** *except*:

(a) Conus medullaris

(b) Filum terminale

(c) Lower part of cauda equina

(d) Spinal meninges

7. **All structures emerge through the sacral hiatus** *except*:

(a) Fifth sacral nerves

(b) Coccygeal nerves

(c) Filum terminale

(d) Spinal meninges

8. **Select the *incorrect statement* about the coccyx:**

(a) Its pelvic surface is related to ganglion impar

(b) Its dorsal surface provides attachment to filum terminale

(c) Its base articulates with the apex of the sacrum

(d) Its pelvic surface provides attachment to sphincter ani externus muscle

Answers

1. *b*, 2. *b*, 3. *a*, 4. *b*, 5. *c*, 6. *a*, 7. *d*, 8. *d*

CHAPTER 3

1. **The membranous layer of superficial fascia of anterior abdominal wall is continuous with all** *except*:

(a) Buck's fascia of penis

(b) Dartos muscle of scrotum

(c) Fascia of Gallaudet

(d) Colles' fascia of perineum

2. **Which of the following structures lie in between the superficial and deep layers of superficial fascia of the anterior abdominal wall?**

(a) Superior epigastric artery

(b) Inferior epigastric artery

(c) Superficial epigastric artery

(d) Lower five intercostal nerves

3. **All the statements about external oblique muscle are correct** *except*:

(a) Its lower-free border forms the inguinal ligament

(b) Its aponeurosis takes part in the formation of rectus sheath

(c) It forms the boundary of lumbar (Petit's) triangle

(d) It takes origin from the outer lip of the iliac crest

4. **The neurovascular plane in the anterior abdominal wall lies between:**

(a) External and internal oblique muscles

(b) Internal and transversus abdominis muscles

(c) Transversus abdominis muscle and fascia transversalis

(d) Fascia transversalis and parietal peritoneum

5. **Anterior wall of rectus sheath below the arcuate line is formed by the aponeurosis of:**

(a) External oblique

(b) Internal oblique

(c) Transversus abdominis

(d) All of the above

6. **Muscle whose aponeurosis forms both anterior and posterior walls of rectus sheath is:**

(a) External oblique

(b) Internal oblique

(c) Transversus abdominis

(d) None of the above

7. **All are the contents of rectus sheath** *except*:

(a) Superior epigastric artery

(b) Rectus abdominis

(c) Superficial epigastric artery

(d) Inferior epigastric artery

8. **Select the *incorrect statement* about the pyramidalis:**

(a) It lies superficial to the rectus abdominis

(b) It is tensor of linea alba

(c) It arises from the body of pubis

(d) It is supplied by the genital branch of the genitofemoral nerve

Answers

1. *c*, 2. *c*, 3. *d*, 4. *b*, 5. *d*, 6. *b*, 7. *c*, 8. *d*

CHAPTER 4

1. **All of the following ligaments are derived from inguinal ligament** *except*:

(a) Lacunar ligament

(b) Interfoveolar ligament

(c) Pectineal ligament

(d) Reflex inguinal ligament

2. **All the statements about cremaster muscle are correct** *except*:

(a) It consists of loops of skeletal muscle fibre, derived from internal oblique muscle

(b) Its function is to pull the testis up toward the superficial inguinal ring

(c) It is supplied by ilioinguinal nerve

(d) Its action is not under voluntary control

3. Cremasteric reflex tests the integrity of spinal segments:
    (a) T11 and T12
    (b) L1 and L2
    (c) L3 and L4
    (d) S1 and S2

4. Select the *incorrect statement* about the conjoint tendon:
    (a) It is formed by the fusion of aponeurosis of internal oblique and transversus abdominis
    (b) It forms the medial half of the posterior wall of the inguinal canal
    (c) It is attached to the pubic crest and pecten pubis
    (d) It is formed by the fusion of aponeurosis of external and internal oblique muscles

5. All the statements about Hesselbach's triangle are correct *except*:
    (a) It lies superficial to the inguinal canal
    (b) It is bounded laterally by inferior epigastric artery
    (c) It is bounded medially by lateral border of rectus abdominis
    (d) It is bounded inferiorly by the inguinal ligament

6. The midinguinal point is a point midway between:
    (a) Pubic tubercle and anterior superior iliac spine
    (b) Pubic tubercle and iliac tubercle
    (c) Pubic symphysis and anterior superior iliac spine
    (d) Pubic symphysis and iliac tubercle

7. Regarding inguinal canal all the statements are true *except*:
    (a) It is an intermuscular slit in the lower part of the anterior abdominal wall
    (b) It is about 4 cm long
    (c) It provides passage to spermatic cord
    (d) The ilioinguinal nerve enters it through deep inguinal ring

8. All the statements about indirect inguinal hernia are true *except*:
    (a) The hernial sac enters the inguinal canal through deep inguinal ring
    (b) It commonly occurs due to persistence of the processus vaginalis
    (c) The neck of hernial sac lies medial to the inferior epigastric vessels
    (d) It is more in young adults than in elderly individuals

9. Select the *incorrect statement* about the direct inguinal hernia:
    (a) The hernial sac enters the inguinal canal pushing the posterior wall of the inguinal canal
    (b) The neck of hernial sac lies medial to the inferior epigastric vessels

    (c) The neck of direct inguinal hernia is narrow as compared to that of indirect inguinal hernia
    (d) It is less commonly strangulated as compared to the indirect inguinal hernia

Answers

1. *b*, 2. *c*, 3. *b*, 4. *d*, 5. *a*, 6. *c*, 7. *d*, 8. *c*, 9. *c*

CHAPTER 5

1. Select the *incorrect statement* about the penis:
    (a) It is a copulatory organ in male
    (b) Its root lies in the superficial perineal pouch
    (c) It is traversed by the urethra
    (d) It is enclosed in the deep fascia

2. All are true about the corpus spongiosum of penis *except*:
    (a) It forms the glans penis
    (b) It forms the bulb of penis
    (c) It lacks cavernous spaces
    (d) It is traversed by the urethra

3. Lymph from the glans penis is drained into:
    (a) External iliac lymph nodes
    (b) Internal iliac lymph nodes
    (c) Deep inguinal lymph nodes
    (d) Superficial inguinal lymph nodes

4. All of the following factors play a role in the erection of penis *except*:
    (a) Psychogenic/cutaneus stimulation
    (b) Parasympathetic stimulation
    (c) Filling of blood in cavernous spaces of corpora cavernosa by the helicine arteries
    (d) Sympathetic stimulation

5. Layer of the anterior abdominal wall that does not continue in the scrotal wall is:
    (a) Skin
    (b) External oblique muscle
    (c) Internal oblique muscle
    (d) Transversus abdominis muscle

6. The innermost covering of the testis is formed by:
    (a) Parietal layer of tunica vaginalis
    (b) Visceral layer of tunica vaginalis
    (c) Tunica vasculosa
    (d) Tunica albuginea

7. All of the following statements about testis are true *except*:
    (a) It develops in the abdominal cavity from a genital ridge derived from the intermediate mesoderm

(b) Testicular pain is carried to T10 and T11 spinal segments through sympathetic fibres

(c) Lymph from the testis is drained into pre- and para-aortic lymph nodes

(d) Testicular veins drain into the renal veins of the corresponding side

8. **Testis normally descends into the lower part of the scrotum at the age of:**

(a) Seventh month of intrauterine life

(b) Eighth month of intrauterine life

(c) Ninth month of intrauterine life

(d) First year of postnatal life

9. **All of the following statements about epididymis are correct *except*:**

(a) It consists of head, body, and tail

(b) Its duct develops from the mesonephric duct

(c) Its duct continues below with the ductus deferens

(d) Its body and tail are applied on to the posteromedial aspect of the testis

10. **The embryological remnants found in relation to the testis and epididymis include all *except*:**

(a) Appendix of the testis

(b) Organ of Giraldes

(c) Paraoöphoron

(d) Appendix of the epididymis

Answers

1. *d*, 2. *c*, 3. *c*, 4. *d*, 5. *d*, 6. *c*, 7. *d*, 8. *c*, 9. *d*, 10. *c*

CHAPTER 6

1. **Select the *incorrect statement* about the peritoneum:**

(a) It is the largest serous membrane in the body

(b) It is lined by endothelial cells

(c) In males it surrounds a closed sac, the peritoneal cavity

(d) In females it surrounds a sac, which has two openings at the ends of uterine tubes

2. **Regarding parietal peritoneum all the statements are correct *except*:**

(a) It forms the innermost layer of the abdominal wall

(b) It is composed of the mesothelial serous membrane

(c) It is insensitive to pain

(d) It develops from the somatopleuric mesoderm

3. **The epiploic foramen (of Winslow) is bounded by:**

(a) Caudate lobe of the liver superiorly

(b) First part of the duodenum inferiorly

(c) Portal vein posteriorly

(d) Right free margin of the lesser omentum anteriorly

4. **Select the *incorrect statement* about the mesentery:**

(a) It suspends the loops of jejunum and ileum from the posterior abdominal wall

(b) Its root extends from the duodenojejunal flexure to the ileocaecal junction

(c) Its root is 6 m long

(d) It crosses in front of the abdominal aorta

5. **Regarding lesser omentum, all the statements are correct *except*:**

(a) It extends between the lesser curvature of stomach and the inferior surface of the liver

(b) Superiorly it is attached to the margins of grooves for ligamentum teres and ligamentum venosum

(c) Its right free margin forms the anterior boundary of epiploic foramen

(d) It contains right and left gastric artery

6. **Select the *incorrect statement* about the sigmoid mesocolon:**

(a) It is a triangular fold of peritoneum suspending the sigmoid colon from pelvic wall

(b) Its apex lies at the division of left common iliac artery

(c) Its attachment extends inferiorly up to the level of S2 vertebra

(d) The left ureter lies behind its apex

7. **Regarding falciform ligament all the statements are correct *except*:**

(a) It is a sickle-shaped fold of peritoneum

(b) It connects the inferior surface of the liver to the anterior abdominal wall

(c) Its concave inferior margin contains ligamentum teres

(d) Its convex superior margin is attached to the inferior surface of the diaphragm and anterior abdominal wall

8. **All are retroperitoneal/extraperitoneal organs *except*:**

(a) Kidneys

(b) Suprarenal glands

(c) Spleen

(d) Descending colon

Answers

1. *b*, 2. *c*, 3. *c*, 4. *c*, 5. *b*, 6. *c*, 7. *b*, 8. *c*

CHAPTER 7

1. **All statements regarding the stomach are correct *except*:**

(a) It is the most dilated part of the alimentary tract

(b) It lies mainly in the left hypochondriac, epigastric, and umbilical regions

(c) Its most fixed part is the pylorus (gastroduodenal junction)

(d) Its most fixed part is the cardiac end (gastroesophageal junction)

2. All of the following arteries supply the stomach *except*:

   (a) Left gastric artery
   (b) Left epiploic artery
   (c) Right gastric artery
   (d) Short gastric artery

3. All of the following structures form the stomach bed *except*:

   (a) Body of pancreas
   (b) Splenic artery
   (c) Right crus and dome of the diaphragm
   (d) Transverse mesocolon

4. All the structures forming the stomach bed are separated from the stomach by the lesser sac *except*:

   (a) Left kidney
   (b) Left suprarenal gland
   (c) Left colic flexure
   (d) Spleen

5. Select the *incorrect statement* about the gastric canal:

   (a) It is located along the lesser curvature of the stomach
   (b) It is also called Magenstrasse
   (c) It is produced due to the absence of longitudinal fold of gastric mucosa
   (d) It is prone to ulceration

6. Select the *incorrect statement* about the spleen:

   (a) It is the largest lymphoid organ in the body
   (b) It filters the microbial agents from the circulation
   (c) It develops in the ventral mesogastrium
   (d) It is located in the left hypochondrium between the fundus of the stomach and diaphragm

7. Regarding spleen all statements are true *except*:

   (a) Its upper pole (medial end) lies 3/4 cm lateral to the spine of T10 vertebra
   (b) Its long axis corresponds to the long axis of the 10th rib
   (c) Its lower pole (lateral end) extends forward up to the midclavicular line
   (d) Its superior border presents one or two notches near its lateral end

8. The hilum of spleen is located on its visceral surface in the region of:

   (a) Renal impression
   (b) Gastric impression
   (c) Colic impression
   (d) Pancreatic impression

Answers

1. *c*, 2. *b*, 3. *c*, 4. *d*, 5. *c*, 6. *c*, 7. *c*, 8. *b*

CHAPTER 8

1. Select the *incorrect statement* about the liver:

   (a) It almost completely occupies right hypochondrium
   (b) It forms about 1/18th of total body weight in a newborn
   (c) It lies largely outside the thoracic cage
   (d) It weighs about 1–2 kg

2. Factors keeping the liver in position include all *except*:

   (a) Hepatic veins
   (b) Intra-abdominal pressure
   (c) Ligaments of liver
   (d) Hepatic pedicle

3. All the statements about the bare area of the liver are correct *except*:

   (a) It is the largest non-peritoneal area of the liver
   (b) It is located on the posterior surface of the right lobe
   (c) It is related to the right spleen
   (d) It is one of the sites of porta systemic anastomosis

4. Select the *incorrect statement* about porta hepatis:

   (a) It is a horizontal fissure on the inferior surface of the liver
   (b) The neck of gallbladder lies at its right end
   (c) The junction of the fissures for ligamentum teres and ligamentum lies at its left end
   (d) The right and left hepatic ducts enter the liver through it

5. Which of the following structures lie anteriorly in the hepatic pedicle just above the termination of the cystic duct?

   (a) Portal vein
   (b) Common hepatic duct
   (c) Right hepatic artery
   (d) Left hepatic artery

6. Select the *incorrect statement* about the gallbladder:

   (a) It lies in an elongated fossa on the inferior surface of the right lobe of liver
   (b) It can store up to 50 ml of bile
   (c) Its body is covered with peritoneum on all sides
   (d) It is distended in extrinsic obstruction of the common bile duct

7. The total number of hepatic segments is:

   (a) 6
   (b) 7

(c) 8

(d) 9

8. **The notable features on the visceral surface of the liver are all *except*:**

(a) Gallbladder

(b) Bare area of liver

(c) Porta hepatis

(d) Fissure of ligamentum teres hepatis

Answers

1. *c*, 2. *d*, 3. *c*, 4. *d*, 5. *b*, 6. *c*, 7. *c*, 8. *b*

CHAPTER 9

1. **All the statements about the duodenum are correct *except*:**

(a) It is the most fixed part of the small intestine

(b) It is about 25 cm long

(c) It extends below the level of umbilicus

(d) It produces an impression on the visceral surface of the liver

2. **Select the *incorrect statement* about the duodenum:**

(a) It is a proximal C-shaped loop of the small intestine

(b) It lies opposite L2, L3, and L4 vertebrae

(c) It extends from the pylorus to the duodenojejunal flexure

(d) It is the most deeply placed part of the gastrointestinal tract

3. **Which part of the duodenum is called duodenal cap by the radiologists?**

(a) First part

(b) Second part

(c) Third part

(d) Fourth part

4. **Regarding duodenum which of the following statements is *not correct*?**

(a) The gastroduodenal artery runs behind its first part

(b) Above the opening of major duodenal papilla, it develops from foregut

(c) Below the opening of major duodenal papilla, it develops from hindgut

(d) The common bile duct opens into its second part

5. **All the statements about the pancreas are correct *except*:**

(a) It lies transversely across the posterior abdominal wall behind the lesser sac

(b) It is an exo-endocrine gland

(c) Its ducts open into the second part of the duodenum

(d) It is mostly intraperitoneal

6. **The posterior surface of the head of pancreas is related to all *except*:**

(a) Inferior vena cava

(b) Aorta

(c) Terminal parts of renal veins

(d) Bile duct

7. **Select the *incorrect statement* about the tail of pancreas:**

(a) It lies within the lienorenal ligament

(b) It comes in contact with the surface of the spleen

(c) It has maximum concentration of islets of Langerhans

(d) It is the most fixed part of the pancreas

8. **All the statements about the neck of pancreas are correct *except*:**

(a) Its anterior surface is related to the pylorus

(b) The portal vein is formed behind it

(c) It lies behind the lesser sac

(d) It presents an upward projection called tuber omentale

Answers

1. *c*, 2. *b*, 3. *a*, 4. *c*, 5. *d*, 6. *b*, 7. *d*, 8. *d*

CHAPTER 10

1. **Select the *incorrect statement* about jejunum:**

(a) It forms the upper two-fifth of the mobile part of the small intestine

(b) It begins at the duodenojejunal flexure

(c) It has more Peyer's patches in its wall than ileum

(d) Its mesentery presents windows

2. **All the statements regarding ileum are correct *except*:**

(a) It forms distal three-fifth of the mobile part of the small intestine

(b) It terminates at the ileocaecal junction

(c) Its mesentery does not present windows

(d) Its proximal part has maximum concentration of Peyer's patches

3. **Meckel's diverticulum is due to persistence of:**

(a) Allantois

(b) Vitello-intestinal duct

(c) Left umbilical vein

(d) Ductus venosus

4. **Select the *incorrect statement* about Meckel's diverticulum:**

(a) It is located about 2 feet proximal to the ileocaecal junction

(b) It is attached to the antimesenteric border

(c) It is usually 20 cm long

(d) It may cause intestinal obstruction

5. The length of the large intestine is about:
   (a) 1 m
   (b) 1.5 m
   (c) 2 m
   (d) 2.5 m

6. All are characteristic features of the large intestine *except*:
   (a) Appendices epiploicae
   (b) Sacculations
   (c) Villi
   (d) Taenia coli

7. Select the *incorrect statement* about the caecum:
   (a) It forms the commencement of the large intestine
   (b) It is ampullary type in most of the cases
   (c) It has greater breadth than length
   (d) It develops from the hindgut

8. The caecum is supplied by:
   (a) Ileocolic artery
   (b) Middle colic artery
   (c) Left colic artery
   (d) Right colic artery

9. The appendix is devoid of all of the following *except*:
   (a) Appendices epiploicae
   (b) Taenia coli
   (c) Sacculations
   (d) Mesentery

10. Select the *incorrect statement* about the appendix:
    (a) The base of appendix corresponds to McBurney's point
    (b) The appendicular artery is a branch of ileocolic artery
    (c) The appendix is innervated by T10 spinal segment
    (d) The commonest position of appendix is subcaecal

Answers

1. *c*, 2. *d*, 3. *b*, 4. *c*, 5. *a*, 6. *c*, 7. *d*, 8. *a*, 9. *d*, 10. *d*

CHAPTER 11

1. Select the *incorrect statement* about the kidneys:
   (a) They are major excretory organs of the body
   (b) They lie on the posterior abdominal wall opposite T12–L3 vertebrae
   (c) Their upper poles are about 5 cm away from the midline
   (d) Their hila are crossed by the transpyloric plane

2. All the muscles are related to the posterior surface of the kidney *except*:
   (a) Transversus abdominis
   (b) Internal oblique
   (c) Psoas major
   (d) Quadratus lumborum

3. Anterior surface of the left kidney is related to all *except*:
   (a) Stomach
   (b) Pancreas
   (c) Left colic flexure
   (d) Left crus of diaphragm

4. In renal colic, the pain is referred from the loin to groin mainly through the spinal segments:
   (a) T9–T12
   (b) T10–L1
   (c) T11–L2
   (d) T12–L3

5. The length of each ureter is about:
   (a) 15 cm
   (b) 20 cm
   (c) 25 cm
   (d) 30 cm

6. All structures form anterior relations of the left ureter *except*:
   (a) Left colic vessels
   (b) Ileocolic vessels
   (c) Left vessels
   (d) Sigmoid mesocolon

7. All the statements are true about renal pelvis *except*:
   (a) It is the upper expanded funnel-shaped part of the ureter
   (b) It receives major calyces
   (c) It lies anterior to renal vessels
   (d) It develops from the ureteric bud

8. All the statements about the right suprarenal gland are true *except*:
   (a) It lies at a lower level than left suprarenal gland
   (b) Partly it lies behind the inferior vena cava
   (c) Superiorly it is related to the bare area of liver
   (d) Right suprarenal vein drains into the inferior vena cava

Answers

1. *c*, 2. *b*, 3. *d*, 4. *c*, 5. *c*, 6. *b*, 7. *c*, 8. *a*

CHAPTER 12

1. All of the following are the muscles of the posterior abdominal wall *except*:
   (a) Psoas major
   (b) Quadratus lumborum

(c) Transversus abdominis

(d) Diaphragm

2. **All the statements about psoas major are correct** *except*:

   (a) It arises from all the lumbar vertebrae
   (b) It contains the lumbar plexus within its substance
   (c) It is pierced by the genitofemoral nerve
   (d) It is the chief extensor of the hip joint

3. Select the *incorrect statement* about the thoraco-lumbar fascia:

   (a) It consists of three layers
   (b) It encloses three muscles between its layers
   (c) It provides origin to psoas major muscle
   (d) It provides attachment to latissimus dorsi muscle

4. Select the *incorrect statement* about the abdominal aorta:

   (a) It extends from T12–L4 vertebrae
   (b) It lies to the right of the inferior vena cava
   (c) It is crossed anteriorly by the pancreas
   (d) Its dorsal aspect gives origin to the median sacral artery

5. All the statements about lumbar plexus are correct *except*:

   (a) It is formed by the ventral rami of upper four lumbar nerves
   (b) It lies within the substance of psoas major muscle
   (c) It communicates with the subcostal nerve
   (d) It divides the psoas major muscle into two planes

6. All of the following branches of lumbar plexus emerge from the lateral border of the psoas major *except*:

   (a) Iliohypogastric
   (b) Ilioinguinal
   (c) Obturator
   (d) Femoral

7. Select the *incorrect statement* about the inferior vena cava:

   (a) It is the largest and widest vein of the body
   (b) It is formed in front of the L5 vertebra
   (c) It drains both gonadal veins
   (d) It is crossed anteriorly by the root of mesentery

8. All of the following veins are tributaries of the inferior vena cava *except*:

   (a) Right suprarenal
   (b) Left suprarenal
   (c) Right renal
   (d) Left renal

Answers

1. *d*, 2. *d*, 3. *c*, 4. *b*, 5. *d*, 6. *c*, 7. *c*, 8. *b*

CHAPTER 13

1. All of the following structures form the boundaries of pelvic inlet *except*:

   (a) Sacral promontory
   (b) Anterior borders of alae of sacrum
   (c) Pecten pubis
   (d) Pubic tubercle

2. Which of the following conjugate diameters of the true pelvis is most important clinically?

   (a) External conjugate
   (b) True conjugate
   (c) Diagonal conjugate
   (d) Obstetrical conjugate

3. Commonest type of female pelvis is:

   (a) Platypelloid type
   (b) Gynecoid type
   (c) Android type
   (d) Anthropoid type

4. The percentage of gynecoid pelvic in females is about:

   (a) 60%
   (b) 42%
   (c) 32%
   (d) 22%

5. Select the *incorrect statement* about the pelvic outlet:

   (a) It is bounded anteriorly by the lower margin of pubic symphysis
   (b) It is bounded anterolaterally by the conjoint ischiopubic rami
   (c) It is bounded posterolaterally by the sacrotuberous ligaments
   (d) Its transverse diameter is maximum

6. Which of the following statements about the true pelvis is incorrect?

   (a) The maximum diameter at its inlet is transverse diameter
   (b) The maximum diameter at its outlet is anteroposterior diameter
   (c) The maximum diameter at its inlet is anteroposterior diameter
   (d) The minimum diameter at its outlet is transverse diameter

7. Which of the following joints is of synovial variety?

   (a) Lumbosacral joint
   (b) Sacroiliac joint
   (c) Pubic symphysis
   (d) Sacrococcygeal joint

8. Which of the following ligaments is the strongest?
   (a) Iliolumbar ligament
   (b) Interosseous sacroiliac ligament
   (c) Sacrospinous ligament
   (d) Sacrotuberous ligament

Answers

1. *d*, 2. *c*, 3. *b*, 4. *b*, 5. *d*, 6. *c*, 7. *b*, 8. *b*

CHAPTER 14

1. The muscles of the true pelvis include all *except*:
   (a) Piriformis
   (b) Obturator internum
   (c) Ischiocavernosus
   (d) Levator ani

2. All are the parts of the levator ani *except*:
   (a) Levator prostate
   (b) Pubococcygeus
   (c) Iliococcygeus
   (d) Coccygeus

3. All are the constituents of pelvic diaphragm *except*:
   (a) Levator ani
   (b) Obturator internus
   (c) Coccygeus
   (d) Pelvic fascia

4. All are the branches of the posterior division of the internal iliac artery *except*:
   (a) Iliolumbar artery
   (b) Lateral sacral arteries
   (c) Superior gluteal artery
   (d) Obturator artery

5. The root value of sacral plexus is:
   (a) L4, L5; S1, S2, S3
   (b) L3, L4, L5; S1, S2
   (c) L5; S1, S2, S3, S4
   (d) L2, L3, L4; S1, S2

6. All the statements about the sacral plexus are correct *except*:
   (a) It is formed by the anterior primary rami of L4 to S4 nerves
   (b) It lies deep to pelvic fascia
   (c) It gives off sciatic nerve
   (d) It gives off femoral nerve

7. All of the following arteries of the pelvis are branches of the internal iliac artery *except*:
   (a) Umbilical artery
   (b) Uterine artery

   (c) Ovarian artery
   (d) Vaginal artery

8. All are the tributaries of internal iliac vein *except*:
   (a) Uterine veins
   (b) Vaginal veins
   (c) Obturator veins
   (d) Umbilical veins

Answers

1. *c*, 2. *d*, 3. *b*, 4. *d*, 5. *a*, 6. *d*, 7. *c*, 8. *d*

CHAPTER 15

1. All of the following structures form deep boundaries of perineum *except*:
   (a) Ischiopubic rami
   (b) Ischial tuberosities
   (c) Sacrospinous ligaments
   (d) Sacrotuberous ligaments

2. All are muscles of superficial perineal pouch *except*:
   (a) Bulbospongiosus
   (b) Ischiocavernosus
   (c) Sphincter urethrae
   (d) Superficial transverse perineal

3. All are the contents of deep perineal pouch in male *except*:
   (a) Membranous urethra
   (b) Cowper's glands
   (c) Root of penis
   (d) Sphincter urethrae muscle

4. Select the *incorrect statement* about the perineal membrane:
   (a) It forms the boundary of both superficial and deep perineal pouches
   (b) Its anterior border thickens to form transverse perineal ligament
   (c) Its posterior border provides attachment to the perineal body in the midline
   (d) It is pierced by the pudendal nerve

5. The gap between the arcuate pubic ligament and transverse perineal ligament in male transmits:
   (a) Spongy urethra
   (b) Dorsal nerves of penis
   (c) Deep dorsal vein of penis
   (d) (b) and (c)

6. All of the following are contents of ischiorectal fossa *except*:
   (a) Posterior scrotal nerve and vessels

(b) Perineal branch of fourth sacral nerve

(c) Sphincter ani externus

(d) Inferior rectal nerve and vessels

7. **All of the following are attached to the perineal body** *except*:

   (a) Bulbospongiosus

   (b) Externus sphincter of anal canal

   (c) External sphincter of urethra

   (d) Ischiocavernosus

8. **All of the following are contents of superficial perineal pouch** *except*:

   (a) Bulbs of the vestibule of vagina

   (b) Bartholin glands

   (c) Bulbourethral glands

   (d) Superficial transverse perineal muscles

Answers

1. *c*, 2. *c*, 3. *c*, 4. *d*, 5. *d*, 6. *c*, 7. *d*, 8. *c*

CHAPTER 16

1. **Select the *incorrect statement* about the urinary bladder:**

   (a) Its neck is its most fixed part

   (b) Its superior surface is the most movable part

   (c) Its trigone is derived from the absorbed parts of the mesonephric ducts

   (d) Its position is abdominopelvic at birth

2. **The bladder structure which serves as a guide to locate the ureteric orifice is:**

   (a) Interureteric crest

   (b) Uvula vesicae

   (c) Trigone

   (d) Uretero-urethral ridge

3. **The female bladder is supplied by all arteries** *except*:

   (a) Superior vesical

   (b) Inferior vesical

   (c) Uterine

   (d) Vaginal

4. **The length of the male urethra is about:**

   (a) 10 cm

   (b) 12 cm

   (c) 16 cm

   (d) 20 cm

5. **All the structures open into the posterior wall of prostatic urethra** *except*:

   (a) Prostatic utricle

   (b) Lacunae of Morgagni

(c) Ejaculatory ducts

(d) Prostatic glands

6. **All the statements about the prostatic part of urethra are correct** *except*:

   (a) It is about 3 cm in length

   (b) It is the widest and most dilatable part

   (c) Its lumen is lined by the stratified squamous epithelium

   (d) It receives the openings of ejaculatory ducts

7. **Select the *incorrect statement* about the female urethra:**

   (a) It is about 4 cm long

   (b) It is embedded in the posterior wall of the vagina

   (c) It pierces the perineal membrane

   (d) It opens into the vestibule of the vagina

8. **All the structures open in the female urethra** *except*:

   (a) Lacunae of Morgagni

   (b) Urethral glands

   (c) Bartholin's glands

   (d) Glands of Skene

9. **All the statements about the female urethra are correct** *except*:

   (a) It is about 4 cm long

   (b) It lies immediately anterior to the vagina

   (c) Its external orifice is situated about 2 inches (5 cm) behind the clitoris

   (d) It pierces the urogenital diaphragm

Answers

1. *d*, 2. *a*, 3. *b*, 4. *d*, 5. *b*, 6. *c*, 7. *b*, 8. *a*, 9. *c*

CHAPTER 17

1. **Select the *incorrect statement* about the prostate gland:**

   (a) It is located in the lesser pelvis below the neck of urinary bladder

   (b) It is devoid of muscular tissue

   (c) Its anterior lobe is devoid of glandular tissue

   (d) Its median lobe is the common site of benign hypertrophy

2. **All the following structures lie within the prostate gland** *except*:

   (a) Ejaculatory ducts

   (b) Prostatic utricle

   (c) Prostatic venous plexus

   (d) Urethra

3. **Which lobe of prostate is responsible for producing** *uvula vesicae*?

   (a) Anterior

   (b) Posterior

(c) Lateral
(d) Median

4. **The surgical approaches of prostatectomy include all** *except*:

(a) Suprapubic
(b) Retropubic
(c) Transrectal
(d) Transurethral

5. **The length of vas deferens is about:**

(a) 15 cm
(b) 25 cm
(c) 35 cm
(d) 45 cm

6. **A *true statement* regarding the vas deferens is:**

(a) It is the principal content of the spermatic cord
(b) It develops from the mesonephric duct
(c) It opens in the membranous part of the urethra
(d) It is extraperitoneal throughout the abdominopelvic part of its course

7. **The secretion of seminal vesicle is rich in:**

(a) Fructose
(b) Prostaglandin
(c) Alkaline phosphatase
(d) (a) and (b)

8. **Select the *incorrect statement* about rectovesical fascia of Denonvilliers:**

(a) It separates the prostate from the rectum
(b) It is formed by the fusion of two layers of the peritoneum intervening between the prostate and the rectum in fetus
(c) It is not adherent to the posterior aspect of the prostate gland
(d) It prevents the backward spread of the prostatic cancer

Answers

1. *b*, 2. *c*, 3. *d*, 4. *c*, 5. *d*, 6. *c*, 7. *d*, 8. *c*

CHAPTER 18

1. **The forward angulations between the long axes of vagina and cervix is called angle of:**

(a) Anteflexion
(b) Anteversion
(c) Retroflexion
(d) Retroversion

2. **When the urinary bladder is empty the angle of anteflexion is about:**

(a) 60°
(b) 90°
(c) 120°
(d) 150°

3. **All are the true ligaments of uterus *except*:**

(a) Transverse cervical ligaments
(b) Round ligaments
(c) Broad ligaments
(d) Uterosacral ligaments

4. **Most important true ligaments providing support to the uterus are:**

(a) Transverse cervical ligaments
(b) Pubocervical ligaments
(c) Uterosacral ligaments
(d) Round ligaments

5. **The lymph from the cervix is drained in all of the following lymph nodes *except*:**

(a) External iliac
(b) Internal iliac
(c) Superficial inguinal
(d) Sacral

6. **Select the *incorrect statement* about the vagina:**

(a) Its anterior wall is shorter than the posterior wall
(b) Its posterior fornix is related to the rectouterine pouch
(c) It is lined by the stratified columnar epithelium
(d) It is lubricated by the cervical mucous

7. **Select the *incorrect statement* about the uterine tube:**

(a) It is about 10 cm long
(b) It conveys ova from the ovary to the uterine cavity
(c) It lies in the attached border of the broad ligament
(d) It provides the site for fertilization of the ovum

8. **All the statements about the ovary are true *except*:**

(a) It is connected to the broad ligament through the mesovarium
(b) It is covered by the peritoneum
(c) Left ovarian vein drains into left renal vein
(d) Lymphatics from the ovary drain into pre-aortic and para-aortic lymph nodes

9. **Select the *incorrect statement* about the clitoris:**

(a) It is homologous to the penis in male
(b) It does not consist of corpus spongiosum
(c) It transmits urethra
(d) It develops from the genital tubercle

Answers

1. *b*, 2. *c*, 3. *c*, 4. *a*, 5. *c*, 6. *c*, 7. *c*, 8. *b*, 9. *c*

CHAPTER 19

1. Select the *true statement* about the rectum:
   (a) It is about 15 cm long
   (b) It is straight in its course
   (c) Its posterior surface is covered by peritoneum
   (d) It presents anteroposterior and lateral curvatures

2. The rectum is characterized by the presence of:
   (a) Taenia coli
   (b) Haustrations
   (c) Permanent transverse mucosal folds within the lumen
   (d) Appendices epiploicae

3. The length of the rectum is about:
   (a) 5 cm
   (b) 7.5 cm
   (c) 12 cm
   (d) 15 cm

4. The middle one-third of the rectum is covered by the peritoneum:
   (a) On all sides
   (b) On the front
   (c) On each side
   (d) On the front and sides

5. The internal hemorrhoids/piles are due to dilatation of the radicles of:
   (a) Superior rectal vein
   (b) Middle rectal vein
   (c) Inferior rectal vein
   (d) (b) and (c)

6. The chief artery supplying the rectum is:
   (a) Superior rectal
   (b) Middle rectal
   (c) Inferior rectal
   (d) Median sacral

7. Select the *incorrect statement* about the anal canal:
   (a) It is situated in the perineum
   (b) It is about 4 cm long
   (c) It is related on each side to the ischiorectal fossa
   (d) It is entirely lined by the stratified squamous epithelium

8. Anorectal ring is formed by all of the following *except*:
   (a) External sphincter
   (b) Internal sphincter
   (c) Coccygeus
   (d) Puborectalis

Answers
1. *d*, 2. *c*, 3. *c*, 4. *b*, 5. *a*, 6. *b*, 7. *d*, 8. *c*

CHAPTER 20

1. All are antigravity muscles of the lower limb *except*:
   (a) Gluteus maximus
   (b) Quadriceps femoris
   (c) Adductor muscles of the thigh
   (d) Calf muscles

2. Line of gravity in the lower limb passes anterior to all *except*:
   (a) Sacrum
   (b) Hip joint
   (c) Knee joint
   (d) Ankle joint

3. Arterial pulses can be felt in the lower limb at all of the following sites *except*:
   (a) At midinguinal point
   (b) In the popliteal fossa
   (c) On the dorsum of the foot
   (d) In the sole of the foot

4. Most preferred site for the intramuscular injection in the lower limb is:
   (a) Gluteal region
   (b) Thigh
   (c) Leg
   (d) Foot

Answers
1. *c*, 2. *b*, 3. *d*, 4. *d*

CHAPTER 21

1. All the statements about the hip bone are correct *except*:
   (a) It consists of three parts: ilium, ischium, and pubis
   (b) In early childhood, three parts are separated from each other by the triradiate fibrocartilage
   (c) Primary centre ossification for the ilium appears first
   (d) It presents a cup-shaped hollow on the lateral aspect of its middle constricted part

2. Ventral segment of the iliac crest provides attachment to all of the following muscles *except*:
   (a) Tensor fascia latae
   (b) External oblique muscle of the abdomen
   (c) Latissimus dorsi
   (d) Erector spinae

3. Medial part of pectin pubis provides attachment to all the structures *except*:
   (a) Lacunar ligament
   (b) Reflected part of the inguinal ligament

(c) Pectineal ligament (of Cooper)
(d) Conjoint tendon

4. **All the statements about the femur are correct *except*:**
   (a) It is the largest and strongest bone of the body
   (b) Its nutrient artery is the largest nutrient artery in the body
   (c) Its angle of anteversion varies from 10° to 15°
   (d) Its neck–shaft angle is less in female

5. **Select the *incorrect statement* about the patella:**
   (a) It is the largest sesamoid bone in the body
   (b) It develops in the tendon of quadriceps femoris
   (c) It has a natural tendency to dislocate medially
   (d) The articular cartilage covering its articular surface is the thickest articular cartilage in the body

6. **Select the *incorrect statement* about the fibula:**
   (a) It is the lateral bone of the leg
   (b) It corresponds to the radius bone of the upper limb
   (c) The law of union of epiphyses is violated in it
   (d) It is commonly used for bone grafting

7. **All the statements about calcaneum are correct *except*:**
   (a) It is the largest tarsal bone
   (b) It starts ossifying after birth
   (c) Anteriorly it articulates with cuboid
   (d) It provides attachment to tendo achillis

8. **Talus provides attachment to:**
   (a) Tibialis posterior
   (b) Tibialis anterior
   (c) Extensor digitorum brevis
   (d) None of the above

9. **Select the *incorrect statement* about the metatarsals:**
   (a) They are miniature long bones
   (b) They ossify from two centres
   (c) Epiphyseal centres of all metatarsals appear at their distal ends
   (d) Second metatarsal is most fixed metatarsal bone

Answers
1. *b*, 2. *d*, 3. *c*, 4. *b*, 5. *c*, 6. *b*, 7. *b*, 8. *d*, 9. *c*

CHAPTER 22

1. **The centre of saphenous opening lies about 3–4 cm below and lateral to:**
   (a) Midinguinal point
   (b) Midpoint of the inguinal ligament
   (c) Pubic tubercle
   (d) Pubic symphysis

2. **Select the *correct statement* about the cribriform fascia:**
   (a) It covers femoral ring
   (b) It covers saphenous opening
   (c) It pierces by the femoral vein
   (d) It forms anterior wall of the femoral sheath

3. **Iliotibial tract provides attachment to:**
   (a) Gluteus maximus
   (b) Gluteus medius
   (c) Tensor fasciae latae
   (d) All the above
   (e) (a) and (c)

4. **Part of quadriceps femoris not attached to femur is:**
   (a) Vastus lateralis
   (b) Vastus medialis
   (c) Vastus intermedius
   (d) Rectus femoris

5. **Select the *incorrect statement* about femoral triangle:**
   (a) It is bounded laterally by the medial border of sartorius
   (b) It is bounded medially by lateral border of adductor longus
   (c) Its base is formed by the inguinal ligament
   (d) Its floor is formed by the muscles

6. **The principal artery supplying the thigh is:**
   (a) Femoral
   (b) Profunda femoris
   (c) Lateral circumflex femoral
   (d) Medial circumflex femoral

7. **All are contents of adductor canal *except*:**
   (a) Femoral artery
   (b) Femoral vein
   (c) Nerve to vastus lateralis
   (d) Saphenous nerve

8. **A stab wound through the apex of femoral triangular can injure all *except*:**
   (a) Femoral artery
   (b) Profunda femoris artery
   (c) Adductor brevis
   (d) Medial cutaneous nerve of the thigh

Answers
1. *c*, 2. *b*, 3. *e*, 4. *d*, 5. *b*, 6. *b*, 7. *c*, 8. *c*

CHAPTER 23

1. **Adductor magnus is supplied by:**
   (a) Femoral nerve
   (b) Obturator nerve

(c) Sciatic nerve

(d) All of the above

(e) (a) and (c)

2. Muscle of the adductor group of thigh not attached to the femur is:

(a) Adductor longus

(b) Adductor brevis

(c) Adductor magnus

(d) Gracilis

3. Adductor of thigh innervated by two different nerves is:

(a) Adductor longus

(b) Adductor brevis

(c) Adductor magnus

(d) Gracilis

4. Which muscle helps in the extension of the hip?

(a) Pectineus

(b) Adductor longus

(c) Adductor brevis

(d) Adductor magnus

5. Most medial muscle of the adductor compartment of thigh is:

(a) Adductor longus

(b) Adductor brevis

(c) Gracilis

(d) Adductor magnus

6. Select the *incorrect statement* about the adductor brevis:

(a) It lies deep to pectineus and adductor longus

(b) It is usually supplied by the anterior division of obturator nerve

(c) It intervenes between anterior and posterior divisions of the obturator nerve

(d) It usually forms the floor of femoral triangle

7. Select the *incorrect statement* about the obturator nerve:

(a) It is derived from L2, L3, L4 spinal nerves

(b) It contributes in the formation of subsartorial plexus of the nerves

(c) It enters the thigh deep to the medial part of inguinal ligament

(d) Its posterior division gives an articular twig to the knee joint

8. All forms cruciate arterial anastomosis on the back of the thigh *except*:

(a) Transverse cervical branch of medial circumference femoral artery

(b) Ascending branch of first perforating artery

(c) Inferior branch of deep division of the inferior gluteal artery

(d) Transverse branch of the lateral circumflex femoral artery

Answers

1. *e*, 2. *d*, 3. *c*, 4. *d*, 5. *c*, 6. *d*, 7. *c*, 8. *c*

CHAPTER 24

1. The key muscle of the gluteal region is:

(a) Gluteus maximus

(b) Gluteus medius

(c) Gluteus minimus

(d) Piriformis

2. All structures enter the gluteal region through greater sciatic foramen *except*:

(a) Sciatic nerve

(b) Pudendal nerve

(c) Tendon of obturator internus

(d) Internal pudendal artery

3. Safe quadrant of the gluteal region for intramuscular injection is:

(a) Upper and inner

(b) Upper and outer

(c) Lower and inner

(d) Lower and outer

4. The gluteal muscle used for intramuscular injection in the gluteal region is:

(a) Gluteus maximus

(b) Gluteus medius

(c) Gluteus minimus

(d) Tensor fasciae latae

5. All the muscles of the gluteal region are supplied by the superior gluteal nerve *except*:

(a) Gluteus maximus

(b) Gluteus medius

(c) Gluteus minimus

(d) Tensor fasciae latae

6. All the statements about sciatic nerve are correct *except*:

(a) It arises from sacral plexus

(b) It enters the gluteal region through greater sciatic foramen

(c) It is related to upper and inner quadrant of the gluteal region

(d) It does not supply any muscle of the gluteal region

7. When standing on one foot the tilting of the pelvis on opposite side is prevented by the contraction of:

(a) Gluteus maximus

(b) Gluteus medius

(c) Gluteus minimus

(d) (b) and (c)

8. All the structures pass through the lesser sciatic foramen *except*:
   (a) Pudendal nerve
   (b) Nerve to quadratus femoris
   (c) Nerve to obturator internus
   (d) Internal pudendal vessels

Answers

1. *d*, 2. *c*, 3. *b*, 4. *b*, 5. *a*, 6. *c*, 7. *d*, 8. *b*

CHAPTER 25

1. All the hamstring muscles:
   (a) Take origin from the ilium
   (b) Are inserted into one of the bones of the leg
   (c) Are supplied by tibial part of the sciatic nerve
   (d) Are extensor of the hip and flexor of the knee

2. Muscle supplied by both common peroneal and tibial parts of the sciatic nerve is:
   (a) Semitendinosus
   (b) Semimembranosus
   (c) Biceps femoris
   (d) Adductor magnus

3. Which of the following is the most deeply located structure in the popliteal fossa?
   (a) Popliteal artery
   (b) Popliteal vein
   (c) Tibial nerve
   (d) Common peroneal nerve

4. Sural nerve is a branch of:
   (a) Sciatic nerve
   (b) Tibial nerve
   (c) Common peroneal nerve
   (d) None of the above

5. Which of the following is not a branch of the common peroneal nerve?
   (a) Sural nerve
   (b) Lateral sural nerve
   (c) Sural communicating nerve
   (d) Lateral inferior genicular nerve

6. Which of the following is not a content of the popliteal fossa?
   (a) Tibial nerve
   (b) Common peroneal nerve
   (c) Posterior cutaneous nerve of the thigh
   (d) Saphenous nerve

7. Select the *incorrect statement* about the oblique popliteal ligament of the knee:
   (a) It is an expansion of the tendon of semitendinosus

(b) It is attached to the lateral condyle of femur
(c) It is pierced by the middle genicular artery
(d) It is pierced by the genicular branch of the posterior division of obturator nerve

8. Sciatic nerve usually terminates:
   (a) At the junction of upper and middle third of the thigh
   (b) At the junction of middle and lower third of the thigh
   (c) In the middle of the thigh
   (d) In the middle of popliteal fossa

Answers

1. *a*, 2. *c*, 3. *a*, 4. *b*, 5. *a*, 6. *d*, 7. *a*, 8. *b*

CHAPTER 26

1. Y-shaped ligament of the hip joint is:
   (a) Ischiofemoral
   (b) Iliofemoral
   (c) Pubofemoral
   (d) Ligament of the head of femur

2. Synovial bursa which communicates with the synovial cavity of the hip joint lies deep to:
   (a) Gluteus maximus
   (b) Gluteal minimus
   (c) Psoas major
   (d) Gluteus medius

3. The pubofemoral ligament of the hip joint becomes tense during:
   (a) Flexion of the thigh
   (b) Extension of the thigh
   (c) Adduction of the thigh
   (d) Abduction of the thigh

4. Nerve likely to be injured in posterior dislocation of the hip joint is:
   (a) Superior gluteal
   (b) Inferior gluteal
   (c) Sciatic
   (d) Pudendal

5. Aseptic avascular necrosis of the head of femur usually occurs due to:
   (a) Subcapital fracture of the neck of femur
   (b) Cervical fracture of the neck of femur
   (c) Basal fracture of the neck of femur
   (d) Intertrochanteric fracture

6. Select the *incorrect statement* about the congenital dislocation of the hip joint:
   (a) It is more common than acquired dislocation

(b) It is usually unilateral

(c) It affects girls more than boys

(d) Its incidence is about 1.5 per 1000 live births

7. Select the *incorrect statement* about the neck shaft angle of the femur:

(a) It is about 125° in adults

(b) It is about 95° in children

(c) Its decrease leads to *coxa vara*

(d) Its increase leads to *coxa valga*

8. The chief source of blood supply to the head and neck of the femur is derived from:

(a) Acetabular branches of the obturator artery

(b) Acetabular branches of the medial circumflex femoral artery

(c) Retinacular branches of the medial circumflex femoral artery

(d) Nutrient artery of the femur

Answers

1. *b*, 2. *c*, 3. *d*, 4. *c*, 5. *a*, 6. *b*, 7. *b*, 8. *c*

CHAPTER 27

1. All are muscles of the anterior compartment of the leg *except*:

(a) Tibialis anterior

(b) Extensor hallucis longus

(c) Peroneus tertius

(d) Peroneus brevis

2. Most medial and superficial muscle of the anterior compartment of the leg is:

(a) Tibialis anterior

(b) Extensor hallucis longus

(c) Extensor digitorum longus

(d) Peroneus tertius

3. Select the *incorrect statement* about the muscles of the anterior compartment of the leg:

(a) They are dorsiflexor of the foot at the ankle

(b) They are supplied by the superficial peroneal nerve

(c) They lie in a tight osseofascial compartment

(d) Most of them arise from the fibula

4. All of the following structures pass beneath the superior extensor retinaculum of the foot *except*:

(a) Anterior tibial artery

(b) Deep peroneal nerve

(c) Dorsal pedis artery

(d) Peroneus brevis

5. All statements regarding the sensory innervation of the dorsum of the foot are correct *except*:

(a) Superficial peroneal nerve supplies most of the dorsum of the foot

(b) Cleft between the first and second toes is supplied by the deep peroneal nerve

(c) Lateral margin of the little toe is supplied by the sural nerve

(d) Medial margin of the big toe is supplied by the saphenous nerve

6. Skin on the medial side of the great toe is supplied by:

(a) Saphenous nerve

(b) Superficial peroneal nerve

(c) Sural nerve

(d) Deep peroneal nerve

7. Select the *incorrect statement* about the deep peroneal nerve:

(a) It is one of the two terminal branches of the sciatic nerve

(b) It is the nerve of the anterior compartment of the leg

(c) It provides sensory innervation to skin in the cleft between the first and second toes

(d) Its lesion results in foot drop

8. All statements regarding dorsalis pedis artery are correct *except*:

(a) It is the continuation of anterior tibial artery at the ankle joint

(b) It helps to form plantar arch by joining with the deep branch of the lateral plantar artery

(c) It lies lateral to the tendon of extensor hallucis longus

(d) It lies medial to the medial terminal branch of the superficial peroneal nerve

Answers

1. *d*, 2. *a*, 3. *b*, 4. *d*, 5. *d*, 6. *b*, 7. *a*, 8. *c*

CHAPTER 28

1. Tendon of which muscle traverses the sole of foot from the lateral to medial side:

(a) Tibialis anterior

(b) Peroneus longus

(c) Peroneus brevis

(d) Peroneus tertius

2. Regarding peroneus longus, which *statement is not correct?*

(a) It arises from the fibula

(b) It passes deep to both superior and inferior peroneal retinacula

(c) It grooves the cuboid bone
(d) It is inserted into the base of the 5th metatarsal

3. Muscles of the lateral compartment are supplied by:
   (a) Deep peroneal nerve
   (b) Superficial peroneal nerve
   (c) Tibial nerve
   (d) Sural nerve

4. Dorsiflexion of the foot is produced by:
   (a) Peroneus longus
   (b) Peroneus brevis
   (c) Peroneus tertius
   (d) None of the above

5. Bursa anserine (anserine bursa) is related to tendons of all of the following muscles *except*:
   (a) Sartorius
   (b) Gracilis
   (c) Semitendinosus
   (d) Semimembranosus

Answers
1. *b*, 2. *d*, 3. *b*, 4. *c*, 5. *d*

CHAPTER 29

1. The muscle "*triceps surae*" is formed by:
   (a) Popliteus and soleus
   (b) Soleus and gastrocnemius
   (c) Plantaris and gastrocnemius
   (d) Flexor digitorum longus and flexor hallucis longus

2. Which muscle is regarded as the '*peripheral heart*'?
   (a) Soleus
   (b) Gastrocnemius
   (c) Tibialis posterior
   (d) Flexor digitorum longus

3 The most deeply placed muscle in the posterior compartment of the leg is:
   (a) Flexor digitorum longus
   (b) Flexor hallucis longus
   (c) Tibialis posterior
   (d) Soleus

4. All the statements about plantaris is correct *except*:
   (a) It lies between soleus and gastrocnemius
   (b) It is absent in about 15–30% of people
   (c) Its tendon is sometimes dubbed as "*freshman nerve*"
   (d) Its tendon can be removed for grafting without causing functional disability

5. Select the *true statement* about posterior tibial artery:
   (a) It is the smaller of the two terminal branches of the popliteal artery
   (b) It runs between gastrocnemius and soleus
   (c) It supplies the muscles of both posterior and lateral compartments of the leg
   (d) Its pulsations can be felt near its origin

6. The tibialis posterior is inserted into all of the following tarsal bones *except*:
   (a) Calcaneum
   (b) Talus
   (c) Navicular
   (d) Cuboid

7. Injury of the tibial nerve can cause loss of:
   (a) Inversion of the foot
   (b) Eversion of the foot
   (c) Plantar flexion of the foot
   (d) Dorsiflexion of the foot

8. Largest and most important branch of the posterior tibial artery is:
   (a) Circumflex fibular artery
   (b) Peroneal artery
   (c) Medial plantar artery
   (d) Lateral plantar artery

Answers
1. *b*, 2. *a*, 3. *c*, 4. *b*, 5. *c*, 6. *b*, 7. *c*, 8. *b*

CHAPTER 30

1. Select the *incorrect statement* about the plantar aponeurosis:
   (a) It is thickening of the central part of the deep fascia of the sole of foot
   (b) It provides insertion to the tendon of plantaris
   (c) It helps to maintain the longitudinal arches of the foot
   (d) It sends slip to all the 5 digits

2. All are muscles of first layer of sole *except*:
   (a) Abductor hallucis
   (b) Flexor hallucis brevis
   (c) Abductor digiti minimi
   (d) Flexor digitorum brevis

3. The medial plantar nerve supply all muscles *except*:
   (a) First lumbrical
   (b) Abductor hallucis
   (c) Flexor digitorum brevis
   (d) Flexor digitorum accessories

4. Select the *incorrect statement* about the interossei of the sole of foot:
   (a) They are seven in number
   (b) Dorsal interossei produce abduction of the toes
   (c) Plantar interossei produce adduction of the toes
   (d) They produce extension of the metatarsophalangeal joints and flexion of the interphalangeal joints

5. All are the muscles of the third layer of sole *except*:
   (a) Flexor hallucis brevis
   (b) Adductor hallucis
   (c) Abductor hallucis
   (d) Flexor digiti minimi brevis

6. Fourth layer of the sole contains:
   (a) Tendon of peroneus longus
   (b) Tendon of flexor hallucis longus
   (c) Tendon of tibialis posterior
   (d) (a) and (c)

7. Which lumbrical muscle in the sole of foot is not supplied by the lateral plantar nerve?
   (a) First lumbrical
   (b) Second lumbrical
   (c) Third lumbrical
   (d) Fourth lumbrical

8. Which muscle of the sole contains two sesamoid bones?
   (a) Abductor hallucis
   (b) Flexor digiti minimi brevis
   (c) Flexor hallucis brevis
   (d) Adductor hallucis

Answers
1. *b*, 2. *b*, 3. *d*, 4. *d*, 5. *c*, 6. *d*, 7. *a*, 8. *c*

CHAPTER 31

1. Bone which is considered as the *keystone* of medial longitudinal arch of foot is:
   (a) Calcaneum
   (b) Cuboid
   (c) Talus
   (d) Navicular

2. Which of the following structures acts as a tie beam of the longitudinal arches of the foot?
   (a) Tendon of tibialis posterior
   (b) Plantar aponeurosis
   (c) Plantar calcaneonavicular ligament
   (d) Interosseous talocalcaneal ligament

3. The most important factor for maintaining the arches of the foot is:
   (a) Shapes of the bones
   (b) Ligaments and plantar aponeurosis
   (c) Tendons of muscles
   (d) Intertarsal joints

4. The main joints of the medial longitudinal arch of foot is:
   (a) Midtarsal
   (b) Talocalcaneonavicular
   (c) Calcaneocuboid
   (d) Cuneonavicular

5. The main joint of the lateral longitudinal arch of foot is:
   (a) Subtalar
   (b) Cuneocuboid
   (c) Calcaneocuboid
   (d) Talocalcaneonavicular

6. In talipes equinus, the patient walks on:
   (a) Toes
   (b) Heel
   (c) Lateral margin of the foot
   (d) Medial margin of the foot

7. All are features of the talipes equinovarus *except*:
   (a) Inversion
   (b) Adduction
   (c) Plantar flexion
   (d) Lateral rotation of the foot

8. The muscle that does not maintain the transverse arch of the foot is:
   (a) Tibialis posterior
   (b) Peroneus longus
   (c) Adductor hallucis
   (d) Extensor digitorum brevis

Answers
1. *c*, 2. *b*, 3. *b*, 4. *b*, 5. *c*, 6. *a*, 7. *d*, 8. *d*

CHAPTER 32

1. All the statements about capsule of the knee join are correct *except*:
   (a) Anteriorly it is replaced by the quadriceps femoris, patella, and ligamentum patellae
   (b) Posteriorly it is strengthened by oblique popliteal ligament
   (c) Posterolaterally it provides passage to the tendon of popliteus
   (d) Inferiorly it encloses the soleus muscle

2. Most important factor to stabilize the knee joint is:

   (a) Muscle
   (b) Ligaments
   (c) Articular surfaces
   (d) Menisci

3. Anteroposterior stability of the knee joint is maintained by:

   (a) Oblique popliteal ligament
   (b) Arcuate popliteal ligament
   (c) Cruciate ligaments
   (d) Medial and lateral collateral ligaments

4. Medial meniscus is more vulnerable to the injury because:

   (a) It is attached to the tibial collateral ligament and allows greater excursion during rotatory movements
   (b) Posterior fibres of its anterior end are continuous with the transverse ligament
   (c) It is larger than the medial lemniscus
   (d) Its anterior posterior ends are attached to the intercondylar area of the tibia

5. Locking of the knee joint is caused by the contraction of:

   (a) Popliteus
   (b) Biceps femoris
   (c) Semimembranosus
   (d) Quadriceps femoris

6. Select the *incorrect statement* about the locking and unlocking of the knee joint:

   (a) Locking occurs at the end of extension
   (b) There is medial rotation of the tibia on femur in locking
   (c) Unlocking occurs during initial phase of flexion
   (d) Locking is essential for standing erect and locomotion

7. Ankle joint is most stable in:

   (a) Plantar flexion
   (b) Dorsiflexion
   (c) Inversion
   (d) Eversion

8. What type of ankle joint is:

   (a) Ellipsoid
   (b) Saddle
   (c) Modified hinge
   (d) Pivot

Answers

1. *d*, 2. *a*, 3. *c*, 4. *a*, 5. *d*, 6. *b*, 7. *b*, 8. *c*

CHAPTER 33

1. The approximate number of superficial inguinal lymph nodes is:

   (a) 2 to 3
   (b) 4 to 5
   (c) 7 to 9
   (d) 15 to 20

2. The commonest cause of swelling in the subinguinal region is:

   (a) Enlargement of inguinal lymph nodes
   (b) Femoral hernia
   (c) Psoas abscess
   (d) Ectopic testis

3. Select the *incorrect statement* about the deep lymphatics of the lower limb:

   (a) They are smaller and fewer in number than the superficial lymphatics
   (b) They drain lymph from all structures deep to deep fascia
   (c) They run along the principal vessels of the lower limb
   (d) They drain mostly into external iliac lymph nodes

4. All the statements about great saphenous vein are correct *except*:

   (a) It is the longest vein in the body
   (b) It is thin-walled and contains only few valves
   (c) It is connected to the deep veins of the leg and thigh by perforating veins (perforators)
   (d) It terminates in the femoral vein after piercing the anterior wall of the femoral sheath

5. All the statements about small saphenous vein are correct *except*:

   (a) It begins as the continuation of the lateral end of the dorsal venous arch
   (b) It possess numerous valves
   (c) It is accompanied by the sural nerve in the leg
   (d) It drains into the great saphenous vein

Answers

1. *a*, 2. *b*, 3. *d*, 4. *b*, 5. *d*

CHAPTER 34

1. Select the *incorrect statement* about the sciatic nerve:

   (a) It arises from the anterior primary rami of L4–S3 spinal nerves
   (b) It is the thickest nerve in the body

(c) It lies superficial to biceps femoris

(d) It undergoes a subfascial course in the angle between the gluteus maximus and long head of the biceps femoris

2. **Complete injury of the sciatic nerve in the gluteal region will not produce:**

   (a) Weakness in the flexion of thigh
   (b) Foot drop
   (c) Complete loss of the skin sensation in the foot
   (d) Paralysis of all the muscles of the leg and foot

3. **All the statements about the femoral nerve are correct** *expect*:

   (a) It is the largest branch of the lumbar plexus
   (b) It arises from the ventral branches of the anterior primary rami of L2, L3, L4 spinal nerves
   (c) It enters the femoral triangle deep to the inguinal ligament

(d) It lies in the groove between psoas major and iliacus

4. **The saphenous nerve is:**

   (a) A branch of the femoral nerve
   (b) The longest cutaneous nerve in the body
   (c) Closely related to great saphenous vein at the ankle
   (d) Thickest cutaneous nerve in the body

5. **All the statements about the obturator nerve are correct** *except*:

   (a) It arises from the ventral branches of the anterior primary rami, of L2, L3, L4 spinal nerves
   (b) It enters the thigh deep to the inguinal ligament
   (c) It supplies all the muscles of the adductor compartment
   (d) It takes part in the formation of subsartorial plexus of the nerves

Answers

1. *c*, 2. *a*, 3. *b*, 4. *d*, 5. *c*

Index